Biologics to Treat Substance Use Disorders

Ivan D. Montoya
Editor

Biologics to Treat Substance Use Disorders

Vaccines, Monoclonal Antibodies, and Enzymes

Springer

Editor
Ivan D. Montoya
National Inst Drug Abuse, Room 4131
National Institutes of Health
Bethesda, MD
USA

ISBN 978-3-319-23149-5 ISBN 978-3-319-23150-1 (eBook)
DOI 10.1007/978-3-319-23150-1

Library of Congress Control Number: 2015957970

Springer Cham Heidelberg New York Dordrecht London

Printed on acid-free paper

Springer International Publishing AG Switzerland is part of Springer Science+Business Media
(www.springer.com)

Foreword

The treatment of drug use disorders (DUDs) is challenging because of the clinical nature of these entities and the limited number and efficacy of available pharmacotherapies. Biologics such as vaccines, monoclonal antibodies, and enzymes offer new alternative therapeutic strategies. The aim for these interventions is to prevent the entry of the drug to the brain and thus interfere with its rewarding and neurotoxic effects.

This book is the first comprehensive compendium of research in the development of biologics to treat DUDs and drug overdose. Most of the preclinical and clinical work on biologics discussed in this book has been supported by NIDA as part of its commitment to the discovery and development of new treatments.

In the development of drug vaccines, a major challenge has been the generation of sufficiently high titers of antibodies to bind to the high concentrations of the drug in the blood of those taking them. As of now, clinical trials with nicotine and cocaine vaccines have been disappointing, but research for the development of vaccines with higher antigenicity is ongoing. Passive immunization with monoclonal antibodies allows the delivery of sufficiently high antibody titers to counteract the drug's effects and thus offers an intervention with which to treat patients who overdose with drugs such as heroin, oxycodone, nicotine, cocaine, or methamphetamine. Research is ongoing for the development of strategies to sustain high levels of monoclonal antibodies so that they can also be used as potential treatments of addiction (methamphetamine, cocaine). Finally, enzymes aimed at accelerating the metabolism of a drug might also be helpful in the treatment of overdoses and when combined with monoclonal antibodies or vaccines might help boost their therapeutic potential.

Similarly as advances emerge on other therapeutic intervention for DUD, one can foresee that their combined use with biologics will help improve clinical outcomes in those afflicted with DUD. This volume will present the reader with a summary of the advances and challenges in the use of biologics for DUD.

Bethesda, MD, USA Nora Volkow National Institute on Drug Abuse (NIDA)

Preface

Substance use disorders (SUDs), including alcohol and drug use disorders (DUDs), are a global public health concern with less than optimal treatment outcomes. There are medications approved by regulatory agencies to treat nicotine (i.e., bupropion, nicotine replacement therapies, and varenicline) and opioid (buprenorphine, methadone, and naltrexone) use disorders. There are no approved medications for cocaine, methamphetamine, and cannabis use disorders, despite more than 25 years of research and multiple medications evaluated (Montoya and Vocci 2008). Moreover, a small proportion of patients with DUDs who received treatment are able to stop using drugs, but most relapse. Therefore, there is a high need to discover safe and effective medications to treat these disorders.

Traditionally, medications development for DUDs has focused on small molecules that cross the blood-brain barrier, have their effect on molecular targets in the brain, and produce changes in brain circuits. These changes are expected to modify the patient's drug use. A new therapeutic approach for DUDs is with biologics such as vaccines, monoclonal antibodies, and enzymes. Biologics are large molecules that do not cross the blood-brain barrier and thus have no CNS effects. The main mechanism of action is a pharmacokinetic antagonism in which the biologic precludes the access of drugs of abuse to the brain. They target the molecule responsible for the DUD peripherally and change its metabolism, distribution, or clearance. As a result, biologics can prevent the reinforcing and neurotoxic effects of drugs and protect against drug use relapse (Montoya 2012).

Biologics have shown an enormous public health benefit and are making a significant impact in many areas of medicine, such as in oncology, rheumatology, dermatology, neurology, and psychiatry, including DUDs. Currently, there are no biologics approved by the FDA to treat DUDs. Potential clinical indications might prevent the initiation of drug use and progression from drug use experimentation to addiction. The current research is focused on treating DUDs and drug overdose (Gorelick 2012).

New products and more efficient methods of production are offering vast opportunities to advance the discovery and development of biologics against drugs of abuse. In addition, as the field expands, more investigators from different areas of expertise are becoming involved in the development of biologics to treat DUDs. Given the rapid progress of this area of research, in 2013 the National Institute on Drug Abuse (NIDA) hosted a meeting that brought together academic investigators, industry representatives, research sponsors, regulators, and government representatives to review the current status of research in the field and to make recommendations to NIDA as to how product development might be accelerated.

The meeting participants identified scientific gaps, opportunities, and directions and developed multiple research collaborations. It became evident that biologics to treat DUDs is a new field with multiple challenges. They include determining the agent's potency, preclinical testing requirements, optimal dosing and schedules, translation from preclinical to clinical, appropriate clinical trial design, and pattern of therapeutic response. The meeting was very successful; most of the authors of this book participated in this meeting and the topics are covered in this book.

This book starts with a general introduction, followed by a review of the research on vaccines against nicotine, cocaine, opioids, and methamphetamine use disorders. Then, there is an introduction to monoclonal antibodies and separate chapters to discuss the anti-cocaine and anti-methamphetamine monoclonal antibodies for the treatment of the respective disorders and drug overdose. The next section discusses the enzyme-based treatments for DUDs, including a butyrylcholinesterase that was recently evaluated to treat cocaine dependence in a phase II/III clinical trial. The fourth section reviews a variety of topics about strategies to optimize the development of biologics to treat DUDs. It includes, for example, adenovirus- and nanoparticle-based vaccines, new adjuvants, hapten design, cell mechanisms of vaccine efficacy, and skin vaccination. The last section includes some practical and ethical considerations for the development of vaccines against drugs of abuse.

This is the first and most comprehensive book about the research and development of biologics to treat DUDs and drug overdose. Its goal is to promote interest and advance the scientific knowledge of anti-drug biologics. The hope is that studies will show that biologics are safe and effective and can be approved by the FDA to treat these challenging medical conditions. Ideally, biologics will be part of the therapeutic armamentarium that health-care providers can prescribe to patients whose brains have been hijacked by drugs and to save the lives of those who overdosed with drugs.

My deepest gratitude goes to all the authors who enthusiastically contributed to this book. Without their support, this book would not have been possible. I want to thank Dr. Jamie Biswas, Chief of the Medications Research Branch of NIDA, for introducing me to the field of biologics to treat DUDs and Dr. Nora Chiang, Chief of the Chemistry and Pharmaceutics Branch of NIDA, for her suggestions to the content and authors of the book. I also want to thank the editors at Springer for their support in developing this book. Finally, I am very grateful to my wife, Martha Velez, and my daughter Lina, who make it all worthwhile.

Bethesda, MD, USA

Iván D. Montoya

References

Gorelick DA. Pharmacokinetic strategies for treatment of drug overdose and addiction. Future Med Chem. 2012;4:227–43.

Montoya ID. Advances in the development of biologics to treat drug addictions and overdose 1. Adicciones. 2012;24:95–103.

Montoya ID, Vocci F. Novel medications to treat addictive disorders. Curr Psychiatry Rep. 2008;10:392–8.

Acknowledgment

To my parents, Eduardo and Magola, who provided unlimited support of my education.

Contents

1 **Introduction: Biologics to Treat Substance Use Disorders: Vaccines, Monoclonal Antibodies, and Enzymes** 1
Phil Skolnick

Part I Vaccines

2 **Therapeutic Vaccines for Treating Nicotine Addiction** 7
Matthew W. Kalnik

3 **Vaccines for Treating Cocaine Use Disorders** 25
Coreen B. Domingo, Daryl Shorter, and Thomas R. Kosten

4 **Vaccines for Opioid Addiction** 37
Michael D. Raleigh and Paul R. Pentel

5 **Vaccines for Methamphetamine Use Disorder** 65
Thomas R. Kosten and Therese A. Kosten

6 **Cocaine and HIV Infection** 75
Timothy Cardozo, Sergey V. Shmelkov, Kenneth Carr, John Rotrosen, Pedro Mateu-Gelabert, and Samuel R. Friedman

Part II Monoclonal Antibodies

7 **Monoclonal Antibodies** 107
S. Michael Owens

8 **Anti-cocaine Monoclonal Antibodies** 109
Hanna N. Wetzel, William J. Ball, and Andrew B. Norman

9 **Discovery and Development of an Anti-methamphetamine Monoclonal Antibody for Use in Treating Methamphetamine Abuse** 119
Michael D. Hambuchen, Misty W. Stevens, Melinda G. Gunnell, W. Brooks Gentry, and S. Michael Owens

Part III Enzymes

10 Enzyme-Based Cocaine Pharmacotherapies: Current Status and Projections for the Future ... 145
James H. Woods and Chang-Guo Zhan

11 Viral Gene Transfer of Enzymes ... 167
W. Stephen Brimijoin

12 Cocaine Hydrolases Designed from Butyrylcholinesterase ... 187
Fang Zheng and Chang-Guo Zhan

Part IV Strategies to Optimize the Development of Biologics to Treat Addictions

13 Adenovirus-Based Vaccines for the Treatment of Substance Use Disorders ... 229
David F. Havlicek, Jonathan B. Rosenberg, Dolan Sondhi, Ronald G. Crystal, and Stephen M. Kaminsky

14 Nanoparticle-Based Nicotine Vaccine ... 249
Petr O. Ilyinskii and Lloyd P.M. Johnston

15 Exploration of DNA Nanostructures for Rational Design of Vaccines ... 279
Xiaowei Liu, Sidney M. Hecht, Hao Yan, Paul R. Pentel, and Yung Chang

16 Adjuvants for Substance Abuse Vaccines ... 295
Frank M. Orson, Berma M. Kinsey, Reetakshi Arora, Muthu Ramakrishnan, and Thomas R. Kosten

17 Skin Vaccination Against Nicotine Addiction ... 309
Xinyuan Chen, Ji Wang, Jeffrey H. Wu, and Mei X. Wu

18 Hapten Design for Anti-addiction Vaccine Development ... 327
Karen C. Collins and Kim D. Janda

19 B Cell Mechanisms Underlying Vaccine Efficacy Against Drugs of Abuse ... 367
Marco Pravetoni

Part V Practical Considerations

20 Practical Considerations for the Development of Vaccines Against Drugs of Abuse ... 397
Oscar B. Torres, Carl R. Alving, Arthur E. Jacobson, Kenner C. Rice, and Gary R. Matyas

21 Ethical Considerations of Biologics to Treat Substance Use Disorders ... 425
Ivan D. Montoya

Index ... 439

Abbreviations

Albu-CocH	Albumin-tagged cocaine hydrolase
AMP	Amphetamine
APC	Antigen-presenting cell
ASC	Antibody-secreting cells
AUC	Area under the concentration-time curve
BCR	B cell receptor
B_{max}	Maximum number of binding sites
cGAMP	Cyclic GMP-AMP
cGAS	Cyclic GMP-AMP synthase
ch	Chimeric
CocE	Cocaine esterase
CocH	Cocaine hydrolase
CpG ODN	Cytosine-phosphodiester-guanine oligonucleotide
DC	Dendritic cells
DM CocE	Double mutant cocaine esterase
DNase	Deoxyribonuclease
ECG	Electrocardiograms
ELISA	Enzyme-linked immunosorbent assay
FcRn	Fc receptor of the neonate
FDC	Follicular dendritic cells
GC	Germinal center
HACA	Human anti-chimeric antibodies
IDO	Indoleamine-2, 3-dioxygenase
IFN	Interferon
IgG	immunoglobulin G
IL	Interleukin
iv	Intravenous
K_d	Dissociation constant
K_I	Inhibition constant
LLPCs	Long-lived plasma cells
mAb	Monoclonal antibody (both singular and plural)

MCV	METH-conjugate vaccine
MDMA	Methylenedioxymethamphetamine
METH	Methamphetamine
MYD88	Myeloid differentiation primary response 88
Nic	Nicotine
Nic-KLH	Nicotine-keyhole limpet hemocyanin conjugates
Nic-SA-CpG	Nicotine-streptavidin-CpG conjugates
Nic-SA-TH-CpG	Tetrahedron DNA assembled with Nic-SA conjugates and CpG
OVA	Ovalbumin
PAMP	Pathogen-associated molecular patterns
PBMC	Peripheral blood mononuclear cells
PBS	Phosphate-buffered saline
PEG CCRQ CocE	Pegylated CocE with the dimer tightly bound
SA	Streptavidin
sc	Subcutaneous
STING	Stimulator of interferon genes
swIg	Switched immunoglobulin B cells
$t_{1/2}$	Half-life
T_{FH}	T follicular helper cells
TH	Tetrahedron DNA
TH-CpG	Tetrahedron DNA assembled with CpG
TLR	Toll-like receptor
VLPs	Virus-like particles

Chapter 1
Introduction: Biologics to Treat Substance Use Disorders: Vaccines, Monoclonal Antibodies, and Enzymes

Phil Skolnick

Traditional, small-molecule approaches have only been marginally successful in developing innovative therapies for substance use disorders (SUDs). For example, there are no FDA-approved medications to treat stimulant (e.g., cocaine and methamphetamine) use disorders, and based on an analysis of trials listed on www.clinicaltrials.gov, no approvals are anticipated during the next 5–7 years. Even when multiple pharmacotherapies are available (e.g., anti-smoking medications), efficacy over the long term is disappointing. Thus, 1-year abstinence rates are less than 20 % for individuals treated with approved products (e.g., nicotine patches and gum, bupropion, and varenicline). There are multiple factors contributing to this dearth of pharmacotherapies, including a high regulatory "bar" for approval (a period of end-of-trial abstinence is currently the only acceptable endpoint measure) (McCann and Li 2012; Winchell et al. 2012; Donovan et al. 2012), low medication compliance during the conduct of clinical trials (Czobor and Skolnick 2011; Anderson et al. 2012, 2014; Somoza et al. 2013), and, with few exceptions, the perception by pharma that developing medications to treat SUDs will not provide a favorable return on investment in real-world practice (Acri and Skolnick 2013). Biological approaches offer an alternative that may resolve some of the drawbacks associated with conventional pharmacotherapies.

Biological approaches are all grounded on a common mechanism: either exclude or retard the entry of an abused substance from the central nervous system. There are currently three means of achieving this objective: (1) vaccines that stimulate the immune system to produce antibodies directed against a specific drug of abuse, (2) passive immunization by administering monoclonal antibodies directed against

---

P. Skolnick, PhD, DSc (hon)
Division of Pharmacotherapies and Medical Consequences of Drug Abuse, National Institute on Drug Abuse, National Institutes of Health, Bethesda, MD, 20892, USA
e-mail: Phil.Skolnick@nih.gov

I.D. Montoya (ed.), *Biologics to Treat Substance Use Disorders: Vaccines, Monoclonal Antibodies, and Enzymes*, DOI 10.1007/978-3-319-23150-1_1

a specific drug of abuse, (3) genetically engineered esterases that catalyze the hydrolysis of cocaine at a rate >3 orders of magnitude higher than the wild-type enzyme.

Positive signals have been reported in proof of principle clinical trials with both a cocaine (TA-CD) and a nicotine vaccine (NicVax®) (Martell et al. 2009; reviewed in Shen and Kosten 2011; Kosten et al. 2014; Hatsukami et al. 2011) in subjects who developed relatively high titers of antidrug antibodies. Perhaps the principal challenge to developing effective vaccines to drugs of abuse is the inability of the immune system to recognize these low molecular weight molecules (e.g., nicotine, cocaine, heroin). These molecules are rendered antigenic through chemical modification, enabling covalent linkage to a protein (e.g., cholera toxin B in the case of the TA-CD cocaine vaccine) (Shen and Kosten 2011; Shen et al. 2012). Nonetheless, despite multiple immunizations, none of the vaccines developed to date resulted in high titers of high affinity antidrug antibodies in a majority of patients. This problem is exemplified in the Martell et al. (2009) report using the TA-CD cocaine vaccine. Robust antibody titers to cholera toxin B were noted in every patient, but far fewer than half of the patients achieved serum antibody levels high enough to affect cocaine use (Martell et al. 2009; Shen and Kosten 2011). Potential strategies to overcome this challenge include the use of more effective adjuvants, alternative vaccine platforms (adenovirus-based vaccines, nanoparticle-based vaccines, DNA scaffolded vaccines), and the design of more effective haptens, topics that will be reviewed in this volume.

In contrast to the vaccines described here that require multiple immunizations to raise therapeutically relevant levels of antibodies (Hatsukami et al. 2011; Martell et al. 2009), monoclonal antibodies provide passive immunization and are thus immediately effective upon administration. Clinical studies have been initiated with a monoclonal antibody directed against methamphetamine (Owens et al. 2011), with first-in-man studies completed in 2013 (Stevens et al. 2014). The limitations of monoclonal antibodies include the potential cost of a commercial product and a limited biological half-life, which could necessitate weekly to monthly administration. Novel technologies that may lower manufacturing costs and the ability to genetically engineer mABs with significantly longer biological half-lives may contribute to the development of a commercially viable treatment for stimulant use disorders. These approaches are also described in this volume.

Also described in this volume is the genetic modification of wild-type enzymes derived from both bacteria and humans that results in an extraordinarily rapid hydrolysis of cocaine. Point mutations in these enzymes can increase the catalytic rate by more than 1000-fold compared to the wild-type enzyme. For example, administration of a mutated butyrylcholinesterase linked to serum albumin dramatically reduces both the toxicological and behavioral effects of cocaine in rodents and nonhuman primates. These effects are attributable to a rapid degradation of cocaine in plasma (and a corresponding rise in a hydrolysis product of cocaine, ecgonine methyl ester) (reviewed in Brimijoin 2011; Schindler et al. 2013). A Phase II facilitation of abstinence study of this product (TV 1380) in cocaine-dependent subjects has recently been completed (www.clinicaltrials.gov). In this study, the enzyme was administered weekly because of its proteolytic degradation. However, recent studies in rodents (Zlebnik et al. 2014) have demonstrated that gene transfer of this enzyme using an adenovirus vector results in a sustained (lasting for the duration of the study, >2 months) reduction in the reinforcing effects of intravenously administered cocaine. Reckitt Benckiser Pharmaceuticals recently reported (Nasser et al. 2014) that a mutated form of bacterial cocaine esterase reduced cocaine plasma exposures by >90 % in response to an intravenous cocaine challenge (50 mg infused over 10 min) in non-treatment seeking volunteers. The sponsor is developing this bacterially derived enzyme as a pharmacotherapy for cocaine intoxication (Nasser et al. 2014).

Biological approaches offer a nontraditional means of treating SUDs, with both advantages and disadvantages compared to conventional pharmacotherapies. Low medication compliance has confounded data interpretation in SUD trials (Anderson et al. 2012, 2014; Somoza et al. 2013) and is also a serious issue in clinical practice (Cutler and Everett 2010). The ability of a biologic to deliver a long-lived effect enables patients to make fewer good decisions (in the ideal, one good decision to receive a vaccine and perhaps a booster immunization) compared to one (or more) good decisions every day to remain compliant with a conventional medication. The specificity of a vaccine (e.g., a heroin vaccine) neither precludes the patient from receiving structurally unrelated molecules as therapy (e.g., methadone, buprenorphine) nor prevents the abuse of either these or other abused drugs. This specificity can be viewed as a potential drawback. Nonetheless, the high incidence of polysubstance abuse is also an issue for conventional therapies, exemplified by a patient abusing cocaine while receiving depot naltrexone to prevent relapse to opiates. The nicotine and cocaine vaccines examined to date require months before meaningful antibody titers are detected (Hatsukami et al. 2011; Martell et al. 2009; Shen and Kosten 2011). This therapeutic "lag" and the apparent requirement for multiple immunizations represent significant barriers to commercialization. However, the very limited success of traditional pharmacotherapies in treating SUDs together with the novel adjuvants, approaches to vaccine design, and delivery systems described in this volume presents biological approaches an appealing alternative that requires additional investment.

References

Acri JB, Skolnick P. Pharmacotherapy of substance use disorders. In: Charney D, Nestler E, Sklar P, Buxbaum J, editors. Neurobiology of mental illness. London: Oxford University Press; 2013. p. 235–45.

Anderson AL, Li SH, Biswas K, McSherry F, Holmes T, et al. Modafinil for the treatment of methamphetamine dependence. Drug Alcohol Depend. 2012;120:135–41.

Anderson AL, Li S-H, Markova D, Holmes T, Chiang N, et al. Bupropion for the treatment of methamphetamine dependence in non-daily users: a randomized, double-blind, placebo-controlled trial. Drug Alcohol Depend. 2014;150:170–4.

Brimijoin S. Interception of cocaine by enzyme or antibody delivered with viral gene transfer: a novel strategy for preventing relapse in recovering drug users. CNS Neurol Disord Drug Targets. 2011;10:880–91.

Cutler DM, Everett W. Thinking outside the pillbox – medication adherence as a priority for health care reform. N Engl J Med. 2010;362:1553–5.

Czobor P, Skolnick P. The secrets of a successful clinical trial: compliance, compliance, and compliance. Mol Interv. 2011;11:107–10.

Donovan DM, Bigelow GE, Brigham GS, Carroll KM, Cohen AJ, et al. Primary outcome indices in illicit drug dependence treatment research: systematic approach to selection and measurement of drug use end-points in clinical trials. Addiction. 2012;107:694–708.

Hatsukami DK, Jorenby DE, Gonzales D, Rigotti NA, Glover ED, et al. Immunogenicity and smoking-cessation outcomes for a novel nicotine immunotherapeutic. Clin Pharmacol Ther. 2011;89:392–9.

Kosten TR, Domingo CB, Shorter D, Orson F, Green C, et al. Vaccine for cocaine dependence: a randomized double-blind placebo-controlled efficacy trial. Drug Alcohol Depend. 2014;140: 42–7.

Martell BA, Orson FM, Poling J, Mitchell E, Rossen RD, et al. Cocaine vaccine for the treatment of cocaine dependence in methadone-maintained patients: a randomized, double-blind, placebo-controlled efficacy trial. Arch Gen Psychiatry. 2009;66:1116–23.

McCann DJ, Li SH. A novel, nonbinary evaluation of success and failure reveals bupropion efficacy versus methamphetamine dependence: reanalysis of a multisite trial. CNS Neurosci Ther. 2012;18:414–8.

Nasser AF, Fudala PJ, Zheng B, Liu Y, Heidbreder C. A randomized, double-blind, placebo-controlled trial of RBP-8000 in cocaine abusers: pharmacokinetic profile of rbp-8000 and cocaine and effects of RBP-8000 on cocaine-induced physiological effects. J Addict Dis. 2014;33(4):289–302.

Owens SM, Atchley WT, Hambuchen MD, Peterson EC, Gentry WB. Monoclonal antibodies as pharmacokinetic antagonists for the treatment of (+)-methamphetamine addiction. CNS Neurol Disord Drug Targets. 2011;10:892–8.

Schindler CW, Justinova Z, Lafleur D, Woods D, Roschke V, et al. Modification of pharmacokinetic and abuse-related effects of cocaine by human-derived cocaine hydrolase in monkeys. Addict Biol. 2013;18:30–9.

Shen X, Kosten TR. Immunotherapy for drug abuse. CNS Neurol Disord Drug Targets. 2011;10: 876–9.

Shen XY, Orson FM, Kosten TR. Vaccines against drug abuse. Clin Pharmacol Ther. 2012;91: 60–70.

Somoza EC, Winship D, Gorodetzky CW, Lewis D, Ciraulo DA, et al. A multisite, double-blind, placebo-controlled clinical trial to evaluate the safety and efficacy of vigabatrin for treating cocaine dependence. JAMA Psychiatry. 2013;70:630–7.

Stevens MW, Henry RL, Owens SM, Schutz R, Gentry WB. First human study of a chimeric anti-methamphetamine monoclonal antibody in healthy volunteers. MAbs. 2014;6:1649–56.

Winchell C, Rappaport BA, Roca R, Rosebraugh CJ. Reanalysis of methamphetamine dependence treatment trial. CNS Neurosci Ther. 2012;18:367–8.

Zlebnik NE, Brimijoin S, Gao Y, Saykao AT, Parks RJ, Carroll ME. Long-term reduction of cocaine self-administration in rats treated with adenoviral vector-delivered cocaine hydrolase: evidence for enzymatic activity. Neuropsychopharmacology. 2014;39:1538–46.

Part I
Vaccines

Chapter 2
Therapeutic Vaccines for Treating Nicotine Addiction

Matthew W. Kalnik

2.1 Devastating Health Impact of Tobacco Smoking

Tobacco use is the leading preventable cause of death today.

Worldwide, tobacco use causes nearly 6 million (M) deaths per year; current trends show that tobacco use will cause > 8 M deaths annually by 2030 (CDC 2015).

For the United States, the epidemic of smoking-caused disease in the twentieth century ranks among the greatest public health catastrophes of the century, while the decline of smoking consequent to tobacco control is surely one of public health's greatest successes. However, the current rate of progress in tobacco control is not fast enough, and much more needs to be done to end the tobacco epidemic. Unacceptably high levels of smoking-attributable disease and death, and the associated costs, will persist for decades without changes in our approach to slowing and even ending the epidemic. If smoking persists at the current rate among young adults in this country, 5.6 million of today's Americans younger than 18 years of age are projected to die prematurely from a smoking-related illness. US Surgeon General (USHHS 2014).

According to the Centers for Disease Control, over 45 million Americans smoke tobacco. The CDC estimates that the direct healthcare costs attributable to treating smoking and smoking-related illness exceed \$170 billion per year and additionally more than \$156 billion in lost productivity (CDC 2015).

M.W. Kalnik, PhD
Antidote Therapeutics, Inc., 22 Firstfield Road, Suite 280, Gaithersburg, MD 20878, USA
e-mail: mkalnik@atibio.com

I.D. Montoya (ed.), *Biologics to Treat Substance Use Disorders: Vaccines, Monoclonal Antibodies, and Enzymes*, DOI 10.1007/978-3-319-23150-1_2

2.2 Efficacy of Currently Available Smoking-Cessation Therapeutics

Current nicotine addiction therapeutics target the nicotinic receptors in the brain either by A) providing replacement nicotine through safer delivery systems such as patches, gums, nasal spray, and others or B) by using small-molecule drugs such as bupropion and varenicline as mimics targeting specific nicotine brain receptors and modification of their downstream action. These therapies have demonstrated efficacy in the short term; however, over 50 % of quitters relapsed within 6 months. Approximately only one in five smokers who quit utilizing the most effective single medication, varenicline, remained abstinent at 1 year (21–23 %; Gonzales et al. 2006; Jorenby et al. 2006). Thus, a clear unmet need exists for new therapies that improve smoking cessation outcomes.

2.3 Nicotine Therapeutic Vaccines

The first conceptualization of using conjugate vaccines to elicit an immune response to morphine as a potential for heroin addiction treatment was reported in the 1970s (Bonese et al. 1974). After a 20-year drought of research activity, progress resurged in the latter half of the 1990s and early 2000s, when the first animal addiction studies testing nicotine conjugate vaccines were conducted. Preclinical proof of concept was demonstrated in animal models of nicotine dependence and withdrawal in several independent academic research laboratories:

(i) The Pentel Lab at the Minnesota Medical Research Foundation (Hieda et al. 1997, 1999; Pentel et al. 2000)
(ii) The Janda Lab at the Scripps Research Institute (Isomura et al. 2001; Carrera et al. 2004)
(iii) The Svensson Lab at the Karolinska Institutet (de Villiers et al. 2002; Lindblom et al. 2002)
(iv) The Cerny and Bachmann Labs at Chilka and Cytos (Cerny et al. 2002; Maurer et al. 2005)

Since then, six nicotine conjugate vaccines have been advanced to clinical testing by biotechnology and pharmaceutical companies (Table 2.1).

2.3.1 More Recent Clinical Progress and a Major Late-Stage Failure

The original promising animal study results (Hartmann-Boyce et al. 2012) led to initially encouraging early-stage clinical studies where NicQβ and NicVAX both demonstrated a significant association between high levels of

Table 2.1 Nicotine vaccines advanced to clinical testing

Vaccine	Biotechnology company	Pharmaceutical codevelopment partner	Development stage attained	Development status
TA-NIC	Celtic (formerly Xenova)	–	Phase II	Halted
NicQβ	Cytos Biotechnology	Novartis	Phase IIb	Halted
NicVAX	Nabi Biopharmaceuticals	GlaxoSmithKline	Phase III	Halted
Niccine	Independent Pharmaceutical	–	Phase II	Halted
SEL-068	Selecta Biosciences	–	Phase I	Reformulation needed
NIC7	Pfizer	n/a	Phase I	Ongoing; results expected 1H 2016

anti-nicotine antibodies (nic · IgG[1]) and long-term abstinence from smoking, when the vaccines were administered in smoking cessation phase II studies in the mid-2000's. The increased long-term abstinence was observed when high-antibody (Ab) responders (approximately the top-third) were compared to the low-Ab responders (the lower two-thirds), and as well when compared to placebo.

In 2010 and 2011, NicVAX was tested as an aid to smoking cessation treatment in two nearly identical 1000-subject randomized, placebo-controlled, multi-center phase III clinical studies. The most promising vaccine at the time and the only nicotine vaccine to reach the Phase III clinical testing stage was shown to have similar efficacy to placebo (Fahim, et al. 2011).

As a consequence of these negative results many of the world's experts and many of the investigators who are authors in this book took a step back and thoroughly assessed the field of therapeutic vaccines for treating nicotine addiction. Several comprehensive and insightful reviews (Moreno and Janda 2009; Hartmann-Boyce et al. 2012; Fahim et al. 2011, 2013; Raupach et al. 2012; Kosten and Domingo 2013; Pentel and LeSage 2014; Kinsey 2014) have generally concluded that the basic scientific principles underlying the PK mechanism are sound. Furthermore, the broad range of preclinical and clinical findings for vaccines and monoclonal antibodies (mAbs) targeting other drugs of abuse, support the continued research and development of therapeutic vaccines for treating addiction, in spite of the NicVAX phase III trial outcomes. Better technologies and platforms aimed at improving the immunogenicity of the vaccines are needed to increase the quantity and quality (high-affinity and high-avidity) nic · IgG elicited by the vast majority of vaccinated smokers.

[1] The IgG class of immunoglobulins are the vast proportion of Ig's elicited by the first generation of nicotine conjugate vaccines.

2.3.2 Mechanism of Action

The molecular mechanism of action of nicotine-specific Abs is best understood as an alteration of the pharmacokinetics of nicotine leading to reduced brain nicotine levels and increased blood levels of nicotine (Gorelick 2012). In general, slower drug delivery to the brain is associated with less intense and less reinforcing effects and thus attenuation of nicotine's addictive potential (Henningfield and Keenan 1993; deWit and Zacny 1995). This is particularly important with respect to nicotine as its greatest reinforcing and subjective effects occur within the first few minutes of smoking (Henningfield et al. 1985).

The nicotine in the blood is the target of the antibody, rather than the nicotinic acetylcholine receptors in the brain current pharmacotherapies target. Antibody binding of nicotine results in a substantial decrease in the rate of rise of nicotine levels in the brain and in lower doses of nicotine accessing neural reward targets, therefore reducing the addictive potential of the drug. Nicotine-specific IgGs have been shown to bind nicotine in the blood: slowing and reducing its distribution to the brain as the antibody-bound nicotine is too large to cross the blood-brain barrier (Hieda et al. 1999).

In summary, nicotine-specific Ab's lead to a lowering of the peak nicotine brain levels (reduced C_{max}) concurrently with a delay of reaching those peak levels (longer T_{max}). This causes blunting of the initial spike of nicotine entering the brain and flattening of the concentration-time course, leading to an overall reduction of the amount of nicotine reaching the brain from a smoked cigarette or other modes of delivery (reduced AUC), thereby reducing the addictive potential of nicotine (the "rate hypothesis" of psychoactive drug addiction) (Porchet et al. 1987; Nelson et al. 2006).

2.3.3 Early Clinical Success (Phase I and II)

The highest vaccine dose group in the NicVAX phase IIb study is the only reported nicotine vaccine treatment arm to demonstrate clinical efficacy prospectively, without stratification by nic · IgG level (NCT00318383). The intent-to-treat analysis indicated that the 5-injection 400 μg NicVAX dose group had significantly higher prolonged abstinence to 6 months as compared to placebo (17.6 % vs. 6.0 %; $p=0.015$; OR of 4.14; 95 % CI, 1.32–13.02) (Hatsukami et al. 2011). The observation of an association between high levels of nic · IgG and long-term abstinence for two independently developed nicotine vaccines provided sufficiently compelling clinical "proof of mechanism" that three global pharmaceutical companies, Novartis, GlaxoSmithKline, and Pfizer, entered the field between 2007 and 2009 (Table 2.1). Novartis and GlaxoSmithKline entered codevelopment partnerships with Cytos and Nabi, respectively, while Pfizer chose to start a new program based upon the learnings from the first generation of vaccine candidates.

2.3.4 *Late-Stage Clinical Setbacks*

Failure to reproduce these results in large pivotal studies has plagued the field since 2010: clinical development of all first-generation nicotine conjugate vaccines has been halted due to the lack of clinical efficacy as compared to placebo, in the intent-to-treat population (TA-NIC, NicQβ, Niccine, and NicVAX). All four of the biotechnology companies developing these four nicotine vaccines no longer exist or have substantially shifted their therapeutic focus. Novartis and GlaxoSmithKline have exited from visible nicotine therapeutic development efforts.

Upon failure of a late-stage clinical study, financial considerations exert a strong influence to rapidly halt the failed effort, particularly in the microcap biotechnology environment where the cost of capital is very high. Unfortunately, this severely limits the availability of resources for exploratory analyses that otherwise could have uncovered new insights into the fundamental biochemical and clinical hurdles encountered. Oftentimes, these pressures prevent the primary study results and postmortem analyses that had been conducted to be published. These insights are what are needed to fuel the next iteration of innovative vaccine designs. In an exception to the rule, exploratory post hoc analyses of the unpublished NicVAX phase III clinic trials have recently entered the public domain via an abandoned patent application (Fahim and Kalnik 2012). These analyses will be described in the following section.

2.4 Correlation of Nicotine-Specific Abs with Abstinence Rates

In spite of these setbacks, insights regarding the putative threshold of high-affinity nicotine-specific Abs needed to support smoking cessation and long-term abstinence have been gained. Elegant preclinical experiments utilizing nicotine-specific mAbs to overcome the inherent variability of biological immune response have provided significant insight into the range of doses and preferred affinities of nic · IgG likely needed vaccination to be effective.

2.4.1 *Dose-Response and Affinity-Response Relationships of Nicotine-Specific mAbs: In Vivo*

Three independent laboratories have generated and characterized nicotine-specific monoclonal antibodies for the treatment of nicotine addiction (Scripps, NIC9D9 from the NIC-KLH vaccine; Pentel/Nabi, Nic311 from NicVAX; and Cytos, Nic12 from NicQβ). Nicotine mAbs (nic · mAbs) can be produced that have uniform affinities and dose amounts, whereas the amount and quality of nic · IgG arising from vaccination are subject to interindividual variability of vaccine response with ranges spanning atleast two orders of magnitude. Furthermore, nic · mAbs can be administered immediately when smokers who want to quit at that moment can begin their smoking cessation efforts when their motivation is highest. Vaccines require a priming series of injections lasting weeks to months before high-affinity nic · IgGs are elicited in high quantities, when the smoker's motivation to quit may have subsided (Hughes and Callas 2011).

Nic · mAbs are precise probes for testing and validating the "rate hypothesis" and the antibody-mediated nicotine-PK mechanism for nicotine addiction as dose levels and affinities can be directly manipulated and controlled. Thus, nic · mAbs afford the opportunity to generate significant insight as to the nicotine affinities and nic · IgG levels required by vaccination for sufficient altering of the PK of the total body burden of nicotine and the commensurate reduction in brain nicotine levels.

The Pentel Lab has ascertained the nic · mAb dose- and affinity-response relationships needed in molecular mechanistic terms and in behavioral terms in vivo. Nic311 is a nic · mAb isolated from mice who were vaccinated with NicVAX using traditional hybridoma techniques (Keyler et al. 2005). In a separate effort (Beerli et al. 2008), B-cells isolated from a human volunteer vaccinated with NicQβ were screened and high-affinity fully human nic · mAbs were isolated and produced (Nic12). Dose-response and affinity-response relationships have been demonstrated with respect to reduction in brain nicotine levels in vivo for both Nic311 and Nic12 for attenuation of nicotine discrimination and self-administration behaviors.

Nic311 (K_d = 60 nM[2]) was dosed from 10 to 160 mg/kg which led to an ~80 % maximal reduction in the amount of nicotine reaching the brain in rats within 3 min of nicotine IV dosing (Fig. 2.1). The dose of nicotine was calculated to be the analogous amount of nicotine absorbed by a smoker from 1 to 2 cigarettes

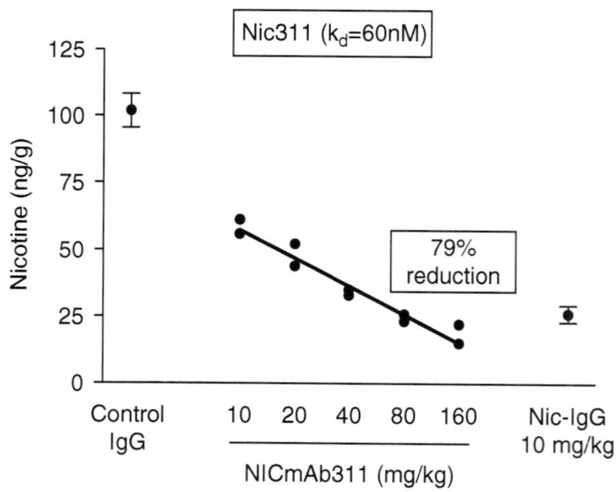

Fig. 2.1 Dose-response relationship for nicotine distribution to the brain after treatment with Nic311 compared with control-mAb in rats (N=2 per dose). Increasing Nic311 dose was associated with decreasing brain nicotine concentration (r = 0.99; p < 0.01) and increasing serum nicotine concentration (data not shown) measured 3 min after a nicotine dose (r = 0.99; p < 0.001) (adapted from Keyler et al. 2005)

[2] The nicotine affinity of the antibody binding to nicotine is expressed throughout this chapter as the equilibrium dissociation rate constant at which 50 % of the nicotine binding sites are saturated (lower values of K_d represent higher affinities).

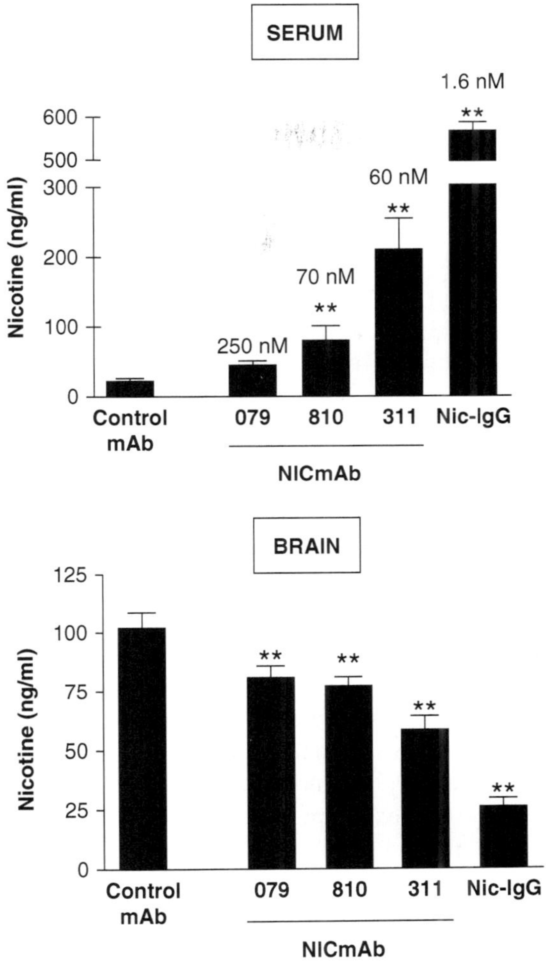

Fig. 2.2 Affinity-response of three (3) Nic · mAbs with affinities (Kd) for nicotine ranging from 60 nM to 260 nM. All three (3) of these Nic · mAbs were derived from hybridomas generated from mice vaccinated with NicVAX. Serum and brain nicotine concentrations were followed after a single nicotine dose in rats pretreated with 10 mg/kg control-mAb, monoclonal Nic · mAbs, or Nic · IgG. Nicotine (0.03 mg/kg) was administered 30 min after the pretreatment and serum and brain collected 3 min after the nicotine dose. Pretreatment with each of the three (3) Nic · mAbs or with Nic · IgG increased nicotine retention in serum and reduced nicotine distribution to brain. Decreasing Kd (values shown above columns in top panel) was associated with increasing nicotine concentration in serum ($r = 0.67$; $p < 0.001$) and decreasing nicotine concentration in brain ($r = 0.69$; $p < 0.001$). ** indicates $p < 0.01$ compared with control-mAb (adapted from Keyler et al. 2005)

(Benowitz 2008). Furthermore, brain nicotine levels were significantly dependent upon the affinity of the nic · mAb. Several nic · mAbs were isolated from mice vaccinated with NicVAX with nicotine K_d's ranging from 60 to 250 nM. This series of nic · mAbs demonstrated a clear affinity-response relationship (Fig. 2.2).

Additionally, for the fully human nic · mAbs isolated from a single human donor (Beerli et al. 2008) in a completely separate, independent laboratory using a different nicotine vaccine (NicQβ), a dose- (Fig. 2.3) and affinity-response relationship was also observed for nic · mAbs with nicotine affinities ranging from 7 nM (Nic12) to over 744 nM. Even though the Nic12 experiments were conducted in mice as opposed to rats, albeit under similar relative nicotine doses and a similar time course to the Nic311 studies, the similarity of the dose-response is striking, with maximal reduction in brain nicotine levels of ~80 % by an ~150 mg/kg nic · mAb dose. Both

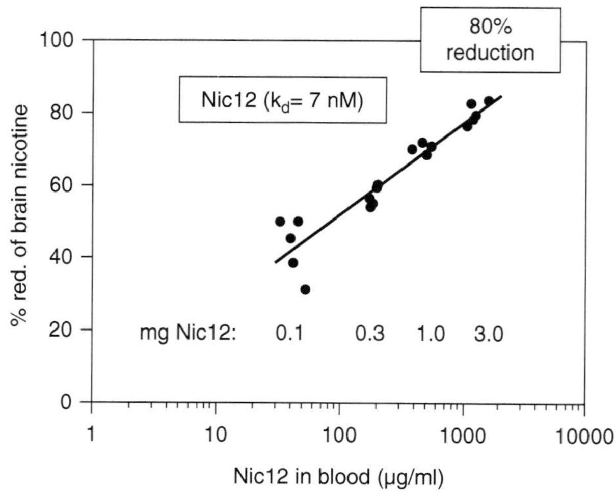

Fig. 2.3 Dose-response of inhibition of nicotine entry into brain by Nic12. Mice were injected i.p. with 0.1, 0.3, 1, or 3 mg of Nic12. One day later, mice were injected i.v. with 750 ng of tritium-labeled nicotine. Mice were sacrificed after 5 min and nicotine concentrations in brains were measured. Antibody concentrations in sera were determined and plotted against the percentage nicotine-reduction in the brain (adapted from Beerli et al. 2008). Copyright (2008) National Academy of Sciences, USA

studies clearly demonstrated statistically significant dose-response and affinity-response relationships in rodent models.

Polyclonal nicotine-specific IgGs elicited by the Nic-Qβ vaccine (alum adjuvant) in humans have nicotine affinities in the 30–70 nM range (Maurer et al. 2005). Rabbits vaccinated with the 3'AmNic-rEPA vaccine in Freund's adjuvant (Pentel et al. 2000) elicited nic · IgG with 1.6 nM affinities to nicotine. Interestingly, since larger vaccine doses and more potent adjuvants can be tested in the preclinical setting not suitable for clinical use, nic · IgG levels upto 500 μg/ml have been readily attained. These very high levels of nic · IgG significantly reduced nicotine levels entering the brain of rodents and attenuated associated nicotine behaviors (Maurer et al. 2005; Keyler et al. 2008).

The 1.6 nM, 10 mg/kg dose of nicotine-specific rabbit IgG lowered brain nicotine levels by an additional 50 % of those attained by the 60 nM Nic311 nic · mAb (10 mg/kg, Fig. 2.1). In theory, a nicotine vaccine which can elicit antibodies with nicotine affinities in the single digit nanomolar range may reduce brain nicotine levels to >90 % compared to controls. Next-generation vaccines will likely benefit from technological improvements (e.g., adjuvants, carriers, haptens/linkers, increased hapten densities, nanoparticles, delivery, etc.) aimed at improving nicotine affinity – possibly even to the sub-nanomolar level, leading to a significant further reduction in brain nicotine levels.

In preclinical studies of the combination of vaccination augmented with nic-mAbs, a functional dose-response relationship was extended to nicotine-specific antibody levels that were higher than either approach was able to attain alone. Figure 2.4 depicts this additive effect where (i) vaccination of rats yielded 166 μg/ml concentration of nic · IgG, (ii) 80 mg/kg dosing of Nic311 yielded a 172 μg/ml levels of nic · mAb, and (iii) combined active and passive immunization yielded nicotine-specific antibody levels of 420 μg/ml nic · IgG and Nic · mAb. The group receiving both nicotine vaccine and nic · mAb demonstrated brain nicotine levels >95 % less than controls. (Roiko et al. 2008).

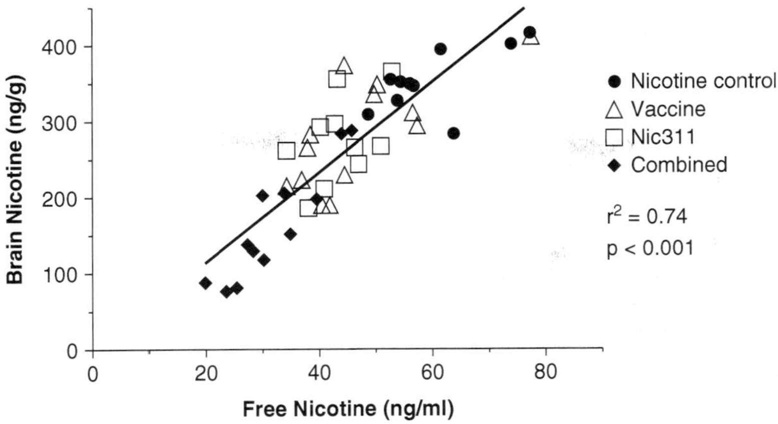

Fig. 2.4 Relationship between free nicotine concentration in serum and the brain nicotine concentrations for rats receiving 0.03 mg/kg doses of nicotine following a four injection regimen of NicVAX and 80 mg/kg nic311 mAb doses according to the locomotor sensitization protocol as described in Roiko et al. 2008. Animals were sacrificed 50 minutes after the final nicotine dose was administered

Table 2.2 Long-term abstinence stratified by post-vaccine Ab level: NicVAX PhIII

Subject group	12-month, 36-week CAR[a] (weeks 17–52)
High Ab (top 33 % by AUC)	13.0 % (n=22/169)
Low Ab (lower 67 %)	5.6 % (n=19/337)
Placebo	6.3 % (n=32/510)
Difference (high Ab vs. low Ab)	7.4 % (p=0.005)
Difference (high Ab vs. placebo)	6.7 % (p=0.006)
Difference (low Ab vs. placebo)	−0.7 % (not significant)

Intent to treat in the first Nabi phase III study (NCT00836199): NicVAX treated N=506, placebo N=510

[a]Continuous abstinence rate similarly measured as the 44-week CAR (Hatsukami et al. 2011), by patient self-reported outcomes in a diary and confirmation by carbon monoxide testing (unpublished)

2.5 Dose-Response Relationships Observed in NicVAX Phase III Studies

In 2012, a patent application from Nabi Biopharmaceuticals was published (WO 2012/07477, PCT/US2011/061229) (Fahim and Kalnik 2012) that contains post hoc exploratory analysis for hypothesis generation of a putative threshold of nic·IgG needed to support long-term abstinence from smoking in an effort to guide future development of nicotine vaccines. Table 2.2 describes the association of nic·IgG in the top 1/3 (33 %) of vaccine responders measured by area under the curve (AUC) with abstinence. Even though non-stratified ITT results were negative in the NicVAX phase III studies (Abstinence rates to one-year: NicVAX = 11 % and placebo = 11 %), a secondary analysis using pre-specified nic · IgG levels defined in the statistical analysis plan to stratify the phase III intent-to-treat (ITT) population and a statistically significant correlation with long-term abstinence was observed (Fahim et al. 2013). Thus, as these stratification analyses were pre-specified prior to unblinding of the phase III results, the observation that high nic · IgG levels support long-term abstinence in the NicVAX phase IIb study (NCT00318383) prospectively confirms the correlation of high nic · IgG with long-term abstinence to 1 year seen in the phase II study.

In the post hoc analyses presented in Table 2.2, the treatment effect of the top 33 % nic · IgG responders by AUC compared to placebo was 6.7 % for 36 weeks of continuous abstinence (CAR weeks 17–52, secondary endpoint). This modest rate of efficacy in the high nic · IgG responder group suggests that other factors beyond inadequate nic · IgG levels may have contributed to the failure of the NicVAX phase III studies (e.g., highly variable nicotine affinities). Unfortunately, one of the main attributes not characterized were the nicotine affinities of nic · IgG due to the rapid wind-down of Nabi Biopharmaceuticals as a result of the phase III failures. Eliciting high-affinity nic · IgG is currently viewed as one of the most important aspects driving functional efficacy and is being actively targeted in the development of second generation of nicotine conjugate vaccines (McCluskie et al. 2013a, b).

Table 2.3 describes a post hoc, pooled, completer analysis of both NicVAX phase III studies (NCT00836199 and NCT01102114) hypothesis generation of the putative threshold level of nic · IgG needed to support long-term abstinence. In a similar post hoc analysis of the NicVAX phase IIb data (unpublished), it was theorized that the nic · IgG level present at the target quit date (TQD) and maintained for the ensuing 4 months would provide insight into the minimum prolonged nic · IgG levels needed to support long-term abstinence. Thus, the

Table 2.3 Antibody dose-response correlation analysis: hypothetical threshold levels

Ab level remained above threshold for all weeks 14–30	12-month 36-week CAR (Wk 17–52)					
Threshold (μg/ml)	≥12.5	≥25	≥50	≥75	≥100	≥125
NicVAX (%)	9.2	10.8	13.1	16.5	18.4	23.3
High Ab	(*n*=54/584)	(*n*=44/407)	(*n*=25/191)	(*n*=16/97)	(*n*=9/49)	(*n*=7/30)
Placebo	7.6 % (*n*=61/807)					
p-value	*p*=0.28	*p*=0.066	*p*=0.021	*p*=0.0061	*p*=0.012	*p*=0.0077
Difference (high Ab above threshold vs. placebo) (%)	1.6	3.2	5.5	8.9	10.8	15.7

Pooled completer analysis of both NicVAX phase III studies (NCT00836199 and NCT01102114)

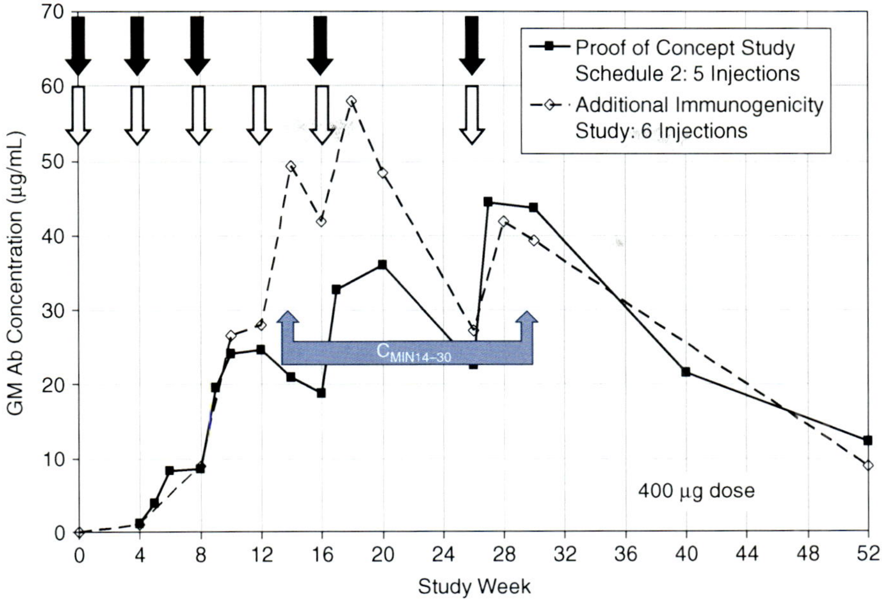

Fig. 2.5 The nic · IgG antibody kinetics from a phase II study of the 6-dose regimen of NicVAX (NCT00598325) and the delineation of weeks 14-30 used to define the Cmin threshold analyses in Table 2.3 (adapted from Fahim et al. 2013)

minimum threshold level of nic · IgG over weeks 14–30 of the study (TQD through one month following the final injection at 6 months; $Cmin_{14-30}$ See Figure 2.5) was used to stratify the ITT population in increments of 25 μg/ml. Notably, this minimum threshold analysis revealed a statistically significant dose-response relationship of nic · IgG levels with long-term abstinence. The statistical analyses were an uncorrected Fisher's exact test for multiple comparisons as this particular stratification analysis had uncovered an association in the phase IIb study. The highest $Cmin_{14-30}$ stratification group with a meaningful group size ($N \geq 30$) had a threshold of ≥125 μg/ml nic · IgG, yielding a long-term abstinence rate of 23.3 % for the completer population in this meta-analysis of both studies. Assuming a 25 % dropout rate, a 17.5 % abstinence rate was achieved for this top ~5 % of IgG responders.

Thus, a nicotine vaccine, with a similar distribution of affinities for nicotine, needs to elicit much higher nic · IgG levels than was predicted based on the NicVAX phase IIb results (>25 μg/ml) (Hatsukami et al. 2011) as well as the NicQβ phase II results (>10 μg/ml) (Bachmann and Jennings 2011). One caveat being that if the affinity-response relationships observed in the preclinical rodent studies of nicotine-specific mAbs (Keyler et al. 2005) (Fig. 2.2) translate to the clinic and then lower levels of nic · IgG with higher nicotine affinities may be sufficient to support long-term abstinence.

2.6 Second-Generation Nicotine Vaccines in the Clinic

Selecta Biosciences and Pfizer are developing the second-generation vaccines SEL-068 and NIC7.001/-003, respectively which have entered early clinical testing. These two vaccines have improvements in hapten, linker, and carrier designs, optimized hapten densities based on functional assays, as well as, in both instances, the addition of promising potent Toll-Like receptor-agonist adjuvants. These improvements are aimed at overcoming the first-generation vaccines' insufficient immune response across the population.

2.6.1 SEL-068

SEL-068 is a novel nanoparticle nicotine vaccine (targeted synthetic vaccine particle, tSVP) (Selecta Biosciences 2015). SEL-068 vaccine has many unique differentiating features. The following is an excerpt from a NIDA-awarded grant (Johnston 2014) –

> Preclinical Development and Clinical Proof of Concept of a Synthetic Nanoparticle [Nicotine Vaccine]:
>
> i) Targeting to antigen presenting cells (APC) to enhance efficacy and reduce off target impact;
> ii) B-cell antigen (nicotine) presentation at high surface density to stimulate robust and rapid B-cell responses;
> iii) T-cell antigen (TCHP) to provide T cell help for affinity maturation of B cell responses and efficient generation of immune memory (Fraser et al. 2014)
> iv) Adjuvant (Toll-like receptor agonist) for APC activation, and
> v) Biocompatible polymers for the time release of active components.

High levels of high-affinity nic · IgG have been elicited by SEL-068 in mice and non-human primates (NHP) (Pittet et al. 2012). Phase I studies of SEL-068 were initiated in 2011 and results have yet to be published. Reformulation of SEL-068 is needed as described (Johnston 2014):

> Selecta conducted a Phase 1 clinical trial of a first generation nicotine vaccine (SEL-068) consisting of a single particle formulation containing all three active components (TLR agonist, TCHP, and nicotine). SEL-068 was well tolerated and generated nicotine-specific antibodies. In this grant we propose to test additional nicotine nanoparticle formulations to further increase the level of anti-nicotine antibodies in humans using a two particle nicotine vaccine in which the TLR agonist and TCHP will be formulated in separate nicotine-containing nanoparticles. The two particles can be mixed and dosed at various ratios and dose levels in the clinic to optimize the human anti-nicotine antibody response. The scope of the grant proposal is formulation, preclinical studies, scale-up and manufacturing and an adaptive design Phase 1 clinical trial.

The need to reformulate SEL-068 to increase the potency of immune response in humans will significantly delay (several years) its advancement into phase II clinical testing.

2.6.2 *NIC7-001*

Based on the published literature, Pfizer has conducted one of the most extensive and systematic preclinical optimization and characterization programs for a nicotine vaccine. Their efforts have provided additional scientific rigor to the field. For example, the Pfizer Vaccines Research group has independently produced analogues of both NicQβ and NicVAX. These analogues have been used as reference benchmarks for the development of their proprietary NIC7 vaccine providing a rich set of research tools to segregate the impact of the different improvements found in NIC7 (carrier, hapten, conjugation chemistry, linker, hapten density, and adjuvant) (Moreno et al. 2010; Pryde et al. 2013; McCluskie et al. 2015).

The Pfizer Vaccines Research group used two different functional assays, (a) reduction of brain nicotine levels in vaccinated animals as compared to placebo and (b) overall binding capacity of nicotine-specific Abs from immunized animals, to guide their lead optimization efforts. Initial investigations suggest that the functional response in mice was influenced more by nic · IgG avidity than by their titers (Davis et al. 2012). Interestingly, a very recent publication suggests that choice of carrier and hapten density may be more significant contributors to the functional activity of a heroin vaccine for treating addiction (Jalah et al. 2015).

Pfizer reported that the addition of the CpG TLR-agonist adjuvant to an analogue of NicVAX – 3'AmNic-DT – increased the reduction of nicotine brain levels in mice to 33 % as compared to placebo approximately tenfold over 3'AmNic-DT with alum only (3 %). Important differences exist between the 3'AmNic-DT utilized in the Pfizer mouse and NHP studies and the 3'AmNic-rEPA (NicVAX) utilized in the clinic:

(a) rEPA is an alternative carrier protein and may lead to an enhanced immune response.
(b) Direct comparison of the hapten density of the two vaccines utilizing the two different carriers was not conducted.
(c) A larger dose of vaccine and alum adjuvant (400 μg and 1.2 mg, respectively) was utilized in the NicVAX (3'AmNic-rEPA) phase III studies (Fahim et al. 2011) as compared to the 10 μg dose of 3'AmNic-DT and 40 μg alum being administered in the mouse and NHP studies (McCluskie et al. 2013a).
(d) NicVAX was administered with six (6) injections and 3'AmNic-DT only 3 injections were administered.

NicVAX dosing regimens were optimized during phase I/II development:

- *Nabi-4503*: 13 μg/ml peak geometric mean concentration (GMC) of nic · IgG attained with a four-dose (100 μg) regimen (Wagena et al. 2008)
- *Nabi-4512*: 44 μg/ml peak GMC attained with a five-dose (400 μg) regimen (Hatsukami et al. 2011)
- *Nabi-4513*: 60 μg/ml peak GMC attained with a six-dose (400 μg) regimen (Fahim et al. 2011)

Although the addition of CpG (500 μg) to the 100 μg dose of 3'AmNic-DT resulted in a tenfold improvement in titers, a direct comparison with the 400 μg dose of 3'AmNic-DT (400 μg Al^{3+})±CpG (500 μg) was not reported. Thus, in the absence of direct experimental comparison, the immune-response improvements due to the 500 μg CpG adjuvant added to the 400 μg dose of 3'AmNic-rEPA (400 μg Al^{3+}) are unknown. A reasonable estimate in the absence of these data is that 500 μg CpG would improve titers of NicVAX by ~2.5-fold. In addition, the NicVAX vaccine manufacturing lots for the phase II and phase III studies were assessed for functional activity in rat models of increased plasma sequestration of nicotine and commensurate decreased brain levels of nicotine, as one of several batch-release criteria (FDA NicVAX IND, unpublished).

In addition, NIC7-001[3] was directly compared to an NicQβ analogue in NHPs. NIC7-001 formulated with alum/CpG adjuvant significantly reduced brain nicotine levels by 81 % compared to controls, whereas only a 7 % reduction was observed for NicQβ/alum ($p<0.0001$). Interestingly, NIC7-001 without the CpG adjuvant elicited tenfold lower nic·IgG levels than the NicQβ analogue, and yet NIC7-001 reduced brain nicotine levels by 33 % compared to placebo – nearly fivefold greater than NicQβ ($P<0.01$) (McCluskie et al. 2013b), suggesting that the NIC7 hapten is functionally more effective.

NIC7-001 has significantly outperformed the first-generation nicotine vaccines based on the high levels of high-affinity nicotine-specific Abs elicited, leading to significant, functionally greater reductions in brain nicotine levels in preclinical mice and NHP studies. In the study of 3'AmNic-DT conjugated with alum/CpG adjuvant in NHP, only about 30 % of nicotine at 100 ng/mL was bound. Strikingly, the authors state that "using a modified conjugate with the same adjuvant combination we have subsequently been able to obtain 100 % binding with a ten-fold higher amount of nicotine (1000 ng/mL)" (McCluskie et al. 2013a) or an ~33-fold increase in nicotine binding for NIC7-001 over the 3'AmNic-DT formulated with the same adjuvant (400 μg Al^{3+} and 500 μg CpG). Even adjusting for the differences estimated between 400 μg NicVAX (3'AmNic-rEPA) and 100 μg 3'AmNic-DT (400 μg Al^{3+}), it is reasonable to conclude that the NIC7-001 alum/CpG formulation will elicit >10–15-fold titers than NicVAX (400 μg vaccine dose with 1.2 μg Al^{3+}). Assuming linearity, these findings suggest that NIC7-001 may induce ~60 % or more of the population to attain nic·IgG levels greater than 125 μg/ml with high affinity.

Well-controlled animal studies of the nic·mAb, Nic311, derived from NicVAX, with nicotine affinity of 60 nM indicated that a 160 mg/kg dose reduced nicotine brain levels by 79 % in a rat PK model and a fully human nic·mAb (Nic12 derived from NicQβ) with nicotine affinity of 7 nM required a 150 mg/kg dose to reduce nicotine levels by 80 % in a mouse PK model. As described above, the hypothetical nic·IgG threshold level of clinical efficacy determined for NicVAX was >125 μg/ml, or 5–10× greater than previously estimated (Maurer et al. 2005; Hatsukami et al. 2011).

[3] NIC7-001 is comprised of a nicotine-hapten antigen (NIC7; pyridine 5C-position linker) conjugated to CRM (~15 haptens/CRM).

In order to bind one to two cigarettes worth of nicotine in the plasma of a smoker and assuming a volume of distribution for the nic·IgG or Nic·mAb of 70 ml/Kg (~2/3 of the Ab resides outside of the bloodstream) that "a serum antibody concentration of 100 μg/ml would provide about 6 μMol of binding sites for nicotine (two binding sites per IgG)" (Pentel and LeSage 2014).

2.7 Basic Research Focused on Improving the Immune Response of Nicotine Conjugate Vaccines

Since its establishment at the National Institutes of Health, the National Institute on Drug Abuse has made a long-term commitment to relieving the burden of smoking and smoking-related illness through sustained sponsorship of basic research, drug discovery, and development of novel biologicals for substance use disorders. Nearly all nicotine conjugate vaccine efforts have been supported by NIDA. Over the last 5 years, NIDA has accelerated dozens of academic and early private sector research efforts by providing tens of millions of dollars to overcome the limitations of first-generation vaccine technology and design (NIDA 2011–2015). Many of these NIDA-sponsored research efforts are aimed at improving adjuvants, formulations, carriers, haptens, hapten density, and synthetic "nanotechnology" vaccine platforms that emphasize high-quality and reproducible production. The rationale and the basis for these fundamentally new approaches will be expanded upon by their investigators in later chapters of this book. Furthermore, a quite novel approach involving gene transfer and prolonged expression of a Nic·mAb (Hicks et al. 2012) promises a single-dose vaccination for the prevention of nicotine addiction/dependency if the preclinical results translate clinically with an acceptable safety profile.

2.8 Summary

Therapeutic vaccines for treating nicotine addiction have been extensively evaluated from the first preclinical "proof of concept" studies in the late 1990s up to and including the recent phase III clinical trials. The disappointing clinical results of the first-generation of candidate vaccines have led to efforts focused on improving vaccine formulations (e.g. TLR agonist adjuvants) and the introduction of novel nicotine-hapten linkers and carriers. Between 2007 and 2010, Novartis and GSK established codevelopment partnerships with Cytos Biotechnology and Nabi Biopharmaceuticals to advance the first generation of nicotine conjugate vaccines into the clinic and both of these programs were halted in late-stage development subsequently both pharmaceutical companies have exited the field, while Pfizer, based on their assessment of the Cytos NicQβ and the Nabi NicVAX programs, coupled with their acquisition of Coley Pharmaceutical and access to a potent proprietary TLR agonist program, decided to pursue independently a second-generation nicotine conjugate vaccine program, NIC7-001. The preclinical results, including NHP studies of NIC7-001, have been sufficiently promising that Pfizer has initiated phase I/II clinical studies with results anticipated in the first half of 2016. Post hoc analyses of the NicVAX phase III studies have provided putative candidate threshold levels of high-affinity nic · IgG > 125 μg/ml (Fahim and Kalnik 2012) and earlier studies of Nic · mAbs (Keyler et al. 2005) demonstrated preclinical efficacy at concentrations of 150 μg/ml. Thus, in conclusion, if the promising NIC7-001 high-affinity immune response and functional results in rodent and NHPs hold true in the clinic, the future could be very bright for this second-generation of nicotine vaccines.

Bibliography

Bachmann M, Jennings G. Therapeutic vaccines for chronic diseases: successes and technical challenges. Phil Trans R Soc B. 2011;366:2815–22.

Beerli R, et al. Isolation of human monoclonal antibodies by mammalian cell display. Proc Natl Acad Sci U S A. 2008;105(38):14336–41.

Benowitz, NL Clinical pharmacology of nicotine: implications for understanding, preventing, and treating tobacco addiction. Clin Pharmacol Ther. 2008 Apr;83(4):531-41.

Bonese K, et al. Changes in heroin self-administration by a rhesus monkey after morphine immunisation. Nature. 1974;252:808–10.

Cahill K, Stead L, Lancaster T. Nicotine receptor partial agonists for smoking cessation. Cochrane Database Syst Rev. 2012;4:CD006103.

Carrera M, et al. Investigations using immunization to attenuate the psychoactive effects of nicotine. Bioorg Med Chem. 2004;12:563–70.

CDC. Smoking & Tobacco Use: Fast Facts. [Online]. 2015. Available at: http://www.cdc.gov/tobacco/data_statistics/fact_sheets/fast_facts/index.htm#cost. Accessed 4 July 2015.

Cerny E, et al. Preclinical development of a vaccine 'against smoking'. Onkologie. 2002;25(5):406–11.

Cornuz J, et al. A vaccine against nicotine for smoking cessation: a randomized controlled trial. PLoS One. 2008;3(6):2547.

Davis H, et al. NIC7-DT, a novel anti-nicotine vaccine, induces better functional antibody responses in mice compares to a Nic-QBeta Mimetic. Society for Research on Nicotine and Tobacco: XIV annual meeting of the SRNT Europe, Helsinki. 2012. p. Abstract O10.

de Villiers S, et al. Active immunization against nicotine suppresses nicotine-induced dopamine release in the rat nucleus accumbens shell. Respiration. 2002;69(3):247–53.

deWit H, Zacny J. Abuse potential of nicotine replacement therapies. CNS Drugs. 1995;4(6):456–68.

Fahim R, Kalnik M. Personlized drug treatment methods. PCT/US, Patent No. PCT/US2011/061229 US20110182918. 2012.

Fahim R, Kessler P, Fuller S, Kalnik M. Nicotine vaccines. CNS Neurol Disord Drug Targets Rev. 2011;8:905–15.

Fahim R, Kessler P, Kalnik M. Therapeutic vaccines against tobacco addiction. Expert Rev Vaccines. 2013;12(3):333–42.

Fraser C, et al. Generation of a universal CD4 memory T cell recall peptide effective in humans, mice and non-human primates. Vaccine. 2014;32(24):2896–903.

Gonzales D, et al. Varenicline, an alpha4beta2 nicotinic acetylcholine receptor partial agonist, vs sustained-release bupropion and placebo for smoking cessation: a randomized controlled trial. JAMA. 2006;296(1):47–55.

Gorelick DA. Pharmacokinetic strategies for treatment of drug overdose and addiction. Future Med Chem. 2012;4(2):227–43.

Hartmann-Boyce J, Cahill K, Hatsukami D, Cornuz J. Nicotine vaccines for smoking cessation. Cochrane Database Syst Rev. 2012;(8):CD007072.

Hatsukami D, et al. Immunogenicity and smoking-cessation outcomes for a novel nicotine immunotherapeutic. Clin Pharmacol Ther. 2011;89(3):392–9.

Henningfield J, Keenan R. Nicotine delivery kinetics and abuse liability. J Consult Clin Psychol. 1993;61(5):743–50.

Henningfield J, Miyasato K, Jasinski D. Abuse liability and pharmacodynamic characteristics of intravenous and inhaled nicotine. J Pharmacol Exp Ther. 1985;234(1):1–12.

Hicks M, et al. AAV-directed persistent expression of a gene encoding anti-nicotine antibody for smoking cessation. Sci Transl Med. 2012;4(140):140ra87.

Hieda Y, et al. Active immunization alters the plasma nicotine concentration in rats. J Pharmacol Exp Ther. 1997;283(3):1076–81.

Hieda Y, et al. Immunization of rats reduces nicotine distribution to brain. Psychopharmacology (Berl). 1999;143(2):150–7.

Hughes J, Callas P. Is delaying a quit attempt associated with less success? Nicotine Tob Res. 2011;13(12):1228–32.

Isomura S, Wirsching P, Janda K. An immunotherapeutic program for the treatment of nicotine addiction: hapten design and synthesis. J Org Chem. 2001;66:4115–21.

Jalah R, et al. Efficacy, but Not antibody titer or affinity, of a heroin hapten conjugate vaccine correlates with increasing hapten densities on tetanus toxoid, but not on CRM197 carriers. Bioconjug Chem. 2015;26:1041–53.

Johnston L. NIH Research Portfolio online reporting tools: project information 1U01DA037592-01. [Online]. 2014. Available at: http://projectreporter.nih.gov/project_info_description.cfm?aid=8707101&icde=25254746&ddparam=&ddvalue=&ddsub=&cr=2&csb=default&cs=ASC. Accessed 5 July 2015.

Jorenby D, et al. Efficacy of varenicline, an alpha4beta2 nicotinic acetylcholine receptor partial agonist, vs placebo or sustained-release bupropion for smoking cessation: a randomized controlled trial. JAMA. 2006;296(1):56–63.

Keyler D, et al. Monoclonal nicotine-specific antibodies reduce nicotine distribution to brain in rats: dose- and affinity-response relationships. Drug Metab Dispos. 2005;33(7):1056–61.

Keyler D, et al. Enhanced immunogenicity of a bivalent nicotine vaccine. Int Immunopharmacol. 2008;8:1589–94.

Kinsey B. Vaccines against drugs of abuse: where are we now? Ther Adv Vaccines. 2014;2(4):106–17.

Kosten T, Domingo C. Can you vaccinate against substance abuse? Expert Opin Biol Ther. 2013;13(8):1093–7.

Lindblom N, et al. Active immunization against nicotine prevents reinstatement of nicotine-seeking behavior in rats. Respiration. 2002;69(3):254–60.

Lockner JW, et al. A conjugate vaccine using enantiopure hapten imparts superior nicotine-binding capacity J Med Chem. 2015 Jan 22;58(2):1005–11.

Maurer P, et al. A therapeutic vaccine for nicotine dependence: preclinical efficacy, and phase I safety and Immunogenicity. Eur J Immunol. 2005;35:2031–40.

McCluskie M, et al. Enhancing immunogenicity of a 3′aminomethylnicotine-DT-conjugate anti-nicotine vaccine with CpG adjuvant in mice and non-human primates. Int Immunopharmacol. 2013a;16(1):50–6.

McCluskie M, et al. A novel anti-nicotine vaccine, shows significantly superior function in non-human primates (NHP) compared to a CYT002-NICQB mimetic. 19th annual meeting of the Society for Research on Nicotine and Tobacco, Boston. 2013b. p. Abstract PA13-4.

McCluskie M, et al. Molecular attributes of conjugate antigen influence function of antibodies induced by anti-nicotine vaccine in mice and non-human primates. Int Immunopharmacol. 2015;16(1):50–6.

Moreno A, Janda K. Immunopharmacotherapy: vaccination strategies as a treatment for drug abuse and dependence. Pharmacol Biochem Behav. 2009;92(2):199–205.

Moreno A, et al. A critical evaluation of a nicotine vaccine within a self-administration behavioral model. Mol Pharm. 2010;7(2):431–41.

Nelson R, et al. Effect of rate of administration on subjective and physiological effects of intravenous cocaine in humans. Drug Alcohol Depend. 2006;82(1):19–24.

NIDA, 2011–2015. NIH Research Online Reporting Tool Query "nicotine vaccines". [Online]. Available at: http://projectreporter.nih.gov/reporter.cfm. Accessed 5 July 2015.

Pentel P, LeSage M. New directions in nicotine vaccine design and use. Adv Pharmacol. 2014;69:553–80.

Pentel PR, et al. A nicotine conjugate vaccine reduces nicotine distribution to brain and attenuates its behavioral and cardiovascular effects in rats. Pharmacol Biochem Behav. 2000;65(1):191–8.

Pittet L, et al. Development and preclinical evaluation of SEL-068, a novel targeted Synthetic Vaccine Particle (tSVP™) for smoking cessation and relapse prevention that generates high titers of antibodies against nicotine. J Immunol. 2012;188(Meeting Abstract Supplement):75.11.

Porchet H, Benowitz N, Sheiner L, Copeland J. Apparent tolerance to the acute effect of nicotine results in part from distribution kinetics. J Clin Invest. 1987;80(5):1466–71.

Pravetoni M, et al. Structurally distinct nicotine immunogens elicit antibodies with non-overlapping specificities. Biochem Pharmacol. 2012;83(4):543–50.

Pryde D, et al. Selection of a novel anti-nicotine vaccine: influence of antigen design on antibody function in mice. PLoS One. 2013;8(10), e76557.

Raupach T, Hoogsteder PHJ, van Schayck C. Nicotine vaccines to assist with smoking cessation: current status of research. Drugs. 2012;72(4):e1–16.

Roiko SA, Harris AC, Keyler DE, Lesage MG, Zhang Y, Pentel PR. Combined active and passive immunization enhances the efficacy of immunotherapy against nicotine in rats. J Pharmacol Exp Ther. 2008;325(3):985–93.

Selecta Biosciences. Selecta biosciences: technology platform. [Online]. 2015. Available at: http://www.selectabio.com/technology-platform/index.cfm. Accessed 5 July 2015.

Stitzer M, de Wit H. Abuse liability of nicotine. In: Benowitz NL, editor. Nicotine safety and toxicity. New York: Oxford University Press; 1998. p. 119–31.

USHHS. The Health Consequences of Smoking—50 years of progress. A Report of the Surgeon General. [Online]. 2014. Available at: http://www.surgeongeneral.gov/library/reports. Accessed 4 July 2015.

Wagena E, de Vos A, Horwith G, van Schayck C. The immunogenicity and safety of a nicotine vaccine in smokers and nonsmokers: results of a randomized, placebo-controlled phase 1/2 trial. Nicotine Tob Res. 2008;10(1):213–8.

Chapter 3
Vaccines for Treating Cocaine Use Disorders

Coreen B. Domingo, Daryl Shorter, and Thomas R. Kosten

3.1 Introduction

Worldwide, the United Nations Office on Drugs and Crime (UNODC) estimates the global annual prevalence of cocaine use to be between .3 and .4 %, affecting 13–20 million individuals between 15 and 64 years of age. North America remains among the top 3 markets for cocaine with more than 5 million past year users and an estimated 3000 deaths annually due to cocaine use (United Nations Office on Drugs and Crime (UNODC) 2012). The impact of cocaine use disorders on our healthcare system is significant, making it a major public health issue. A recent US National Survey on Drug Use and Health noted that cocaine use disorders accounted for 8 % of all patients who entered substance abuse treatment programs (SAMHSA 2012a, b). Further, of patients 21 years or older, cocaine was found to be the most common illicit drug involved in drug-related emergency department (ED) visits, accounting for almost half of the approximately one million illicit drug-related ED visits annually (NIH-NIDA 2011). These drug-related ED visits cover a wide range of brain and cardiovascular-related disorders (Kosten et al. 2011). Brain disorders include seizures, strokes, movement disorders, more general neuropsychiatric impairment, and psychoses. Movement disorders associated with stimulants include chorea, dystonia, akathisia, and choreoathetosis. While cocaine-induced psychosis is uncommon, users can experience delusions of persecution and hallucinations of virtually any type. Cocaine's profound effects on the cardiovascular system can

C.B. Domingo, DrPH • D. Shorter, MD • T.R. Kosten, MD (✉)
Michael E DeBakey Veterans Affairs Medical Center, Houston, TX, USA

Menninger Department of Psychiatry and Behavioral Sciences, Baylor College of Medicine, Houston, TX, USA
e-mail: cdomingo@bcm.edu; shorter@bcm.edu; kosten@bcm.edu

I.D. Montoya (ed.), *Biologics to Treat Substance Use Disorders: Vaccines, Monoclonal Antibodies, and Enzymes*, DOI 10.1007/978-3-319-23150-1_3

result in serious and often lethal complications including myocardial ischemia and infarction, cardiomyopathy, myocarditis, arrhythmias, endocarditis, and aortic dissection. Within the first hour after cocaine intake, the risk of myocardial infarction (MI) is significant and is 23.7 times greater compared to 3 h following intake in individuals who are otherwise at low risk for MI (Mittleman et al. 1991). Chest pain is commonly experienced by cocaine users that present to emergency departments and is associated with acute MI in upward of 6 % of these patients (Mukherjee 2008). Obstructive coronary artery disease has been found in 35–40 % in patients that experience cocaine-induced chest pain that underwent diagnostic angiography (Dressler et al. 1990). Thus, developing a medication that would not only reduce the reinforcing properties of cocaine but also its many medical complications is a critical need. Although research is advancing, there are presently no FDA-approved pharmacotherapies for cocaine dependence (Kosten et al. 2011; Haile et al. 2012).

In terms of optimal pharmacotherapeutic interventions for the treatment of cocaine use disorder, characteristics such as agent duration of action and frequency of administration are primary considerations. Immunotherapies present a relevant and timely intervention, since they can be long-acting agents to prevent relapse as well as blocking a broad range of cocaine's effects, including those in the central nervous system (e.g., reward, reinforcement, neuropsychiatric sequelae) as well as cardiovascular system. Active vaccines against cocaine have a substantial history of development and can potentially reduce reinforcement and some acute toxicity from cocaine (Kosten and Owens 2005; Orson et al. 2008; Haney and Kosten 2004). These vaccine-induced antibodies are meant to bind to cocaine molecules in the circulation, preventing their ability to traverse the blood–brain barrier, and prevent activation of the brain's reinforcement pathways (e.g., dopamine activation of the nucleus accumbens) and thus blunt the addictive liability of cocaine. An important component of this capture of cocaine by the antibody is that bound cocaine molecules are metabolized into inactive compounds which minimally bind to the antibody and are subsequently excreted (Fox et al. 1996). The cocaine is broken down by pseudocholinesterase in the circulation or by nonenzymatic hydrolysis into inactive metabolites such as benzoylecgonine, ecgonine methylester, and benzoic acid body (Stewart et al. 1979). In theory, these inactive metabolites do not bind to the antibody. Therefore, free antibody is available to bind more cocaine, rather than remaining attached to metabolites. This detachment from inactive metabolites likely prolongs and potentiates the antibodies' capacity for blocking more cocaine from entering the brain (Kosten et al. 2012).

This simple "sponge" model of anti-cocaine antibodies probably describes a significant component of their actions (Shen and Kosten 2011). However, these antibodies cannot indefinitely soak up the abused drugs since the total number of antibody binding sites is necessarily limited. Furthermore, not every cocaine molecule of a bolus dose can be tightly bound. The additional actions of the anti-cocaine antibodies act as pharmacokinetic buffers against the rapid transit of cocaine into the brain. The rapid brain accumulation within seconds from a bolus cocaine dose delivered by either smoked or intravenous cocaine administration is prevented by the relatively slower equilibrium developed between free and antibody-bound cocaine in the blood. Smoked cocaine administration is highly reinforcing while cocaine powder for intranasal administration has much less reinforcement for an equivalent dose (Nelson et al. 2006; Cornish and O'Brien 1996; Walsh et al. 2009; Smith et al. 2001; Rush et al. 1999). Furthermore, oral cocaine requires considerably larger doses to be as reinforcing as the intravenous route of administration. This need for an increased dose in part reflects that oral cocaine reaches the brain relatively slowly, and although high blood and brain levels can be attained, much higher levels are needed to produce euphoria or other reinforcing effects. The kinetic effects of a pool of antibodies in circulation may act in a similar way by slowing drug entry into the brain and reducing the reinforcing effects of this drug. Thus, the specificity and ability of antibodies to slow cocaine entry from the blood vessels into the brain, heart, and other key organs can be a more effective blocker of reinforcement and perhaps toxicity than a transporter-based antagonist. However, any antibody strategy will be a competitive antagonism that can be overridden by sufficient doses of cocaine. Overall, these immunotherapies are aids to prevent relapse among patients motivated to become and remain abstinent and are less likely to be successful for inducing abstinence among current heavily cocaine-dependent individuals. Vaccines also will be most successful in conjunction with other behavioral and pharmacological therapies (Kosten et al. 2012).

3.2 Development of Cocaine Immunotherapy

The first report of an anti-cocaine vaccine was made by Bagasra in 1992 (Bagasra et al. 1992) and during that same time period other investigators tried to create cocaine catalytic antibodies (Chandrakumar et al. 1993; Landry et al. 1993; Basmadjian et al. 1995; Berkman et al. 1996). The simple anti-cocaine vaccine linked a cocaine derivative such as norcocaine to an antigenic carrier protein, since the cocaine alone was too small to elicit an immune response. The more complex catalytic antibodies attempted to imitate normal esterases in tissue such as butyrylcholinesterase (Lynch et al. 1997) that hydrolyze cocaine at its phenyl ester to give ecgonine methyl ester and benzoic acid. Because these metabolites have little if any pharmacological activity, the cocaine would be rendered inactive. The concept with catalytic antibodies was to create transition state analogs as haptens that would mimic the intermediate and unstable chemical structures that lead to the hydrolysis reaction. Thus, these antibodies would act as enzymes to catalyze the release of the benzoyl group from cocaine. One vaccination approach produced polyclonal antibodies that were reported to have this effect, although the potential superiority to the already existing normal cholinesterase in human blood was not clear (Chandrakumar et al. 1993). Landry (Landry et al. 1993) produced monoclonal antibodies that had the potential for selection of a high-activity enzyme-like antibody, but this never reached clinical testing. Berkman (Berkman et al. 1996) chemically prepared a hapten that induced antibodies when conjugated to keyhole limpet hemocyanin (KLH) and reported this hapten as being chemically stable and long lived rather than spontaneously breaking down from its seemingly unstable transition state conformation. Monoclonal antibodies were developed from this KLH vaccine in mice, but were not subjected to definitive behavioral testing for efficacy in reducing cocaine actions or reinforcement. Furthermore, although catalytic antibodies would allow a relatively small number of antibodies from a vaccine or monoclonal to destroy cocaine molecules and rapidly take on more cocaine, the quantity, affinity, and behavioral efficacy of these antibodies were not addressed.

At about the same time as these catalytic antibodies were being developed, a significant discovery advanced the development of cocaine vaccines for making antibodies against the cocaine itself rather than making antibodies as catalysts for metabolism of cocaine (Matsushita et al. 2001). This discovery involved the linker molecule between the carrier protein and the cocaine hapten. The structure of this linker had typically included a string of three to eight carbons between the attachment to the carrier protein and the cocaine molecule. Another important variation was in the position on the cocaine molecule for attaching this linker chain. Janda reported that having an amide group in the carbon chain of the linker and having that linker attached at the methyl ester position rather than at the tropane nitrogen of cocaine gave better results than other linkage structures and linking positions on the cocaine. Among the other linking positions, a photoactivation method inserted a linker between one of the carbon-carbon bonds of cocaine rather than the methyl ester or the tropane nitrogen of cocaine (Ettinger et al. 1997). However, this method did not allow control over which bond or how many of the carbon-carbon bonds of the cocaine would get these linker attachments. In spite of this limitation for commercial application of such a vaccine, the resulting vaccine appeared to produce functional antibodies based on both place preference conditioning assays and attenuation of the discriminative stimulus properties of cocaine (Johnson and Ettinger 2000).

Janda's anti-cocaine vaccine used a hapten named GNC that had a six-carbon linker terminating in a carboxylic acid group and conjugated to KLH on its free lysines (Carrera et al. 1995). Vaccinated rats showed suppression of cocaine-induced locomotor activity and lower brain levels of cocaine. Using this same vaccine, he then showed prevention of cocaine reinstatement of self-administration in rats (Carrera et al. 2000). Jhanda and colleagues then developed a second hapten called GND that replaced the two ester groups of GNC with two amide groups. Similar to GNC, vaccinated rats displayed suppression of cocaine's locomotor activity (Carrera et al. 2001).

A similar anti-cocaine vaccine was created consisting of succinyl norcocaine (SNC) conjugated to bovine serum albumin (BSA) (Fox et al. 1996). This vaccine reduced cocaine brain levels of vaccinated mice after a cocaine dose. Furthermore, rhesus monkeys vaccinated with SNC-BSA had suppressed operant responding to a food reward (Koetzner et al. 2001). A commercial version of this same vaccine conjugated SNC to cholera toxin B. This commercial vaccine called TA-CD elicited antibody levels sufficient to antagonize self-administration of cocaine in rats (Kantak et al. 2000, 2001). Cocaine-specific antibodies generated in response to TA-CD also reduced early cocaine distribution to the brain by 25–80 % compared to controls. Both TA-CD and the KLH-related vaccines were used subcutaneously in mice. However, one study vaccinated mice both intranasally and subcutaneously with SNC–KLH and measured serum and brain cocaine levels after a challenge with cocaine (Hrafnkelsdottir et al. 2005). The brain levels were less for all cocaine-immunized groups than for controls, but brain levels of cocaine were 2 times higher in the intranasally vaccinated mice than in the subcutaneously vaccinated mice. Because the serum level of antibodies was fivefold higher in the intranasally than in the subcutaneously vaccinated mice, the investigators suggested that mucosal antibodies could sequester the cocaine and that intranasal vaccination could be useful for smoked or snorted cocaine. This intranasal route of administration was never moved to clinical trials, however, and intramuscularly administered TA-CD, which conjugated SNC to inactivated cholera toxin B, is the only cocaine vaccine so far that has made it into clinical trials.

3.3 Clinical Studies of the Cocaine Vaccine TA-CD

Human dosing of the TA-CD cocaine vaccine initially tested three different ascending doses with a dosing schedule based on the rodent work. In the rodents, a dosing schedule of an initial vaccination followed by two additional boosts had produced cocaine-specific antibodies at relatively high titers (Kantak et al. 2000, 2001). The schedule of human dosing therefore was three times over a 12-week period, although one rather than two booster vaccinations are typically given in humans for cholera protection (Svennerholm et al. 1984). The dose of TA-CD in the first human cohort started at 10 ug, because this dose was the standard used for cholera vaccination and was therefore considered relatively safe (Jertborn et al. 1992). Subsequent cohorts of subjects had dosing escalated 10- and 100-fold to 100 ug and 1000 ug per dose.

The phase I trial of TA-CD enrolled formerly cocaine-dependent subjects who were residing in a drug-free residential program without access to cocaine (Kosten et al. 2002). The 34 subjects were allocated to placebo ($n=6$), 10 ug ($n=8$), 100 ug ($n=10$), and 1000 ug ($n=10$). The TA-CD-induced cocaine-specific antibodies in all vaccinated subjects, but the peak antibody levels were quite variable across subjects within each of the three dose groups. The average of these peak levels also showed no difference between the 10 ug and 100 ug doses. However, the 1000 ug dose showed a clear doubling in antibody levels compared to these other two doses. These antibody levels declined by fourfold within 3 months after the final vaccination and did not persist beyond 1 year. Overall, the safety profile for the vaccine was quite favorable. Almost all recipients (33 of 34) reported local pain and/or tenderness at the injection site, with no difference between experimental and placebo groups or across the three different vaccine doses. This side effect profile was consistent with what might be expected from the alum adjuvant (Grabenstein 1994). Treatment-related systemic adverse effects that occurred in all groups included mild tachycardia, elevated temperature, and hypertension (Kosten et al. 2002). However, no serious adverse effects occurred during vaccination or the 12 months of follow-up.

Further studies examined the effects of smoked cocaine administration in vaccinated humans (Haney et al. 2010). Ten cocaine-dependent men were assessed for 13 weeks for the effects of cocaine (0, 25, 50 mg) prior to vaccination and at weekly intervals thereafter. Two doses of TA-CD (82 μg, $n = 4$; 360 μg, $n = 6$) were administered at weeks 1, 3, 5, and 9. The peak antibody titers ranged from 200 to 2300 units with a mean of 800 units. This mean antibody titer of 800 units corresponded to a 20 μg/ml level of anti-cocaine IgG and based on this study was considered the minimal level needed in order for the TA-CD vaccine to substantially decrease the intoxicating effects of a single smoked cocaine dose. A split of subjects on the mean peak plasma antibody levels showed that those in the upper half had an immediate and robust (55–81 %) reduction in subjective ratings of cocaine effects. However, those in the lower half showed no significant reduction. Higher plasma antibody levels were associated with higher peak heart rate after smoking cocaine at 50 mg, but no other potential toxicities were reported including no allergic or inflammatory responses to the vaccinations. Since cocaine primarily increases heart rate by peripheral rather than central activation of the sympathetic nervous system, higher plasma cocaine levels in the peripheral circulation probably accounted for the enhanced heart rate in the high-antibody group. Plasma cocaine levels significantly correlated with heart rate after being fully vaccinated and taking cocaine. Thus, increased plasma cocaine probably contributed to the greater cocaine-induced tachycardia in the subjects with high antibody levels.

A phase IIa outpatient trial randomized 18 subjects to two dose levels of TA-CD: 100 μg given for 4 injections and 400 μg given for 5 injections. These injections were administered over 3 months, and 16 of 18 subjects (89 %) successfully completed the 14-week study. Both vaccine dosages elicited an immunological response with cocaine-specific antibodies that persisted for at least 6 months (Martell et al. 2005). Mean antibody levels were three times higher in the high-dose group, but both groups showed substantial variability in antibody levels across subjects. The high-dose group was more likely to achieve and remain abstinent during the study (71 % vs 44 %). However, a substantial number of patients in both groups relapsed at 6 months (89 % in the low-dose and 43 % in the high-dose group), when the antibody levels had dropped to very low levels. No subjects had serious adverse events including the two subjects who did not complete the study and had received only one vaccination. These two did not discontinue due to side effects. Vaccination boosters between 9.5 and 12.5 months after initial vaccination resulted in substantial antibody titer responses in all vaccines.

An initial phase IIb trial enrolled 115 cocaine-dependent, methadone-maintained subjects who completed 5 injections of TA-CD at 360 μg or placebo (Cornish and O'Brien 1996). The actively vaccinated subjects were stratified into high- and low-antibody-producing groups based on a cutoff above 43 μg/ml. This cutoff level was calculated to be a sufficient antibody level to block three to four expected doses of cocaine that cocaine addicts might take in order to try to override the antibody blockade. The cutoff antibody level that was considered the level needed to block a single smoked cocaine dose was determined from the previous cocaine administration study as above 20 μg/ml (Haney et al. 2010). About one-third of the vaccinated subjects did not attain this peak antibody level of 20 ug/ml, and about one-third attained levels above 43 ug/ml, which was the high-antibody group. This high-antibody group showed a greater percentage of cocaine-free urines than either the placebo or low-antibody groups during weeks 9–16 (45 % vs 35 %), when the antibody levels were considered to be in the therapeutic range for the high-antibody group. Furthermore, the proportion of subjects having a 50 % reduction in cocaine use from the baseline 8 weeks compared to weeks 9–16 also was significantly greater in the high-IgG than low-IgG subjects (0.53 vs 0.23) ($P<0.04$). The high antibody levels remained elevated at the 25-week follow-up, 3 months after the last vaccination. The safety profile of the vaccine was favorable with the most common side effects being injection site induration and tenderness, and no severe adverse events were related to the vaccine. In summary, while attaining high (≥43 μg/mL) IgG anti-cocaine antibody levels was associated with significantly reduced cocaine use, only 38 % of the vaccinated attained these IgG levels and they had only 2 months of adequate cocaine blockade. Thus, any practical use of this vaccine will require bimonthly boosters in order to maintain these high-IgG levels, as well as getting better vaccines and adjuvants so that a greater proportion of those vaccinated can attain these potentially therapeutic antibody levels.

Although these actively immunized subjects showed no significant difference from the placebo subjects in complete abstinence, their reduction in cocaine use may be therapeutically meaningful. Over half (0.53) of the high-IgG group showed no new episodes of cocaine use at least 50 % of the time (Preston criteria). Furthermore, they doubled their cocaine-free urines from a baseline below 20 to 45 % between weeks 8 and 16, and doubling of cocaine-free urines has been associated with a significant improvement in social functioning in a previous study. This previous meta-analysis of 368 subjects in two 25-week randomized, controlled trials of behavioral abstinence reinforcement in methadone-maintained cocaine abusers found that social functioning was substantially improved with a doubling of cocaine-free urines (Ghitza et al. 2007).

The cholera toxin B produced substantial IgG antibody responses to the cholera protein in every patient, but reasons for the lower levels of anti-cocaine antibodies in as many as one-third of these patients appear to be complex. This poor vaccine response in some patients was associated with the presence of IgM antibodies capable of binding cocaine prior to the initial vaccination of those subjects. Immunological recognition of cocaine before vaccination could represent a response to cocaine that is T-cell independent. One possibility may be adduct formation by the cocaine to native proteins in vivo (Deng et al. 2002) that results in inhibition of the desired T-dependent response to the conjugate vaccine (Lindroth et al. 2004).

The antibody levels appear to decline substantially over about 3 months after the peak antibody response, and a booster vaccination is needed to restimulate a rise in the antibody levels to their peak and maintain therapeutic levels for an additional 3 months. Thus, patients may need to get additional boosters every 3 months for a period of protection lasting 2 years, since exposure to cocaine alone will not provoke an increase in antibodies. However, after boosting with the conjugate vaccine, sufficient quantities of newly produced antibodies will be available for binding the cocaine in the circulation where it can be metabolized and the metabolites excreted (Stewart et al. 1979).

The success of these studies led to the development of a larger phase II multisite study to compare the effect of TA-CD to placebo on the degree of modulation of cocaine use in cocaine-dependent individuals who were motivated to quit or reduce use of cocaine (Kosten et al. 2014). The primary objective of this study was to evaluate the effect of 5 doses of TA-CD 400 μg compared to placebo on cocaine dependence over 8 weeks (weeks 9–16 inclusive). Subjects were recruited from 6 centers in the United States and included only subjects with a principal diagnosis of cocaine dependence without comorbid other drug dependences except for marijuana and nicotine. Following the initial vaccination, four boosters were given at study weeks 3, 5, 9, and 13 with at least 10 days between vaccinations. Three times per week visits were scheduled through study week 16 to collect the urine specimens and self-report on cocaine use.

Nationally 300 subjects were randomized, 152 to the active vaccine and 148 to placebo. The two groups were well matched and had equivalent baseline cocaine and alcohol use. The therapeutic peak antibody level of greater than 42/ug IgG was attained by 67 % of the 130 vaccine subjects receiving five vaccinations, which was twice the rate found in the previous single-site study (Martell et al. 2009). In the actively vaccinated group, those with peak antibody levels greater than 42/ug had almost 3-times fewer subjects dropout (7 % vs 20 %). Although for the full 16-week cocaine-positive urine rates showed no significant difference between the three groups (placebo, high IgG, low IgG), after week 8, more vaccinated than placebo subjects attained abstinence for at least 2 weeks of the trial (24 % vs 18 %), and the high-IgG group had the most cocaine-free urines for the last 2 weeks of treatment (OR = 3.02). Side effects also did not distinguish the two groups and the most common side effects reported were pain at the vaccination site and musculoskeletal aches. There were no sustained fevers or other signs of vaccination-related toxicities. There were also no differences in side effects related to peak antibody levels.

The adequately immunized subjects in this larger study may have increased their cocaine use to overcome the competitive anti-cocaine antibody blockade, since these antibody levels were only sufficient to block modest doses of cocaine. In contrast to the intent of this vaccine as a relapse prevention agent, these study patients were using cocaine several times per week and rarely attempted abstinence during the clinical trial. This difference in patient populations was reflected in much higher rate of cocaine-free urines during weeks 9–16 among the high-antibody-level patients, which was 48 % in the single-site study compared to only 25 % in the national multisite study. The difference outcome between the two studies may reflect several non-pharmacological differences in design and programmatic structure. First, the single-site study setting involved a daily methadone program with monitoring 6 days per week vs three times weekly monitoring in the national study. Second, delivery of cognitive behavioral therapy was mandated in the single-site methadone study and optional in the national study. Third, the single study site patient group was more homogenous than the primary cocaine users drawn from six sites in different regions of the country. Fourth, financial incentives of $55 per week plus $65 for each of the five vaccinations were approximately three times higher in the national than the single-site study, and this compensation may have been used to trade for cocaine.

3.4 Conclusions and Future Directions

Learning from these two clinical trials, future trials should consider a more structured study setting such as a day-treatment program to attain initial abstinence and obtain a more homogeneous population of patients who have been at least 2 weeks cocaine-free prior to starting the TA-CD vaccinations. Initial abstinence will take advantage of a key pharmacological component for which these vaccines can help in sustaining abstinence and preventing relapse to drug abuse and which is called the "priming effect" (de Wit 1996). Priming involves markedly intensified drug craving, rather than reduced craving after exposure to even a single small dose of cocaine during abstinence. This priming increases the risk for falling into a binge pattern of abuse and relapse. Finally, all of these cocaine vaccine clinical trials were most likely to succeed in patients who had a strong and sustained antibody response combined with the special advantage of the spontaneous and enzymatic hydrolysis of cocaine into inactive metabolites while still in the bloodstream, an advantage that vaccines for other abused drugs do not share.

Greater integration of CBT would facilitate the maintenance and initiation of abstinence. Any successful vaccination program needs to have 2–3 months where the patient can be brought to a treatment site for five vaccinations. During these 2–3 months, the patients could be vulnerable to relapse if they have already discontinued drug use. While continued drug abuse during the 3 months of vaccination does not interfere with the vaccine's ability to stimulate the required antibody production, continued drug abuse may lead to the patient dropping out before the full five vaccinations can be completed. To ensure compliance with the schedule of vaccinations, interventions could vary from residential substance abuse care to outpatient contingency management.

Acknowledgments Research support was provided by NIH grant P50-DA18197. Additionally, in part, this material is the result of work supported with resources and the use of facilities at the Michael E. DeBakey VA Medical Center, Houston, Texas. The views expressed in this article are those of the authors and do not necessarily reflect the position or policy of the Department of Veterans Affairs or the US government.

References

Bagasra O, Forman LJ, Howeedy A, Whittle P. A potential vaccine for cocaine abuse prophylaxis. Immunopharmacology. 1992;23:173–9.

Basmadjian GP, Singh S, Sastrodjojo B, Smith BT, Avor KS, Chang F, Mills SL, Seale TW. Generation of polyclonal catalytic antibodies against cocaine using transition state analogs of cocaine conjugated to diphtheria toxoid. Chem Pharm Bull (Tokyo). 1995;43(11):1902–11. PMID 8575031.

Berkman CE, Underiner GE, Cashman JR. Synthesis of an immunogenic template for the generation of catalytic antibodies for (–)-cocaine hydrolysis. J Org Chem. 1996;61:5686–9.

Carrera MR, Ashley JA, Parsons LH, Wirsching P, Koob GF, Janda KD. Suppression of psychoactive effects of cocaine by active PMID immunization. Nature. 1995;378:727–30.

Carrera MR, Ashley JA, Zhou B, Wirsching P, Koob GF, Janda KD. Cocaine vaccines: antibody protection against relapse in a rat model. Proc Natl Acad Sci. 2000;97:6202–6.

Carrera MR, Ashley JA, Wirsching P, Koob GF, Janda KD. A second-generation vaccine protects against the psychoactive effects of cocaine. Proc Natl Acad Sci. 2001;98:1988–92.

Chandrakumar NS, Carron CP, Meyer DM, Beardsley PM, Nash SA, Tam LL, Rafferty M. Phenylphosphonate monoester analogs of cocaine. Potential haptens for the generation of catalytic antibodies. Bioorg Med Chem Lett. 1993;3:309–12.

Cornish JW, O'Brien CP. Crack cocaine abuse: an epidemic with many public health consequences. Annu Rev Public Health. 1996;17:259–73.

de Wit H. Priming effects with drugs and other reinforcers. Exp Clin Psychopharmacol. 1996;4:5–10.

Deng SX, de Prada P, Landry DW. Anticocaine catalytic antibodies. J Immunol Methods. 2002;269(1–2):299–310.

Dressler FA, Malekzadeh S, Roberts WC. Quantitative analysis of amounts of coronary arterial narrowing in cocaine addicts. Am J Cardiol. 1990;65:303–8.

Ettinger RH, Ettinger WF, Harless WE. Active immunization with cocaine-protein conjugate attenuates cocaine effects. Pharmacol Biochem Behav. 1997;58:215–20.

Fox BS, Kantak KM, Edwards MA, Black KM, Bollinger BK, Botka AJ, French TL, Thompson TL, Schad VC, Greenstein JL, Gefter ML, Exley MA, Swain PA, Briner TJ. Efficacy of a therapeutic cocaine vaccine in rodent models. Nat Med. 1996;2(10):1129–32.

Ghitza UE, Epstein DH, Preston KL. Psychosocial functioning and cocaine use during treatment: strength of relationship depends on type of urine-testing method. Drug Alcohol Depend. 2007;911(2–3):169–77.

Grabenstein JD. ImmunoFacts: vaccines and immunological drugs. St. Louis: Facts and Comparisons Inc; 1994. p. 487b.

Haile CN, Mahoney 3rd JJ, Newton TF, De La Garza 2nd R. Pharmacotherapeutics directed at deficiencies associated with cocaine dependence: focus on dopamine, norepinephrine and glutamate. Pharmacol Ther. 2012;134:260–77.

Haney M, Kosten TR. Therapeutic vaccines for substance dependence. Expert Rev Vaccines. 2004;3:11–8.

Haney M, Gunderson EW, Jiang H, Collins ED, Foltin RW. Cocaine-specific antibodies blunt the subjective effects of smoked cocaine in humans. Biol Psychiatry. 2010;67(1):59–65.

Hrafnkelsdottir K, Valgeirsson J, Gizurarson S. Induction of protective and specific antibodies against cocaine by intranasal immunisation using a glyceride adjuvant. Biol Pharm Bull. 2005;28:1038–42.

Jertborn M, Svennerholm A-M, Holmgren J. Safety and immunogenicity of an oral recombinant cholera B subunit-whole cell vaccine in Swedish volunteers. Vaccine. 1992;10(2):130–2.

Johnson MW, Ettinger RH. Active cocaine immunization attenuates the discriminative properties of cocaine. Exp Clin Psychopharmacol. 2000;8:163–7.

Kantak KM, Collins SL, Lipman EG, Bond J, Giovanoni K, Fox BS. Evaluation of anti-cocaine antibodies and a cocaine vaccine in a rat self-administration model. Psychopharmacology (Berl). 2000;148:251–62.

Kantak KM, Collins SL, Bond J, Fox BS. Time course of changes in cocaine self-administration behavior in rats during immunization with the cocaine vaccine IPC-1010. Psychopharmacology (Berl). 2001;153:334–40.

Koetzner L, Deng S, Sumpter TL, Weisslitz M, Abner RT, Landry DW, Woods JH. Titer-dependent antagonism of cocaine following active immunization in rhesus monkeys. J Pharmacol Exp Ther. 2001;296:789–96.

Kosten T, Owens SM. Immunotherapy for the treatment of drug abuse. Pharmacol Ther. 2005;108(1):76–85.

Kosten TR, Rosen M, Bond J, Settles M, Roberts JS, Shields J, Jack L, Fox B. Human therapeutic cocaine vaccine: safety and immunogenicity. Vaccine. 2002;20:1196–204.

Kosten TR, Newton TF, De La Garza R, Haile CN. Cocaine and methamphetamine dependence: advances in treatment. 1st ed. Washington, DC: American Psychiatric Publishing; 2011.

Kosten T, Domingo C, Orson F, Kinsey B. Vaccines against stimulants: cocaine and MA. Br J Clin Pharmacol. 2012;77(2):368–74.

Kosten TR, Domingo CB, Shorter D, Orson F, Green C, Somoza E, Sekerka R, Levin FR, Mariani JJ, Stitzer M, Tompkins DA, Rotrosen J, Thakkar V, Smoak B, Kampman K. Vaccine for cocaine dependence: a randomized double-blind placebo-controlled efficacy trial. Drug Alcohol Depend. 2014;140:42–7.

Landry DW, Zhao K, Yang GX, Glickman M, Georgiadis TM. Antibody-catalyzed degradation of cocaine. Science. 1993;259:1899–901.

Lindroth K, Mastache EF, Roos I, Fernández AG, Fernández C. Understanding thymus-independent antigen-induced reduction of thymus-dependent immune responses. Immunology. 2004;112(3): 413–9.

Lynch TJ, Mattes CE, Singh A, Bradley RM, Brady RO, Dretchen KL. Cocaine detoxification by human plasma butyrylcholinesterase. Toxicol Appl Pharmacol. 1997;145:363–71.

Martell BA, Mitchell E, Poling J, Gonsai K, Kosten TR. Vaccine pharmacotherapy for the treatment of cocaine dependence. Biol Psychiatry. 2005;58:158–64.

Martell BA, Orson FM, Poling J, Mitchell E, Rossen RD, Gardner T, Kosten TR. Cocaine vaccine for the treatment of cocaine dependence in methadone-maintained patients: a randomized, double blind, placebo-controlled efficacy trial. Arch Gen Psychiatry. 2009;66(10):1116–23.

Matsushita M, Hoffman TZ, Ashley JA, Zhou B, Wirsching P, Janda KD. Cocaine catalytic antibodies: the primary importance of linker effects. Bioorg Med Chem Lett. 2001;11:87–90.

Mittleman MA, Mintzer D, Maclure M, Tofler GH, Sherwood JB, Muller J. Clinical investigation and reports. CrossMark. 1991;99:2737–41. http://circ.ahajournals.org/content/99/21/2737.full. Accessed 05/25/2015.

Mukherjee D. Management of cocaine-associated chest pain and myocardial infarction: a scientific statement from the American Heart Association Acute Cardiac Care Committee of the Council on Clinical Cardiology. Cardiosource-The American College of Cardiology. 2008. http://www.medscape.com/viewarticle/572723. Accessed 06/21/15.

Nelson RA, Boyd SJ, Ziegelstein RC, Herning R, Cadet JL, Henningfield JE, Schuster CR, Contoreggi C, Gorelick DA. Effect of rate of administration on subjective and physiological effects of intravenous cocaine in humans. Drug Alcohol Depend. 2006;82(1):19–24.

NIH-NIDA. Drug facts: drug related hospital emergency room visits. 2011. http://www.drugabuse.gov/publications/drugfacts/drug-related-hospital-emergency-room-visits. Accessed 01/15/2015.

Orson FM, Kinsey BM, Singh RA, Wu Y, Gardner T, Kosten TR. Substance abuse vaccines. Ann N Y Acad Sci. 2008;1141:257–69.

Rush CR, Baker RW, Wright K. Acute physiological and behavioral effects of oral cocaine in humans: a dose–response analysis. Drug Alcohol Depend. 1999;55(1–2):1–12.

SAMHSA. Substance Abuse and Mental Health Services Administration, Center for Behavioral Health Statistics and Quality. Treatment Episode Data Set (TEDS): 2000–2010. National Admissions to Substance Abuse Treatment Services. DASIS Series S-61, HHS Publication No. (SMA) 12-4671. Rockville, MD: 2012a.

SAMHSA. The DAWN report: highlights of the 2010 drug abuse warning network (DAWN) findings on drug-related emergency department visits. 2012b. http://www.samhsa.gov/data/sites/default/files/DAWN096/DAWN096/SR096EDHighlights2010.htm. Accessed 11/02/2014.

Shen X, Kosten TR. Immunotherapy for drug abuse. CNS Neurol Disord Drug Targets. 2011; 10(8):876–9.

Smith BJ, Jones HE, Griffiths RR. Physiological, subjective and reinforcing effects of oral and intravenous cocaine in humans. Psychopharmacology (Berl). 2001;156(4):435–44.

Stewart DJ, Inaba T, Lucassen M, Kalow W. Cocaine metabolism: cocaine and norcocaine hydrolysis by liver and serum esterases. Clin Pharmacol Ther. 1979;25:464–8.

Svennerholm A, Gothefors L, Sack D, Bardhan P, Holmgren J. Local and systemic antibody responses and immunological memory after immunization with cholera B subunit by different routes. Bull World Health Organ. 1984;62:909–18.

United Nations Office on Drugs and Crime (UNODC). 2012 Report. http://www.unodc.org/documents/data-and-analysis/WDR2012/WDR_2012_web_small.pdf. Accessed 05/10/2015.

Walsh SL, Stoops WW, Moody DE, Lin SN, Bigelow GE. Repeated dosing with oral cocaine in humans: assessment of direct effects, withdrawal, and pharmacokinetics. Exp Clin Psychopharmacol. 2009;17(4):205–16.

Chapter 4
Vaccines for Opioid Addiction

Michael D. Raleigh and Paul R. Pentel

4.1 Introduction

4.1.1 Rationale for Pursuing a Vaccine Strategy for Opioid Addiction Treatment

Opioid addiction is an unlikely target for treatment with a vaccine because effective agonist and antagonist treatments are already available. The motivation to consider additional approaches such as vaccines stems from the real as well as the perceived limitations of currently available medications and the resulting reluctance of both providers and opioid addicts to consider their use. Less than one in five candidates for agonist or antagonist medications in the USA are currently receiving them (NSDUH 2013).

Agonists (methadone, buprenorphine) have side effects such as constipation, require careful titration to avoid excessive sedation, and are themselves abusable and therefore subject to tight regulation and restricted availability (Appel et al. 2004; Rosenberg and Phillips 2003). Apart from the challenges posed by these considerations, the infrastructure needed to adequately regulate and administer agonist therapy is not currently feasible in many developing or politically unstable countries. Many opioid abusers, as well as prescribers, object to using an addictive

M.D. Raleigh, PhD (✉)
Pharmacology and Toxicology, Minneapolis Medical Research Foundation, Minneapolis, MN 55415, USA
e-mail: rale0011@umn.edu

P.R. Pentel, MD
Department of Medicine, Hennepin County Medical Center, Minneapolis Medical Research Foundation, Minneapolis, MN 55415, USA

Department of Medicine, University of Minnesota, Minneapolis, MN, USA
e-mail: pentel@umn.edu

I.D. Montoya (ed.), *Biologics to Treat Substance Use Disorders: Vaccines, Monoclonal Antibodies, and Enzymes*, DOI 10.1007/978-3-319-23150-1_4

medication as therapy. Although data strongly suggest that long-term use of agonist therapy is preferable, many opioid abusers on methadone opt to discontinue it at some point and have a very high risk of relapse (D'Aunno and Vaughn 1992; Nosyk et al. 2012). Antagonists (naltrexone) are less attractive to some opioid addicts because they do not directly suppress craving (Minozzi et al. 2006). Naltrexone blocks the action of all opioids and complicates treatment when those receiving it legitimately need opioids for analgesia. As with agonist therapy, it is common for those receiving naltrexone to periodically go off of it, either to see if it's still needed or to enable the abuse of their opioid of choice (Krupitsky et al. 2013).

Given these limitations, additional medication options could be helpful as alternatives for those who reject agonist or antagonist therapy, to protect patients when they opt to discontinue agonist or antagonist therapy, or to use in combination with agonists or antagonists. Opioid vaccines offer all of these options. The long duration of action of opioid vaccines is an additional potential benefit as it would require less frequent dosing and presumably improve compliance.

4.1.2 Mechanism of Action of Addiction Vaccines

This chapter focuses on issues specific to opioid vaccines: those directed against heroin as well as those directed against commonly abused prescription opioids. Comprehensive reviews of addiction vaccine design and mechanism of action are available elsewhere (Pentel and LeSage 2014; Kosten et al. 2014a; Stowe et al. 2011a). For the purposes of the current chapter, pertinent aspects of addiction vaccine action include the following.

Goal The goal of addiction vaccines is to generate drug-specific antibodies that can bind the target drug in serum and extracellular fluid and reduce or slow its distribution to the brain. Through these action vaccines can reduce the effects of the targeted drug(s), including addiction-relevant behaviors such as drug self-administration. In some but not all cases, these antibodies also alter drug elimination (Keyler et al. 1999). Because the abused doses of most drugs can exceed the binding capacity of the antibodies generated by vaccination, the most tractable clinical setting for vaccine use may be relapse prevention (blocking the action of a single or limited drug dose) rather than cessation (blocking the action of continuous high-dose drug use).

Vaccine design Addictive drugs, including opioids, are not by themselves immunogenic and will not elicit antibodies, but can be rendered immunogenic by linking either the target drug or a structurally related compound (hapten) to a foreign carrier protein through a linker. The resulting immunogen is generally mixed or covalently attached to an adjuvant, a class of compounds or mixtures that nonspecifically enhance the antibody response.

Antibody specificity Antibodies produced by such vaccines are generally highly specific for the targeted drug and do not bind even closely related drugs or most drug metabolites. No binding of antibodies to endogenous compounds or structures has been found.

Duration of action The half-life of drug-specific antibodies in rodents has not been carefully studied but has been estimated at 1–2 months for nicotine (Maurer et al. 2005) or heroin (Anton and Leff 2006) vaccines. Antibody levels can be restored by booster doses of vaccine. A study of the effects of the heroin vaccine M(gly)$_4$-KLH on locomotor activity in rats showed efficacy as long as 50 days after the last vaccine dose (Raleigh et al. 2013). Human data are not available for heroin vaccines, but phase II studies of nicotine or cocaine vaccines estimated drug-specific antibody half-lives of about 2 months (Maurer et al. 2005; Hatsukami et al. 2005; Kosten et al. 2002; Haney et al. 2010).

Vaccine safety No side effects beyond local irritation or transient minor systemic symptoms, similar to those associated with many infectious disease vaccines, have been seen to date in either animals or humans (Hatsukami et al. 2011; Kosten et al. 2014b).

Vaccine efficacy Vaccines for nicotine, cocaine, methamphetamine, and heroin/morphine have shown considerable efficacy for blocking or attenuating drug effects in rodents and primates. Nicotine and cocaine vaccines have progressed to phase III clinical trials (Hatsukami et al. 2011; Kosten et al. 2014b), but none have shown efficacy for reducing use of the targeted drug. The main limitation of this approach appears to be the lower serum antibody levels generated by these vaccines in humans compared to animals. Phase II clinical trials suggest that those individuals generating higher antibody levels may have benefited from vaccination, while those with lower antibody responses did not (Martell et al. 2009).

Combining addiction vaccines with other treatment medications Because their mechanisms of action differ and are complementary, it may be possible to use addiction vaccines in combination with other treatment medications. This has been demonstrated in principle for the use of a nicotine-specific monoclonal antibody along with the nicotinic receptor antagonist mecamylamine in rats (LeSage et al. 2012).

Efforts to improve addiction vaccines Second-generation vaccines using optimized hapten or linker structures, novel carrier proteins, nanoparticles as scaffolds or delivery systems, and newer adjuvants appear promising. It is likely that second-generation vaccines will provide the efficacy needed to study the therapeutic potential of addiction vaccines.

4.1.3 History of Opioid Vaccine Exploration

The first addiction vaccines studied were directed against opioids. Radioimmunoassays for morphine were developed in the early 1970s consisting

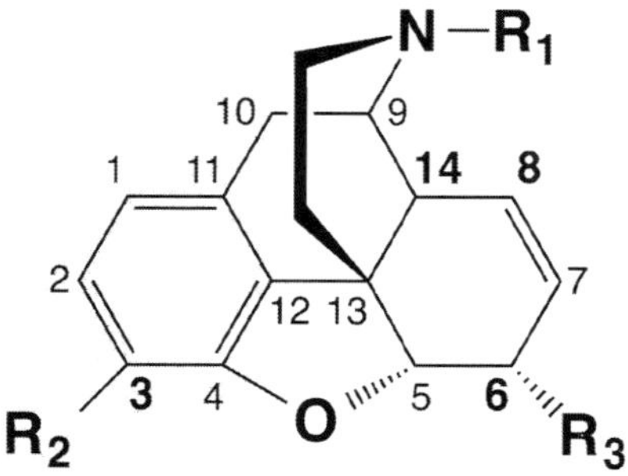

Fig. 4.1 Morphine structure. C3, C6, and the bridgehead nitrogen are the most common sites of linker (R_1, R_2, R_3) attachment for the synthesis of haptens used in heroin/morphine vaccines. Immunogen structures are provided in Table 4.2

of morphine linked via C6 or C3 (Fig. 4.1) to bovine serum albumin (Wainer et al. 1972a; Spector and Parker 1970; Adler and Liu 1971; Spector 1971). The intent of these assays was to allow the sensitive measurement of morphine concentrations in biological fluids. Realizing that IgG antibodies are largely confined to serum and extracellular fluid, it was soon shown that animals immunized with this conjugate would bind and sequester morphine or heroin in serum and that the distribution of morphine to the brain could be reduced (Hill et al. 1975). Opioid analgesia was likewise reduced by vaccination (Berkowitz and Spector 1972; Torten et al. 1975). The therapeutic potential of vaccines directed against morphine/heroin for treating addiction was consequently appreciated and investigated.

One such heroin vaccine was studied in a single monkey that had been trained to self-administer either heroin or cocaine (Bonese et al. 1974). (Note: Most vaccines intended to target either morphine or heroin have used haptens derived from modifications of morphine because of its greater stability in solution compared to heroin. The antibodies produced by such vaccines generally recognize or cross-react with and bind both morphine and heroin with high affinity. Because heroin is of greater interest as a target for addiction therapy, we will use the term heroin vaccines in this chapter for those derived from either heroin or morphine.) Subsequent vaccination against heroin reduced heroin, but not cocaine, self-administration. Similar results were obtained with the passive administration of heroin-specific antibodies (Killian et al. 1978). The attenuation of heroin self-administration by vaccination was substantial but could be overcome by greatly increasing the heroin unit dose. Because of this potential limitation, as well as increasing interest in methadone or naltrexone as treatment options, further efforts to develop heroin vaccines were not pursued at the time. It was not until nearly 25 years later that interest in opioid vaccines was rekindled by (1) the limited utilization of methadone and naltrexone, suggesting the need for additional types of pharmacotherapies; (2) an alarming increase in prescription opioid abuse and addiction (Dart et al. 2015); and (3) advances in addiction vaccine design owing to efforts with nicotine, cocaine, and infectious disease vaccines (Koff et al. 2013; Pentel et al. 2009).

4.1.4 Challenges in Developing Opioid Vaccines

The challenges posed by developing effective opioid vaccines are in part common to all addiction vaccines, and in part unique to opioid vaccines. The dominant shared challenge is reliably producing high concentrations of antibody in serum. This is important because the molar doses of these abused drugs are large and can easily exceed the binding capacity of serum antibody generated by vaccination (Table 4.1). Drug-specific antibody levels of up to 500 ug/ml, occasionally higher, can be elicited in rodents with nicotine (Cornish et al. 2013), cocaine (Kantak et al. 2000), or heroin (Kosten et al. 2014a; Anton and Leff 2006; Raleigh et al. 2013) vaccines. However, antibody levels achieved in clinical trials of nicotine or cocaine vaccines have been an order of magnitude or more lower, only rarely exceeding 100 ug/ml (Hatsukami et al. 2011; Martell et al. 2009; Esterlis et al. 2013). Vaccination of rodents generates higher antibody levels in part because higher immunogen doses can be administered. In humans, the largest tolerable volume of the injected solution is lower, and, in the case of alum adjuvant, the maximum allowable adjuvant dose is lower (because of concerns about aluminum toxicity) so that the maximum adsorbed dose of immunogen is also lower. For example, preclinical studies of the nicotine vaccine NicVAX (3'-aminonicotine conjugated to recombinant *Pseudomonas* endotoxin A) in rats used immunogen doses of up to 300 ug/kg (Cornish et al. 2013), while the highest dose used in clinical trials was approximately 6 ug/kg (Hatsukami et al. 2011). However, it is not clear whether the higher immunogen doses used in

Table 4.1 Estimated single and daily doses of commonly abused drugs. The ratio of drug dose to antibody-binding capacity is calculated using a theoretical drug-specific antibody concentration of 200 µg/ml in serum

Drug	Dose (mg/kg)	Molar ratio of drug to antibody-binding capacity
Nicotine		
Single dose	0.015	0.5
Daily dose	0.3	10
Cocaine		
Single dose	0.5	9
Daily dose	10	160
Methamphetamine		
Single dose	1	40
Daily dose	5	200
Heroin		
Single dose	3	40
Daily dose	9	120
Oxycodone		
Single dose	1	18
Daily dose	6	100

rodents are also needed in humans. Some animal studies have used adjuvants or dosing routes that are highly immunogenic but not appropriate or approved for humans, such as Freund's adjuvant administered intraperitoneally. In both animals and humans, there is also considerable individual variability in antibody levels.

Challenges specific to opioid vaccines are that (1) most opioids have one or more active metabolites; (2) many different opioids are abusable, and opioid abusers often switch among opioids when their drug of choice is not available. It has not so far been possible to design a single immunogen that elicits antibodies which bind all of these opioids and metabolites; (3) some opioids have legitimate medical uses (analgesia, treatment of opioid addiction), and it is desirable for this option to be preserved; and (4) opioids are immunosuppressive and might impair an individual's vaccine response.

Active metabolites Heroin is a prodrug that is rapidly and sequentially converted in serum to its active metabolites 6-acetylmorphine (6-AM), morphine, and morphine-6-glucuronide (Fig. 4.2) (Rook et al. 2006a). Heroin is considered a prodrug because of its extremely rapid conversion to 6-AM (half-life 7 min in humans) resulting in

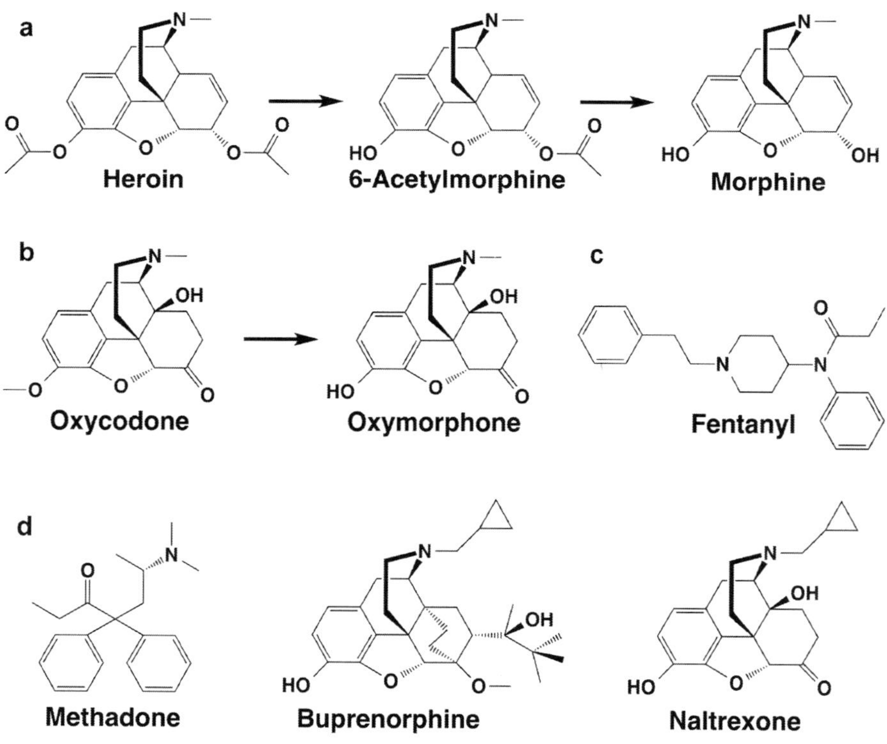

Fig. 4.2 Commonly abused opioids and their active metabolites. (**a**) Heroin and active metabolites. The downstream metabolite morphine-6-glucuronide, which is not formed in mice or rats, is not shown. (**b**) Oxycodone and its metabolite oxymorphone. Hydrocodone and hydromorphone (not shown) have analogous structures but lack a C14 hydroxyl group. (**c**) Fentanyl. (**d**) Nontargeted opioids: methadone, buprenorphine, and naltrexone

very low serum and brain levels (Rook et al. 2006b) and because its affinity for the mu opioid receptor is substantially lower than that of its active metabolites (Inturrisi et al. 1983). Heroin is more lipophilic than these metabolites, enters the brain more readily, and may undergo some conversion to 6-AM within the brain, but the quantitative contribution of this pathway to heroin action is unclear (Andersen et al. 2009). Heroin's immediate rewarding effects, those occurring within the first few minutes of a heroin dose, are probably attributable in greatest measure to 6-AM (Raleigh et al. 2013; Bogen et al. 2014). Conversion of 6-AM to morphine in serum is somewhat slower (half-life 22 min) but still rapid enough that morphine may contribute to the early behavioral effects of heroin (Rook et al. 2006b).

It is not entirely clear to what extent vaccines targeting heroin owe their efficacy to binding heroin per se, its active metabolites, or both (Fig. 4.3). Even though heroin is a prodrug, the binding of heroin by antibody could potentially slow or block its conversion to 6-AM and downstream metabolites. However, this is unlikely because immunization of rats with vaccines that bind and retain substantial heroin in serum does not prevent the rapid accumulation of 6-AM in serum, within minutes of a heroin dose. One such vaccine was shown to reduce 6-AM but not heroin distribution to the brain in rats after a single heroin dose, yet it markedly attenuated heroin analgesia and self-administration (Raleigh et al. 2013). Additional data argue against the binding of morphine being important, at least for blocking the very early

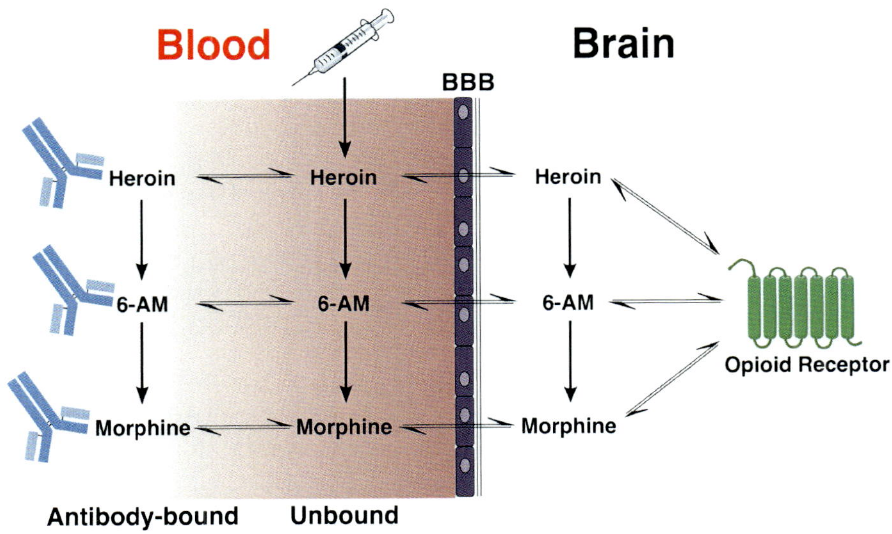

Fig. 4.3 Possible fates of heroin and active metabolites in the blood and brain in the presence of morphine-specific antibodies. Heroin administered to a vaccinated individual may undergo (1) distribution directly into the brain, (2) conversion to its more active metabolites, or (3) binding to antibody. 6-AM and morphine share these outcomes. Antibody generated by heroin vaccines can bind each of these compounds in serum and potentially slow or reduce their entry into the brain. It is also possible that the binding of heroin to antibody slows its conversion to the more active 6-AM, but initial data in rats suggests this is not a major contributor to vaccine efficacy

effects of heroin; a "dynamic" heroin vaccine (see Sect. 4.2), which selectively retains heroin and 6-AM but not morphine in serum, is effective in blocking heroin self-administration (Schlosburg et al. 2013). Together, these studies implicate 6-AM in serum as the primary vaccine target for altering the early effects of heroin. The role of morphine-6-glucuronide (M-6-G) has not been studied in the context of vaccines because rodents do not produce this metabolite (Antonilli et al. 2005), but morphine-specific antibodies have been shown to bind M-6-G in vitro (Anton and Leff 2006; Raleigh et al. 2013; Kosten et al. 2013).

Oxycodone and hydrocodone, the most commonly abused prescription opioids, also have active metabolites (Fig. 4.2). Fortunately, antibodies directed at oxycodone or hydrocodone also bind these metabolites with comparable affinities (Pravetoni et al. 2012a, 2013).

Many abusable opioids: the specificity of opioid vaccines The abuse of prescription opioids such as oxycodone and hydrocodone increased dramatically in the first decade of this century and rose to more than ten times the prevalence of heroin abuse in the USA (Dart et al. 2015). Those abusing prescription opioids may switch among them depending on availability and cost, or transition to heroin. Addressing this complex epidemiology may require vaccines that can target each of the most commonly abused opioids.

It does not appear feasible to design a single immunogen that will elicit antibodies that bind all of the commonly abused opioids. The commonly abused opioids, as well as the most commonly used therapeutic opioids, differ sufficiently in structure that antibodies generally do not appreciably cross-react among them (Fig. 4.2). For example, antibodies generated using haptens based on morphine generally bind heroin and its active metabolites avidly but have orders of magnitude lower affinities for oxycodone or hydrocodone (Pravetoni et al. 2012b; Stowe et al. 2011b). Targeting a wide range of abusable opioids will require a different approach such as coadministering heroin and oxycodone vaccines, as discussed below (Sect. 4.6).

The prescription opioid fentanyl is less commonly abused. Antibodies elicited by heroin or oxycodone vaccines do not appreciably bind fentanyl (Raleigh et al. 2013; Pravetoni et al. 2013), but fentanyl-based haptens can generate such antibodies and block fentanyl analgesia in rodents (Torten et al. 1975).

There is a beneficial aspect to the selectivity of antibodies elicited by heroin or oxycodone vaccines in that their much lower affinities for the addiction treatment medications methadone, buprenorphine, and naltrexone should allow these medications to retain their clinical efficacy for treating opioid addiction. It should be possible, in principle, to combine opioid vaccines with these opioid addiction treatment medications without compromising the efficacy of either. The role of vaccines in this setting could be to (1) enhance blockade of the effects of heroin or prescription opioids that are abused despite maintenance on treatment medications, (2) provide blockade of abused opioid effects during periods of noncompliance with treatment medications, or (3) provide blockade of opioid effects when patients transition off their treatment medications.

4.2 Heroin Vaccine Design

4.2.1 Opioid Scaffold and Linker Position

Most opioid haptens use C6 or the bridgehead (piperidinyl) nitrogen for linker attachment (Fig. 4.1, Table 4.2). Two of the earliest reports described haptens derived from morphine with linkers at C3 that elicited antibodies with activity against both morphine and heroin. The more extensively studied of these was later reported to have been analyzed incorrectly and to actually have the linker at C6 (Wainer et al. 1972a, b). Findlay et al. (1981) analyzed a range of opioid haptens based on morphine or oxycodone and concluded that haptens using the C6 linker position showed greatest recognition of structural differences around the bridgehead nitrogen and C14, while haptens using the bridgehead nitrogen linker position showed greatest recognition of structural differences at C3 or C6. This is consistent with the general principle that structural recognition by antibodies is greatest for aspects of a hapten distant from the site of linker attachment, because linker attachment hides the linker position and its immediate environment from presentation to B-cell receptors (Matyas et al. 2014).

Heroin vaccines Heroin vaccines with C6 linkers are generally synthesized from morphine. Although these lack both the 3- and 6-acetyl groups present on heroin, the elicited antibodies bind heroin, 6-AM and morphine with comparable affinities, consistent with the notion that these positions are not a critical component of the hapten face interacting with antibody (Anton and Leff 2006; Raleigh et al. 2013; Kosten et al. 2013). However, alterations at C8 or C14 are recognized so that these antibodies have little affinity for oxycodone or hydrocodone (Findlay et al. 1981).

Several reports describe heroin vaccines using the bridgehead nitrogen linker position (Schlosburg et al. 2013; Findlay et al. 1981; Matyas et al. 2014). A "dynamic" hapten placed a linker at this position on heroin, rather than morphine, to retain the acetyl groups at C3 and C6 and allow the hapten to be converted in vivo sequentially from the diacetyl to the monoacetyl and then the non-acetylated analogs (Stowe et al. 2011b). This sequence was intended to mimic in vivo heroin metabolism and expose the vaccinated animal to immunogen analogs of each of the active heroin metabolites. Although the rapid deacetylation of this hapten in vivo precluded measuring the presumed conversion, the antibodies produced by vaccination bound 6-AM with higher affinity than heroin or morphine, and blocked heroin analgesia better than the analogous hapten with OH groups at C3 and C6. An additional study of the bridgehead nitrogen linker position using stable substituents on C3 and/or C6, so that sequential exposure to acetylated analogs was not a feature, showed that this immunogen structure was also capable of generating antibodies against heroin, 6-AM, and morphine (Matyas et al. 2014). It appears, therefore, that a variety of approaches involving either C6 or the bridgehead nitrogen are available to generate antibodies of interest for therapeutic applications. These approaches have not been extensively compared so it is unclear which, if any, is best.

Table 4.2 Heroin immunogen structures and specificities determined by ELISA

R_1: bridgehead nitrogen	Opioid	Relative specificity (%)	Reference
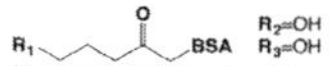 *N*-carboxypropylnormorphine-BSA, **1**	1. Morphine Normorphine Hydromorphone Dihydromorphine	100 90 79 34	Findlay et al. (1981)
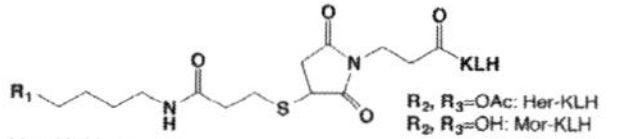 Her-KLH, **2** Mor-KLH, **3**	2. Morphine Heroin 6-AM	100 267 32,000	Schlosburg et al. (2013), Stowe et al. (2011b), Bremer et al. (2014), Bremer and Janda (2012)
	3. Morphine Heroin 6-AM	100 8.5 <1.2	
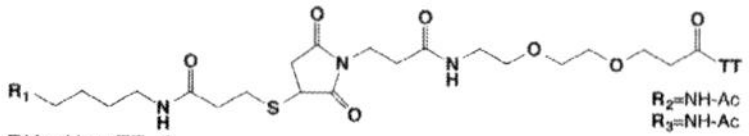 DiAmHap-TT, **4**	4. Morphine Heroin 6-AM	100 1033 425	Matyas et al. (2014)
R_2: C3			
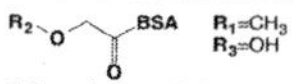 3-O-carboxymethylmorphine-BSA, **5**	5. Morphine Heroin Normorphine	100 133 100 (relative to dihydromorphone)	Spector and Parker (1970), Adler and Liu (1971), Spector (1971), Berkowitz and Spector (1972), Berkowitz et al. (1974)

R_3: C6			
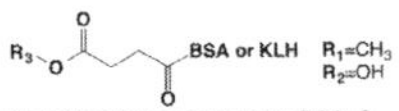 Morphine-6-hemisuccinate-BSA, **6** Morphine-6-hemisuccinate-KLH, **7**	6. Morphine Heroin Codeine Hydromorphone	100 110 70 22	Wainer et al. (1972a, b, 1973), Hill et al. (1975), Bonese et al. (1974), Killian et al. (1978), Kosten et al. (2013), Akbarzadeh et al. (1999), Ma et al. (2006)
	7. Morphine 6-AM	100 173	
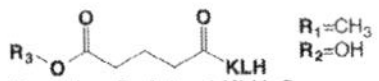 Morphine-6-glutaryl-KLH, **8**	8. Morphine Heroin	100 0.46	Li et al. (2011)
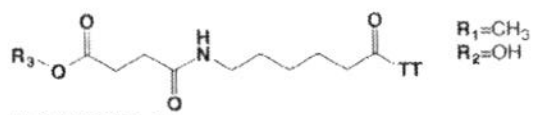 M-TFCS-TT, **9**	9. Morphine Heroin 6-AM	Described as "equivalent specificity"	Anton and Leff (2006)
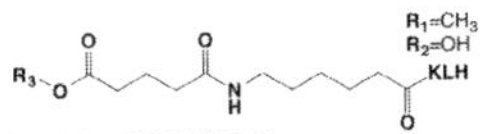 Morphine-TFCS-KLH, **10**	10. Morphine Heroin 6-AM	100 12 40	Li et al. (2014)
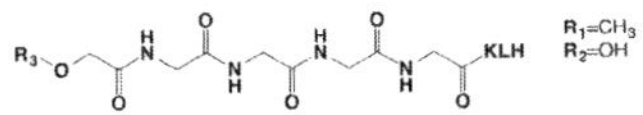 M(Gly)$_4$-KLH, **11**	11. Morphine Heroin 6-AM M-6-G	100 167 125 50	Raleigh et al. (2013, 2014), Pravetoni et al. (2012b)
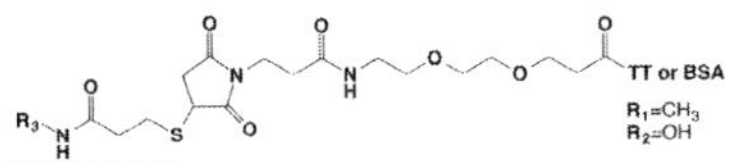 MorHap-TT, **12** MorHap-BSA, **13**	12. Morphine Heroin 6-AM	100 <3.6 54	Matyas et al. (2014), Torres et al. (2014)

See Fig. 4.1 for linker attachment positions R_1, R_2, *and* R_3

Oxycodone vaccines Vaccines directed against oxycodone use the C6 linker position, analogous to its use in heroin vaccines. Use of C8 was less effective and the bridgehead nitrogen position has not, to our knowledge, been studied (Pravetoni et al. 2012a, 2013).

4.2.2 Linker Structure

A surprisingly wide variety of linkers have been used for heroin or oxycodone vaccines and found to be satisfactory. Linker length has varied from 2 to 24 atoms (Table 4.2). In general, linkers have been designed to be flexible and to have low structural complexity. This reflects an attempt to make the linker itself less immunogenic, so that the immune response is focused more on the hapten.

It is not apparent that any one linker length or structure is superior to all others, and this is a challenging question to address. Linker length and composition may affect not just the ability of a hapten to engage B-cell receptors, they may also affect the density of hapten that can be attached to its carrier protein, which is known to be a critical determinant of immunogenicity (Carroll et al. 2011). Hapten density on its carrier (the haptenation ratio) is often not measured or, in the case of very large protein carriers such as KLH, is difficult to measure accurately. As a result, the influence of the linker on haptenation chemistry is difficult to separate from its influence on the ability of immunogen to engage B-cell receptors. In addition, reported heroin vaccines have used many different carrier proteins and adjuvants, and their efficacy has been analyzed using different in vitro or in vivo assays, further confounding the ability to compare vaccines across or even within studies.

4.2.3 Carrier and Hapten Density

Opioid vaccines have used many of the same carrier proteins known to be most effective for other types of haptens including nicotine and cocaine (Table 4.2). These include bovine serum albumin (BSA, not suitable for human use because of dietary exposure to this protein), tetanus toxoid, and keyhole limpet hemocyanin (KLH). As with linkers, direct comparisons are few but tetanus toxoid and KLH were found equally effective for an oxycodone vaccine. When measured (using BSA conjugates as models), molar ratios of 15–22 haptens/protein have been effective (Pravetoni et al. 2012b; Stowe et al. 2011b; Matyas et al. 2014), and more so than lower ratios (unpublished data). More extensive experience with other hapten-protein conjugate vaccines suggests that optimization of carrier haptenation is a critical aspect of conjugate vaccine design, regardless of the carrier (Carroll et al. 2011).

4.2.4 *Adjuvant*

Adjuvants used in opioid vaccines reflect those used for other types of immunizations. The most common is alum because of its acceptability for human use and long track record of efficacy and safety. Other adjuvants used clinically or experimentally, for unrelated vaccines, have unsurprisingly also shown efficacy with opioid vaccines. A combination of alum and CpG was more effective than either one alone for a heroin vaccine (Bremer et al. 2014), consistent with a previous report with a nicotine vaccine (McCluskie et al. 2013). Monophosphoryl lipid A (MPLA) embedded in a liposome, mixed with a heroin hapten-tetanus toxoid conjugate so that the MPLA liposome functioned as an adjuvant, elicited high titers of opioid antibodies (Matyas et al. 2013). Surprisingly little is known about the extent to which adjuvant potencies in rodents or even primates are predictive of results in humans, and this question will likely require clinical trials to identify the best options.

4.3 Heroin Vaccine Immunogenicity

4.3.1 *Affinity and Specificity*

The amount of drug that can be bound by antibody is a function of both the amount of antibody available and the affinity, or strength of binding, between antibody and drug. Opioid antibody affinity has been measured for morphine rather than heroin due to heroin's instability in serum. Using equilibrium dialysis or radioimmunoassay, Kd values of 24.5, 16.6 (Stowe et al. 2011b), and 2.5–4.0 (Anton and Leff 2006) were reported for three vaccines (immunogens 2, 3, and 9 of Table 4.2). These values compare favorably with Kd's measured for nicotine or cocaine vaccines. Competition ELISA methods, which are simpler and less expensive, can be used in lieu of equilibrium dialysis or radioimmunoassay to compare relative affinities and specificities of various ligands for antibody but cannot generate accurate Kd values for free drug (see following paragraph).

4.3.2 *Antibody Concentration*

Serum antibody titers measured by ELISA are often used as a surrogate for concentration, because their measurement is quick and inexpensive. However, ELISA titers actually measure antibody binding to the coating antigen, which includes linker and carrier protein, rather than to free drug alone. ELISA titers are also sensitive to assay conditions, making comparisons between laboratories uninformative. ELISA assays can be calibrated to provide an estimate of serum antibody concentration using a monoclonal opioid antibody (Raleigh et al. 2013) or nonspecific IgG (Kosten et al. 2013). Concentrations can also be obtained by equilibrium dialysis or radioimmunoassay, which avoid the potential confounding effects of linker or carrier protein.

Estimates of serum anti-morphine antibody concentrations obtained by equilibrium dialysis or a suitably calibrated ELISA range from 200 to 800 ug/ml, (Anton and Leff 2006; Raleigh et al. 2013; Kosten et al. 2013; Stowe et al. 2011b) similar to those reported with other addiction vaccines (although one very high value of 2840 ug/ml was also reported (Stowe et al. 2011b). This range can be verified by measuring the concentrations of opioids retained in serum in vaccinated animals, to provide an estimate of the minimum serum antibody concentration that would have to be present to bind them. This calculation gives similar estimates, e.g., 300–400 ug/ml in rats receiving heroin or 6-AM (unpublished calculation based on (Raleigh et al. 2014)). To put these serum antibody concentrations in perspective, most infectious disease vaccines produce serum neutralizing antibody concentrations that are several orders of magnitudes lower (Scott et al. 2011). It can be argued that efforts to optimize the immunogenicity of heroin vaccines have already been quite successful and that the limitations of vaccine efficacy stem from the difficulty of the task: the need to bind the large heroin doses used by opioid addicts.

4.3.3 Vaccination During Opioid Administration

It is likely that opioid abusers will need to be vaccinated before they become abstinent from using opioids, so that high antibody levels are present when abstinence is attempted. In animals, concurrent exposure to drugs such as nicotine or methamphetamine during vaccination does not impair the immune response to the corresponding addiction vaccines (Hieda et al. 2000; Byrnes-Blake et al. 2001). Similarly, in rats vaccinated against heroin, subsequent exposure to heroin does not impair their antibody response to booster doses of vaccine (Raleigh et al. 2014). These data suggest that vaccination against heroin will not be impaired by concurrent heroin use.

An additional issue is that morphine is known to be immunosuppressive, and heroin addicts have been reported to have a lower antibody response to hepatitis B vaccines than controls (Rodrigo et al. 1992). Many heroin addicts also have chronic infections such as HIV or hepatitis C that can impair immune responses (Quaglio et al. 2002). The opioid-abusing population may require different or more aggressive vaccination regimens to achieve the highest possible antibody levels from opioid vaccines.

4.4 Heroin Vaccine Efficacy

4.4.1 Opioid Doses

Clinical laboratory investigations show rewarding effects of heroin in addicts at doses as low as 0.4 mg/kg administered i.v. (Comer et al. 2008), but abused doses are generally much larger. Studies of heroin maintenance as a therapeutic option, which allow heroin addicts to adjust their dose, report mean daily doses of 500–600 mg (7–9 mg/kg) typically injected i.v. in 1–3 doses (Reuter 2009; Haemmig and Tschacher 2001; Rentsch et al. 2001). Doses used likely vary depending upon heroin price and purity and degree of opioid tolerance. Thus, the target dose that must be addressed by a vaccine is unclear but by any estimate it is considerable.

Animal models of heroin abuse often differ from the doses or manner in which addicts use these drugs (Table 4.3). Heroin or morphine self-administration protocols typically use relatively low i.v. unit doses, e.g., 0.06 mg/kg/infusion although they may achieve a substantial total dose, up to 2 mg/kg, over a 1–2 h session (Bonese et al. 1974; Schlosburg et al. 2013; Raleigh et al. 2014). Higher heroin or morphine doses are used to study vaccine effects on opioid analgesia or locomotor activity, but these are usually administered s.c. and are absorbed more slowly than with i.v. dosing. These differences between dosing regimens in animals and humans add to the difficulty of predicting the clinical impact of opioid vaccines.

4.4.2 Vaccine Effects on Heroin and Metabolite Pharmacokinetics

Behaviorally active doses of opioids often exceed the expected binding capacity of antibody that can be generated by vaccination (Table 4.1). This is also true for nicotine or cocaine, yet vaccines targeting these drugs have been repeatedly shown to alter their behavioral effects in animals. One key to this apparent paradox is that addiction vaccines can slow the early distribution of drug to the brain, in the first few minutes after drug dosing, even when large drug doses are involved (Pentel et al. 2006; Fox et al. 1996). This is important because the rewarding and reinforcing effects of addictive drugs are also greatest shortly after drug is administered. For this reason, studies of vaccine effects on drug pharmacokinetics have focused on drug levels measured shortly after a dose.

Relatively few data are available regarding vaccine effects on opioid and metabolite levels in the serum or brain. The methods required are cumbersome because of the instability of heroin and, to a lesser extent 6-AM, in serum even after removal from the experimental animal, owing to serum pH and cholinesterase activity (Jones et al. 2013).

The best studied vaccine with regard to its effects on opioid pharmacokinetics is M(Gly)$_4$-KLH, which elicits antibodies that bind heroin as well as 6-AM and morphine with comparable affinities (Raleigh et al. 2013). Vaccinated rats receiving a single dose of heroin 0.26 mg/kg i.v. retained high levels of all three opioids in serum 4 min after heroin administration, which were 10–100 times higher than in non-vaccinated controls (Fig. 4.4). Brain 6-AM levels were reduced by 44 % in vaccinated rats. Brain levels of heroin and morphine were not reduced, but were tenfold or more lower than those of 6-AM in both vaccinated and control rats, supporting the dominant role of 6-AM in mediating the early effects of heroin. The reduction in brain 6-AM concentration was closely correlated with the serum antibody concentration. Substantial reductions in brain 6-AM were seen primarily in animals that had serum opioid-specific antibody concentrations of >200 ug/ml.

Repeated administration of heroin was studied by the administration of 8 heroin doses i.v. over 1 h to rats vaccinated against heroin (Raleigh et al. 2014). Brain 6-AM concentration was reduced by 48 % in rats receiving a cumulative heroin dose of 0.5 mg/kg, but the decrease was smaller and not significant in those receiving

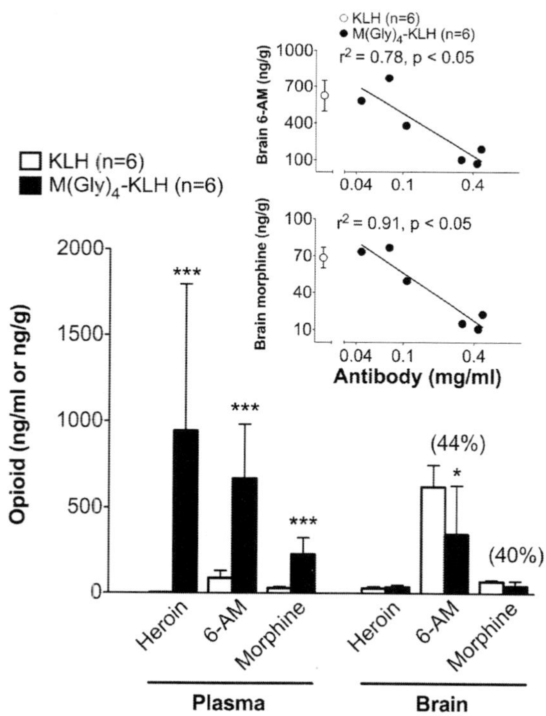

Fig. 4.4 Effect of vaccination with M(Gly)$_4$-KLH on heroin and metabolite distribution in the plasma and brain in rats. Heroin, 6-AM, and morphine were significantly retained in plasma 4 min after 0.26 mg/kg heroin i.v. Brain 6-AM, but not heroin or morphine, concentrations were significantly reduced compared to controls. $^{*}p<0.05$, $^{***}p<0.001$ compared to KLH controls. Numbers in parentheses are the percent decrease compared to controls. (*Inset*) Higher serum antibody concentrations were associated with lower brain 6-AM and morphine concentrations ($n=5$–6) (Adapted from Raleigh et al. (2013))

1.0 mg/kg heroin. Morphine concentrations in the brain were reduced at both heroin doses, while heroin concentrations were not but were also very low. These data support the ability of vaccination to reduce the early distribution of 6-AM to the brain, but also suggest lesser efficacy with higher heroin doses. A caveat is that vaccine was administered i.p. in Freund's adjuvant.

Several additional studies using other heroin vaccines found generally similar results. Vaccination of rats with the Her-KLH vaccine led to substantial retention of heroin and 6-AM in serum after a heroin dose of 0.5 mg/kg i.v. (Schlosburg et al. 2013), and a vaccine using the C6 linker position reduced morphine brain concentration by 24 % after an i.p. heroin dose of 4 mg/kg (Kosten et al. 2013).

These pharmacokinetic data are not by themselves sufficient to predict how well opioid vaccines will block the effects larger or more chronic doses of heroin, but the behavioral data discussed below provide additional evidence that altering the effects of clinically relevant heroin doses is feasible.

4.4.3 Vaccine Effects on Heroin or Morphine-Associated Behaviors in Animals

Opioid vaccines have been shown to block or attenuate many opioid addiction-relevant behaviors in animals, some involving single opioid doses but others using repeated or chronic dosing.

Opioid analgesia is among the simplest behavioral assays to perform so it has been examined with many opioid vaccines. While this is not an addictive behavior, it reflects the ability of antibody to bind active drug or metabolites, and hot-plate analgesia is centrally mediated so that it depends upon the ability of antibodies to reduce brain opioid exposure. Studies using either mice or rats show suppression of opioid analgesia at s.c. heroin or morphine doses of up to 2 mg/kg (Table 4.3). In general, the specificity of vaccines for particular opioids measured by ELISA assay is reflected by their potency in blocking analgesia from the same opioids.

A variety of opioid vaccines also attenuate opioid-induced locomotor activation at doses of up to 10 mg/kg s.c. morphine (Li et al. 2011) or 0.25 mg/kg s.c. heroin (Raleigh et al. 2013). Efficacy has been shown to persist for at least 2 weeks of every other day heroin dosing. For the M(Gly)$_4$-KLH vaccine, the magnitude of blockade correlates with serum opioid-specific antibody levels and is most prominent in animals with antibody levels of >200 ug/ml (Raleigh et al. 2013). This is the same antibody concentration range found to be most effective in reducing 6-AM distribution to the brain.

Heroin vaccines also reduce heroin or morphine self-administration in rats and, in one older report, in one monkey. Protocols have examined either the acquisition (Stowe et al. 2011b; Raleigh et al. 2014) or reacquisition (Anton and Leff 2006; Schlosburg et al. 2013) of self-administration at unit heroin doses of up to 0.1 mg/kg/infusion and total doses per session of up to 2 mg/kg. Two studies showed heroin dose dependence. A rat study found a reduction in heroin self-administration with

Table 4.3 Effects of heroin/morphine vaccines on opioid addiction-relevant behaviors in rats

Immunogen	Behavior attenuated/ blocked	Opioid	Dose and route	Reference
Her-KLH, **2**	CPP Hot-plate von Frey acquisition reacquisition reinstatement	Morphine Heroin	4 mg/kg, s.c. 0.4 mg/kg, s.c. 1 mg/kg, s.c. 1 mg/kg, s.c. 0.06 mg/kg/inf, i.v. 0.06 mg/kg/inf, i.v. up to 6.5 mg/kg/6-h 0.18 mg/kg, i.v.	Schlosburg et al. (2013), Stowe et al. (2011b)
DiAmHap-TT, **4** MorHap-TT, **12**	Hot-plate	Heroin	0.75 mg/kg, s.c.	Matyas et al. (2014)
3-O-carboxymethyl-morphine-BSA, **5**	PPQ writhing test[a]	Morphine	0.5–1.0 mg/kg, s.c.	Berkowitz and Spector (1972)
Morphine-6-hemisuccinate-BSA, **6**	Tail-flick reacquisition[b]	Morphine Heroin	2 mg/kg, s.c. 0.006–0.1 mg/kg/inf, i.v. up to 1–2 mg/kg/2-h	Bonese et al. (1974), Ma et al. (2006)
Morphine-6-hemisuccinate-KLH, **7**	CPP Tail-flick Hot-plate	Morphine	1–2 mg/kg, s.c. 2 mg/kg, s.c. 2 mg/kg, s.c.	Kosten et al. (2013)
Morphine-6-glutaryl-KLH, **8** Morphine-TFCS-KLH, **10**	Locomotor activity reinstatement	Morphine Heroin	10 mg/kg s.c. 0.5 mg/kg s.c.	Li et al. (2011, 2014)
M-TFCS-TT, **9**	reacquisition	Heroin	0.06 mg/kg, i.v.	Anton and Leff (2006)
M(Gly)4-KLH, **11**	Hot-plate Locomotor activity acquisition reinstatement dose reduction	Heroin	1 mg/kg, s.c. 0.25 mg/kg, s.c. 0.06 mg/kg, i.v. up to 2 mg/kg/2-h 0.6 mg/kg, s.c. 0.003–0.06 mg/kg/inf, i.v. up to 2 mg/kg/2-h	Raleigh et al. (2013, 2014)

Abbreviations: *CPP* conditioned place preference, *HSA* heroin self-administration, *inf* infusion, *PPQ* p-phenylquinone

[a]Indicates experiment performed in mice

[b]Indicates experiment performed in rhesus monkey

heroin unit doses of 0.003–0.01 mg/kg but small compensatory increases at unit doses of 0.03 or 0.06 mg/kg (Fig. 4.5) (Raleigh et al. 2014). The monkey study used progressively escalating heroin doses and found resumption of heroin self-administration when unit doses reached 1–2 mg/kg (Bonese et al. 1974). A limitation of these studies is that human opioid abusers administer substantially larger unit doses of heroin, albeit far few times daily. This is difficult to model in rats that are not already tolerant to high doses of opioid because these large doses cause sedation and respiratory depression.

Several studies also showed marked suppression of the reinstatement of heroin responding in rats after extinction of self-administration. The heroin doses used were large (up to 0.6 mg/kg) but administered s.c. (Raleigh et al. 2014; Li et al. 2014).

Although these models are imperfect, the data clearly establish the ability of heroin vaccines to block opioid addiction-relevant behaviors in animals despite opioid doses at times exceeding the binding capacity of the available antibody. They also underscore the need to generate very high antibody levels to achieve this.

Clinical trials A heroin vaccine developed in Iran reached Phase I clinical trials (Scott et al. 2011). This morphine BSA conjugate, shown to generate morphine-specific antibodies in animals, was administered unblinded to 347 opioid users. No adverse effects were noted but the reported experimental and methodological detail was limited. This vaccine is not well suited to clinical use because BSA was used as the carrier.

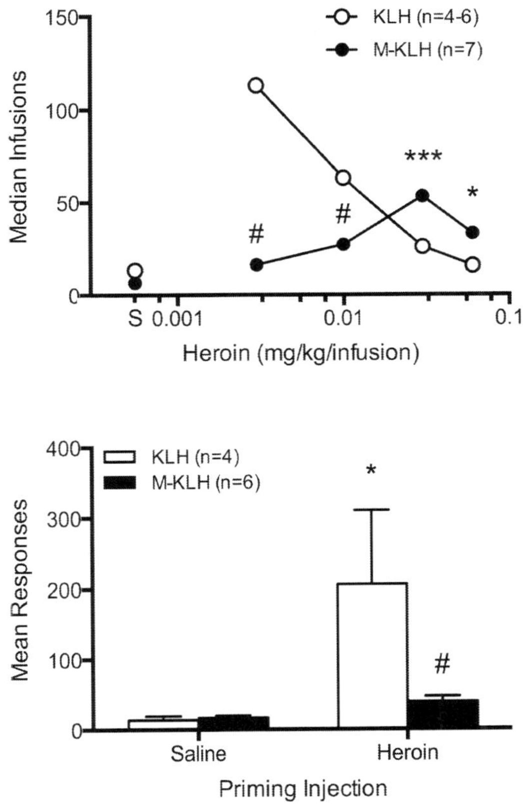

Fig. 4.5 Effect of vaccination with M(Gly)$_4$-KLH on heroin self-administration (HSA) during heroin dose reduction and reinstatement. (*Top*) Heroin dose reduction: infusions/session in rats that acquired HSA and completed the dose-reduction protocol. Rats were trained at a heroin unit dose of 0.06 mg/kg/inf. The heroin dose was then sequentially decreased every 5 days to 0.03, 0.01, 0.003, and 0 mg/kg. *$p<0.05$, ***$p<0.001$, higher number of infusions compared to KLH. #$p<0.05$, higher proportion of rats with HSA below baseline compared to KLH. (*Bottom*) Blockade of reinstatement of heroin responding in vaccinated rats. Mean (± SEM) active lever presses during extinction in vaccinated and control rats after a s.c. priming injection of saline or 0.6 mg/kg heroin. *$p<0.05$, heroin reinstated HSA compared to saline in KLH rats. #$p<0.05$, heroin failed to reinstate HSA in M-KLH rats compared to KLH controls (Adapted from Raleigh et al. (2014))

4.5 Oxycodone Vaccines

Oxycodone is the most commonly abused prescription opioid, and oxycodone abusers often transition to heroin (Dart et al. 2015). Based on the preclinical efficacy of heroin vaccines and in particular M(Gly)$_4$-KLH, an analogous oxycodone immunogen was developed using the C6 linker position: OXY(Gly)$_4$-KLH (Pravetoni et al. 2012a). With a haptenation ratio (measured using the model protein BSA) of 16, this immunogen elicited antibodies in mice or rats with specificity for oxycodone and its active metabolite oxymorphone (also marketed as an analgesic and subject to abuse), but no appreciable binding to morphine, methadone, buprenorphine, or naltrexone. There was significant cross-reactivity with hydrocodone, which differs from oxycodone only by the absence of a hydroxyl group at C14 (Pravetoni et al. 2013). Cross-reactivity with hydrocodone adds substantially to the clinical potential of this immunogen because hydrocodone is also commonly abused. A pertinent negative is that there was no cross-reactivity with the (Gly)$_4$ linker alone in competition ELISA.

Several alternative hapten designs proved less immunogenic than OXY(Gly)$_4$-KLH (Pravetoni et al. 2013). The analogous hydrocodone(Gly)$_4$-KLH was less effective in binding either hydrocodone or oxycodone, and placing the linker at C8 was also less effective. Oxy(Gly)$_4$-KLH was equally immunogenic when conjugated to tetanus toxoid, native KLH (a didecamer), or KLH dimer (Pravetoni et al. 2014a). OXY(Gly)$_4$-KLH was somewhat less immunogenic when administered s.c. in alum compared to i.p. in Freund's adjuvant, but even with s.c. administration in alum, it retained the ability to reduce the distribution of either oxycodone or hydrocodone to brain and block hot-plate analgesia. Pharmacokinetic effects were oxycodone dose related but appreciable even at an oxycodone dose of 0.5 mg/kg i.v. which is within the range abused by humans (Pravetoni et al. 2012a). Vaccination of rats also attenuated the acquisition of oxycodone self-administration (Pravetoni et al. 2014b).

4.6 Multivalent Opioid Vaccines

Recognizing that opioid abusers may switch among opioids, there may be a clinical advantage to administering several opioid vaccines at once in order to broaden the range of opioids targeted. This approach is feasible because the immune system has the capacity to respond to multiple immune challenges simultaneously. Responses to the individual vaccine components are generally preserved. With this goal, one study examined the coadministration of M(Gly)$_4$-KLH and OXY(Gly)$_4$-KLH immunogens to rats (Pravetoni et al. 2012b). Serum antibody titers to the component immunogens were the same as when each immunogen was administered alone. When animals received a single challenge dose of the active heroin metabolite 6-AM along with oxycodone, the distribution of each of these drugs to the brain was reduced to the same extent as when each immunogen was administered alone. There was a trend toward a greater reduction in brain oxycodone in the combined immunogen group because M(Gly)$_4$-KLH shows some cross-reactivity with oxycodone. This study supports the feasibility of combining opioid vaccines to extend their range of coverage. Immunogens covering additional opioids could, in principle, be added if clinical abuse patterns made this necessary.

4.7 Combining Opioid Vaccines with Existing Pharmacotherapies

If effective, the likely clinical role of opioid vaccines would be to complement rather than replace existing pharmacotherapies. The key features of opioid vaccines that would encourage their use include their long duration of action (booster doses might be needed every 2–3 months), lack of side effects, lack of addiction or diversion potential, and novel mechanism of action.

Enhance the efficacy of pharmacotherapies Some patients on agonist or antagonist maintenance, even at recommended doses, continue to periodically use heroin (Krupitsky et al. 2013; Belding et al. 1998). A vaccine could enhance the blockade of any abused heroin and thereby minimize its use.

Provide additional coverage during medication noncompliance Some patients on buprenorphine maintenance intentionally skip one or more doses in order to restore opioid sensitivity and then abuse their opioid of choice. The long duration of action of vaccines could provide "backup" coverage to block the effects of the abused opioids.

Provide coverage when patients transition off agonist or antagonist therapy Many opioid abusers receiving methadone, buprenorphine, or naltrexone will choose to stop therapy at some point (Nosyk et al. 2012; Bentzley et al. 2015). The risk of relapse to opioid abuse is very high, as is the risk of opioid overdose from use of high opioid doses when opioid tolerance is not yet fully developed. A vaccine could provide protection during this vulnerable period.

A nonaddictive and well-tolerated alternative Despite the established benefits of agonist medications, some opioid abusers, or those involved in their care, object to the use of addictive medications as treatments (Rosenberg and Phillips 2003). Vaccines would add a nonaddictive option. Side effects of agonist medications are generally minimal but, for those troubled by side effects or the potential for side effects, vaccines might be appealing since they have no sustained side effects.

Less need for regulation Vaccines would not require the tight regulation and oversight needed for the safe dispensing of agonist medications. This might encourage their use in locations that lack programs or facilities for safe opioid dispensing.

Ease of changing treatment modalities Opioid abusers who are vaccinated would have no difficulty switching to agonist or antagonist medications if they chose to, since vaccines do not interfere with their actions. Similarly, those wishing to switch from agonist or antagonist medications to a vaccine could be vaccinated while still receiving their medication, so that high antibody levels are present when the medications are stopped.

4.8 Feasibility and Translation

Vaccine components Most opioid vaccines studied in animals are protein conjugates assembled using carrier proteins (KLH, tetanus toxoid) and adjuvants (alum, MPLA, CpG oligonucleotides) that are either approved or in experimental use in humans (Table 4.2).

Cessation v. relapse prevention Vaccines are likely to be most effective in clinical settings where the opioid doses used are few and intermittent, rather than settings involving regular use of consistently high daily doses. For this reason, vaccines are likely to be more effective for relapse prevention than cessation. For relapse prevention, the goal of vaccination would be to diminish the effect of a "slip" where a single or at most a few opioid doses are used. If those opioid doses were rendered less rewarding, the risk of the "slip" progressing to relapse might be lower. By contrast, cessation would involve vaccinating a current opioid abuser as a means of helping to initiate abstinence. In this case, the opioid dose presented to circulating antibodies would be much higher than in the setting of relapse, and vaccination might have less impact.

In practice, opioid abusers could be vaccinated while still using opioids, prior to or at the same time as entering a treatment program, so that high levels of antibody are available within a few months, when abstinence has been established through standard treatment approaches, to assist with relapse prevention.

Drug switching Drug switching among opioids can be addressed in part by the use of multivalent vaccines (Pravetoni et al. 2012b) that target a wider range of abusable opioids (Sect. 4.6). The use of non-opioid drugs would of course need to be addressed through other means. These considerations are not unique to vaccines; patients on methadone or buprenorphine maintenance commonly use other classes of drugs as well, and this is managed through counseling and other social supports.

Treatment of pain in vaccinated individuals Methadone or buprenorphine could be used to treat acute pain in patients who have received heroin or oxycodone vaccines. Some additional prescription opioids such as fentanyl are not bound by the vaccines developed to date and would also be available for pain relief.

Preexisting antibodies The existence of low levels of opioid antibodies in non-vaccinated opioid users has been reported (Biagini et al. 1990; Gamaleya 1993;

Ryan et al. 1972; Gamaleya et al. 1993). Their specificity and potential impact on opioid action have not been well studied. A clinical trial of a cocaine vaccine found preexisting anti-cocaine IgM in some subjects prior to vaccination and these subjects had a blunted response to the vaccine (Orson et al. 2013). Further exploration of this possibility in opioid users would be of interest.

4.9 Summary

There are abundant challenges to be addressed in developing opioid vaccines. These include (1) generating sufficient levels of antibodies to bind the large doses of opioids abused and (2) targeting the wide variety of abused opioids and their active metabolites while preserving the activity of methadone, buprenorphine, and naltrexone. Nevertheless, a variety of candidate heroin or oxycodone vaccines show considerable promise in clinically relevant animal models of opioid addiction. Advances in vaccine design and the development of new adjuvants are likely to make next-generation opioid vaccines even more effective. Because there is little experience with addiction vaccines in humans, translation to clinical use is likely to require the careful evaluation of a variety of vaccine candidates and vaccination strategies. The potential to administer vaccines along with existing opioid addiction pharmacotherapies is particularly attractive and presents many potential ways that opioid vaccines could be used to improve treatment outcomes.

Acknowledgments The authors would like to acknowledge funding received from the National Institute of Health National Institute on Drug Abuse (grants DA026300, DA030715).

References

Adler FL, Liu CT. Detection of morphine by hemagglutination-inhibition. J Immunol. 1971;106(6):1684–5.

Akbarzadeh A, Mehraby M, Zarbakhsh M, Farzaneh H. Design and synthesis of a morphine-6-succinyl-bovine serum albumin hapten for vaccine development. Biotechnol Appl Biochem. 1999;30(Pt 2):139–46.

Andersen JM, Ripel A, Boix F, Normann PT, Morland J. Increased locomotor activity induced by heroin in mice: pharmacokinetic demonstration of heroin acting as a prodrug for the mediator 6-monoacetylmorphine in vivo. J Pharmacol Exp Ther. 2009;331(1):153–61.

Anton B, Leff P. A novel bivalent morphine/heroin vaccine that prevents relapse to heroin addiction in rodents. Vaccine. 2006;24(16):3232–40.

Antonilli L, Petecchia E, Caprioli D, Badiani A, Nencini P. Effect of repeated administrations of heroin, naltrexone, methadone, and alcohol on morphine glucuronidation in the rat. Psychopharmacology (Berl). 2005;182(1):58–64.

Appel PW, Ellison AA, Jansky HK, Oldak R. Barriers to enrollment in drug abuse treatment and suggestions for reducing them: opinions of drug injecting street outreach clients and other system stakeholders. Am J Drug Alcohol Abuse. 2004;30(1):129–53.

Belding MA, McLellan AT, Zanis DA, Incmikoski R. Characterizing "nonresponsive" methadone patients. J Subst Abuse Treat. 1998;15(6):485–92.

Bentzley BS, Barth KS, Back SE, Book SW. Discontinuation of buprenorphine maintenance therapy: perspectives and outcomes. J Subst Abuse Treat. 2015;52:48–57.

Berkowitz B, Spector S. Evidence for active immunity to morphine in mice. Science. 1972;178(67):1290–2.

Berkowitz BA, Ceretta KV, Spector S. Influence of active and passive immunity on the disposition of dihydromorphine-H[3]. Life Sci. 1974;15:1017–28.

Biagini RE, Klincewicz SL, Henningsen GM, MacKenzie BA, Gallagher JS, Bernstein DI, et al. Antibodies to morphine in workers exposed to opiates at a narcotics manufacturing facility and evidence for similar antibodies in heroin abusers. Life Sci. 1990;47(10):897–908.

Bogen IL, Boix F, Nerem E, Morland J, Andersen JM. A monoclonal antibody specific for 6-monoacetylmorphine reduces acute heroin effects in mice. J Pharmacol Exp Ther. 2014;349(3):568–76.

Bonese KF, Wainer BH, Fitch FW, Rothberg RM, Schuster CR. Changes in heroin self-administration by a rhesus monkey after morphine immunization. Nature. 1974;252:708–10.

Bremer PT, Janda KD. Investigating the effects of a hydrolytically stable hapten and a Th1 adjuvant on heroin vaccine performance. J Med Chem. 2012;55(23):10776–80.

Bremer PT, Schlosburg JE, Lively JM, Janda KD. Injection route and TLR9 agonist addition significantly impact heroin vaccine efficacy. Mol Pharm. 2014;11:1075–80.

Byrnes-Blake KA, Carroll FI, Abraham P, Owens SM. Generation of anti-(+)methamphetamine antibodies is not impeded by (+)methamphetamine administration during active immunization of rats. Int Immunopharmacol. 2001;1(2):329–38.

Carroll FI, Blough BE, Pidaparthi RR, Abraham P, Gong PK, Deng L, et al. Synthesis of mercapto-(+)-methamphetamine haptens and their use for obtaining improved epitope density on (+)-methamphetamine conjugate vaccines. J Med Chem. 2011;54(14):5221–8.

Comer SD, Sullivan MA, Whittington RA, Vosburg SK, Kowalczyk WJ. Abuse liability of prescription opioids compared to heroin in morphine-maintained heroin abusers. Neuropsychopharmacology. 2008;33(5):1179–91.

Cornish KE, de Villiers SH, Pravetoni M, Pentel PR. Immunogenicity of individual vaccine components in a bivalent nicotine vaccine differ according to vaccine formulation and administration conditions. PLoS One. 2013;8(12):e82557.

D'Aunno T, Vaughn TE. Variations in methadone treatment practices. Results from a national study. JAMA. 1992;267(2):253–8.

Dart RC, Surratt HL, Cicero TJ, Parrino MW, Severtson SG, Bucher-Bartelson B, et al. Trends in opioid analgesic abuse and mortality in the United States. N Engl J Med. 2015;372(3):241–8.

Esterlis I, Hannestad JO, Perkins E, Bois F, D'Souza DC, Tyndale RF, et al. Effect of a nicotine vaccine on nicotine binding to beta2*-nicotinic acetylcholine receptors in vivo in human tobacco smokers. Am J Psychiatry. 2013;170(4):399–407.

Findlay JW, Butz RF, Jones EC. Relationships between immunogen structure and antisera specificity in the narcotic alkaloid series. Clin Chem. 1981;27(9):1524–35.

Fox BS, Kantak KM, Edwards MA, Black KM, Bollinger BK, Botka AJ, et al. Efficacy of a therapeutic cocaine vaccine in rodent models. Nat Med. 1996;2:1129–32.

Gamaleya NB. Antibodies to drugs as indicators of chronic drug use. An alternative to toxicological hair analysis. Forensic Sci Int. 1993;63(1–3):285–93.

Gamaleya N, Tagliaro F, Parshin A, Vrublevskii A, Bugari G, Dorizzi R, et al. Immune response to opiates: new findings in heroin addicts investigated by means of an original enzyme immunoassay and morphine determination in hair. Life Sci. 1993;53(2):99–105.

Haemmig RB, Tschacher W. Effects of high-dose heroin versus morphine in intravenous drug users: a randomised double-blind crossover study. J Psychoactive Drugs. 2001;33(2):105–10.

Haney M, Gunderson EW, Jiang H, Collins ED, Foltin RW. Cocaine-specific antibodies blunt the subjective effects of smoked cocaine in humans. Biol Psychiatry. 2010;67(1):59–65.

Hatsukami DK, Rennard S, Jorenby D, Fiore M, Koopmeiners J, de Vos A, et al. Safety and immunogenicity of a nicotine conjugate vaccine in current smokers. Clin Pharmacol Ther. 2005;78(5):456–67.

Hatsukami DK, Jorenby DE, Gonzales D, Rigotti NA, Glover ED, Oncken CA, et al. Immunogenicity and smoking-cessation outcomes for a novel nicotine immunotherapeutic. Clin Pharmacol Ther. 2011;89(3):392–9.

Hieda Y, Keyler DE, Ennifar S, Fattom A, Pentel PR. Vaccination against nicotine during continued nicotine administration in rats: immunogenicity of the vaccine and effects on nicotine distribution to brain. Int J Immunopharmacol. 2000;22(10):809–19.

Hill JH, Wainer BH, Fitch FW, Rothberg RM. Delayed clearance of morphine from the circulation of rabbits immunized with morphine-6-hemisuccinate bovine serum albumin. J Immunol. 1975;114(4):1363–8.

Inturrisi CE, Schultz M, Shin S, Umans JG, Angel L, Simon EJ. Evidence from opiate binding studies that heroin acts through its metabolites. Life Sci. 1983;33 Suppl 1:773–6.

Jones JM, Raleigh MD, Pentel PR, Harmon TM, Keyler DE, Remmel RP, et al. Stability of heroin, 6-monoacetylmorphine, and morphine in biological samples and validation of an LC-MS assay for delayed analyses of pharmacokinetic samples in rats. J Pharm Biomed Anal. 2013;74:291–7.

Kantak KM, Collins SL, Lipman EG, Bond J, Giovanoni K, Fox BS. Evaluation of anticocaine antibodies and a cocaine vaccine in a rat self-administration model. Psychopharmacology (Berl). 2000;148(3):251–62.

Keyler DE, Hieda Y, St. Peter J, Pentel PR. Altered disposition of repeated nicotine doses in rats immunized against nicotine. Nicotine Tob Res. 1999;1:241–9.

Killian A, Bonese K, Rothberg RM, Wainer BH, Schuster CR. Effects of passive immunization against morphine on heroin self-administration. Pharmacol Biochem Behav. 1978;9:347–52.

Koff WC, Burton DR, Johnson PR, Walker BD, King CR, Nabel GJ, et al. Accelerating next-generation vaccine development for global disease prevention. Science. 2013;340(6136):1232910.

Kosten TR, Rosen M, Bond J, Settles M, Roberts JS, Shields J, et al. Human therapeutic cocaine vaccine: safety and immunogenicity. Vaccine. 2002;20(7–8):1196–204.

Kosten TA, Shen XY, O'Malley PW, Kinsey BM, Lykissa ED, Orson FM, et al. A morphine conjugate vaccine attenuates the behavioral effects of morphine in rats. Prog Neuropsychopharmacol Biol Psychiatry. 2013;45:223–9.

Kosten T, Domingo C, Orson F, Kinsey B. Vaccines against stimulants: cocaine and methamphetamine. Br J Clin Pharmacol. 2014a;77:368–74.

Kosten TR, Domingo CB, Shorter D, Orson F, Green C, Somoza E, et al. Vaccine for cocaine dependence: a randomized double-blind placebo-controlled efficacy trial. Drug Alcohol Depend. 2014b;140:42–7.

Krupitsky E, Nunes EV, Ling W, Gastfriend DR, Memisoglu A, Silverman BL. Injectable extended-release naltrexone (XR-NTX) for opioid dependence: long-term safety and effectiveness. Addiction. 2013;108(9):1628–37.

LeSage MG, Shelley D, Pravetoni M, Pentel PR. Enhanced attenuation of nicotine discrimination in rats by combining nicotine-specific antibodies with a nicotinic receptor antagonist. Pharmacol Biochem Behav. 2012;102(1):157–62.

Li QQ, Luo YX, Sun CY, Xue YX, Zhu WL, Shi HS, et al. A morphine/heroin vaccine with new hapten design attenuates behavioral effects in rats. J Neurochem. 2011;119(6): 1271–81.

Li Q, Sun C, Luo Y, Xue Y, Meng S, Xu L, et al. A conjugate vaccine attenuates morphine- and heroin-induced behavior in rats. Int J Neuropsychopharmacol. 2014;18(5):1–11.

Ma LX, Zhou Q, Zheng HB, Li SB. [Preparation and characterization of anti-morphine vaccine antibody]. Xi Bao Yu Fen Zi Mian Yi Xue Za Zhi. 2006;22(3):368–70.

Martell BA, Orson FM, Poling J, Mitchell E, Rossen RD, Gardner T, et al. Cocaine vaccine for the treatment of cocaine dependence in methadone-maintained patients: a randomized, double-blind, placebo-controlled efficacy trial. Arch Gen Psychiatry. 2009;66(10):1116–23.

Matyas GR, Mayorov AV, Rice KC, Jacobson AE, Cheng K, Iyer MR, et al. Liposomes containing monophosphoryl lipid A: a potent adjuvant system for inducing antibodies to heroin hapten analogs. Vaccine. 2013;31(26):2804–10.

Matyas GR, Rice KC, Cheng K, Li F, Antoline JF, Iyer MR, et al. Facial recognition of heroin vaccine opiates: type 1 cross-reactivities of antibodies induced by hydrolytically stable haptenic surrogates of heroin, 6-acetylmorphine, and morphine. Vaccine. 2014;32(13):1473–9.

Maurer P, Jennings GT, Willers J, Rohner F, Lindman Y, Roubicek K, et al. A therapeutic vaccine for nicotine dependence: preclinical efficacy, and Phase I safety and immunogenicity. Eur J Immunol. 2005;35(7):2031–40.

McCluskie MJ, Pryde DC, Gervais DP, Stead DR, Zhang N, Benoit M, et al. Enhancing immunogenicity of a 3'aminomethylnicotine-DT-conjugate anti-nicotine vaccine with CpG adjuvant in mice and non-human primates. Int Immunopharmacol. 2013;16(1):50–6.

Minozzi S, Amato L, Vecchi S, Davoli M, Kirchmayer U, Verster A. Oral naltrexone maintenance treatment for opioid dependence. Cochrane Database Syst Rev. 2006;1:CD001333.

Nosyk B, Sun H, Evans E, Marsh DC, Anglin MD, Hser YI, et al. Defining dosing pattern characteristics of successful tapers following methadone maintenance treatment: results from a population-based retrospective cohort study. Addiction. 2012;107(9):1621–9.

NSDUH. Results from the 2013 national survey on drug use and health: mental health findings. U.S. Department of Health and Human Services; 2013. Available from: http://www.samhsa.gov/data/sites/default/files/NSDUHmhfr2013/NSDUHmhfr2013.pdf.

Orson FM, Rossen RD, Shen X, Lopez AY, Wu Y, Kosten TR. Spontaneous development of IgM anti-cocaine antibodies in habitual cocaine users: effect on IgG antibody responses to a cocaine cholera toxin B conjugate vaccine. Am J Addict. 2013;22(2):169–74.

Pentel PR, LeSage MG. New directions in nicotine vaccine design and use. Adv Pharmacol. 2014;69:553–80.

Pentel PR, Dufek MB, Roiko SA, Lesage MG, Keyler DE. Differential effects of passive immunization with nicotine-specific antibodies on the acute and chronic distribution of nicotine to brain in rats. J Pharmacol Exp Ther. 2006;317(2):660–6.

Pentel PR, Keyler DE, Kosten TR. Immunotherapies to treat drug addiction. In: Levine MM, editor. New generation vaccines. 4th ed. New York: Dekker; 2009. p. 982–92.

Pravetoni M, Le Naour M, Harmon TM, Tucker AM, Portoghese PS, Pentel PR. An oxycodone conjugate vaccine elicits drug-specific antibodies that reduce oxycodone distribution to brain and hot-plate analgesia. J Pharmacol Exp Ther. 2012a;341(1):225–32.

Pravetoni M, Raleigh MD, Le Naour M, Tucker AM, Harmon TM, Jones JM, et al. Coadministration of morphine and oxycodone vaccines reduces the distribution of 6-monoacetylmorphine and oxycodone to brain in rats. Vaccine. 2012b;30(31):4617–24.

Pravetoni M, Le Naour M, Tucker AM, Harmon TM, Hawley TM, Portoghese PS, et al. Reduced antinociception of opioids in rats and mice by vaccination with immunogens containing oxycodone and hydrocodone haptens. J Med Chem. 2013;56(3):915–23.

Pravetoni M, Vervacke JS, Distefano MD, Tucker AM, Laudenbach M, Pentel PR. Effect of currently approved carriers and adjuvants on the pre-clinical efficacy of a conjugate vaccine against oxycodone in mice and rats. PLoS One. 2014a;9(5):e96547.

Pravetoni M, Pentel PR, Potter DN, Chartoff EH, Tally L, LeSage MG. Effects of an oxycodone conjugate vaccine on oxycodone self-administration and oxycodone-induced brain gene expression in rats. PLoS One. 2014b;9(7):e101807.

Quaglio G, Talamini G, Lugoboni F, Lechi A, Venturini L, Jarlais DC, et al. Compliance with hepatitis B vaccination in 1175 heroin users and risk factors associated with lack of vaccine response. Addiction. 2002;97(8):985–92.

Raleigh MD, Pravetoni M, Harris AC, Birnbaum AK, Pentel PR. Selective effects of a morphine conjugate vaccine on heroin and metabolite distribution and heroin-induced behaviors in rats. J Pharmacol Exp Ther. 2013;344(2):397–406.

Raleigh MD, Pentel PR, LeSage MG. Pharmacokinetic correlates of the effects of a heroin vaccine on heroin self-administration in rats. PLoS One. 2014;9(12):e115696.

Rentsch KM, Kullak-Ublick GA, Reichel C, Meier PJ, Fattinger K. Arterial and venous pharmacokinetics of intravenous heroin in subjects who are addicted to narcotics. Clin Pharmacol Ther. 2001;70(3):237–46.

Reuter P. Can heroin maintenance help Baltimore? 2009. Available from: http://www.abell.org/sites/default/files/publications/cja_HeroinMaintenance_0209.pdf.

Rodrigo JM, Serra MA, Aparisi L, Escudero A, Gilabert MS, Garcia F, et al. Immune response to hepatitis B vaccine in parenteral drug abusers. Vaccine. 1992;10(11):798–801.

Rook EJ, Huitema AD, van den Brink W, van Ree JM, Beijnen JH. Pharmacokinetics and pharmacokinetic variability of heroin and its metabolites: review of the literature. Curr Clin Pharmacol. 2006a;1:109–18.

Rook EJ, Huitema AD, van den Brink W, van Ree JM, Beijnen JH. Population pharmacokinetics of heroin and its major metabolites. Clin Pharmacokinet. 2006b;45(4):401–17.

Rosenberg H, Phillips KT. Acceptability and availability of harm-reduction interventions for drug abuse in American substance abuse treatment agencies. Psychol Addict Behav. 2003;17(3):203–10.

Ryan JJ, Parker CW, Williams Jr RC. Globulin binding of morphine in heroin addicts. J Lab Clin Med. 1972;80(2):155–64.

Schlosburg JE, Vendruscolo LF, Bremer PT, Lockner JW, Wade CL, Nunes AA, et al. Dynamic vaccine blocks relapse to compulsive intake of heroin. Proc Natl Acad Sci U S A. 2013;110(22):9036–41.

Scott JA, Ojal J, Ashton L, Muhoro A, Burbidge P, Goldblatt D. Pneumococcal conjugate vaccine given shortly after birth stimulates effective antibody concentrations and primes immunological memory for sustained infant protection. Clin Infect Dis. 2011;53(7):663–70.

Spector S. Quantitative determination of morphine in serum by radioimmunoassay. J Pharmacol Exp Ther. 1971;178(2):253–8.

Spector S, Parker CW. Morphine: radioimmunoassay. Science. 1970;168(3937):1347–8.

Stowe GN, Schlosburg JE, Vendruscolo LF, Edwards S, Misra KK, Schulteis G, et al. Developing a vaccine against multiple psychoactive targets: a case study of heroin. CNS Neurol Disord Drug Targets. 2011a;10(8):865–75.

Stowe GN, Vendruscolo LF, Edwards S, Schlosburg JE, Misra KK, Schulteis G, et al. A vaccine strategy that induces protective immunity against heroin. J Med Chem. 2011b;54(14):5195–204.

Torres OB, Jalah R, Rice KC, Li F, Antoline JF, Iyer MR, et al. Characterization and optimization of heroin hapten-BSA conjugates: method development for the synthesis of reproducible hapten-based vaccines. Anal Bioanal Chem. 2014;406(24):5927–37.

Torten M, Miller CH, Eisele JH, Henderson GL, Benjamini E. Prevention of the effects of fentanyl by immunological means. Nature. 1975;253(5492):565–6.

Wainer BH, Fitch FW, Rothberg RM, Fried J. Morphine-3-succinyl – bovine serum albumin: an immunogenic hapten-protein conjugate. Science. 1972a;176(4039):1143–5.

Wainer BH, Fitch FW, Rothberg RM, Fried J. The structure of morphine monohemisuccinate. Science. 1972b;178(4061):647–8.

Wainer BH, Fitch FW, Fried J, Rothberg RM. A measurement of the specificities of antibodies to morphine-6-succinyl-BSA by competitive inhibition of 14 C-morphine binding. J Immunol. 1973;110(3):667–73.

Chapter 5
Vaccines for Methamphetamine Use Disorder

Thomas R. Kosten and Therese A. Kosten

5.1 Introduction

5.1.1 Problem of Methamphetamine Abuse

Methamphetamine (MA) abuse poses a serious health problem in the United States (Gonzales et al. 2010; Hunt et al. 2006) and in many parts of Asia (McKetin et al. 2008). There are no effective pharmacotherapies for this addiction, although much research has been directed toward it (Haile et al. 2009; Karila et al. 2010).

5.1.2 Effects of MA on Behavior and Physiology

MA can be highly addictive, meaning that use of the drug increases over time and becomes out of control. The MA addict, like other drug addicts, may begin to use MA due to its euphoria-producing effects. Then, drug use can become compulsive and done at the exclusion of other behaviors, such as those necessary to maintain

---

T.R. Kosten, MD (✉)
Menninger Department of Psychiatry and Behavioral Sciences, Baylor College of Medicine, Houston, TX, USA

The Michael E DeBakey Veteran's Affairs Medical Center, Houston, TX, USA
e-mail: kosten@bcm.edu

T.A. Kosten, VAMC
Menninger Department of Psychiatry and Behavioral Sciences, Baylor College of Medicine, Houston, TX, USA

Department of Psychology, University of Houston, Houston, TX, USA

The Michael E DeBakey Veteran's Affairs Medical Center, Houston, TX, USA

I.D. Montoya (ed.), *Biologics to Treat Substance Use Disorders: Vaccines, Monoclonal Antibodies, and Enzymes*, DOI 10.1007/978-3-319-23150-1_5

their basic needs (Kosten et al. 2012). The initial euphoric effects of drugs and the addictive effects are ascribed to their ability to increase levels of the neurotransmitter, dopamine (DA), in specific brain areas, including the nucleus accumbens (DiChiara 1999; Volkow et al. 2004; Wise 2004). Indeed, MA does increase DA levels as wells as enhance levels of other neurotransmitters, including norepinephrine, serotonin, and gamma-aminobutyric acid, among others (Sulzer et al. 2005). MA is sympathomimetic; it stimulates a number of bodily processes related to stress responses. These include increasing heart rate and body temperature, among others. Thus, MA use has multiple peripheral and central effects (Kosten et al. 2012).

5.1.3 Outline of Chapter

In this chapter, we will first describe what immunotherapy for MA abuse is, what its advantages are over standard pharmacotherapeutic approaches, and what its hypothetical mechanism is. Next, we describe how vaccines can be constructed and administered. Then, we explain how the efficacy of a vaccine is assessed. Finally, we present the results of some of our research as well as those from other laboratories in which MA vaccines have been tested in animals.

5.2 Approach of Immunotherapy

5.2.1 How Immunotherapy Differs from Pharmacotherapy

Like research for addiction treatment in general, the typical approach in the development of medications for MA abuse is to test agents that act at similar sites of action in the brain as the abused drug. However, such pharmacotherapies can also cause many untoward effects that likely reduce compliance. For example, disulfiram treatment for cocaine abuse can enhance cocaine-induced paranoia in humans and cocaine-induced seizures in mice (Gaval-Cruz et al. 2008) in addition to the aversive effects caused by alcohol ingestion (Towell et al. 1983). An alternative treatment approach for addiction that we, and others, have used is immunotherapy (Janda and Trewwek 2012; Owens et al. 2011; Shen et al. 2012). It should be noted that the purpose of immunotherapy is to augment psychological interventions similar to the use of pharmacotherapies. And, because the main obstacle to treatment success is preventing relapse to drug use, this is the goal of the immunotherapeutic approach.

5.2.2 Advantages of Immunotherapy

One advantage of this approach is a potential increase in compliance because treatments could consist of obtaining only a few injections over a long period of time. This contrasts with the typical pharmacotherapeutic intervention that usually requires taking a medication daily or several times a week. And, immunotherapy would have fewer side effects than a pharmacotherapy that could affect several other functions in addition to the targeted effects related to reducing addictive behaviors. Another advantage of immunotherapy is that the vaccine would generate antibodies, and these antibodies would target and sequester the drug molecules in circulation. The result would be preventing or slowing the actions of MA (or other vaccine-specific targets) in the brain. This should reduce the adverse effects of the MA, which are not typically blocked with administration of most pharmacological treatments. Indeed, results from clinical studies that tested anti-cocaine and anti-nicotine vaccines have shown some effectiveness (Hatsukami et al. 2005, 2011; Martell et al. 2009).

5.2.3 *Hypothetical Mechanism*

The mechanism of action for these anti-MA antibodies certainly involves holding the MA in the bloodstream after ingestion. That is, a vaccine that targets a specific abused drug should, in theory, block or attenuate the psychological and physiological effects that support addiction. Although drug-specific vaccination should theoretically prevent entry of the drug into the brain, the antibodies will, at least, buffer the capacity of the drug to cross the blood-brain barrier and affect the areas of the brain related to its addictive actions. Indeed, MA antibodies might have an important pharmacokinetic effect of slowing entry of the MA into the brain. Slowing entry alone reduces the reinforcing effects of the drug as seen in human and nonhuman primate self-administration studies (deWit et al. 1992; Marsch et al. 2001; Woolverton and Wang 2004). While no study has measured the rate of the rise of brain MA levels with and without MA antibodies in the blood, several studies have found reduced MA brain levels after MA administration in vaccinated compared to non-vaccinated animals (Shen et al. 2013a); (Laurenzana et al. 2009; Miller et al. 2013). Some studies also have reported that anti-MA vaccinated rats show increased MA blood levels after an MA challenge, which may be important for enhancing some aversive actions of MA such as nervousness, anxiety, and even paranoia in human MA abusers.

5.3 Vaccine Construction and Administration

5.3.1 *Construction*

The construction of a vaccine to target a specific drug of abuse has several steps and involves various parameters. These include the choice of what carrier protein to chemically attach to the hapten, the small molecule, such as MA, that is needed to induce immunogenicity. And which chemical part of the small molecule that will be the target of this attachment can vary. In addition, the vaccine may not only consist of the haptenated carrier protein but can also include an adjuvant. An adjuvant is used to help boost the immune response in order to induce the body to produce a greater amount of antibodies. Numerous choices are available at these various steps in the vaccine construction. It is necessary to test these variations in constructs empirically; the chemical composition does not reliably predict the body's immune responsivity. Typically, these tests are performed in mice first. Once the most efficacious vaccine construct is determined, further tests in higher species may be done, and then, they can be tested in humans. However, only some carrier proteins and adjuvants are acceptable for use in humans. Thus, it would be practical to conduct such studies with agents that are already approved for use in humans.

We have tested a number of different MA vaccine constructs in mice. Other laboratories have also conducted studies in mice and other nonhuman species. Most of these MA vaccines used keyhole limpet hemocyanin (KLH) as the carrier protein, although the hapten design and adjuvant differed across these studies. For example, we tested an anti-MA vaccine in mice that was made by attaching the hapten, succinyl methamphetamine (SMA), to KLH and administering it with monophosphoryl lipid A (MPL) as the adjuvant (Shen et al. 2013b). Although we found this vaccine generated antibodies and blocked the conditioned rewarding effects of MA, its potential for manufacturing an equivalent human vaccine could be improved by altering the carrier protein and the adjuvant.

Because the goal is not only to develop a more effective vaccine but also to design one that can be given to humans, we expanded upon our previous work by testing a vaccine made from the same MA hapten, SMA, attached to a tetanus toxoid (TT) carrier protein using aluminum (alum) as the primary adjuvant and conducted further studies adding the Toll-like receptor 4 (TRL4) adjuvant E6020 or the Toll-like receptor 5 (TRL5) adjuvant entolimod. Entolimod, a salmonella flagellin derivative and a TLR5 agonist, has demonstrated efficacy for a medical radiation countermeasure in pivotal animal studies, but its immunoadjuvant properties, which are characteristic of flagellin and its derivatives, have not yet been tested (Mizel and Bates 2010). A number of improved vaccines containing a fusion of an antigen (typically viral) with complete or truncated versions of flagellin have been successfully engineered. As an example, a series of seasonal flu vaccines designed using this approach (Kalnin et al. 2014; Song et al. 2014) are in the advanced stage of clinical development by VaxInnate (Cranbury, NJ) (http://clinicaltrials.gov/show/NCT02015494). These data suggest that the use of entolimod, a flagellin derivative capable of activating TRL5 signaling (Burdelya et al. 2008), may improve the efficacy of methamphetamine conjugate vaccine. All of these agents can be given to humans and so are ideal for development of a human vaccine, although the immunogenicity of the TT carrier protein may not be as good as KLH due to its smaller size (Dagan et al. 2010).

5.3.2 Administration

Both active vaccines and passive anti-MA antibodies have been tested in animals. Active immunization refers to the administration of the vaccine construct to the animal that will be tested. Often, there are two or more "booster" administrations of the same vaccine given across several weeks. This is done to increase antibody production. Passive immunization means that some animals will be vaccinated, and the sera that contain the antibodies are collected and administered to other, non-vaccinated animals. These passively administered antibodies are not monoclonal antibodies, in which all the antibodies have the same affinity and molecular structure because they are derived from a single clone of antibody-producing B cells. Monoclonal anti-MA antibodies have been produced by Owens et al. (2011) and have advantages over the simple vaccination approach, which produces a polyclonal response of multiple types of anti-MA antibodies with differing affinities and cross-reactivity to binding related compounds besides MA.

There are advantages and specific purposes for monoclonal versus direct vaccine approaches. Administration of monoclonal antibodies could be useful in an acute situation, such as in an emergency overdose. The duration of effect is short-lasting with the monoclonal antibody approach compared to the active immunization approach. In addition, it would be more costly to manufacture monoclonal antibodies. The active immunization approach is less costly to manufacture, but it would take some time for the person to generate antibodies in response to the vaccinations. In both cases, antibodies would be fairly specific to the targeted drug of abuse. If the addict ingested a different drug that might have similar effects but differs in chemical structure, neither vaccination approach would be effective. Both approaches have been used in tests of MA immunotherapy in animals as described below.

5.4 Measuring the Efficacy of a Vaccine in Preclinical Studies

5.4.1 Antibody Titers and Affinity

The first step in research on the development of vaccines targeted at a drug of abuse is to measure antibody titers in sera. This can be done at multiple time points after the initial vaccination and the booster administrations using enzyme-linked immunosorbent assay (ELISA). Levels are usually determined by measurements of optical density (OD) obtained using a microplate reader coated with specific anti-MA antibody. An increase in titer levels over days and weeks indicates that antibodies were generated.

We vaccinated 60 female BALB/c mice with SMA-TT prepared with alum as the adjuvant (Haile et al., in submission). A second administration of the vaccine (i.e., booster) was given at week 3. Antibody titers were assessed from pooled sera samples taken at several times over a 22-week period. As seen in Fig. 5.1, antibody levels increase over time particularly after the second vaccination. Two observations are that boosters are clearly substantially elevating the initially produced antibody levels and that these anti-MA antibody levels decline over time, when an additional booster is needed to again elevate these antibody levels.

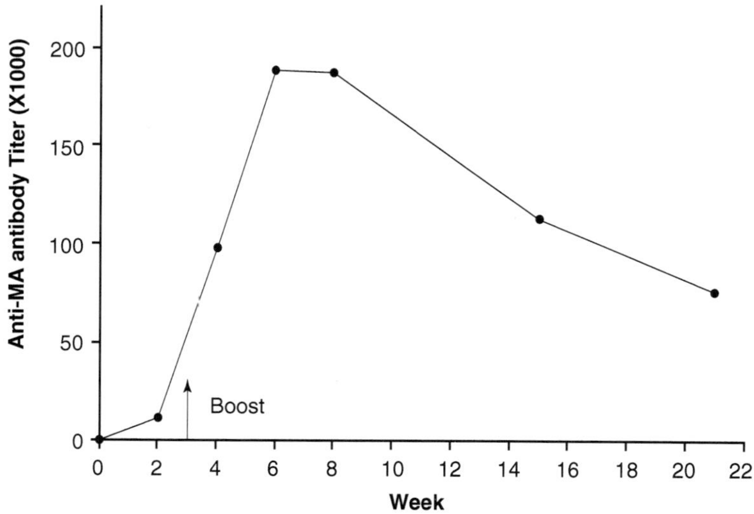

Fig. 5.1 Pooled antibody titer levels measured by ELISA on sera samples obtained from weeks 2 through 21 after the initial vaccination with SMA-TT with alum alone as adjuvant are presented. The *arrow* at week 3 indicates the time that a vaccination boost was administered

While high antibody levels are critical for efficacy, they are not sufficient to establish whether a vaccine construct has good potential for further study. The affinity of the antibodies should also be assessed. That is, it is important to know how well the antibodies bind to the antigen, such as MA. This affinity of the polyclonal antibody response can be assessed by a variety of techniques, but the important concepts are that these polyclonal antibodies will have multiple affinities rather than a single affinity and the amount of each of these antibodies together will determine the efficacy of this mix of antibodies. In our studies, we have found that our vaccines produce up to 20% high-affinity antibodies and 80% moderate-affinity. From our calculations these moderate-affinity antibodies are sufficient to bind the MA before it can enter the brain, and our assessment of brain levels of MA after vaccination indicates a fourfold reduction in MA levels, as blood levels rise (Haile et al., in submission).

5.4.2 *Functional Tests*

The next step in preclinical research on vaccines for addiction is to test if there are functional effects. That is, it is important to see that vaccinated animals show different, often seen as attenuated, behavioral or physiological responses to the administration of the target drug. While this may seem straightforward, it is often not. Drugs of abuse have multiple effects and most of these can differ by the dose administered. In addition, many of these responses will change with repeated drug administration.

When an increase in a response to a drug is seen with repeated administration, this is considered sensitization. Sensitization is also seen by demonstrating that lower doses produce a response that would be seen in a drug-naive animal given a higher dose under acute conditions. Conversely, some drug responses decrease with repeated administration, a phenomenon called tolerance. Tolerance is also seen by demonstrating that higher doses are needed to produce a response that would be seen in a drug-naive animal given a lower dose under acute conditions. Further complicating the picture is that the dose-response function of a specific drug rarely appears to be linear with increasing response levels induced by increasing doses. In some cases, an increase in dose produces an effect that masks or interferes with the expression of the response under study. The net effect will look like a response to a lower dose. Thus, it is very important to test the function of a vaccine with multiple doses of the drug and include the appropriate control groups or conditions.

Various functional assays have been used in the preclinical assessments of MA vaccines. Since MA affects locomotor activity and this is easily measured in a standard, commercially available apparatus, it is usually the first behavior to examine. Other tests can be used to evaluate the addictive properties of MA. These include conditioned place preference (CPP) and operant self-administration. And both of these procedures can be used to assess acquisition and reinstatement of the behavior. The latter effect is particularly significant because it is thought to be a model of relapse to drug use after abstinence in humans (Shaham et al. 2003). Other functional assessments of the efficacy of MA vaccines that have been used include measuring body temperature and the discriminative stimulus effects of MA.

5.5 Results of Studies with MA Vaccines

We have assessed antibody titers in response to various conjugate MA vaccine preparations. In one study (Shen et al. 2013a), we found good levels of antibodies in response to SMA-KLH prepared with MPL as the adjuvant. Mice were vaccinated and given boosters at 3 and 20 weeks after the initial vaccination. Measures of antibody titers were at a peak level by 6 weeks and remained at about this level through week 18 post-initial vaccination. The levels increased after the second booster and remained high through week 35. In another study, we prepared SMA with another carrier protein, TT, and used aluminum as the adjuvant (Haile et al., in submission). Mice were vaccinated and given a booster at week 3. The antibody titers were measured at several time points for 21 weeks following the first vaccination with a single booster at week 3. The antibody levels increase greatly after the boost given at week 3 to 100K at week 4 and to their highest levels of about 200K from weeks 6 to 8. The levels then modestly declined to 125K at week 15 and to 100K at week 21.

We find that about 3–4% of mice do not produce antibodies to MA with these vaccines even when the TLR4 or TLR5 adjuvants are included. In humans this challenge of immunological non-response has also occurred, and our cocaine vaccine produced very poor antibody responses in 10–25% of subjects (Kosten et al. 2014;

Martell et al. 2009). However, these human studies only had aluminum as an adjuvant, and with these newer TLR4 and TLR5 adjuvants added to the aluminum, we expect fewer of these poorly responsive subjects.

We examined the functional effects of an SMA-KLH vaccine and an SMA-TT vaccine in mice on locomotor activity and in CPP using active immunization procedures. Mice vaccinated with SMA-KLH showed reduced conditioned effects of MA (e.g., approach behaviors) and reduced locomotor activity in response to MA but did not show a decrease in acquisition of MA CPP (Shen et al. 2013a). In our unpublished study with active immunization using SMA-TT in mice, we also did not find a significant decrease in the acquisition of MA CPP. However, reinstatement of the behavior was significantly altered (Haile et al., in submission). In fact, the vaccine appeared to have enhanced the aversive effects of repeated exposures to higher doses of MA because these mice actually showed a significant avoidance of the MA-paired environment. This enhanced aversion may reflect a more sustained MA effect from the buffering and retention of the MA in the blood from its binding to the anti-MA antibodies. Stated differently, the acute surge in relatively lower levels of MA produces preference and reinforcing effects, while the sustained increase in higher MA levels produces aversion and the negative effects described by humans as anxiety, nervousness, and even paranoia (Kosten et al. 2012).

Monoclonal MA antibodies passively administered to rats or pigeons decreased the locomotor activating and discriminative stimulus effects of MA as well as reduced self-administration behavior (Byrnes-Blake et al. 2005; McMillan et al. 2002, 2004). However, in another study with rats, an anti-MA vaccine linked to KLH did not alter the locomotor effects of a 3 mg/kg dose of MA (Byrnes-Blake et al. 2001), and another study reported enhanced the acquisition of MA self-administration (Duryee et al. 2009).

Anti-MA vaccines may be effective for specific behavioral or physiological responses to MA within certain dose ranges. A different anti-MA vaccine also linked to KLH did not affect rectal temperature or locomotor activity unless a very high dose (5.6 mg/kg) was administered (Miller et al. 2013). Additionally, in the locomotor assay, the stereotypic effects of MA were blocked; but no group differences were seen at MA doses of 3.2 mg/kg or less. It is possible that the discrepancies across studies are due to a species difference or perhaps to differences in vaccine preparations or even due to behavioral assessment procedures. Nonetheless, data from our studies support the ability of anti-MA vaccine to attenuate conditioned reward in mice.

5.6 Conclusions and Future Directions

Overall, several animal studies suggest that immunotherapy for MA abuse is a viable treatment approach. Further research is needed to determine the most effective anti-MA vaccine construct by using multiple behavioral and physiological assays. In particular, tests using MA self-administration would provide important information on whether the vaccine can attenuate the reinforcing effects of MA that maintain addictive behavior or block drug-induced reinstatement of extinguished self-administration behavior, an important model of relapse.

Acknowledgments This research was supported by grant DP1DA033502 from the National Institute on Drug Abuse (TRK), the Alkek Foundation for Experimental Therapeutics (TAK), and the Department of Veterans Affairs (TRK).

References

Burdelya LG, Krivokrysenko VI, Tallent TC, Strom E, Gleiberman AS, Gupta D, Kurnasov OV, Fort FL, Osterman AL, Didonato JA, Feinstein E, Gudkov AV. An agonist of toll-like receptor 5 has radioprotective ability in mouse and primate models. Science. 2008;320: 226–30.

Byrnes-Blake KA, Carroll FI, Abraham P, Owens SM. Generation of anti-(+)methamphetamine antibodies is not impeded by (+)methamphetamine administration during active immunization of rats. Int Immunopharmacol. 2001;1:329–38.

Byrnes-Blake KA, Laurenzana EM, Landes RD, Gentry WB, Owens SM. Monoclonal IgG affinity and treatment time alters antagonism of (+)-methamphetamine effects in rats. Eur J Pharmacol. 2005;521:86–94.

Dagan R, Poolman J, Siegrist C-A. Glycoconjugate vaccines and immune interference: a review. Vaccine. 2010;28:5513–23.

deWit H, Bodker B, Amber J. Rate of increase of plasma drug level influences subjective response in humans. Psychopharmacology (Berl). 1992;107:352–8.

DiChiara G. Drug addiction as dopamine-dependent associative learning disorder. Eur J Pharmacol. 1999;375:13–30.

Duryee MJ, Bevins RA, Reichel CM, Murray JE, Dong Y, Thiele GM, Sanderson SD. Immune responses to methamphetamine by active immunization with peptide-based, molecular adjuvant-containing vaccines. Vaccine. 2009;27:2981–8.

Gaval-Cruz M, Schroeder JP, Liles LC, Javors MA, Weinshenker D. Effects of disulfiram and dopamine beta-hydroxylase knockout on cocaine-induced seizures. Pharmacol Biochem Behav. 2008;89:556–62.

Gonzales R, Mooney L, Rawson RA. The methamphetamine problem in the United States. Ann Rev Pub Health. 2010;31:385–98.

Haile CN, Kosten TA, Shen XY, O'Malley PW, Winoske KJ, Kinsey BM, Huang Z, Lykissa ED, Naidu N, Arora R, Kosten TR, Orson FM Altered methamphetamine place conditioning in mice vaccinated with a succinyl-methamphetamine-tetanus-toxoid vaccine. Amer J Addictions (in press)

Haile CN, Kosten TR, Kosten TA. Pharmacogenetic treatments for drug addiction: cocaine, amphetamine and methamphetamine. Am J Drug Alcohol Abuse. 2009;35:161–77.

Hatsukami DK, Jorenby DE, Donzales G, Aigotti RN, Glover ED, Oncken CA, Tashkin DP, Reus VI, Akhavain RC, Fahim RE, Kessler PD, Niknian M, Kalnik MW, Rennard SI. Immunogenicity and smoking-cessation outcomes for a novel nicotine immunotherapeutic. Clin Pharmacol Therap. 2011;89:392–9.

Hatsukami DK, Rennard S, Jorenby D, Fiore M, Koopmeiners J, deVos A, Horwith G, Pentel PR. Safety and immunogenicity of a nicotine conjugate vaccine in current smokers. Clin Pharmacol Therap. 2005;78:456–67.

Hunt D, Kuck S, Truitt L. Methamphetamine use: lessons learned. In: National Institute of Justice. Cambridge, MA: Abt Associates; 2006.

Janda KD, Trewwek JB. Vaccines targeting drugs of abuse: is the glass half-empty or half-full? Nat Rev Immunol. 2012;12:67–72.

Kalnin K, Tibbitts T, Yan Y, et al. Low doses of flagellin-L2 multimer vaccines protect against challenge with diverse papillomavirus genotypes. Vaccine. 2014;32:3540–7.

Karila L, Weinstein A, Aubin HJ, Benyamina A, Reynaud M, Batki SL. Pharmacological approaches to methamphetamine dependence: a focused review. Br J Clin Pharmacol. 2010;69:1365–2125.

Kosten TR, Domingo CB, Shorter D, Orson F, Green C, Somoza E, Sekerka R, Levin FR, Mariani JJ, Stitzer M, Tompkins DA, Rotrosen J, Thakkar V, Smoak B, Kampman K. Vaccine for cocaine dependence: a randomized double-blind placebo-controlled efficacy trial. Drug Alcohol Depend. 2014;140:42–7.

Kosten TR, Newton TF, DeLaGarza R, Haile CN. Cocaine and methamphetamine dependence: advances in treatment. Arlington: Arlington. American Psychiatric Publishing; 2012.

Laurenzana EM, Hendrickson HP, Carpenter D, Peterson EC, Gentry WB, West M, Che Y, Carroll FI, Owens SM. Functional and biological determinants affecting the duration of action and efficacy of anti-(+)-methamphetamine monoclonal antibodies in rats. Vaccine. 2009;27:7011–20.

Marsch LA, Bickel WK, Badger GJ, Rathmell JP, Swedberg MDB, Jonzon B, Norsten-Hoog C. Effects of infusion rate of intravenously administered morphine on physiological, psychomotor, and self-reported measures in humans. J Pharmacol Exp Therap. 2001;299:1056–65.

Martell BA, Orson FM, Poling J, Mitchell E, Rossen RD, Gardner T, Kosten TR. Cocaine vaccine for the treatment of cocaine dependence in methadone-maintained patients: a randomized, double-blind, placebo-controlled efficacy trial. Arch Gen Psychiatry. 2009;66:1116–23.

McKetin R, Kozel N, Doublas J, Ali R, Vicknasingam B, Lund J, Li JH. The rise of methamphetamine in Southeast and East Asia. Drug Alcohol Rev. 2008;27:220–8.

McMillan DE, Hardwick WC, Li M, Gunnell MG, Carroll FI, Abraham P, Owens SM. Effects of murine-derived anti-methamphetamine monoclonal antibodies on (+)-methamphetamine self-administration in the rat. J Pharmacol Exp Therap. 2004;309:1248–55.

McMillan DE, Hardwick WC, Li M, Owens SM. Pharmacokinetic antagonism of (+) -methamphetamine discrimination by a low-affinity monoclonal anti-methamphetamine antibody. Behav Pharmacol. 2002;13:465–73.

Miller ML, Moreno AY, Aarde SM, Creehan KM, Vandewater SA, Vaillancourt BD, Wright MJ, Janda KD, Taffe MA. A methamphetamine vaccine attenuates methamphetamine-induced disruptions in thermoregulation and activity in rats. Biol Psychiatry. 2013;73:721–8.

Mizel SB, Bates JT. Flagellin as an adjuvant: cellular mechanisms and potential. J Immunol. 2010;185:5677–82.

Owens SM, Atchley WT, Hambuchen MD, Peterson EC, Gentry WB. Monoclonal antibodies as pharmacokinetic antagonists for the treatment of (+)-methamphetamine addiction. CNS Neurol Disord Drug Targets. 2011;10:892–8.

Shaham Y, Shalev U, Lu L, DeWit H. The reinstatement model of drug relapse: history, methodology and major findings. Psychopharmacology (Berl). 2003;168:3–20.

Shen X, Orson FM, Kosten TA, Kinsey BM, Yan W, Wang X, Kosten TR. Anti-methamphetamine vaccine attenuates brain levels and locomotor activity of methamphetamine in mice. San Diego: College on the Problems of Drug Dependence; 2013a.

Shen XY, Kosten TA, Lopez AY, Kinsey BM, Kosten TR, Orson FM. A vaccine against methamphetamine attenuates its behavioral effects in mice. Drug Alcohol Depend. 2013b;129:41–8.

Shen XY, Orson FM, Kosten TR. Vaccines against drug abuse. Clin Pharmacol Ther. 2012;91:60–70.

Song L, Liu G, Umlauf S, Liu X, et al. A rationally designed form of the TLR5 agonist, flagellin, supports superior immunogenicity of Influenza B globular head vaccines. Vaccine. 2014;32:4317–23.

Sulzer D, Sonders MS, Poulsen NW, Galli A. Mechanisms of neurotransmitter release by amphetamines: a review. Prog Neurobiol. 2005;75:406–33.

Towell JF, Cho JK, Roh BL, Wang RI. Disulfiram and erythrocyte aldehyde dehydrogenase inhibition. Clin Pharmacol Ther. 1983;33:517–21.

Volkow ND, Fowler JS, Wang GJ, Swanson JM. Dopamine in drug abuse and addiction: results from imaging studies and treatment implications. Mol Psychiatry. 2004;9:557–69.

Wise RA. Dopamine, learning and motivation. Nat Rev Neurosci. 2004;5:483–94.

Woolverton WL, Wang Z. Relationship between injection duration, transporter occupancy and reinforcing strength of cocaine. Eur J Pharmacol. 2004;486:251–7.

Chapter 6
Cocaine and HIV Infection

Timothy Cardozo, Sergey V. Shmelkov, Kenneth Carr, John Rotrosen, Pedro Mateu-Gelabert, and Samuel R. Friedman

6.1 Brief Review of Prior Cocaine Vaccine Trials

This area is reviewed in depth in a previous chapter. The earliest PubMed reference to a cocaine vaccine is a 1992 citation from Bagasra et al. (1992) describing immunization of inbred Fischer rats either with cocaine emulsification in complete Freund adjuvant or with cocaine conjugated with keyhole-limpet hemocyanin as carrier plus CFA. Both immunizations were effective in raising antibodies that protected the animals from the CNS effects of cocaine. Antibody (Ab) levels and CNS protection were highly correlated. Two years later, the National Institute on Drug Abuse funded a $700,000 grant to ImmuLogic Pharmaceutical Corporation (Waltham, MA) to complete animal testing and to develop a plan for clinical trials (Nadis 1996). The ImmuLogic product also raised antibodies that restricted cocaine access to the brain and reduced both the CNS effects of cocaine and cocaine self-administration (Fox 1997; Wise and Ranaldi 1996). Subsequent work has

T. Cardozo (✉)
Department of Biochemistry and Molecular Pharmacology, NYU School of Medicine, New York, NY, USA
e-mail: timothy.cardozo@nyumc.org

S.V. Shmelkov
Departments of Neuroscience and Physiology and Psychiatry, NYU School of Medicine, New York, NY, USA

K. Carr
Departments of Psychiatry and Biochemistry and Molecular Pharmacology, NYU School of Medicine, New York, NY, USA

J. Rotrosen
Department of Psychiatry, NYU School of Medicine, New York, NY, USA

P. Mateu-Gelabert • S.R. Friedman
Institute for Infectious Disease Research, National Development and Research Institutes, Inc., New York, NY, USA

I.D. Montoya (ed.), *Biologics to Treat Substance Use Disorders: Vaccines, Monoclonal Antibodies, and Enzymes*, DOI 10.1007/978-3-319-23150-1_6

largely focused on cholera toxin B-based vaccines (Kosten et al. 2013, 2014a, b, c; Kosten and Domingo 2013; Brimijoin et al. 2013; Orson et al. 2013; Haney et al. 2010; Martell et al. 2009), on adenovirus-based vaccines (Rosenberg et al. 2012; Koob et al. 2011; Wee et al. 2012; Cai et al. 2013), and on approaches using these vaccines in combination with other biologics, such as viral vector delivery of the cocaine hydrolase gene (Gao et al. 2013; Carroll et al. 2012).

The cholera toxin B-based vaccine has been tested in human subjects (Kosten et al. 2014b; Haney et al. 2010; Martell et al. 2009; Stitzer et al. 2010). In a human laboratory study involving ten cocaine-dependent men, Haney et al. (2010) established that the TA-CD vaccine elicited Abs that were highly effective in reducing the subjective effects of smoked cocaine. Abs levels varied greatly, and those with more Abs showed greater attenuation of cocaine effects. Study participants also reported less cocaine use while they were outside of the human laboratory setting, and this phenomenon was associated with higher Abs titers.

Martell et al. (2009) conducted a large placebo-controlled clinical trial, involving 115 methadone-maintained subjects most of whom smoked crack cocaine. The goals of the study were to evaluate immunogenicity, safety, and efficacy of the TA-CD vaccine administered five times in reducing cocaine use. As in the Haney study, Ab production varied significantly across subjects and those subjects who produced IgG antibody levels of 43 μg/ml or greater used less cocaine than those with lower IgG levels. Only 38 % of subjects produced the higher Abs titers. Subsequently, Kosten et al. (2014b) conducted a larger, multicenter, randomized placebo-controlled trial involving 300 cocaine-dependent subjects (who were not in methadone programs). The same TA-CD vaccine was used, and five vaccinations administered at weeks 1, 3, 5, 9, and 13 with subjects followed through week 24. In this study, 67 % of the vaccinated subjects achieved titers of 42 μg/ml or greater, and these subjects had lower dropout rates and more frequent abstinence during the final 2 weeks of the trial. Overall, there were no significant differences between the placebo group and the high and low IgG groups in terms of cocaine-positive urines. The major findings of these clinical trials are (1) the vaccine is effective in generating anti-cocaine Abs; (2) anti-cocaine Ab production is highly variable; (3) anti-cocaine Abs and Abs titers are associated with reduced subjective responses to cocaine and reduction of cocaine use, though the magnitude of the latter is limited; and (4) the vaccine appears to be extremely safe and well tolerated, minor injection site reactions being the most frequent adverse event. Overall, these studies suggest that anti-cocaine vaccines have potential benefits but need to be improved in order to have meaningful clinical utility.

6.1.1 Bioethical, Legal, and Policy Issues

Despite the very limited success to date and the amount of work remaining to be done before an effective vaccine could be available, a number of reports have already focused on bioethical, legal, and policy issues around vaccinating against addiction (Cohen 1997, 2000; Hall and Carter 2004; Hall and Gartner 2011; Katsnelson 2004; Young et al. 2012). Issues include loss of privacy, stigmatization, voluntary vs. coerced or compelled use, use within the criminal justice system and by drug courts, for whom should a vaccine be targeted (i.e., addicts vs. the drug naïve who are at risk), and intended vs. unintended consequences. These are compelling issues that are only tangentially part of the scope of this chapter.

6.2 Review of Prior HIV Vaccine Trials

The 30-year evolution of HIV vaccine strategies has been guided in large part by vaccine clinical trial failures that disabused incorrect notions. These failures confirmed that many research and development concepts borrowed from prior successful, licensed vaccines would not work against HIV. Prior to the HIV vaccine effort, the limiting step in viral vaccine development was usually isolation of the pathogenic virus and development of a method to culture it in the laboratory. The clinical success of prior non-HIV vaccines (polio, measles, hepatitis B, tetanus, etc.) firmly established that immunization with the right protein antigen was capable of generating a protective Ab (usually IgG) response in humans. (Notably, although neutralizing antibodies are often associated with protection, several vaccines do not elicit neutralizing Abs and still protect (Excler et al. 2014))

Current vaccines in clinical use elicit a variety of responses that may correlate with their efficacy, but these vaccines were developed empirically, so the mechanisms by which they confer protection remain poorly understood. Nevertheless, the vaccine responses include serum Ab (IgG), mucosal Abs (IgG and IgA), and T-cell responses (Siegrist 2013). Currently licensed vaccines target a variety of pathogens that infect via different mechanisms. Although general conclusions for any vaccine correlates are always hotly debated, when only subunit-based vaccines bearing viral epitopes are considered, a host serum IgG response is the common feature of vaccine-induced immunity (Table 6.1). Furthermore, although immune regulatory

Table 6.1 Correlates of vaccine-induced immunity for viral subunit vaccines

Vaccines	Vaccine type	Serum IgG	Mucosal IgG	Mucosal IgA	T cells
Hepatitis A	Killed	++			
Japanese encephalitis	Killed	++			
Polio Salk	Killed	++	+		
Rabies	Killed	++			
Influenza	Killed, subunit	++	(+)		
Hepatitis B (HBsAg)	Protein	++			
Papillomavirus (human)	VLPs	++	++		
Rotavirus	VLPs	(+)	(+)	++	

Adapted from Siegrist (2013)

mechanisms posit an opposition between cellular and humoral immunity, many reports suggest that B- and certain T-cell responses coordinate to produce the best overall vaccine-induced immunity and that innate immunity can shape these responses (reviewed in Siegrist 2013).

In retrospect, the historical approach to viral vaccine development succeeded against viruses that exhibit minimal antigenic variation (antigenic variation may be conceptualized as the variation in reactivity of the virus with human antibodies). By contrast, HIV may be the most antigenically variable pathogenic virus known. The first randomized placebo-controlled phase III clinical trial of the traditional vaccine strategy, consisting of immunization with repeated boosting injections of recombinant HIV surface envelope proteins, took place in the 1990s. The trial was known as the VaxGen trial, and the vaccine was trademarked as AIDSVAX®. This vaccine successfully elicited autologous-strain-specific, anti-HIV neutralizing antibodies but failed to protect human subjects from HIV acquisition.

One conclusion that became better appreciated as a result of the VaxGen trial was that the degree of antigenic variation exhibited by circulating HIV strains was too great to overcome with existing vaccine technology, namely, that immunization could protect only against the strains comprising the vaccine, but vaccinated individuals were very unlikely to encounter those strains among the thousands circulating in the real world. Accordingly, a paradigm shift took hold in the HIV vaccine field: some thought leaders advocated acknowledging the inability of antibodies elicited by vaccination to protect against HIV infection and instead supported developing methods to stimulate cell-mediated immunity against the virus in the hope of clearing the virus successfully upon encounter. Cell-mediated immunity stimulation is generally achieved through delivery of an intact, functional, but attenuated and engineered viral vector, such as adenovirus.

The known efficacy of licensed live, attenuated viral vaccines, e.g., against polio, seemed consistent with this approach. Promising preclinical data on an adenovirus construct advanced this alternative approach toward a second randomized placebo-controlled phase III HIV vaccine clinical trial. Unfortunately, this approach, too, failed and, worse, appeared to have increased infection risk for certain subsets of the vaccinated subjects (STEP study) (Kim et al. 2010). The failure of both the traditional and the major alternative approach to HIV vaccination left the field at a loss over the first decade of the twenty-first century. Fortunately, a third randomized placebo-controlled phase III clinical trial, the RV144 trial, had already started and finally resulted in the observation, in 2009, of statistically significant protection from HIV acquisition by a vaccine (Rerks-Ngarm et al. 2009). Interestingly, the RV144 trial was formulated as a hybrid of the two prior failed approaches, consisting of both a viral vector prime intended to stimulate cell-mediated immunity and the same AIDSVAX® protein immunogen boosts from the VaxGen trial. This recipe was highly controversial, if simply from a "two-wrongs-don't-make-a-right" point-of-view, to the point that many major thought leaders in the field objected to the trial in a letter published in *Science* (Burton et al. 2004).

Ironically, this "flawed" recipe turned out to be the only one that has ever resulted in any evidence that human subjects can be protected from HIV acquisition by vaccination

(Haynes et al. 2012). In this study, HIV infection was reduced by approximately 30 %. Although RV144 provided the first evidence of HIV vaccine efficacy, the effect was not strong enough to justify development of its ALVAC canarypox prime-AIDSVAX recombinant protein boost vaccine into a commercial product. Unfortunately, the protective effect was transient, disappearing after 6 months in the study population. Sub-analyses suggest that the antibody response did not endure (Haynes et al. 2012).

6.2.1 *Human Immune Correlates of Protection in HIV*

The RV144 case-control study was specifically designed to correlate protection from HIV infection with vaccine-induced immune factors (Haynes et al. 2012). More than 270 assays were performed for the RV144 immune correlates case-control study. Of these 270 measurements of host immune molecular function, only three were associated with an odds ratio (OR) of less than 0.6 of being infected with HIV. Thus, only these three detected a host molecular entity, high levels of which were significantly associated with low levels of infection. The common viral antigen used in all three assays was a short peptide fragment from position 166 to 179 of the V2 loop of HIV's surface envelope glycoprotein ($V2^{166-179}$; Fig. 6.1).

The superset of the viral antigens of all three assays was the entire V1V2 glycoprotein domain of HIV's surface envelope glycoprotein (two of the viral antigens were fragments of the largest one; see Fig. 6.1). These three viral antigens detected vaccine-elicited host antibodies that DIRECTLY led to protection (the low OR suggests that these antibodies directly blocked infecting viruses) (Haynes et al. 2012). These are the only three assays to detect such molecules, as the only other protection-associated OR was a significantly *high* OR for plasma IgA, which can only be

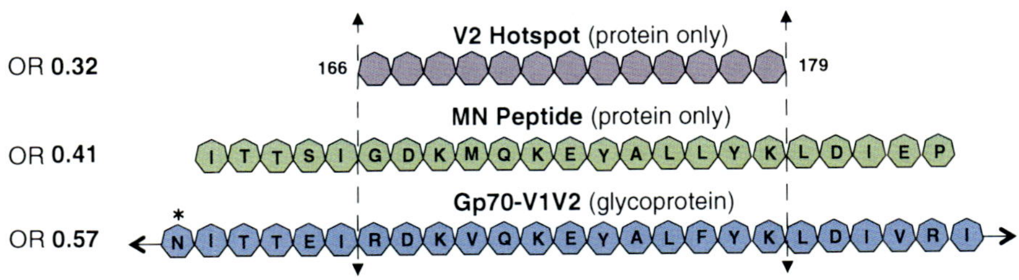

Fig. 6.1 Protection maps to $V2^{166-179}$. Of the approximate 270 assays performed in the RV144 immune correlates analysis, only Abs binding three reagents showed an odds ratio (*OR*) of 0.57 or lower (Haynes et al. 2012) (OR shown at the left of the above figure). These reagents were the gp70-V1V2 fusion glycoprotein (sequence for a portion of the V1V2 domain of gp70 shown in blue heptagons with glycosylation sites indicated by an asterisk), the MN peptide (sequence shown as green heptagons from positions 161–183), and the V2 Hotspot (shown as purple heptagons spanning positions 166–179). All three of these reagents include an unglycosylated portion of the V2 domain spanning positions 166–179 (Adapted from Tassaneetrithep et al. *PLoS One*. 2013; Creative Commons Attribution)

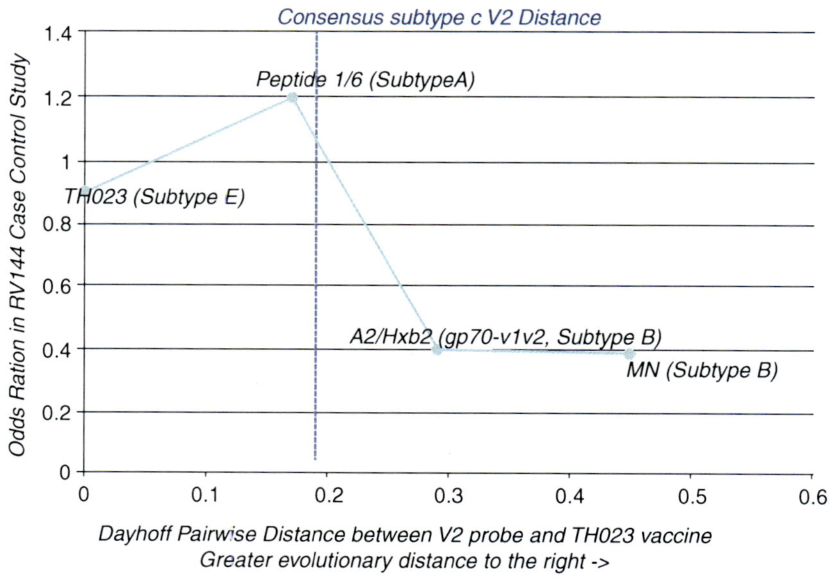

Fig. 6.2 Protective Abs need to be elicited by the subtype AE strain TH023 and yet cross-react with subtype B strains. Plotting the OR (Y-axis) of diverse V2 loop peptides tested in the RV144 case-control study against the evolutionary distance of each peptide from the TH023 immunogen (X-axis) shows that protection (low OR) only appears at the distance of subtype B. Thus, only those Abs elicited from subtype AE but cross-reacting with evolutionary distant subtype B strains were associated with protection. Abs that cross-reacted with less distant heterologous viruses (e.g., subtype A) were not associated with protection

explained by indirect mechanisms (Haynes et al. 2012). The protection observed in the RV144 trial did not correlate with broadly neutralizing antibody levels measured in vaccinated subjects. Thus, anti-V1V2 Abs, and perhaps only anti-V2$^{166–179}$ human antibodies, are the only molecular entities with direct evidence of association with protection from HIV infection. Interestingly, protection against neutralization-resistant viruses was also recently correlated with anti-V2 Abs in a nonhuman primate (NHP) model (Barouch et al. 2012).

A sieve analysis of the RV144 data *independently* found only two amino acid positions in the HIV genome that were statistically associated with vaccine efficacy and both positions are within or near the same common region identified in Fig. 6.1 (position 169 and position 181) (Rolland et al. 2012). Furthermore, a plot of the OR of a series of V1V2 domain antigens tested in the RV144 immune correlates analysis containing the 169–179 region of HIV's V2 loop shows that protection only appears when the antibodies in vaccinated subjects, which were likely elicited from a subtype AE HIV strain, cross-react with strains from subtype B (Fig. 6.2). These are the two most evolutionarily distant HIV subtypes among circulating strains, suggesting that the protective antibodies may be targeting accessible, functionally important epitopes in the virus that are conserved across most circulating strains. This observation extracted directly from the RV144 case-control analysis of human subjects has been partly confirmed by an independent, follow-up study

(Zolla-Pazner et al. 2014). Thus, integration of *all* the detailed protection data from the RV144 trial points to Abs elicited by the ALVAC-AIDSVAX vaccine targeting epitope(s) composed of amino acids located approximately in $V2^{165-179}$ and conserved across circulating HIV strains as being the most likely molecular entities associated with protection from HIV acquisition in human subjects. While these may not be the only epitopes responsible for the protection observed in the RV144 trial, these are the only ones for which such specific molecular detail can be inferred directly and exclusively from the primary RV144 trial human subject data. Most importantly, for the first time, an approximate, but very specific, location and composition of antibody-targeted epitopes on HIV-1's viral envelope have been associated with protection from HIV acquisition in human subjects.

6.3 Molecular Opportunity of a Combined Cocaine and HIV Immunogen

The above recent history of the parallel cocaine and HIV vaccine immunogen development efforts shows some striking parallels.

1. Both efforts have resulted at the present time in the identification of defined immunogens that have demonstrated partial efficacy of around 30 % in human subjects. In both cases, these starting points are promising, but not sufficient for product development on their own merits.
2. Both immunogens are highly "epitope focused," with epitope in this sense referring to antibody-targeted epitopes (as opposed to T-cell-targeted epitopes). This means that protective antibodies need to target a small, highly specific molecular shape. For the cocaine immunogen, cocaine itself is the epitope, as are all haptens that are successfully immunogenic when conjugated to carrier proteins. For the HIV vaccine, although the immunogen used in the RV144 trial was not epitope focused by design, the immune correlates analysis clearly suggests that at least one very specific epitope was responsible for protection.

Accordingly, from this starting point, one can envision a combined cocaine and HIV vaccine, provided that its nature is to be "epitope focused" or preferentially exhibiting the specific protective epitopes in a highly immunogenic configuration. For the purposes of the following discussion, we will refer to the cocaine hapten-protein conjugate as "epitope focused."

6.3.1 *Concept of Epitope Focusing*

The term epitope is used interchangeably in the scientific literature to refer to a single molecular entity at different spatial scales. An antibody-targeted epitope is defined as a three-dimensional chemical surface and shape bound by the

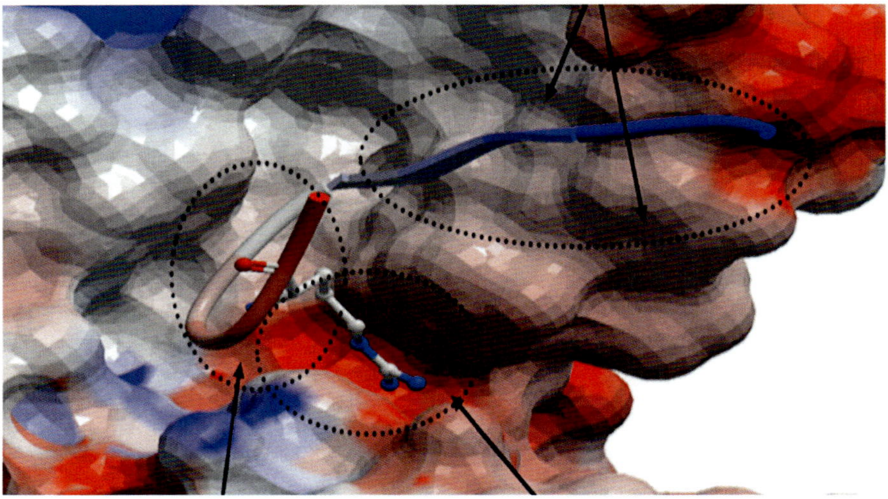

Fig. 6.3 The real definition of an antibody-targeted epitope: the molecular surface of the anti-HIV monoclonal 447-52D (PDB 1Q1J) is shown as a geometric object colored by electrostatics (*red* negative charge, *blue* positive). The backbone of the bound HIV antigen is shown in ribbon diagram with the single most strongly bound side chain shown in stick diagram. The amino acids in the *circles* all make contact with the antibody and thus, only their contacting atoms, in aggregate, form a chemical entity that is the epitope targeted by this antibody. This entity is poorly represented by any amino acid sequence because only a few atoms from any of the participating amino acids may actually make contact with the antibody while many noncontacting atoms enable or restrict the contacting atoms by van der Waals interactions, steric hindrance, or electrostatic interactions

antigen-combining site of an antibody. Historically, antibodies have been proven to be highly specific, so one can infer that the shape and chemistry of the epitope are also highly unique among the nearly infinite variety of such shapes and chemistries in biology. Nevertheless, many years of immunologic measurements were made with antibodies and peptide antigens before the availability of atomic detail structural information on these complexes.

The term "antibody-targeted epitope" in the literature, when it refers to peptide epitopes, has been equated to a short peptide segment within a protein (also termed a "linear epitope") or an entire protein domain. Similarly, the antibodies in question often referred to a polyclonal collection of monoclonal antibodies that targeted these segments or domains. Now that crystallographic structures of monoclonal antibodies bound to their cognate antigens are available, it is clear that individual antibody-targeted epitopes are best defined by the amino acids seen to be contacting a monoclonal antibody in a crystallographic complex, be they continuous or discontinuous in the sequence of the protein antigen (Fig. 6.3).

For the purposes of this discussion, a single antibody-targeted epitope in HIV's surface envelope glycoprotein is a single unique defined chemical entity decorating the surface of this protein, no different from cocaine decorating the surface of its carrier protein as a hapten conjugate. Protein chemistry is sufficiently robust that epitopes targeted by one monoclonal antibody can be directly adjacent to and

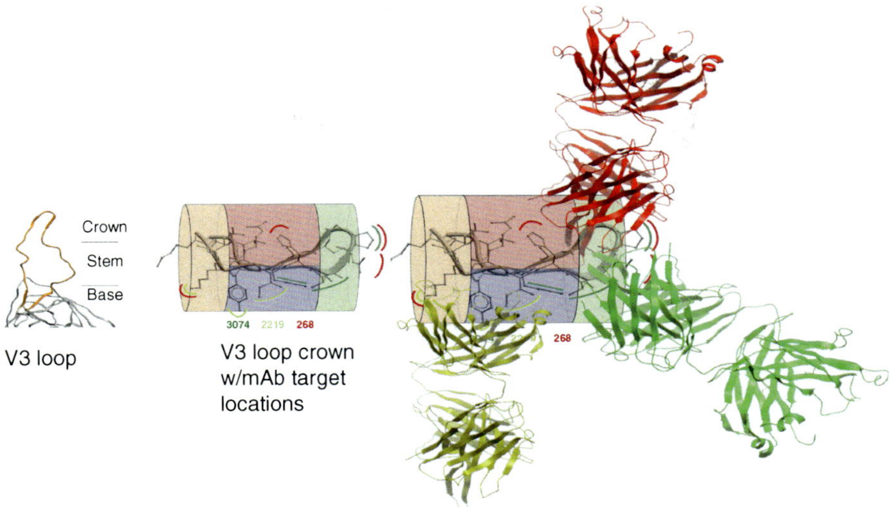

Fig. 6.4 Epitopes are often closely adjacent and overlapping discrete 3D shapes in a short peptide segment. *Left*: HIV's V3 loop (*orange*) emerging from gp120 (*gray*). *Middle*: locations on V3 crown of monoclonal antibody (mAb)-targeted epitopes (*curved lines*: mAb 268 = *red*, mAb 3074 = *green*, mAb 2219 = *yellow*). The V3 crown is divided into four zones: stem, *orange*; turn, *green*; and two faces of ß-sheet, red and blue to assist depiction of the three-dimensional space. *Right*: mAb structures are depicted to illustrate distribution of their epitopes around the V3 crown (Adapted from Zolla-Pazner and Cardozo (2010))

actually overlapping that targeted by a different monoclonal antibody (from a different B cell and with a different amino acid sequence), yet be unrecognized by the other monoclonal antibody (Fig. 6.4). Accordingly, one can strictly theorize that a clonal antibody response can be elicited by immunization with an immunogen that presents only the unique chemical entity representing an individual epitope. In practice, eliciting by immunization a functional polyclonal response narrowly focused on individual viral epitopes has been achieved (Correia et al. 2014), but only in one report for an HIV epitope (Cardozo et al. 2014).

Epitope-focusing technology may be a particularly acute need for HIV vaccine research. HIV protein immunogens designed to elicit broadly neutralizing antibodies (bNAbs) have failed to do so. These immunogens have often been variations of modifications of natural gp120 sequences. A big reason for the failure may be that HIV is highly antigenically variable and all naturally occurring gp120 sequences have evolved to display an abundance of immunodominant "decoy" epitopes that are type specific or elicit Abs that are otherwise advantageous to viral fitness (Tobin et al. 2008). Nevertheless, hidden among these decoy epitopes are epitopes that are true sites of vulnerability for the virus and that are conserved across strains, for example, those epitopes that are a structural component of host receptor binding sites or the epitopes identified in the RV144 trial.

Epitope focusing seeks to isolate these vulnerable epitopes and present them exclusively or preferentially on a non-HIV scaffold to form an epitope-focused

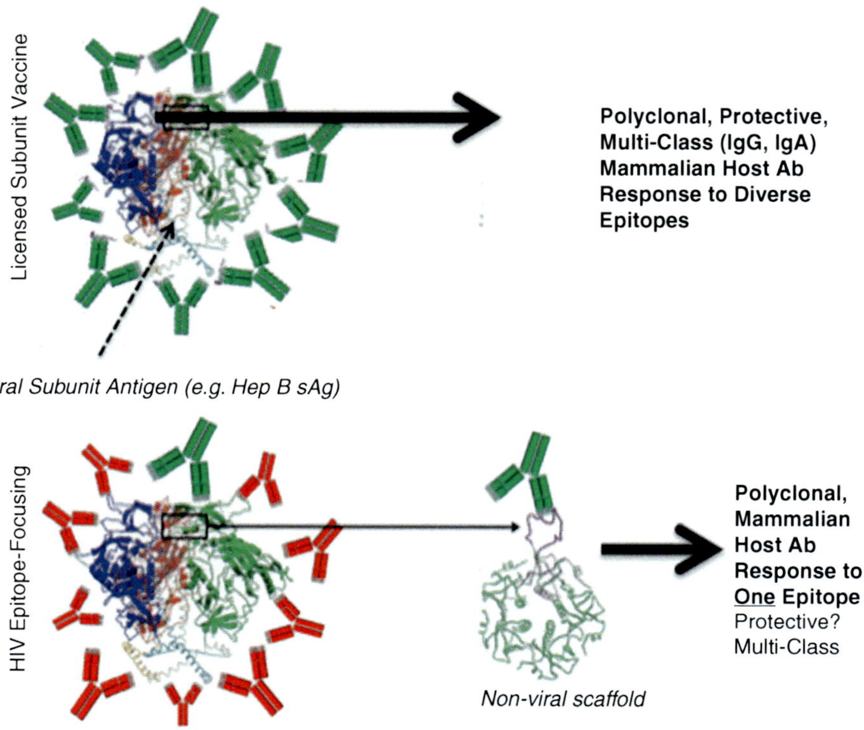

Fig. 6.5 How epitope vaccines differ from current viral vaccines. *Upper panel*: Currently licensed viral subunit vaccines are illustrated in the upper panel, wherein the major viral antigen is used to immunize subjects, resulting in protective IgG +/– IgA Abs (green Ab cartoons) elicited to many different sites on the antigen. *Lower panel*: Immunization with HIV's gp120 antigen results almost entirely in the elicitation of Abs that do not protect against acquisition of circulating HIV viruses (red Ab cartoons). Nevertheless, the RV144 trial demonstrated that rare Abs to specific epitopes are hidden in this response that can protect against HIV acquisition. Epitope focusing seeks to "splice" out the epitopes targeted by these useful Abs and present them on non-HIV scaffolds

immunogen (Fig. 6.5). The advantage of this approach is the ability to concentrate and potentially amplify the antibody response to known protective epitopes. Since, as previously discussed, specific peptide regions associated with protection in human subjects have been strongly implicated by RV144 clinical trial data, epitope focusing to these regions can be theorized as a straightforward method to optimize the existing RV144 vaccine.

6.3.2 Cholera Toxin B: The Common Scaffold

Interestingly, the only cocaine immunogen tested in a randomized placebo-controlled clinical trial (Shen et al. 2012) and the only epitope-focused HIV immunogen to successfully elicit functional, broadly cross-strain anti-HIV antibodies

(Cardozo et al. 2014) both used the identical protein scaffold to present their epitopes: cholera toxin B. Cholera toxin B (CTB) is the inert mucosa ganglioside binding subunit of the cholera toxin, so it is not toxic by itself but elicits a protective serum and mucosal anti-cholera toxin response upon immunization. It is highly immunogenic and elicits high antibody titers. Furthermore, each CTB gene product forms a pentamer, so its antigenicity is multivalent.

It is the central immunogen in a licensed cholera vaccine that has been widely and successfully used with an excellent safety record in humans. These properties of CTB make it an attractive carrier protein for vaccine investigations of cocaine and HIV at the discovery level. Notably, the cocaine vaccine showed no safety issues in humans, and the HIV construct differs from the licensed, safe-in-humans CTB protein by a short (<30 amino acid) peptide insert, so the safety concerns in humans of currently envisioned forms of CTB-based epitope-focused HIV and cocaine immunogens are very likely to be minimal.

6.4 The Concept of a Combined Cocaine and HIV Vaccine

Neither of the biologically active, specific anti-cocaine and anti-HIV immunogens is sufficiently protective in human subjects at the present time to be developed into a licensed product. Nevertheless, the existence of these two medicinal prototypes raises the theoretical possibility of a vaccine or immunotherapy available in the near future that can simultaneously raise anti-cocaine and anti-HIV Abs. Such a medicinal intervention has no precedent.

For the purposes of this text, we clarify the difference between the term "vaccine" and "immunotherapy." An immunogen that raises Abs against antigens to which the individual has never been exposed is, in traditional terms, a vaccine. Since the desired activity of anti-cocaine Abs is more commonly envisioned to take place in individuals who have previously been exposed to cocaine, the cocaine immunogens are technically a form of immunotherapy while their use in naïve individuals constitutes vaccination. The above-envisioned HIV immunogen is a true vaccine. HIV immunotherapy is potentially feasible, including via the administration of broadly neutralizing anti-HIV monoclonal antibodies to HIV-positive individuals.

6.4.1 *Combination Vaccination/Vaccine Coadministration*

A combination vaccine consists of two or more different vaccines that have been combined into a single shot. Combination vaccines have been in use in the United States since the mid-1940s. Examples of combination vaccines in current use target DTaP (diphtheria-tetanus-pertussis) (Papaevangelou 1998), trivalent IPV (three strains of inactivated polio vaccine) (Faden et al. 1993), MMR (measles-mumps-rubella) (Bart et al. 1986), and DTaP-Hib (Fritzell and Plotkin 1992). The combination vaccine concept has been so successful clinically that greater combinations of immunogens (DTaP-Hep B-IPV-Hib) in a single vaccination have been introduced (Esposito et al. 2014). Simultaneous vaccination, or coadministration, is when more than one vaccine shot is administered during the same doctor's visit, usually in separate limbs (e.g., one in each arm). An example of simultaneous vaccination might be administering DTaP in one arm or leg and IPV in another arm or leg during the same visit. Studies with the recently licensed HPV vaccine showed that coadministration did not reduce efficacy or safety of the individual vaccines (Noronha et al. 2014), although deleterious vaccine interactions have been theorized infrequently (Dagan et al. 2008).

Giving an at-risk individual several vaccinations during the same visit offers a practical advantage, and a combination vaccine promises even more benefit. Penetrance of treatment programs, treatment adherence, and use of public health resources for health maintenance and disease prevention is poor for adults in many of the communities afflicted by concurrent cocaine use and HIV infection. Coadministration of a cocaine-HIV vaccine could maximize compliance and afford protection more quickly than sequentially delivered vaccines. Given the history of safety and efficacy of coadministration of vaccines, this is a desirable aspect of the combined cocaine and HIV vaccine strategy. Furthermore, a combination vaccine affords the minor pain reduction advantage of a single injection instead of two. Nevertheless, a critical subject for future research is to confirm that a combined or coadministered cocaine and HIV vaccine are safe and effective compared to the coadministered version and with other commonly administered vaccines. This may be an especially interesting question if the first versions of cocaine and HIV vaccines are only partially effective.

6.4.2 HIV Prevention

HIV prevention methods are existing alternatives to vaccines. Although they present implementation difficulties compared to vaccines, these interventions are clinically proven, so they must be taken into account in theorizing about the impact of a combined cocaine-HIV vaccine (WHO Guidelines Approved by the Guidelines Review Committee 2014). Syringe exchange is highly effective at preventing HIV transmission among PWIDs (Abdul-Quader et al. 2013). Preexposure prophylaxis (PreP) is defined as the use of highly active antiretroviral therapy (HAART) prior to HIV exposure in HIV-negative subjects who are at high risk for exposure. The O52 study showed that PreP was over 95 % effective in preventing HIV acquisition in discordant couples. Other PrEP trials were much less effective, but theoretically, the effectiveness of such an approach could be very high for a small defineable group of individuals at risk in the population (reviewed in Wilton et al. (2015)). Circumcision also appears to be highly effective in preventing HIV transmission in non-US populations, where circumcision rates are low (reviewed in Tobian et al. (2014)).

6.4.3 *Alternative Promising Approaches Lacking Primary Evidence in Humans*

The only biologic medicinal interventions supported by activity observed in randomized placebo-controlled phase III clinical trials (TA-CD for cocaine and RV144 for HIV) are for a CTB-cocaine conjugate immunogen and a V2 loop-based epitope-focused HIV vaccine immunogen. While these are the only truly clinical-evidence-based biologics that can be inferred at the present time, technologies in both cocaine and HIV immunotherapies have continued to advance in the years since these trials were commenced.

The advances in the area of cocaine immunogens are reviewed in a previous chapter. Briefly, newer generations of cocaine hapten moieties with improved immunogenic and cross-reactive properties have been produced and studied. Similarly, alternative delivery approaches, including viral vector-based delivery of cocaine conjugates, cocaine-hydrolyzing enzymes, and anti-cocaine monoclonal antibodies, have been reported.

Similarly, in the HIV vaccine arena, a large number of broadly neutralizing monoclonal antibodies (bNAbs) have been isolated from HIV-positive individuals and characterized in detail in the past few years. Some of these antibodies neutralize more than 80 % of circulating viruses and antibodies targeting CD4 neutralize close to 100 % of viruses *in vitro* (Pace et al. 2013), so theoretically, if they can be elicited by vaccination, these monoclonal antibodies, or their polyclonal analogs, could be very promising. Unfortunately, only one functional (e.g., neutralizing) polyclonal antibody response in a mammal has ever been rationally elicited that specifically recapitulated the breadth and specific activity of an individual monoclonal anti-HIV neutralizing antibody (Cardozo et al. 2014), and this was an anti-V3 loop antibody targeting a very different epitope chemical entity than those targeted by the bNAbs.

Protection in RV144 did not correlate with antibody-mediated neutralization activity, so it is unlikely that any neutralizing antibody with significant breadth of specificity was responsible for the only known HIV protective effect observed in human subjects. Nevertheless, as an exploratory approach, much work has been reported on strategies to elicit such antibodies, including, as with the cocaine area, the use of viral vectors as immunogens, and to directly express the bNAbs in a sustained fashion rather than elicit them. Indeed, this latter approach has recently led to its logical conclusion that immunogenic viral epitopes need not be targeted at all: a CD4 mimic that neutralizes 100 % of viral isolates can instead be expressed in a sustained fashion using an adenovirus-associated virus vector (Gardner et al. 2015).

DNA vaccine approaches also offer a similar opportunity to viral vector approaches, as many aspects are conceptually parallel (Mossman et al. 1999; Haigwood et al. 1999). All viral vector/DNA approaches, although promising in their exploration beyond the constraints of natural antibody elicitation via immunization, in turn, however, suffer from the poor historical track record of such gene therapy-related approaches in human subjects, including the STEP study itself that previously failed unexpectedly (Kim et al. 2010).

6.4.4 Molecular Interactions in Common to HIV and Cocaine Use

Understanding common molecular targets affected by HIV infection and cocaine use may provide some further insight into the theoretical impact of a combination vaccine in specific US populations. Generally, HIV-1 cell entry is mediated by gp120 interaction with its receptor CD4 and its coreceptors CCR5 and CXCR4. Cocaine acts on cells via its effect on the dopamine transporter and σ-1receptor. *In vivo* evaluation of the interaction between HIV and cocaine was performed in huPBL-SCID mouse. This mouse model was initially developed by Mosier et al. to assess HIV pathogenesis *in vivo*. This is a hybrid human-mouse model in which human PBL are implanted into the peritoneal cavity of SCID mice (Mosier et al. 1991). Roth et al. have demonstrated that concurrent administration of cocaine and HIV results in a high rate of HIV-infected huPBL (Roth et al. 2002). This group also showed that *in vitro* exposure of PBL to cocaine increased expression of chemokine receptors CCR5 and CXCR4. Expression of CCR5 was also shown to increase *in vivo* preceding the boost in viral infection. Furthermore, a selective σ-1 antagonist, BD1047, blocked the effects of cocaine on HIV replication in the huPBL-SCID mouse, suggesting the role of σ-1 receptors in the modulation of the expression of HIV coreceptors (Roth et al. 2005).

In fact, σ-1R was shown to be one of cocaine's main molecular targets (Matsumoto et al. 2002). σ-1R is a receptor chaperone at the mitochondrion-associated endoplasmic reticulum membrane that plays an important role in the ER-mitochondrial Ca^{2+} signaling and in cell survival (Hayashi and Su 2007). Cocaine upregulates the expression of σ-1R (Liu et al. 2005) and induces its translocation to the plasma membrane (Yao et al. 2010) and cocaine is able to bind σ-1R (Sharkey et al. 1988). In microglia, binding of cocaine to the translocated σ-1R leads to the activation of signaling cascade resulting in the induction of MCP-1 expression. MCP-1 in turn results in enhanced transmigration of monocytes leading to neuroinflammation (Yao et al. 2010). This could be one of the molecular mechanisms that explain how cocaine may increase susceptibility of HIV-infected individuals to HIV-1-associated neurocognitive disorder (HAND).

Additionally, this effect of cocaine can be mediated through its direct action on brain microvasculature. This is achieved via cocaine induction of the expression of cytokines (Yao et al. 2010), adhesion molecules (Yao et al. 2011a), and PDGF (Yao et al. 2011b). Thus, cocaine increases molecular permeability of the blood-brain barrier and HIV viral invasion by the induction of cytokines IL-8, interferon-inducible protein-10, MIP-1alpha, MCP-1, and TNF-alpha (Zhang et al. 1998). Cocaine was also shown to promote the induction of the adhesion molecules ALCAM, VCAM, ICAM, and E-selectin in both *in vitro* and *in vivo* experiments, and at least in case of ALCAM, it was mediated by the activation of σ-1R (Yao et al. 2011a; Gan et al. 1999). Cocaine induces PDGF-BB in human brain microvascular endothelial cells through the binding to σ receptor and activation of downstream signaling pathways (Yao et al. 2011b). The effect of cocaine on permeability of the blood-brain barrier is abrogated *in vivo* by PDGF-BB neutralizing antibody (Yao et al. 2011b).

Another important player in cocaine/HIV-1 interaction is the NMDA receptor. HIV-1 gp120 and Tat induce NMDAR-dependent neuronal death (Pattarini et al. 1998; Haughey et al. 2001). The mechanism of this phenomenon is not well understood. HIV infection results in release of excess glutamate by glia resulting in excitotoxicity via activation of glutamate receptors. NMDA receptor antagonists prevent gp120 neurotoxicity *in vitro* (Lipton et al. 1991). It was shown that gp120 directly binds to mouse NMDAR heterodimer subunits NR1/NR2A and NR1/NR2B (Xin et al. 1999) and that Tat binds to NR1/NR2A (Li et al. 2008). Moreover, gp120, through release of IL-1, and Tat, by recruitment of active src, increase tyrosine phosphorylation of NMDARs, which result in overactivation of the receptors by increasing delivery and potentiation of NMDAR currents (Haughey et al. 2001; Viviani et al. 2006; King et al. 2010). In addition, gp 120-activated glia release cytokines and other mediators, which may inhibit the reuptake of glutamate and induce its release (Barbour et al. 1989; Vesce et al. 1997). As such, NMDAR mediates damaging effects of HIV in the brain. Similarly, NMDAR is a target of cocaine.

Cocaine has complex influence on NMDARs in brain regions involved in reward circuitry (Ortinski 2014). Cocaine alters subunit composition of NMDARs and their synaptic distribution. NMDA receptor function can also be affected by D1 dopamine receptors. Interestingly, it was shown that σ-1R forms heteromers with D1 dopamine receptor (Navarro et al. 2010). As the effect of cocaine is mediated by the dopamine system, this interaction may explain cocaine action on NMDARs. Therefore, NMDAR is a common target of HIV-1 and cocaine and, thus, it could be the intersection point where cocaine and HIV-1 may exert their reciprocal effect on HIV progression and cocaine addiction.

Taken together, cocaine promotes HIV-1 infection and replication by upregulating HIV-1 coreceptors and inducing cytokine production. Via its effect on brain microvasculature and NMDAR, cocaine enhances neurotoxicity, therefore exacerbating HAND. In light of the described molecular interactions between HIV-1 and cocaine, the impact of a combined cocaine-HIV vaccine or immunotherapies on cocaine- and HIV-associated phenotypes has the promise of synergy at the molecular level.

6.4.5 Cocaine, High-Risk Sexual Behavior, and HIV

Cocaine produces short-lived, intense euphoric effects in human subjects along with an immediate profound craving for more (Breiter et al. 1997). Human neuroimaging and rodent neurobehavioral studies point to a shared neural substrate for sexual arousal and orgasm and cocaine's motivating and rewarding effects (Carboni et al. 1989; Childress et al. 2008; Frascella et al. 2010; Meisel et al. 1993; Pfaus et al.

1990). Further, the same molecular and morphological changes in brain reward circuitry that mediate transition from psychostimulant use to addiction are induced by certain patterns of “excessive” sexual behavior (Hedges et al. 2010; Meisel and Mullins 2006; Nestler 2008). It is therefore unsurprising that behavioral cross-sensitization between repeated psychostimulant exposure and sexual behavior has been demonstrated in animal models (Levens and Akins 2004; Fiorino and Phillips 1999; Bradley and Meisel 2001).

Although the determinants of human behavior are more complex than those isolated in controlled animal studies, the basic science findings suggest a neurobiological basis for the relationship between cocaine abuse and sexual promiscuity. It is not uncommon for individuals to use cocaine strategically to facilitate sexual activity (Volkow et al. 2007), and stimulant-induced increase in sexual desire has been identified as a potential contributing factor to HIV transmission (Volkow et al. 2007). In general, cocaine use is strongly associated with high-risk sexual behavior (Kopetz et al. 2014; Lejuez et al. 2005), and crack cocaine appears to pose a unique risk. Increasing rates of HIV infection are consistently associated with crack use (Marx et al. 1991) and individuals who continue to use crack after HIV diagnosis report a high prevalence of unprotected sex, multiple partners, and exchanging sex for drugs or money (Harzke et al. 2009). An exacerbating factor in this destructive spiral is prefrontal cortical dysfunction in cocaine users, leading to a loss of self-control (Garavan et al. 2008). Moreover, recent evidence suggests that prefrontal function may be further degraded by interactive neurotoxic effects of cocaine and HIV (Meyer et al. 2014).

6.4.6 The Impact of a Combination Medicinal Intervention for Cocaine and HIV

With a molecular picture of a combination cocaine-HIV vaccine, HIV prevention and treatment, and the pathophysiological overlap between HIV and cocaine in mind, we now turn our attention to the impact of these molecular and/or pharmacologic elements on cocaine use and HIV infection in real populations. Theoretically, in populations affected by both HIV and cocaine use, a combination cocaine-HIV vaccine could synergize to profoundly lower HIV acquisition rates, even if each component of the vaccine were only partly effective as the current prototypes. The reality of HIV transmission networks might predict a very different outcome, however.

One target population might be amenable to a combination cocaine and HIV vaccine while another is more suitable for cocaine and HIV immunotherapies. A true combination vaccine would only physiologically make sense for administration to HIV-negative individuals who have never used cocaine. For HIV-positive individuals who have never used cocaine, the physiological parallel to a combination vaccine at this point in time, if any, would be cocaine vaccine administration in combination with proven HIV prevention measures.

For HIV-negative, cocaine users, the parallel would be HIV vaccine administration and/or proven HIV prevention measures, cocaine use interventions, and, possibly, cocaine immunotherapies. For HIV-positive, cocaine users, HIV treatment in combination with cocaine use treatment may include either or both cocaine and HIV immunotherapies. These different modes of prevention and treatment matched to the status of the individuals have divergent indications at both the population and individual levels (prevention in some cases and treatment in others). This is an additional complexity in considering the medicinal impact of a combined cocaine and HIV vaccine on the complex landscape of cocaine use and HIV infection in the United States.

6.5 Networks

Networks of cocaine use and networks of individuals at high risk for HIV are both diverse and poorly understood, so the overlap between them in specific populations is exceptionally complex (Friedman et al. 2009). In addition, the presence of comorbidities complicates the expected impact of a combination cocaine-HIV vaccine or matched immunotherapies, e.g., a cocaine user may simply switch to another drug. Finally, the various US populations at risk for or experiencing significant cocaine use, at various risks for HIV infection, or at various risks/incidences of both are highly diverse, ranging from young to middle-aged African-American women in rural North Carolina to white suburban teenagers in affluent communities to concentrated, ethnically diverse urban individuals using "speedballs" to many other geographically, socially, or economically stratified groups.

Some minority groups may be particularly positioned at the intersection of cocaine use and HIV/AIDS: African Americans account for the majority of individuals in the United States who use crack cocaine, and HIV is spreading faster among African Americans as compared to other US populations. Although this may be primarily due to the epidemic among African-American men who have sex with men rather than being directly tied to cocaine use, some studies are clearly suggestive of a general connection between cocaine use and HIV in this population (Harzke et al. 2009; Fothergill et al. 2009). In each and every one of these groups, the dynamics of cocaine use, HIV infection, and comorbidities may be dramatically different. Nevertheless, for illustrative purposes, we explore here a systematic way of thinking about the predicted impact of a combination cocaine-HIV vaccine or immunotherapy on certain well-known US populations.

6.5.1 *Comorbidities*

A major confounding factor in theorizing multivalent medicinal interventions such as a combined cocaine and HIV vaccine, or vaccine/prevention/treatment combinations, is the presence of comorbidities with both afflictions. Generally, people who live in disadvantaged neighborhoods, people with mental illnesses, and people with a history of trauma, persecution, or abuse, including individuals with less common sexual orientations, exhibit greater rates of substance abuse (Boardman et al. 2001; Lipton and Johnson 1998). How does the presence of concurrent alcohol or heroin use, for example, alter the picture? Many cocaine users are frequent users of alcohol, heroin, nicotine, and/or other drugs. Similarly, the frequency of mental disorders such as bipolar disorder and schizophrenia is higher in habitual drug users. The effects of concurrent cocaine and alcohol use appear to be additive (Pennings et al. 2002), so it is possible that they are relatively independent afflictions biologically within the same individual, even if their triggers are inextricable within the individual's social environment. Notably, medications exist for many of the comorbidities, such as HIV infection and alcohol, nicotine, and mental disorders, while none exists for cocaine.

6.5.2 Predicting Individual Behavior in Response to Combined Cocaine-HIV Intervention

Despite the complexity of the situation, some individual responses to a cocaine vaccine or immunotherapy or an HIV vaccine or immunotherapy can be predicted based on first principles. In the general population characterized by people who do not habitually use illegal (cocaine, heroin, etc.) or legal drugs (alcohol, cigarettes, marijuana) and who do not have prominent HIV risk factors (frequent unprotected sex with multiple partners, etc.), a combination cocaine-HIV vaccine could be expected to synergize to reduce HIV spread, as every HIV exposure would have a lower probability of HIV acquisition and the blunted effect of cocaine use would be expected to lead to fewer risky behaviors (Fig. 6.6). However, increased risky behavior due to confidence in the HIV vaccine and the use of other stimulants in place of cocaine could lead to increases in other public health problems.

In individuals who are already cocaine users or part of HIV transmission networks, the situation may be very different. First, let us consider the response to an *ideal* cocaine vaccine or immunotherapy. By ideal, we posit that the anti-cocaine antibodies introduced by the intervention completely or almost completely blunt the euphoric effect of cocaine upon administration. In response to this intervention, a cocaine user can be expected to respond in one of four ways that affects the network, in addition to increasing dosage until they give up (Fig. 6.7):

- They may change their route of administration. This may mean, in some individuals, engaging in intravenous cocaine delivery (PWID) or smoking crack. Based on population observations, this change would be expected to immediately increase the risk of HIV acquisition in an HIV-negative individual.
- They may reduce cocaine use. This could be theorized to decrease their HIV risk.

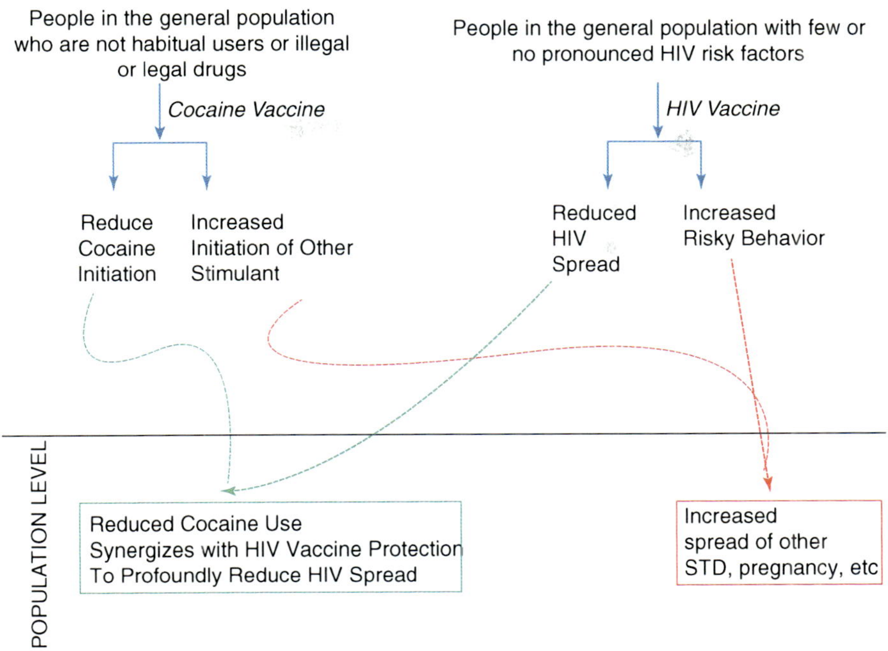

Fig. 6.6 Schematic of how individual cocaine and HIV vaccines may impact individuals and how these effects may combine into an overall effect in the general population

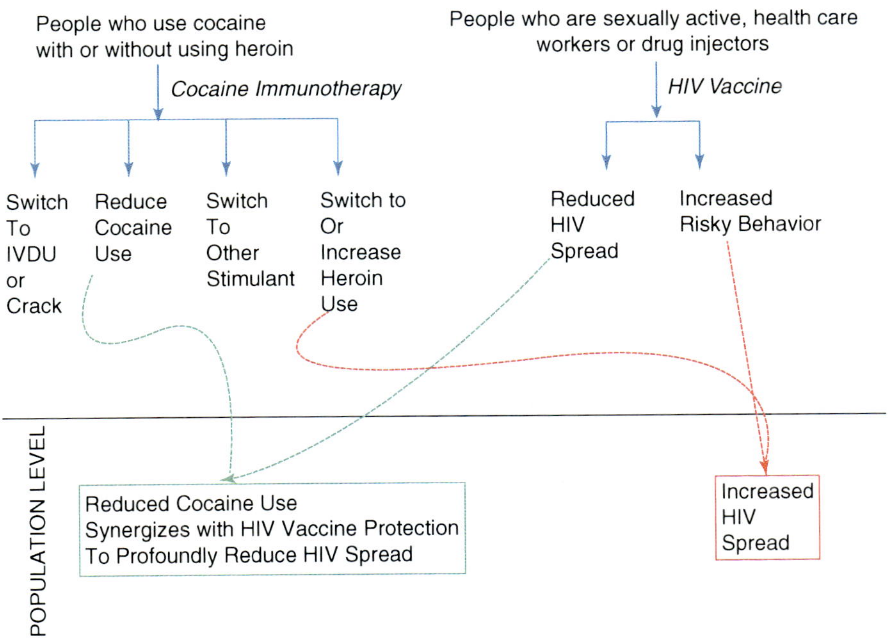

Fig. 6.7 Schematic of how individual cocaine immunotherapy and an HIV vaccine may impact individuals and how these effects may combine into an overall effect in certain populations

- They may switch to another stimulant drug. This has variable effects on their HIV risk, depending on the stimulant.
- They may switch to or increase their use of heroin. This immediately increases their HIV risk if they choose to inject. This may be more likely to occur for people who use both cocaine and heroin.

Now, let us consider independently the response to an *ideal* HIV vaccine. By ideal, we posit that the vaccine is 90–100 % effective in preventing HIV infection upon either parenteral or mucosal exposure. By definition, one response is a certainty: the probability of acquisition in the vaccinated population will dramatically be reduced. However, an indirect consequence in the longer term that was already observed with the success of HAART is that individuals will increase their risk behavior as their confidence in the vaccine grows.

Finally, we try to consider what the effect would be in certain populations if, as is closer to reality at present, either vaccine/immunotherapy is not ideal, e.g., only 30 % effective at blunting cocaine's effect or preventing HIV infection upon exposure and/or that the HIV vaccine is differentially efficacious for mucosal (sexual transmission) as opposed to parenteral (PWID) exposure. The following discussion is a theoretical exercise in physiological and behavioral modeling that assumes acceptance of vaccination for addiction and HIV. *This assumption is not intended to, in any way, diminish the very real bioethical, policy, and legal issues of implementing these vaccines.*

6.5.3 Illustrative Population #1: The General Population at Low Risk for Either HIV or Cocaine Initiation

The prototype cocaine and HIV vaccines are already proven to be extremely safe, with few if any detectable adverse effects. For this reason, it is not unimaginable (although unlikely at this time due to the bioethical, policy, and legal issues) that a combination cocaine-HIV vaccine could become part of the standard, universal childhood vaccination schedule in the United States eventually. If this were the case, the HIV risk and the risk for problematic cocaine use could potentially be significantly reduced in the general population over time. For example, 10 % of young adults self-report having tried cocaine (Administration, S. A. a. M. H. S. 2014). If a significant fraction of these individuals experience a blunted effect, it would not be surprising for overall cocaine use in the population to trend downward over time. Furthermore, if a significant proportion of these individuals are at increased risk for HIV acquisition because of their cocaine use, the overall HIV incidence in the population would be reduced as a result of the combination vaccine being widely administered. Nevertheless, the confidence in these vaccines may lead to increased risk behavior and actually increase HIV spread in certain populations. For this reason, the HIV vaccine component would need to be much more effective than current prototypes to entertain this scenario.

6.5.4 *Illustrative Population #2: Speedballers or Cocaine Injectors*

Speedballing is the simultaneous injection of both heroin and cocaine in the same syringe. It is a common practice among people who inject drugs (PWID). Thus, in the 2009 National HIV Behavioral Surveillance study of approximately 10,000 PWID recruited by respondent-driven sampling in 20 US metropolitan areas, the more commonly injected drugs during the prior 12 months were heroin (90 %), speedball (58 %), and cocaine or crack (49 %). Like other PWID, speedball injectors are at high risk for HIV and hepatitis C (Administration, S. A. a. M. H. S. 2014; Broz et al. 2014).

The conditions under which a combination cocaine-HIV vaccine would be administered to speedballers are unclear. Some might seek this as a way to decrease drug use and/or HIV risk. On the other hand, it is not unimaginable that, in some US jurisdictions, some PWID might be compelled to undergo such vaccination. In either case, both the HIV transmission and the behavioral outcomes of such vaccination are very hard to predict. It is possible that those who were vaccinated might increase their frequency of heroin injection and/or take up the use of other stimulants either by injection or by other routes. Such changes might increase or decrease the frequency of sharing of injection equipment and/or of unsafe sex. They might also lead vaccine recipients to change their injection or sexual networks (e.g., to interact with other amphetamine injectors), which might affect both their individual risk of becoming infected and the vulnerability of the community networks to the spread of HIV (and hepatitis C). Again, available data do not let us estimate whether these changes would increase or decrease individual or community risk-of-infection levels. Prudence would suggest that considerable research be done on these issues before such a vaccination program was put into effect for speedball users. As with all people who inject drugs, maintenance or expansion of other services, such as syringe exchange, drug use treatment of various (effective) modalities, and other harm reduction services, would be advisable. Since we do not know at present whether PrEP is effective at preventing parenteral HIV transmission, it is unclear whether it should also be used for this purpose, although its use to prevent sexual transmission in the networks of PWID seems reasonable.

It should also be noted that any HIV vaccine that is to be used for PWID populations needs to be effective for parenteral exposure. Any vaccine that is only effective for mucosal exposure, or which has been tested only in sexual transmission studies, might well find its protective effects overwhelmed by behavior disinhibition effects.

6.5.5 *Illustrative Population #3: Primarily Middle Class Nonmedical Users of Prescription Opioids*

The prevalence and incidence of nonmedical prescription opioid (PO) use have increased markedly in the United States during the past 20 years, particularly among young adults (SAMHSA 2014). Users of these drugs have included a larger proportion of suburban youth than is generally true of studies of people who inject drugs, although there is some evidence that they are at high risk of becoming injectors if they do not do so already (Cleland et al. 2011; Jones 2013; Lankenau et al. 2012; Mars et al. 2014; Rosenblum et al. 2007; Davis and Johnson 2008). These subjects also are likely to engage in high-risk sexual behavior (Argento et al. 2015; Benotsch et al. 2011).

Another important question is the extent to which they use cocaine, its form, and whether or not they inject it. To the extent that they do so, they are potentially appropriate targets for a theoretical combined vaccine against cocaine and HIV.

An ongoing study of mostly middle class young (18–29 year old) residents of New York City who have used opiates outside of prescribed contexts may be informative. The subjects were recruited through respondent-driven sampling (RDS), which is a form of sampling in which respondents are given coupons to recruit additional respondents who meet the criteria—in this case, they were instructed to give coupons to people they know and had seen in the prior 30 days who were 18–29 years old, who lived in New York, and who use prescription opioids in non-medical ways and/or who use heroin. Respondents were given remuneration for recruiting other participants in this way. Figure 6.8 provides a picture of the RDS recruitment chains together with other information discussed below. Of 164 participants, 66 % were men; 72 % white non-Hispanics, 8 % white Hispanics, and 11 % multiracial/ethnic; and 2 % each Black or African American and Asian. They were recruited in three New York boroughs, Manhattan (32 %), Staten Island (24 %), and Brooklyn (35 %), with 4 % each living in Bronx and Queens. Only 12 % report themselves as poor, with others reporting they are lower middle class (30 %), middle class (40 %), upper middle class (14 %), and affluent (4 %). 86 % have health insurance and 84 % have seen a doctor in the last year. Thus, they can be classed as a primarily middle class New York City sample. Two of the subjects are HIV infected. Both of these are current cocaine users. In addition, 45 (27 %) are infected with hepatitis C.

Among these participants, 96 % have used cocaine at least once in their lifetime (including 71 % who have used crack) and 67 % have used cocaine together with speedball. About half (48 %) have used cocaine on a "regular" basis (three times a week or more) for at least a month at some time in their lives; 52 % have injected drugs at least once; and 24 % have had at least 1 month of regular injected cocaine use. In the last 30 days, 19 % of the sample injected cocaine on more than 1 day. Figure 6.8a provides information about the recruitment chain in terms of which respondents reported using and injecting cocaine in the last 30 days. What is clear is that in many cases, young adults knew and recruited other young adults who differed from themselves in terms of whether they used cocaine and/or injected drugs of any kind. This suggests that their friendship groups pose many opportunities for cross-group injection or sexual transmission of HIV.

A number of them face significantly elevated social and behavioral sexual risks for HIV infection. They had a mean of 3.06 sexual partners in the last 90 days (men 3.44, women 2.34) with a range of 0–70 partners. As seen in Fig. 6.8b, 13 of the participants, including 8 current cocaine users, have taken part in a group sex event in the last 90 days.

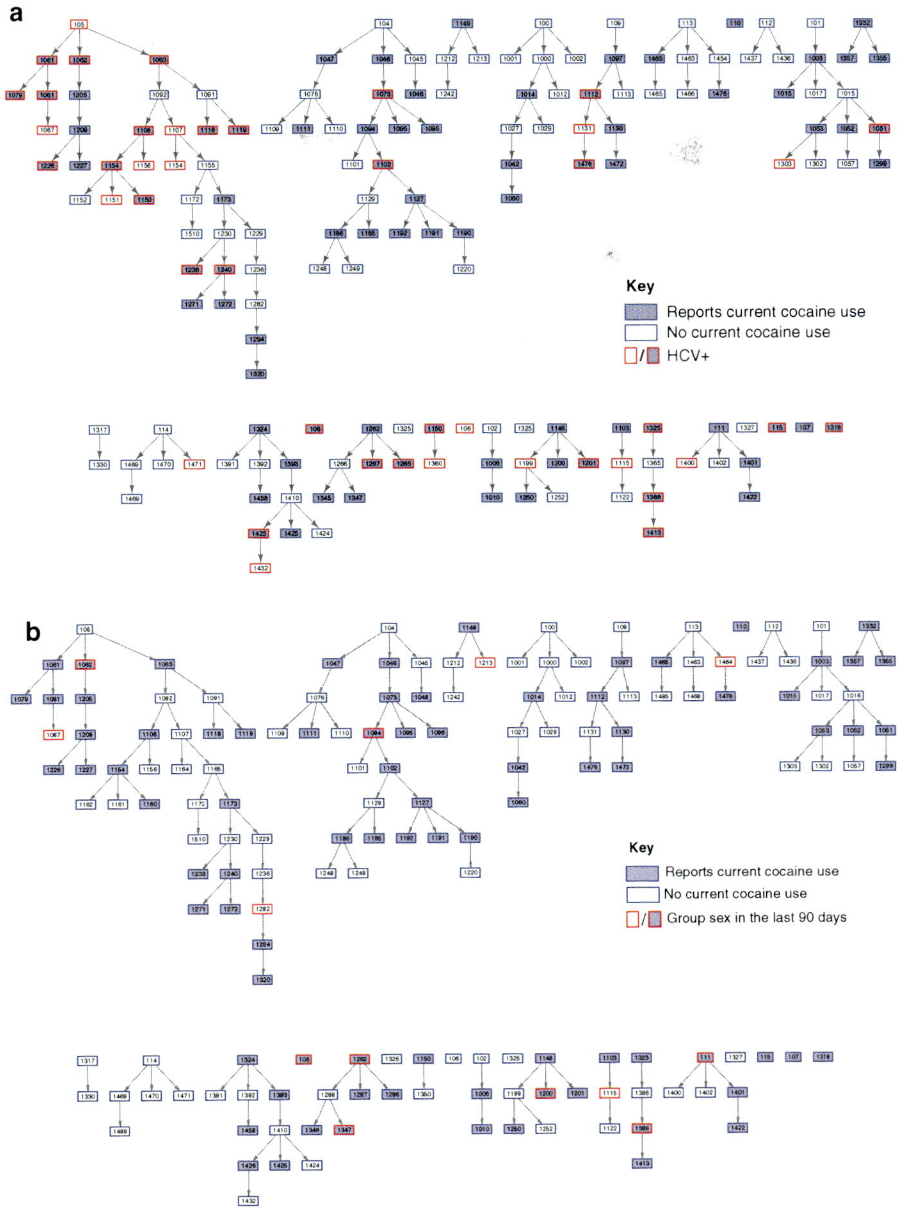

Fig. 6.8 Cocaine Use, HCV Infection (**a**) and Group Sex Participation (**b**) in Recruitment Chains

These youth face several current and future HIV risks. At the current time, those who do not inject drugs face primarily sexual risk. The presence of a nontrivial proportion of youth in the recruitment networks who report taking part in group sex, together with the likelihood that this behavior is underreported, suggests that their sexual networks may be highly interconnected—which means that HIV could spread rapidly through their networks (as does the presence of people who inject drugs in the recruitment networks). For these non-injecting youth, a mucosal HIV vaccine would be useful. Since many of them will begin to inject drugs within a period of a few years, however, an HIV vaccine that is also effective against parenteral exposure will clearly be much more valuable.

For those who do not currently use cocaine, a partially effective preventive cocaine vaccine is likely to reduce their risk of becoming problematic cocaine users in the future or of becoming cocaine injectors. This would prevent the problems that cocaine use can cause them and others in itself. It also can decrease the increased sexual risk of HIV exposure that many cocaine users face and, if they inject drugs, prevent them from the particularly high risks of infection that PWID who inject cocaine face in the United States.

6.6 Conclusions

Based on the existing prototypes, the prospects are good for the eventual availability of a combination cocaine and HIV vaccine or the matched concept of either of these vaccines implemented in combination with highly effective HIV prevention methods and cocaine immunotherapies. Putting bioethical, legal, and policy aspects aside for now, these types of interventions may have profound beneficial synergistic effects physiologically in individuals comorbid for HIV infection and cocaine use, based on the molecular overlap of these two conditions. Although a highly efficacious HIV vaccine would be incontrovertibly beneficial in the general population, predicting the impact of a combination HIV and cocaine vaccine in specific populations is more complex, especially if either vaccine is not ideally efficacious. The impact of a combination cocaine-HIV vaccine or immunotherapy may be synergistic and dramatically beneficial to certain existing populations in the United States and synergistic and detrimental or undetectable to other populations. Many intermediate or multiphasic outcomes in the short and long term are also likely. This uncertainty should be weighed against the benefits and deficiencies of existing HIV prevention measures should a combination cocaine and HIV vaccine become available. Meeting the challenge of better understanding cocaine use and HIV risk networks could be just as important for enhancing the utility or implementation strategy of a combination cocaine-HIV vaccine as meeting the molecular challenges of developing such a vaccine.

Acknowledgments P30 DA11041 (Center for Drug Use and HIV Research)

DP1 DA034989 (Preventing HIV Transmission by Recently Infected Drug Users)

R01 DA035146 (HIV, HCV, and STI Risk Associated with Nonmedical Use of Prescription Opioids)

DP1 DA036478 (Combined Cocaine and HIV Vaccine)

Bibliography

Abdul-Quader AS, et al. Effectiveness of structural-level needle/syringe programs to reduce HCV and HIV infection among people who inject drugs: a systematic review. AIDS Behav. 2013;17:2878–92. doi:10.1007/s10461-013-0593-y.

Argento E, Chettiar J, Nguyen P, Montaner J, Shannon K. Prevalence and correlates of nonmedical prescription opioid use among a cohort of sex workers in Vancouver, Canada. Int J Drug Policy. 2015;26:59–66. doi:10.1016/j.drugpo.2014.07.010.

Bagasra O, Forman LJ, Howeedy A, Whittle P. A potential vaccine for cocaine abuse prophylaxis. Immunopharmacology. 1992;23:173–9.

Barbour B, Szatkowski M, Ingledew N, Attwell D. Arachidonic acid induces a prolonged inhibition of glutamate uptake into glial cells. Nature. 1989;342:918–20. doi:10.1038/342918a0.

Barouch DH, et al. Vaccine protection against acquisition of neutralization-resistant SIV challenges in rhesus monkeys. Nature. 2012;482:89–93. doi:10.1038/nature10766.

Bart KJ, Orenstein WA, Hinman AR. The virtual elimination of rubella and mumps from the United States and the use of combined measles, mumps and rubella vaccines (MMR) to eliminate measles. Dev Biol Stand. 1986;65:45–52.

Benotsch EG, Koester S, Luckman D, Martin AM, Cejka A. Non-medical use of prescription drugs and sexual risk behavior in young adults. Addict Behav. 2011;36:152–5. doi:10.1016/j.addbeh.2010.08.027.

Boardman JD, Finch BK, Ellison CG, Williams DR, Jackson JS. Neighborhood disadvantage, stress, and drug use among adults. J Health Soc Behav. 2001;42:151–65.

Bradley KC, Meisel RL. Sexual behavior induction of c-Fos in the nucleus accumbens and amphetamine-stimulated locomotor activity are sensitized by previous sexual experience in female Syrian hamsters. J Neurosci. 2001;21:2123–30.

Breiter HC, et al. Acute effects of cocaine on human brain activity and emotion. Neuron. 1997;19:591–611.

Brimijoin S, Shen X, Orson F, Kosten T. Prospects, promise and problems on the road to effective vaccines and related therapies for substance abuse. Expert Rev Vaccines. 2013;12:323–32. doi:10.1586/erv.13.1.

Broz D, et al. HIV infection and risk, prevention, and testing behaviors among injecting drug users -- National HIV Behavioral Surveillance System, 20 U.S. cities, 2009. Morb Mortal Wkly Rep Surveill Summ. 2014;63:1–51.

Burton DR, et al. Public health. A sound rationale needed for phase III HIV-1 vaccine trials. Science. 2004;303:316. doi:10.1126/science.1094620.

Cai X, et al. Probing active cocaine vaccination performance through catalytic and noncatalytic hapten design. J Med Chem. 2013;56:3701–9. doi:10.1021/jm400228w.

Carboni E, Imperato A, Perezzani L, Di Chiara G. Amphetamine, cocaine, phencyclidine and nomifensine increase extracellular dopamine concentrations preferentially in the nucleus accumbens of freely moving rats. Neuroscience. 1989;28:653–61.

Cardozo T, et al. Vaccine focusing to cross-subtype HIV-1 gp120 variable loop epitopes. Vaccine. 2014. doi:10.1016/j.vaccine.2014.07.026.

Carroll ME, et al. Combined cocaine hydrolase gene transfer and anti-cocaine vaccine synergistically block cocaine-induced locomotion. PLoS One. 2012;7, e43536. doi:10.1371/journal.pone.0043536.

Childress AR, et al. Prelude to passion: limbic activation by "unseen" drug and sexual cues. PLoS One. 2008;3, e1506. doi:10.1371/journal.pone.0001506.

Cleland CM, Rosenblum A, Fong C, Maxwell C. Age differences in heroin and prescription opioid abuse among enrolees into opioid treatment programs. Subst Abuse Treat Prev Policy. 2011;6:11. doi:10.1186/1747-597X-6-11.

Cohen PJ. Immunization for prevention and treatment of cocaine abuse: legal and ethical implications. Drug Alcohol Depend. 1997;48:167–74.

Cohen P. No more kicks: there are treatments on the way that promise to destroy the allure of addictive drugs for good. Problem solved? New Sci. 2000;166:22–6.

Correia BE, et al. Proof of principle for epitope-focused vaccine design. Nature. 2014;507:201–6. doi:10.1038/nature12966.

Dagan R, Poolman JT, Zepp F. Combination vaccines containing DTPa-Hib: impact of IPV and coadministration of CRM197 conjugates. Expert Rev Vaccines. 2008;7:97–115. doi:10.1586/14760584.7.1.97.

Davis WR, Johnson BD. Prescription opioid use, misuse, and diversion among street drug users in New York City. Drug Alcohol Depend. 2008;92:267–76. doi:10.1016/j.drugalcdep.2007.08.008.

Esposito S, et al. Hexavalent vaccines for immunization in paediatric age. Clin Microbiol Infect. 2014;20 Suppl 5:76–85. doi:10.1111/1469-0691.12444.

Excler JL, Ake J, Robb ML, Kim JH, Plotkin SA. Nonneutralizing functional antibodies: a new 'old' paradigm for HIV vaccines. Clin Vaccine Immunol. 2014. doi:10.1128/CVI.00230-14.

Faden H, Duffy L, Sun M, Shuff C. Long-term immunity to poliovirus in children immunized with live attenuated and enhanced-potency inactivated trivalent poliovirus vaccines. J Infect Dis. 1993;168:452–4.

Fiorino DF, Phillips AG. Facilitation of sexual behavior and enhanced dopamine efflux in the nucleus accumbens of male rats after D-amphetamine-induced behavioral sensitization. J Neurosci. 1999;19:456–63.

Fothergill KE, Ensminger ME, Green KM, Robertson JA, Juon HS. Pathways to adult marijuana and cocaine use: a prospective study of African Americans from age 6 to 42. J Health Soc Behav. 2009;50:65–81.

Fox BS. Development of a therapeutic vaccine for the treatment of cocaine addiction. Drug Alcohol Depend. 1997;48:153–8.

Frascella J, Potenza MN, Brown LL, Childress AR. Shared brain vulnerabilities open the way for nonsubstance addictions: carving addiction at a new joint? Ann N Y Acad Sci. 2010;1187: 294–315. doi:10.1111/j.1749-6632.2009.05420.x.

Friedman SR, Sterk C, Sufian M, Des Jarlais DC. Will bleach decontaminate needles during cocaine binges in shooting galleries? JAMA. 1989;262:1467.

Friedman SR, Cooper HL, Osborne AH. Structural and social contexts of HIV risk Among African Americans. Am J Public Health. 2009;99:1002–8. doi:10.2105/AJPH.2008.140327.

Fritzell B, Plotkin S. Efficacy and safety of a Haemophilus influenzae type b capsular polysaccharide-tetanus protein conjugate vaccine. J Pediatr. 1992;121:355–62.

Gan X, et al. Cocaine enhances brain endothelial adhesion molecules and leukocyte migration. Clin Immunol. 1999;91:68–76. doi:10.1006/clim.1998.4683.

Gao Y, et al. Effects of anti-cocaine vaccine and viral gene transfer of cocaine hydrolase in mice on cocaine toxicity including motor strength and liver damage. Chem Biol Interact. 2013;203:208–11. doi:10.1016/j.cbi.2012.08.006.

Garavan H, Kaufman JN, Hester R. Acute effects of cocaine on the neurobiology of cognitive control. Philos Trans R Soc Lond B Biol Sci. 2008;363:3267–76. doi:10.1098/rstb.2008.0106.

Gardner MR, et al. AAV-expressed eCD4-Ig provides durable protection from multiple SHIV challenges. Nature. 2015;519:87–91. doi:10.1038/nature14264.

Haigwood NL, et al. Protection from pathogenic SIV challenge using multigenic DNA vaccines. Immunol Lett. 1999;66:183–8.

Hall W, Carter L. Ethical issues in using a cocaine vaccine to treat and prevent cocaine abuse and dependence. J Med Ethics. 2004;30:337–40.

Hall W, Gartner C. Ethical and policy issues in using vaccines to treat and prevent cocaine and nicotine dependence. Curr Opin Psychiatry. 2011;24:191–6. doi:10.1097/YCO.0b013e328345922b.

Haney M, Gunderson EW, Jiang H, Collins ED, Foltin RW. Cocaine-specific antibodies blunt the subjective effects of smoked cocaine in humans. Biol Psychiatry. 2010;67:59–65. doi:10.1016/j.biopsych.2009.08.031.

Harzke AJ, Williams ML, Bowen AM. Binge use of crack cocaine and sexual risk behaviors among African-American, HIV-positive users. AIDS Behav. 2009;13:1106–18. doi:10.1007/s10461-008-9450-9.

Haughey NJ, Nath A, Mattson MP, Slevin JT, Geiger JD. HIV-1 Tat through phosphorylation of NMDA receptors potentiates glutamate excitotoxicity. J Neurochem. 2001;78:457–67.

Hayashi T, Su TP. Sigma-1 receptor chaperones at the ER-mitochondrion interface regulate Ca(2+) signaling and cell survival. Cell. 2007;131:596–610. doi:10.1016/j.cell.2007.08.036.

Haynes BF, et al. Immune-correlates analysis of an HIV-1 vaccine efficacy trial. N Engl J Med. 2012;366:1275–86. doi:10.1056/NEJMoa1113425.

Hedges VL, Staffend NA, Meisel RL. Neural mechanisms of reproduction in females as a predisposing factor for drug addiction. Front Neuroendocrinol. 2010;31:217–31. doi:10.1016/j.yfrne.2010.02.003.

Jones CM. Heroin use and heroin use risk behaviors among nonmedical users of prescription opioid pain relievers – United States, 2002–2004 and 2008–2010. Drug Alcohol Depend. 2013;132:95–100. doi:10.1016/j.drugalcdep.2013.01.007.

Katsnelson A. Ethical quagmire awaits vaccine for cocaine addiction. Nat Med. 2004;10:1007. doi:10.1038/nm1004-1007a.

Kim JH, Rerks-Ngarm S, Excler JL, Michael NL. HIV vaccines: lessons learned and the way forward. Curr Opin HIV AIDS. 2010;5:428–34. doi:10.1097/COH.0b013e32833d17ac.

King JE, Eugenin EA, Hazleton JE, Morgello S, Berman JW. Mechanisms of HIV-tat-induced phosphorylation of N-methyl-D-aspartate receptor subunit 2A in human primary neurons: implications for neuroAIDS pathogenesis. Am J Pathol. 2010;176:2819–30. doi:10.2353/ajpath.2010.090642.

Koob G, et al. Anti-cocaine vaccine based on coupling a cocaine analog to a disrupted adenovirus. CNS Neurol Disord Drug Targets. 2011;10:899–904.

Kopetz C, et al. Gender and social rejection as risk factors for engaging in risky sexual behavior among crack/cocaine users. Prev Sci. 2014;15:376–84. doi:10.1007/s11121-013-0406-6.

Kosten TR, Domingo CB. Can you vaccinate against substance abuse? Expert Opin Biol Ther. 2013;13:1093–7. doi:10.1517/14712598.2013.791278.

Kosten TR, Domingo CB, Hamon SC, Nielsen DA. DBH gene as predictor of response in a cocaine vaccine clinical trial. Neurosci Lett. 2013;541:29–33. doi:10.1016/j.neulet.2013.02.037.

Kosten TA, Shen XY, Kinsey BM, Kosten TR, Orson FM. Attenuation of cocaine-induced locomotor activity in male and female mice by active immunization. Am J Addict. 2014a;23:604–7. doi:10.1111/j.1521-0391.2014.12152.x.

Kosten TR, et al. Vaccine for cocaine dependence: a randomized double-blind placebo-controlled efficacy trial. Drug Alcohol Depend. 2014b;140:42–7. doi:10.1016/j.drugalcdep.2014.04.003.

Kosten T, Domingo C, Orson F, Kinsey B. Vaccines against stimulants: cocaine and MA. Br J Clin Pharmacol. 2014c;77:368–74. doi:10.1111/bcp.12115.

Lankenau SE, et al. Initiation into prescription opioid misuse amongst young injection drug users. Int J Drug Policy. 2012;23:37–44. doi:10.1016/j.drugpo.2011.05.014.

Lejuez CW, Bornovalova MA, Daughters SB, Curtin JJ. Differences in impulsivity and sexual risk behavior among inner-city crack/cocaine users and heroin users. Drug Alcohol Depend. 2005;77:169–75. doi:10.1016/j.drugalcdep.2004.08.013.

Levens N, Akins CK. Chronic cocaine pretreatment facilitates Pavlovian sexual conditioning in male Japanese quail. Pharmacol Biochem Behav. 2004;79:451–7. doi:10.1016/j.pbb.2004.08.021.

Li W, et al. NMDA receptor activation by HIV-Tat protein is clade dependent. J Neurosci. 2008;28:12190–8. doi:10.1523/JNEUROSCI.3019-08.2008.

Lipton DS, Johnson BD. Smack, crack, and score: two decades of NIDA-funded drugs and crime research at NDRI 1974–1994. Subst Use Misuse. 1998;33:1779–815.

Lipton SA, Sucher NJ, Kaiser PK, Dreyer EB. Synergistic effects of HIV coat protein and NMDA receptor-mediated neurotoxicity. Neuron. 1991;7:111–8.

Liu Y, Chen GD, Lerner MR, Brackett DJ, Matsumoto RR. Cocaine up-regulates Fra-2 and sigma-1 receptor gene and protein expression in brain regions involved in addiction and reward. J Pharmacol Exp Ther. 2005;314:770–9. doi:10.1124/jpet.105.084525.

Mars SG, Bourgois P, Karandinos G, Montero F, Ciccarone D. "Every 'never' I ever said came true": transitions from opioid pills to heroin injecting. Int J Drug Policy. 2014;25:257–66. doi:10.1016/j.drugpo.2013.10.004.

Martell BA, et al. Cocaine vaccine for the treatment of cocaine dependence in methadone-maintained patients: a randomized, double-blind, placebo-controlled efficacy trial. Arch Gen Psychiatry. 2009;66:1116–23. doi:10.1001/archgenpsychiatry.2009.128.

Marx R, Aral SO, Rolfs RT, Sterk CE, Kahn JG. Crack, sex, and STD. Sex Transm Dis. 1991;18:92–101.

Matsumoto RR, McCracken KA, Pouw B, Zhang Y, Bowen WD. Involvement of sigma receptors in the behavioral effects of cocaine: evidence from novel ligands and antisense oligodeoxynucleotides. Neuropharmacology. 2002;42:1043–55.

Meisel RL, Mullins AJ. Sexual experience in female rodents: cellular mechanisms and functional consequences. Brain Res. 2006;1126:56–65. doi:10.1016/j.brainres.2006.08.050.

Meisel RL, Camp DM, Robinson TE. A microdialysis study of ventral striatal dopamine during sexual behavior in female Syrian hamsters. Behav Brain Res. 1993;55:151–7.

Meyer VJ, et al. Crack cocaine use impairs anterior cingulate and prefrontal cortex function in women with HIV infection. J Neurovirol. 2014;20:352–61. doi:10.1007/s13365-014-0250-x.

Mosier DE, et al. Human immunodeficiency virus infection of human-PBL-SCID mice. Science. 1991;251:791–4.

Mossman SP, et al. Immunization against SIVmne in macaques using multigenic DNA vaccines. J Med Primatol. 1999;28:206–13.

Nadis S. Drugs institute gives grant for cocaine vaccine. Nature. 1996;382:568. doi:10.1038/382568b0.

Navarro G, et al. Direct involvement of sigma-1 receptors in the dopamine D1 receptor-mediated effects of cocaine. Proc Natl Acad Sci U S A. 2010;107:18676–81. doi:10.1073/pnas.1008911107.

Nestler EJ. Review. Transcriptional mechanisms of addiction: role of DeltaFosB. Philos Trans R Soc Lond B Biol Sci. 2008;363:3245–55. doi:10.1098/rstb.2008.0067.

Noronha AS, Markowitz LE, Dunne EF. Systematic review of human papillomavirus vaccine coadministration. Vaccine. 2014;32:2670–4. doi:10.1016/j.vaccine.2013.12.037.

Orson FM, et al. Spontaneous development of IgM anti-cocaine antibodies in habitual cocaine users: effect on IgG antibody responses to a cocaine cholera toxin B conjugate vaccine. Am J Addict. 2013;22:169–74. doi:10.1111/j.1521-0391.2013.00314.x.

Ortinski PI. Cocaine-induced changes in NMDA receptor signaling. Mol Neurobiol. 2014;50: 494–506. doi:10.1007/s12035-014-8636-6.

Pace CS, et al. Bispecific antibodies directed to CD4 domain 2 and HIV envelope exhibit exceptional breadth and picomolar potency against HIV-1. Proc Natl Acad Sci U S A. 2013;110:13540–5. doi:10.1073/pnas.1304985110.

Papaevangelou G. Current combined vaccines with hepatitis B. Vaccine. 1998;16(Suppl):S69–72.

Pattarini R, Pittaluga A, Raiteri M. The human immunodeficiency virus-1 envelope protein gp120 binds through its V3 sequence to the glycine site of N-methyl-D-aspartate receptors mediating noradrenaline release in the hippocampus. Neuroscience. 1998;87:147–57.

Pennings EJ, Leccese AP, Wolff FA. Effects of concurrent use of alcohol and cocaine. Addiction. 2002;97:773–83.

Pfaus JG, et al. Sexual behavior enhances central dopamine transmission in the male rat. Brain Res. 1990;530:345–8.

Rerks-Ngarm S, et al. Vaccination with ALVAC and AIDSVAX to prevent HIV-1 infection in Thailand. N Engl J Med. 2009;361:2209–20. doi:10.1056/NEJMoa0908492.

Rolland M, et al. Increased HIV-1 vaccine efficacy against viruses with genetic signatures in Env V2. Nature. 2012;490:417–20. doi:10.1038/nature11519.

Rosenberg JB, et al. AAVrh.10-mediated expression of an anti-cocaine antibody mediates persistent passive immunization that suppresses cocaine-induced behavior. Hum Gene Ther. 2012;23:451–9. doi:10.1089/hum.2011.178.

Rosenblum A, et al. Prescription opioid abuse among enrollees into methadone maintenance treatment. Drug Alcohol Depend. 2007;90:64–71. doi:10.1016/j.drugalcdep.2007.02.012.

Roth MD, et al. Cocaine enhances human immunodeficiency virus replication in a model of severe combined immunodeficient mice implanted with human peripheral blood leukocytes. J Infect Dis. 2002;185:701–5. doi:10.1086/339012.

Roth MD, Whittaker KM, Choi R, Tashkin DP, Baldwin GC. Cocaine and sigma-1 receptors modulate HIV infection, chemokine receptors, and the HPA axis in the huPBL-SCID model. J Leukoc Biol. 2005;78:1198–203. doi:10.1189/jlb.0405219.

SAMHSA (Substance Abuse and Mental Health Services Administration), *Results from the 2013 National Survey on Drug Use and Health: Summary of National Findings*, NSDUH Series

H-48, HHS Publication No. (SMA) 14-4863. Rockville, MD: Substance Abuse and Mental Health Services Administration, 2014.

Sharkey J, Glen KA, Wolfe S, Kuhar MJ. Cocaine binding at sigma receptors. Eur J Pharmacol. 1988;149:171–4.

Shen XY, Orson FM, Kosten TR. Vaccines against drug abuse. Clin Pharmacol Ther. 2012;91: 60–70. doi:10.1038/clpt.2011.281.

Siegrist CA. Vaccine immunology. Plotkin SA, Orenstein SA, Offit PA (eds)., Vaccines (6th ed.), Philapelphia: Elsevier Saunders; 2013. p. 14–32.

Stitzer ML, Polk T, Bowles S, Kosten T. Drug users' adherence to a 6-month vaccination protocol: effects of motivational incentives. Drug Alcohol Depend. 2010;107:76–9. doi:10.1016/j.drugalcdep.2009.09.006.

Tobian AA, Kacker S, Quinn TC. Male circumcision: a globally relevant but under-utilized method for the prevention of HIV and other sexually transmitted infections. Annu Rev Med. 2014;65:293–306. doi:10.1146/annurev-med-092412-090539.

Tobin GJ, et al. Deceptive imprinting and immune refocusing in vaccine design. Vaccine. 2008;26:6189–99. doi:10.1016/j.vaccine.2008.09.080.

Vesce S, Bezzi P, Rossi D, Meldolesi J, Volterra A. HIV-1 gp120 glycoprotein affects the astrocyte control of extracellular glutamate by both inhibiting the uptake and stimulating the release of the amino acid. FEBS Lett. 1997;411:107–9.

Viviani B, et al. Interleukin-1 beta released by gp120 drives neural death through tyrosine phosphorylation and trafficking of NMDA receptors. J Biol Chem. 2006;281:30212–22. doi:10.1074/jbc.M602156200.

Volkow ND, et al. Stimulant-induced enhanced sexual desire as a potential contributing factor in HIV transmission. Am J Psychiatry. 2007;164:157–60. doi:10.1176/appi.ajp.164.1.157.

Wee S, et al. Novel cocaine vaccine linked to a disrupted adenovirus gene transfer vector blocks cocaine psychostimulant and reinforcing effects. Neuropsychopharmacology. 2012;37: 1083–91. doi:10.1038/npp.2011.200.

WHO Guidelines Approved by the Guidelines Review Committee. Consolidated guidelines on HIV prevention, diagnosis, treatment and care for key populations. Geneva: World Health Organization; 2014.

Wilton J, Senn H, Sharma M, Tan DH. Pre-exposure prophylaxis for sexually-acquired HIV risk management: a review. HIV/AIDS. 2015;7:125–36. doi:10.2147/HIV.S50025.

Wise RA, Ranaldi R. Cocaine vaccines revisited. Nat Med. 1996;2:1073–4.

Xin KQ, et al. Evidence of HIV type 1 glycoprotein 120 binding to recombinant N-methyl-D-aspartate receptor subunits expressed in a baculovirus system. AIDS Res Hum Retroviruses. 1999;15:1461–7. doi:10.1089/088922299309973.

Yao H, et al. Molecular mechanisms involving sigma receptor-mediated induction of MCP-1: implication for increased monocyte transmigration. Blood. 2010;115:4951–62. doi:10.1182/blood-2010-01-266221.

Yao H, et al. Cocaine hijacks sigma1 receptor to initiate induction of activated leukocyte cell adhesion molecule: implication for increased monocyte adhesion and migration in the CNS. J Neurosci. 2011a;31:5942–55. doi:10.1523/JNEUROSCI.5618-10.2011.

Yao H, Duan M, Buch S. Cocaine-mediated induction of platelet-derived growth factor: implication for increased vascular permeability. Blood. 2011b;117:2538–47. doi:10.1182/blood-2010-10-313593.

Young MJ, Sisti DA, Rimon-Greenspan H, Schwartz JL, Caplan AL. Immune to addiction: the ethical dimensions of vaccines against substance abuse. Nat Immunol. 2012;13:521–4. doi:10.1038/ni.2321.

Zhang L, et al. Cocaine opens the blood–brain barrier to HIV-1 invasion. J Neurovirol. 1998;4: 619–26.

Zolla-Pazner S, Cardozo T. Structure-function relationships of HIV-1 envelope sequence-variable regions refocus vaccine design. Nat Rev Immunol. 2010;10:527–35. doi:10.1038/nri2801.

Zolla-Pazner S, et al. Vaccine-induced IgG antibodies to V1V2 regions of multiple HIV-1 subtypes correlate with decreased risk of HIV-1 infection. PLoS One. 2014;9, e87572. doi:10.1371/journal.pone.0087572.

Part II
Monoclonal Antibodies

Chapter 7
Monoclonal Antibodies

S. Michael Owens

7.1 Introduction

The discovery of a hybridoma technology to generate monoclonal antibodies from immunized mice was first reported by George Köhler and César Milstein in 1975. To make this discovery, they developed a lymphocyte fusion technique that allowed selection of monoclonal antibodies of refined specificity and affinity. They received a Noble Prize in Physiology or Medicine in 1984 for this breakthrough innovation.

The use of monoclonal antibodies as drugs has advanced significantly over the last three decades particularly in the treatment of cancer and autoimmune diseases. The precise and reproducible specificity of these antibodies against disease targets allows them to act as high-affinity antagonists to neutralize or block molecular events leading to the attenuation or prevention of disease processes.

The first generation of monoclonal antibodies was derived from mouse B-cell hybridomas, but the antigenicity of these foreign proteins prevented their direct use as medication for treating human disease. The next significant step toward the safe use of monoclonal antibodies for treating human disease came with the development of a process for chimerization of the antibodies to reduce antigenicity. Replacing the heavy- and light-chain immunoglobulin constant domains of the mouse antibodies with the corresponding human amino sequences generated these so-called "chimeric" antibodies. This reduced the mouse protein content to about 34 % of the sequence, without significant changes in the antibody-binding specificity. Replacing the constant domains with human sequences also allowed improved effectiveness of activation of effector cell functions (e.g., macrophages and T cells) that are important for treating some types of cancers.

S.M. Owens
Department of Pharmacology and Toxicology, College of Medicine,
University of Arkansas for Medical Sciences, Little Rock, AR, 72205, USA
e-mail: mowens@uams.edu

I.D. Montoya (ed.), *Biologics to Treat Substance Use Disorders: Vaccines, Monoclonal Antibodies, and Enzymes*, DOI 10.1007/978-3-319-23150-1_7

In the next breakthrough, the antigen binding site framework V regions were replaced with human sequences. This generated "humanized" monoclonal antibodies. After this molecular change, only the original mouse complementary determining region sequences remained. This meant only about 5–10 % of the total humanized sequence of the new immunoglobulin was from the mouse. The third clinically important type of monoclonal antibody is fully human in their protein sequence. These proteins are generated through screening of antibody display libraries derived from human immune cells or by screening antibody libraries using transgenic mice that are engineered to produce human antibodies. Chimeric, humanized and fully human antibodies are all potentially antigenic when used in humans, but chimeric followed by humanized antibodies are the most antigenic.

The first report of the treatment of adverse effect from a drug of abuse using a monoclonal antibody was in Valentine et al. 1996. In these preclinical studies, a high-affinity anti-phencyclidine antigen-binding fragment derived from a mouse monoclonal antibody was used to treat phencyclidine effects in a rat model of phencyclidine overdose. The first report of an FDA clinical trial of a monoclonal antibody for the treatment of addiction was by Stevens et al. in 2014 (ClinicalTrials.gov Identifier: NCT01603147). This clinical trial was a first in kind Phase 1a study of an anti-methamphetamine chimeric monoclonal antibody in healthy adult female and male subjects. Other investigators have reported treatment of addiction or overdose in rodent models using monoclonal antibodies against cocaine and nicotine.

Therapeutic monoclonal antibodies offer the potential for a high degree of specificity. This specificity can include binding recognition for a single molecule (methamphetamine but not amphetamine) or recognition of a family of drugs of abuse (phencyclidine and structurally similar arylcyclohexylamines). Through protein engineering, intact monoclonal antibodies or antibody fragments (e.g., single-chain antibodies) can be created to increase or decrease their duration of action, route of elimination, reduce their risk of immunogenicity, or improve their affinity or specificity for the target drug of abuse.

The critical next step is to test monoclonal antibodies against drugs of abuse in humans for safety and efficacy. The two chapters in this section will discuss the preparation for and conducting of clinical trials for methamphetamine and cocaine abuse.

References

Stevens MW, Henry RL, Owens SM, et al (2014) First human study of a chimeric anti-methamphetamine monoclonal antibody in healthy volunteers. MAbs 6:1649–1656. doi: 10.4161/19420862.2014.976431

Valentine JL, Owens SM (1996) Antiphencyclidine monoclonal antibody therapy significantly changes phencyclidine concentrations in brain and other tissues in rats. J Pharmacol Exp Ther 278:717–724.

Chapter 8
Anti-cocaine Monoclonal Antibodies

Hanna N. Wetzel, William J. Ball, and Andrew B. Norman

8.1 Introduction to Anti-cocaine Monoclonal Antibodies

The use of an anti-cocaine monoclonal antibody (mAb) is similar to the concept of cocaine vaccines, discussed elsewhere in this book. Although vaccines have many advantages as an immunotherapy for cocaine abuse, the use of anti-cocaine mAbs addresses the limitations of cocaine vaccines: the polyclonal response that produces between-patient variability of affinities of the antibodies raised, the amount of antibodies raised, and the delay in the production of antibodies. Directly injecting therapeutically relevant doses of antibodies with known high affinity and selectivity avoids the between-patient variability in response to active immunization. Anti-cocaine mAbs could be used as a stand-alone treatment or as a supplement to patients treated with cocaine vaccines who do not produce adequate levels of high-affinity antibodies. Additionally, the antibodies are active immediately upon injection, whereas vaccines require time to elicit an immune response. Therefore, mAbs are better suited to mitigating relapse upon release from rehabilitation facilities and to overdose rescue than are the vaccines. Clearly, the active and passive immunotherapy approaches could be used together in individual patients. As there appears to be a minimum concentration of high-affinity anti-cocaine antibodies in order to be effective in relapse prevention, in those patients that produce sub-therapeutic concentrations the anti-cocaine mAb would augment their cocaine binding capacity to above therapeutic concentrations.

The proposed mechanism of action of these mAbs is that the cocaine-mAb complex is too large to cross the blood-brain barrier, and thus the distribution of cocaine to the brain is inhibited. Since the site of action of cocaine related to abuse is in the

H.N. Wetzel • W.J. Ball • A.B. Norman (✉)
Department of Pharmacology and Cell Biophysics, College of Medicine,
University of Cincinnati, 231 Albert Sabin Way, Cincinnati, OH 45267-0575, USA
e-mail: andrew.norman@uc.edu

I.D. Montoya (ed.), *Biologics to Treat Substance Use Disorders: Vaccines, Monoclonal Antibodies, and Enzymes*, DOI 10.1007/978-3-319-23150-1_8

brain, this cocaine is rendered pharmacodynamically inert. Anti-cocaine mAbs have characteristics of both chemical antagonism (defined as a compound that binds to and inactivates a drug) and pharmacokinetic antagonism (defined as a compound that decreases drug concentration at the site of action) (Rang et al. 2007). Presumably, these mAbs have no effect on the receptors mediating addiction, so the risk of side effects associated with targeting cocaine's site of action (the dopamine transporter) is avoided. However, the high specificity is also a potential disadvantage of this approach. Because antibodies remain in the periphery and have no effect on cocaine's pharmacodynamics in the brain, these therapies do not treat the underlying mechanisms that cause addiction. Consequently, environment-induced cocaine-seeking behavior ("craving") that could lead to relapse would not be affected by the immunotherapy. In the future, a centrally active pharmacotherapy may help alleviate this initial relapse event by targeting the pharmacodynamic mechanisms underlying relapse. This strategy is viable because the high specificity of the anti-cocaine antibodies (Paula et al. 2004) makes the likelihood of interactions between the pharmacotherapy and the immunotherapy minimal.

This review seeks to summarize the generation, binding properties, pharmacokinetics, effects on the disposition of cocaine, and the behavioral effects of the anti-cocaine mAbs that have been investigated with emphasis on those that are at an advanced stage of preclinical development.

8.2 Anti-cocaine Monoclonal Antibodies

8.2.1 Murine and Human/Chimeric mAbs

The first generation of anti-cocaine mAbs was murine, such as GNC92H2 (Carrera et al. 2000) and MO240 (Fox et al. 1996). Establishing that these mAbs significantly modified the effects and the pharmacokinetics of cocaine in rodents (see below) provided impetus to produce anti-cocaine antibodies that had humanized structures that would be more suitable for clinical use. The second generation of anti-cocaine mAbs was designed to have human IgG sequences, and the production methods employed were unique from traditional mAb production techniques in that double-transgenic/double-deletion mouse lines were used. These mice were engineered with the genes encoding the murine heavy (H) and light (L) IgG1 chains deleted and substituted with their human variants. Consequently, these mice generate human IgG1 antibodies in response to vaccination (Lonberg et al. 1994), and standard hybridoma technology can be used to produce human antibodies. When these mice were immunized with a cocaine-based hapten-carrier conjugate, human anti-cocaine antibodies were raised. As a result of this technology, an anti-cocaine mAb, with the preclinical designation 2E2, was generated that has a fully human sequence $\gamma 1$ heavy (H) chain but the light chain proved to be a murine λ light (L) chain.

The mixed chain mAb 2E2 has the highest affinity for cocaine (Kd=4 nM) out of a series of anti-cocaine antibodies that were generated from these transgenic mice and also had specificity for cocaine over its inactive metabolites, with 10-,

1,500-, and 25,000-fold lower binding affinities for the three most prevalent cocaine metabolites benzoylecgonine, ecgonine methyl ester, and ecgonine, respectively. This antibody also has higher affinity for the active metabolite cocaethylene than for cocaine (Paula et al. 2004). Though murine/chimeric anti-cocaine mAbs had great success in preclinical studies, there were safety concerns associated with their clinical use. It has been shown that nonhuman antibodies are more likely to induce anti-antibody responses, which can decrease the efficacy of the therapy and cause adverse side effects. These are less likely to occur when the therapeutic antibody is humanized (Hwang and Foote 2005). Therefore, efforts have been made to humanize murine and chimeric anti-cocaine antibodies or generate fully human mAbs.

The recently developed humanized anti-cocaine mAb h2E2 is the humanized successor to 2E2. 2E2 was originally produced from murine hybridoma cell lines in ascites fluid from severe combined immunodeficiency (SCID) mice (nude mice). SCID mice were used to avoid the production of anti-human IgG antibodies in the host mice. However this method is expensive and had low production yields and high variability in production between batches. Furthermore, in vivo production using ascites fluid is not suitable for human use as there were concerns about murine viruses and other contaminants. For this reason, the constructed genes encoding the H and L chains of this mAb were cloned into Chinese hamster ovary (CHO) cells using proprietary GPEx technology (Bleck 2012). During this process of cloning the 2E2 human H chain and the murine L chain, the murine λ_c L chain constant region was replaced with the λ_c human chain constant region, whereas the variable region of the L chain was unmodified. This modified mAb (h2E2) is now produced in gram quantities using this stable CHO cell line (Kirley and Norman 2015). The humanization process did not compromise the binding properties of this mAb. In fact, h2E2 has a similar Kd for cocaine than the chimeric/mixed chain mAb 2E2. It also retained specificity for cocaine over its inactive metabolite BE and has high affinity for the active metabolite cocaethylene (Kirley and Norman 2015).

A fully human anti-cocaine mAb, GNCgzk, has also been disclosed. This mAb was generated using a method similar to that used to create the chimeric 2E2 using transgenic mice. It was then transfected into CHO cells for production of the recombinant mAb protein (Eubanks et al. 2014). This mAb has extremely high affinity for cocaine (Kd = 0.18 nM; Eubanks et al. 2014) and is very selective for cocaine over inactive metabolites (Treweek and Janda 2012) with approximately 1,000-fold lower affinity for BE relative to cocaine compared to the approximately tenfold lower relative binding affinity for BE displayed by h2E2.

8.2.2 Fab Fragments of Anti-cocaine mAbs

Though the properties of the mAbs are ideal for long-term treatment, it has been suggested that the Fab fragments of these antibodies would be more ideal for treatment of cocaine overdose. Fab fragments retain binding affinity and specificity for cocaine but have faster distribution and elimination kinetics. The Fab fragment of chimeric GNC92H2 (Kd = 100 nM), for example, was more effective in preventing

Table 8.1 The affinity and catalytic efficiency of anti-cocaine mAbs and cocaine esterases

Enzyme/antibody	Km (μM)	Kcat
3B9	490	0.11 min^{-1}
15A10	220	2.3 min^{-1}
BChE	38	1.2 min^{-1}
Bacterial cocaine esterase	0.640	7.8 s^{-1}

seizures, lethality, and premorbid ataxia in a mouse model of overdose (Treweek et al. 2011) than the intact IgG. A Fab fragment of h2E2 has also been reported (Kirley and Norman 2015), which has approximately 100-fold higher affinity for cocaine (Kd = 1.6–3.7 nM) than the Fab fragment of GNC92H2, making it likely that the Fab fragment of h2E2 will also be effective in mitigating the effects of cocaine overdose.

8.2.3 Catalytic Antibodies

A series of antibodies have been designed with the ability to catalyze the hydrolysis of cocaine to inactive metabolites. These antibodies were the conceptual precursors to the extensively studied cocaine esterases, which are discussed elsewhere in this book, which also metabolize cocaine to its inactive metabolites. It was found that antibodies against the transition-state analogs between a molecule and its metabolite could be catalytic (Tramontano et al. 1986). This is because the antibody binds to and stabilizes the transition state, which lowers the activation energy, thus speeding the reaction (Landry et al. 1993). One such mAb, called 3B9, was directed against an analog of the transition state between cocaine and ecgonine methyl ester, with catalytic activity approaching that of the natural human butyrylcholinesterase (BChE) (Table 8.1).

The catalytic antibody that received the most attention was 15A10 (Yang et al. 1996). This mAb has an improved Km and Kcat over 3B9, but none of the catalytic antibodies have near the efficiency of the more recently developed cocaine esterases (Howell et al. 2014) (discussed elsewhere in this book). A summary of the characteristics of these antibodies compared to the natural and artificial enzymes is provided in Table 8.1.

8.3 Pharmacokinetics of Anti-cocaine mAbs

Like other antibodies, the pharmacokinetics of anti-cocaine mAbs is generally characterized by a slow elimination and a small volume of distribution. This profile is ideal for an immunotherapy for drug abuse. Long elimination means that less frequent dosing will be needed, and a low volume of distribution means that the mAb will likely remain in the plasma to bind to cocaine and prevent its distribution.

The pharmacokinetics of 2E2, h2E2, and GNC92H2 has been evaluated in multiple species. The elimination half-life of mAb GNC92H2 in mice was reported to be 12.1 days (Treweek et al. 2011). The mAbs 2E2 and h2E2 also had half-lives in mice of more than a week and also had a low volume of distribution of approximately 0.3 l/kg after i.v. administration (Norman et al. 2007; Wetzel et al. 2014). Similarly, in rats, 2E2 had a long terminal elimination half-life of more than a week and a low volume of distribution (Norman et al. 2009). The long half-life in rodents indicates that these mAbs, especially the humanized h2E2, could have long-lasting effects in humans if used clinically for the prevention of relapse in cocaine abusers.

8.4 Effects of Anti-cocaine mAbs on the Distribution of Cocaine and Cocaethylene

Though the effects of active immunization on cocaine distribution have been investigated on multiple occasions (Fox et al. 1996; Fox 1997; Carrera et al. 2000), studies on the effects of anti-cocaine mAbs on cocaine distribution are limited to 2E2 and h2E2. Again, it is thought that these antibodies act by preventing cocaine from crossing the blood-brain barrier and sequestering it in the plasma. Therefore, it is expected that in the presence of the mAb, cocaine concentrations will be lower in the brain and higher in the plasma compared to control animals. This effect is, in fact, observed in both mice and rats.

8.4.1 Cocaine

In mice, the mAb 2E2 was shown to decrease the brain area under the time-concentration curve (AUC) by 78 %. This was accompanied by an increase in plasma concentrations (Norman et al. 2007). Similarly, in mice, when cocaine was injected i.v. one hour after i.v. administration of h2E2, there was a dramatic decrease in the brain cocaine AUC and an increase in plasma cocaine concentrations (unpublished data). These results support the proposed mechanism of action and indicate that these antibodies will be clinically efficacious.

8.4.2 Cocaethylene

The effectiveness of h2E2 against cocaethylene was tested in mice. Cocaethylene is an active metabolite of cocaine that is formed in the presence of ethanol. The mAb dramatically decreased the area under the cocaethylene time-concentration curve in the brain, consistent with h2E2's high affinity for cocaethylene. This indicates that h2E2 will be effective in addicts that co-abuse cocaine and alcohol (Wetzel et al. 2014).

It may be expected that binding of cocaethylene to a large protein would slow its elimination by preventing enzymatic degradation. Indeed, the terminal elimination half-life of cocaethylene may have been decreased in the presence of h2E2. However, plasma cocaethylene concentrations did decline quite rapidly in the presence of h2E2 over the first hour after i.v. injection (Wetzel et al. 2014). More work is needed to see if this represents distribution to other compartments, metabolism, or clearance.

8.5 The Effects of Anti-cocaine mAbs on Behavior

8.5.1 *Toxic Effects*

The murine antibody GNC92H2 has been shown to decrease premorbid behavior (convulsions, loss of righting posture, Straub tail response, agitation, and tonic seizures) (Carrera et al. 2005; Treweek and Janda 2012). The human antibody GNCgzk and its F(ab')2 fragment prevented premorbid ataxia (Eubanks et al. 2014). Both these antibodies also decreased the lethality of cocaine.

8.5.2 *Self-Administration*

Self-administration of cocaine in rats is the most commonly used model of addiction. The effects of four different anti-cocaine mAbs on self-administration have been characterized (Fox et al. 1996; Carrera et al. 2000; Kantak et al. 2000; Norman et al. 2009). Depending on the schedule of cocaine delivery, dose of antibody, and unit dose of cocaine, opposite effects on the rate of self-administration were observed both between and within studies. Our proposed explanation for this phenomenon is achieved by applying the compulsion zone theory to the observed results.

This theory states that self-administration events (lever presses) will only occur when cocaine concentrations are between two set points (Norman and Tsibulsky 2006). The upper limit of this zone is called the satiety threshold (Tsibulsky and Norman 1999), and the lower limit is the priming threshold (Norman et al. 1999). Therefore, rats will only press the lever when cocaine concentrations are above the priming threshold but below the satiety threshold. Reinstatement occurs when cocaine concentration is above the priming threshold. At this point, the rat will rapidly press the lever until concentrations cross the satiety threshold at which point self-administration will be very regular as concentrations periodically rise above and then fall to satiety threshold as the dose of cocaine is eliminated. An important feature of this model is that there are two important parameters: priming threshold, which is a measure of reinstatement probability, and satiety threshold, which is the pharmacodynamic parameter regulating maintained self-administration. Any study that only reports the number of presses or rate of pressing during a session does not differentiate these two parameters, making meaningful interpretation difficult, especially when the limited schedule of delivery potentially interferes with priming. Therefore, all studies conducted in the Norman lab separate reinstatement from maintenance and use an FR-1 schedule (Norman et al. 1999, 2002, 2009; Tsibulsky and Norman 1999; Norman and Tsibulsky 2006).

The simplest way to explain the potentially contradictory effects of mAbs on self-administration is in the context of the effects of the mAb 2E2 on priming threshold and satiety threshold (Norman et al. 2009). In this study, priming threshold was measured by giving non-contingent programmed injections of cocaine until self-administration was reinstated. This is a model of relapse and essentially measures the amount of cocaine needed to adequately raise plasma concentrations of the antibody to allow enough cocaine to cross into the brain and raise concentrations above the priming threshold. By this method of measurement, 2E2 initially raised the cocaine priming threshold threefold. In a human, this would mean that the patient is less likely to relapse after a given dose of cocaine. This increase in priming threshold accounts for the decrease in self-administration observed after treatment with the catalytic antibody 15A10 and the murine mAb GNC92H2. These results are consistent with each other, in that 15A10 decreased cocaine intake only at lower cocaine unit doses (Baird et al. 2000), while GNC92H2 only decreased intake at high antibody unit doses (Carrera et al. 2000). In both these cases, it is likely that the stoichiometric relationship between cocaine and antibody more favored the antibody, preventing enough cocaine to induce priming from ever reaching the brain. The mAb MO240 was shown to decrease self-administration, regardless of cocaine unit dose or mAb dose (Fox et al. 1996; Kantak et al. 2000).

Once priming has occurred, the animal moves into maintenance phase. Here, the animal will press the lever only when cocaine concentrations drop by first-order kinetics below satiety threshold. The mAb 2E2 was shown to accelerate the rate of self-administration during this phase. The effect is explained by the much higher peripheral concentrations in the presence of the antibody. Since cocaine is cleared through first-order kinetics, it falls faster at higher concentrations causing cocaine concentrations to reach the satiety threshold faster at any given unit dose in the presence of 2E2. This effect was more pronounced at lower unit doses, as the stoichiometric relationship between 2E2 and cocaine was, on average, smaller during this phase. This increase in self-administration diminished over time as antibody concentrations decreased. This decrease in inter-injection intervals during the maintenance phase likely accounts for the reported increase in the rate of self-administration caused by the mAbs 15A10 and GNC92H2, which were both observed when high cocaine unit doses (Baird et al. 2000) or low mAb doses (Carrera et al. 2000) were used. Therefore, the stoichiometric relationship more favors cocaine, which likely allowed the animals to prime quickly and spend most of the session in maintenance, making the total number of presses per session higher in the presence of a mAb. The only mAb that was not reported to increase self-administration under any conditions is MO240. However, these studies used extremely low antibody doses (4–12 mg) and a delivery schedule that severely limited cocaine access (FR-5 for the stimulus light and FI-5 for cocaine) which could interfere with rats' ability to prime even in the presence of very little antibody (Fox et al. 1996; Kantak et al. 2000). Additionally, it was shown that after an i.v. injection of 4 mg of mAb, the maximum effect on self-administration is not observed until 2 days postinjection (Fox et al. 1996).

8.6 Summary

Despite these relatively minor discrepancies between studies, it is clear that anti-cocaine mAbs produce a measurable and often dramatic reduction of the magnitude of cocaine-induced responses in vivo. It is likely that by antagonizing cocaine-induced responses in humans, anti-cocaine mAbs will provide a useful contribution to the treatment of cocaine abuse in human addicts/abusers.

References

Baird TJ, Deng SX, Landry DW, Winger G, Woods JH. Natural and artificial enzymes against cocaine. I. Monoclonal antibody 15A10 and the reinforcing effects of cocaine in rats. J Pharmacol Exp Ther. 2000;295:1127–34.

Bleck GT. Consistent production of genetically stable mammalian cell lines. Biopharm Int. 2012;25:56–9.

Carrera MR, Ashley JA, Zhou B, Wirsching P, Koob GF, Janda KD. Cocaine vaccines: antibody protection against relapse in a rat model. Proc Natl Acad Sci U S A. 2000;97:6202–6.

Carrera MR, Trigo JM, Wirsching P, Roberts AJ, Janda KD. Evaluation of the anticocaine monoclonal antibody GNC92H2 as an immunotherapy for cocaine overdose. Pharmacol Biochem Behav. 2005;81:709–14.

Eubanks LM, Ellis BA, Cai X, Schlosburg JE, Janda KD. A human recombinant monoclonal antibody to cocaine: preparation, characterization and behavioral studies. Bioorg Med Chem Lett. 2014;24:4664–6.

Fox BS. Development of a therapeutic vaccine for the treatment of cocaine addiction. Drug Alcohol Depend. 1997;48:153–8.

Fox BS, Kantak KM, Edwards MA, Black KM, Bollinger BK, Botka AJ, et al. Efficacy of a therapeutic cocaine vaccine in rodent models. Nat Med. 1996;2:1129–32.

Howell LL, Nye JA, Stehouwer JS, Voll RJ, Mun J, Narasimhan D, et al. A thermostable bacterial cocaine esterase rapidly eliminates cocaine from brain in nonhuman primates. Transl Psychiatry. 2014;4, e407.

Hwang WY, Foote J. Immunogenicity of engineered antibodies. Methods. 2005;36:3–10.

Kantak KM, Collins SL, Lipman EG, Bond J, Giovanoni K, Fox BS. Evaluation of anti-cocaine antibodies and a cocaine vaccine in a rat self-administration model. Psychopharmacology (Berl). 2000;148:251–62.

Kirley TL, Norman AB. Characterization of a recombinant humanized anti-cocaine monoclonal antibody and its Fab fragment. Hum Vacc Immunother. 2015;11(2):458–67.

Landry DW, Zhao K, Yang GX, Glickman M, Georgiadis TM. Antibody-catalyzed degradation of cocaine. Science. 1993;259:1899–901.

Lonberg N, Taylor LD, Harding FA, Trounstine M, Higgins KM, Schramm SR, et al. Antigen-specific human antibodies from mice comprising four distinct genetic modifications. Nature. 1994;368:856–9.

Norman AB, Tsibulsky VL. The compulsion zone: a pharmacological theory of acquired cocaine self-administration. Brain Res. 2006;1116:143–52.

Norman AB, Norman MK, Hall JF, Tsibulsky VL. Priming threshold: a novel quantitative measure of the reinstatement of cocaine self-administration. Brain Res. 1999;831:165–74.

Norman AB, Welge JA, Tsibulsky VL. Characterization of the distribution of the cocaine priming threshold and the effect of SCH23390. Brain Res. 2002;946:253–61.

Norman AB, Tabet MR, Norman MK, Buesing WR, Pesce AJ, Ball WJ. A chimeric human/murine anticocaine monoclonal antibody inhibits the distribution of cocaine to the brain in mice. J Pharmacol Exp Ther. 2007;320:145–53.

Norman AB, Norman MK, Buesing WR, Tabet MR, Tsibulsky VL, Ball WJ. The effect of a chimeric human/murine anti-cocaine monoclonal antibody on cocaine self-administration in rats. J Pharmacol Exp Ther. 2009;328:873–81.

Paula S, Tabet MR, Farr CD, Norman AB, Ball Jr WJ. Three-dimensional quantitative structure-activity relationship modeling of cocaine binding by a novel human monoclonal antibody. J Med Chem. 2004;47:133–42.

Rang HP, Dale MM, Ritter JM, Flower RM. Rang and Dale's pharmacology. Philadelphia: Elsevier; 2007.

Tramontano A, Janda KD, Lerner RA. Catalytic antibodies. Science. 1986;234:1566–70.

Treweek JB, Janda KD. An antidote for acute cocaine toxicity. Mol Pharm. 2012;9:969–78.

Treweek JB, Roberts AJ, Janda KD. Immunopharmacotherapeutic manifolds and modulation of cocaine overdose. Pharmacol Biochem Behav. 2011;98:474–84.

Tsibulsky VL, Norman AB. Satiety threshold: a quantitative model of maintained cocaine self-administration. Brain Res. 1999;839:85–93.

Wetzel HN, Tabet MR, Ball WJ, Norman AB. The effects of a humanized recombinant anti-cocaine monoclonal antibody on the disposition of cocaethylene in mice. Int Immunopharmacol. 2014;23:387–90.

Yang G, Chun J, ArakawaUramoto H, Wang X, Gawinowicz MA, Zhao K, et al. Anti-cocaine catalytic antibodies: a synthetic approach to improved antibody diversity. J Am Chem Soc. 1996;118:5881–90.

Chapter 9
Discovery and Development of an Anti-methamphetamine Monoclonal Antibody for Use in Treating Methamphetamine Abuse

Michael D. Hambuchen, Misty W. Stevens, Melinda G. Gunnell, W. Brooks Gentry, and S. Michael Owens

Abbreviations

AMP	(+)-amphetamine (unless denoted as other stereoisomer)
AUC	area under the concentration-time curve
B_{max}	maximum number of binding sites
ch	chimeric
C_{ss}, C_{min}, C_{max}	denotes the steady-state, minimum, and maximum concentrations during chronic administration of a drug
ECG	electrocardiograms
ELISA	enzyme-linked immunosorbent assay
FcRn	Fc receptor of the neonate
HACA	human anti-chimeric antibodies
IgG	immunoglobulin G
iv	intravenous
K_d	dissociation constant
mAb	monoclonal antibody (both singular and plural)

M.D. Hambuchen • M.G. Gunnell • S.M. Owens (✉)
Department of Pharmacology and Toxicology, College of Medicine, University of Arkansas for Medical Sciences, Little Rock, AR 72205, USA
e-mail: hambuchenmichaeld@uams.edu; mgunnell@uams.edu; mowens@uams.edu

M.W. Stevens
InterveXion Therapeutics, LLC, Little Rock, AR 72205, USA
e-mail: misty.stevens@intervexion.com

W.B. Gentry
Department of Pharmacology and Toxicology, College of Medicine, University of Arkansas for Medical Sciences, Little Rock, AR 72205, USA

Department of Anesthesiology, College of Medicine, University of Arkansas for Medical Sciences, Little Rock, AR 72205, USA
e-mail: GentryWilliamB@uams.edu

I.D. Montoya (ed.), *Biologics to Treat Substance Use Disorders: Vaccines, Monoclonal Antibodies, and Enzymes*, DOI 10.1007/978-3-319-23150-1_9

K_I	inhibition constant
MCV	METH-conjugate vaccine
MDMA	(+/−)-methylenedioxymethamphetamine (unless denoted as other stereoisomer)
METH	(+)-methamphetamine (unless denoted as other stereoisomer)
$t_{1/2}$	half-life
sc	subcutaneous

9.1 Introduction

Methamphetamine (METH) is a highly addictive drug that is commonly abused. In 2005, a study by the RAND Corporation estimated the economic impact of METH abuse in the USA was 23.4 billion dollars (Nicosia et al. 2009). Quest Diagnostics (2014) reports that positive workplace screens for (METH) are the highest since 2007, with a ten percent increase from 2012 to 2013. The Treatment Episode Data Set (TEDS, a nationwide database of substance abuse treatment admissions) shows 7 % of substance abuse treatment is for amphetamines (mostly METH), but in 20 states >10 % of admissions are for METH abuse treatment (SAMHSA 2012). For example, in California and Hawaii, METH treatment comprises 27 % and 31 %, respectively, of all reported substance abuse treatments.

Addiction to METH involves drug-induced modification of neuronal circuits leading to a repetitive cycle of binge use and intoxication, abstinence and withdrawal, craving, and relapse to use (Koob and Volkow 2010). Clinical trials of more traditional small-molecule agonist and antagonist medications for METH abuse report these potential medications have limited effects, poor compliance, or success in a limited population or even lead to increased METH use (Brensilver et al. 2013). For example, treatment with the selective serotonin reuptake inhibitor sertraline, and the atypical antipsychotic aripiprazole, can lead to increased METH use (Shoptaw et al. 2006; Tiihonen et al. 2007). Because of the wide-ranging actions of METH in the central nervous system (CNS), finding a specific pharmacological target in the CNS is proving difficult.

At the neuronal level, METH use results in increased synaptic cleft concentrations of norepinephrine and dopamine with some effect on serotonin release (Cruickshank and Dyer 2009). Both the reward and stimulant effects of METH are related to dopamine release in the nucleus accumbens (Sellings and Clarke 2003). METH enters the neuron by reverse action of monoamine transporters and passive diffusion resulting in interaction with the vesicular monoamine transporter and release of monoamines to the cytoplasm and then the synaptic cleft (Sulzer et al. 2005). Examples of other METH mechanisms of action in the brain include inhibition of monoamine oxidase, increased dopamine (and therefore norepinephrine) synthesis, and alteration of dopamine transporter and vesicular monoamine transporter trafficking.

Table 9.1 Advantages of treating METH addiction with antibody therapy

Can decrease or block METH exposure in the brain
Can be combined with behavioral therapy and other medications to:
Increase patient "willpower" to quit abusing METH
Aid in the initiation and continuation of more positive behaviors (i.e., not using drugs)
Longer term therapeutic effects compared to small-molecule medications due to lengthy half-life of IgG

Considering the known executive control impairment, withdrawal, and situational and stress-related craving in METH-addicted individuals (Koob and Volkow 2010), it is likely that patients in addiction treatment will relapse to METH use during their treatment and comply poorly with the treatment regimen (Hillhouse et al. 2007). Medications that are continuously effective and function during the long time periods when addicted patients are not in behavioral counseling could offer a significant compliance advantage. An ideal medication for treating relapse would not be addictive or produce additive or synergistic effects in the presence of binge METH use. Ultimately, a medication should improve the general health of the patient (e.g., improved appetite) while not negatively interacting with medical treatments for METH-related comorbidities (e.g., depression) or other unrelated disease states (Kresina et al. 2004).

While meeting all these potential medication design criteria is extremely challenging, many of these criteria are met by anti-METH antibody-based medications. Table 9.1 lists the potential advantages for the use of antibody therapy in METH-addicted patients.

9.2 Anti-METH Monoclonal Antibody Compared to Active Immunization with a METH-Conjugate Vaccine for the Treatment of METH Abuse

Medical treatment with anti-METH antibodies could be accomplished in several ways, but the two major methods currently in clinical testing or being prepared for testing are the administration of preformed anti-METH monoclonal antibodies (mAb, both singular and plural) or active vaccination with a METH-conjugate vaccine (MCV). Anti-METH IgG antibodies are large-molecular-weight proteins (~150 kDA) with two high-affinity METH binding sites (e.g., 7 nM K_d for METH). After intravenous administration of anti-METH mAb to animals, results show the antibody remains mainly confined to the blood plasma (not red blood cells) and extracellular fluid space of the body. For this reason it is not surprising that in vivo mAb binding of METH is very high in the blood plasma (Gentry et al. 2009; Owens et al. 2011).

Compared to production of anti-METH polyclonal antibodies generated by active immunization, mAb can provide protective effects against METH immediately after mAb treatment. Acute studies in rats show that the administration of anti-METH mAb immediately decreases METH-induced stimulant effects

(Byrnes-Blake et al. 2003; Laurenzana et al. 2014). Active immunization with a MCV, however, requires approximately 9–12 weeks before the antibody titers and affinity for METH are high enough to offer meaningful pharmacological protection (Rüedi-Bettschen et al. 2013). Compared to MCVs, anti-METH mAb treatment can produce predictable and reproducible serum antibody concentrations. Because they can be administered intravenously in known doses, they circumvent the inherent individual patient variability in polyclonal immune response after immunization with a MCV. In humans taking immunosuppression medications (e.g., glucocorticoids) or with immune-compromised disease states (e.g., AIDS), it may not be possible to use active immunization for developing an anti-METH antibody response. This problem would not occur with mAb therapy since the antibodies are preformed and could be administered to most patients as needed. MAb therapy could also achieve much higher concentrations than produced by active vaccination and could provide the opportunity to dose to a desired effect level. Unfortunately, the much higher cost of a mAb is a significant factor in the amount that can be administered. In addition to the immediate and controllable anti-METH antibody concentrations, a mAb medication is a homogenous solution of the same high-affinity anti-METH antibody. Rather than the polyclonal antibody response from a MCV that generates antibodies with a variety of affinities and specificities for METH, each mAb has exactly the same amino acid sequence, affinity, and specificity for METH. This assures a more consistent treatment among patients.

Each type of immunotherapy has advantages and disadvantages, which will require testing in humans before they can be adequately judged. However, it is also possible that in certain clinical scenarios, mAb and vaccination could be used in combination (Carrera et al. 2000; Roiko et al. 2008; Cornish et al. 2011).

While our scientific team is working on both types of antibody-based therapy, we think anti-METH mAb therapy has the most advantages for treating patient addiction. These advantages and possible disadvantages will be discussed in detail in upcoming sections. Table 9.2 summarizes some of the key advantages and disadvantages of mAb therapy.

Table 9.2 Potential advantages and disadvantages of anti-METH mAb therapy

Advantages
Immediate protection from METH overdose and METH-induced relapse to addiction
Well-defined pharmaceutical preparation
Dosing by established principles of clinical pharmacology
Therapeutic levels are easily maintained
MAb duration of action and affinity can be modified by protein engineering
Because the biological half-life is very long in humans (e.g., 3 weeks), patient compliance and use are likely to be improved
Nonaddictive
Disadvantages
Cost of the medications is high
Eventual immune response against mAb could limit length of treatment

9.3 The Mechanism of Action for Anti-METH mAb-Mediated Reductions in METH Effects

The most common reason suggested by patients for their persistent METH use and relapse to METH use is the positive-reinforcing effects of METH (Newton et al. 2009). This makes METH a disease target for antibody medications. Anti-METH mAb therapy is predicted to reduce the overall METH-induced effects including the reward type effects associated with continued or renewed use in addicted patients. Anti-METH mAb treatment shows efficacy in a variety of preclinical rat models of METH abuse including the reduction of METH brain concentrations, reduction of METH-induced locomotor effects, decreases in the duration of these effects (Byrnes-Blake et al. 2003; Laurenzana et al. 2014; Hambuchen et al. 2014), and the reduction of METH self-administration (McMillan et al. 2004).

Anti-METH mAb has dramatic effects on the disposition of in vivo METH. The apparent METH volume of distribution in humans is very high, at about 3.73 L/kg or 261 L in a 70 kg human (Cook et al. 1993), indicating extensive extravascular METH distribution. In stark contrast, the apparent volume of distribution of chimeric anti-METH mAb7F9 (ch-mAb7F9, to be discussed later in the chapter) is only 5–6 L in healthy adult male or female subjects following a single ch-mAb7F9 dose of 0.2–20 mg/kg (Stevens et al. 2014a, ClinicalTrials.gov Identifier: NCT01603147).

In an adult male or female of 70 kg, this is a volume of distribution of about 0.08 L/kg. This means that when METH is bound by high-affinity ch-mAb7F9 (METH $K_d = 6.9$ nM), the distribution of METH out of the bloodstream will be substantially reduced (Stevens et al. 2014b). In rat studies of a 1 mg/kg METH dose in the presence of a mouse anti-METH mAb, there was a substantial increase in area under the METH serum concentration-time curve relative to control rats without antibody treatment (Laurenzana et al. 2003). Binding of METH to the antibody also alters the clearance of METH. The effects on METH clearance will be discussed later in this chapter.

As depicted in Fig. 9.1, anti-METH mAb binding decreases entry of METH across the blood-brain barrier to active sites in the brain (Byrnes-Blake et al. 2003; Laurenzana et al. 2003, 2009). For example, a continuous subcutaneous METH infusion of 5.6 mg/kg/day in rats followed by anti-METH mAb administration results in immediate reductions in brain METH concentrations (Laurenzana et al. 2009). As another component of the mechanism of action, these antibodies are thought to decrease the rate of entry of METH into the brain. Human subjective responses to cocaine (e.g., "high" and "liking") are significantly lower when the drug is infused more slowly (Abreu et al. 2001). Based on data from tissue distribution studies in rats, anti-METH mAb reduces METH entry into a variety of other critical organs, including the fetal brain in utero (Laurenzana et al. 2003; White et al. 2014). These tissue changes in METH disposition lead to decreases in METH-induced pharmacological (e.g., psychomotor and cardiovascular) effects in animal models (Gentry et al. 2006; Laurenzana et al. 2014; Hambuchen et al. 2014).

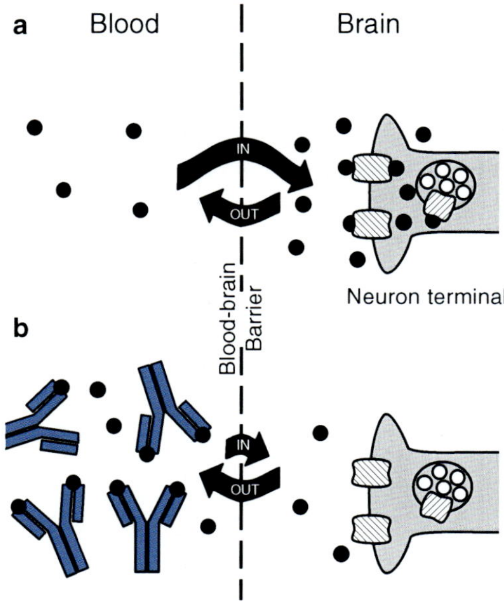

Fig. 9.1 Anti-METH mAb effects on METH brain concentrations. (**a**) METH (*black circles*) brain entry before anti-METH antibody administration leads to interaction with neurons resulting in the release of monoamines (*open circles*) and production of stimulant actions. (**b**) Anti-METH antibody ("Y"-shaped symbols) binds METH in the bloodstream and reduces the amount and rate (as denoted by the direction and length of the *curved arrows*) of METH brain entry

Anti-METH polyclonal antibodies resulting from active vaccination can block high-dose METH (3 mg/kg) inhibition of food-maintained behavior (Rüedi-Bettschen et al. 2013) despite the lower titers, affinity, and consistency of response compared to mAb treatment.

Inhibition of METH-induced locomotor activity is a frequently used preclinical measure of the effectiveness of candidate anti-METH mAb by our research group. It is often combined and correlated with pharmacokinetic changes in METH serum and brain concentrations in the same set of animals. Repeated METH administration, however, can produce sensitization and shifting baseline effects from dose to dose (despite complete elimination of METH between doses). While higher stimulant doses produce increased incidence of early locomotor activity suppressing stereotypic effects (Schiorring 1971), these effects also increasingly occur with repetitive administration of even low stimulant doses (Segal and Mandell 1974). While decreasing locomotor activity with an antibody is not a direct measurement of decreasing METH addiction, it does show the inhibition of a METH-induced effect which results from METH-induced dopamine release in the CNS (Sellings and Clarke 2003). Considering that anti-METH mAb act by restricting the entry of METH to the brain, this is likely a suitable measurement of an overall decrease in METH effects. The measurement is also noninvasive compared to directly measuring brain drug or neurotransmitter concentrations. Since it can be performed without significant training of animals, it allows for higher throughput testing of multiple key time points during an anti-METH mAb treatment regimen.

9.4 Anti-METH mAb Has Prolonged Duration of Action

An important potential therapeutic advantage of mAb over small-molecule medications is the extended duration of action and the likely long time periods between required mAb administrations. This is due to the very long elimination half-lives of mAb, which range from approximately 2–4 weeks in humans. The long half-life of these therapeutic proteins results from in vivo FcRn (Fc receptor of the neonate) recycling of IgG mAb proteins. This process protects IgG molecules from intracellular catabolism (Lobo et al. 2004; Wang et al. 2008).

Most small-molecule drugs used for the treatment of chronic diseases like high blood pressure or depression require patients to take their medication 1–3 times a day for extended or indefinite periods of time. This is manageable with self-motivated, compliant patients. However, patients being treated for METH addiction would likely have difficulty complying with frequent dosing on a daily basis.

Most small-molecule medications are dosed based on the drug's half-life. For example, a drug with a 10 h half-life might be effectively dosed in patients twice a day. Assuming the same pharmacological principles apply to the dosing of anti-METH mAb medications, the mAb could be administered by an intravenous infusion once every 3 weeks if the half-life of the mAb is in the range of 18–24 days. We think this would offer patients a significant advantage because the protective anti-METH mAb medication would be present in the bloodstream during the extended periods of time when they are not under direct medical care or counseling for their addiction. The disadvantage would be that the patient might forget to be treated with such infrequent scheduled treatment periods.

While dosing with an anti-METH mAb could offer immediate therapeutic benefits, one of the many unknowns concerning the use of mAb to treat addiction is how long it will take to reach maximum effects. For most small-molecule medications, well-established principles of clinical pharmacokinetics show that the time needed to reach maximum steady-state concentrations in the body is only dependent on the half-life of the drug (Rowland and Tozer 1995). After 1, 2, 3, or 4 half-lives of the drug, 50, 75, 87.5, and 94 %, respectively, of the final steady-state concentrations are reached. Most clinical pharmacologists agree that after four half-lives of a medication, the maximum effects (and side effects) would be achieved. Thus, if the patient is dosed with an anti-METH mAb medication once every mAb half-life (e.g., once every 3 weeks), after 12 weeks the patient's steady-state value of mAb concentration would be at ~94 % of the final value. To achieve steady-state concentrations more rapidly, a higher loading dose could be used at the start of the treatment. This treatment strategy will be demonstrated in a later section of this review.

9.5 Regeneration of METH Binding Capacity by In Vivo METH Elimination Processes

Another important aspect of the duration of action and efficacy of anti-METH antibodies is related to the fate of the antibody-METH complex. In vivo elimination processes play a major role in maintaining the functional capacity of the mAb to neutralize METH effects. As illustrated, METH is cleared in the male rat primarily by metabolism and in male humans primary by renal passive filtration along with some metabolism (Cook et al. 1993; Mendelson et al. 1995; Rivière et al. 1999). The pharmacokinetic values for the male rat and male human are, respectively, volume of distribution, 9.0 and 3.73 L/kg; clearance, 126 and 3.2 ml/min/kg; and $t_{1/2}$, 63 min and 13.1 h. As discussed earlier, a mAb IgG is cleared by intracellular catabolism (Lobo et al. 2004; Wang et al. 2008). Pharmacokinetic analysis of METH concentration-time data in the absence and presence of anti-METH ch-mAb7F9 (to be discussed later in this chapter) in male Sprague-Dawley rats shows the following results for the terminal elimination $t_{1/2}$ of ch-mAb7F9, METH, and ch-mAb7F9 plus METH (Table 9.3).

In the studies summarized in Table 9.3, the elimination half-life of METH in the presence of an anti-METH mAb (i.e., 2.3–6.5 h) is much closer to the value for the half-life of METH alone (1.1 h) than to the mAb half-life (9.8–13.1 days). We also find that even though METH binding in the presence of anti-METH murine mAb is very high, the unbound METH concentrations are also relatively high (Laurenzana et al. 2009). Considered together, these data show the capacity for mAb binding of METH in vivo can be regenerated (or restored) through mammalian in vivo METH elimination processes (see Fig. 9.2) in the rat. It is likely that the high-affinity binding of METH continuously works to redistribute the drug by lowering the volume of distribution of METH (discussed earlier). This redistribution makes greater amounts of unbound METH available in the systemic circulatory system for metabolic and renal clearance.

Table 9.3 Ch-mAb7F9 and METH $t_{1/2}$ values in the absence and presence of two different doses of anti-METH ch-mAb7F9 in male Sprague-Dawley rats

Rat treatment group ($n=12$)	Saline or METH Dose (sc)	Ch-mAb7F9 Dose (iv)	$t_{1/2}$ ch-mAb7F9 (Days)	$t_{1/2}$ METH (h)
Ch-mAb7F9 only	Saline	15 mg.kg	10.9	
Ch-mAb7F9 only	Saline	150 mg/kg	11.5	
METH only	1 mg/kg			1.1
METH + Ch-mAb7F9	1 mg/kg	15 mg/kg	13.1	2.3
METH + Ch-mAb7F9	1 mg/kg	150 mg/kg	9.8	6.5

All data are from (Stevens et al. 2014b), except for the studies of METH only which are from (Rivière et al. 1999).
Please note the units for $t1/2$ for ch-mAb7F9 and METH are in days and hours, respectively.

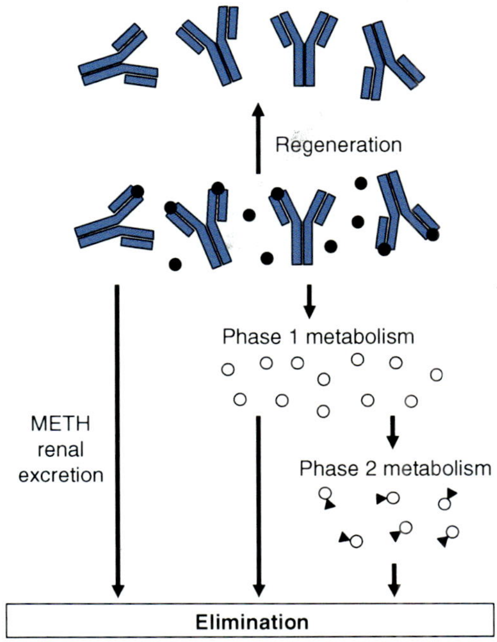

Fig. 9.2 Regeneration of anti-METH antibody binding capacity through continuous elimination of METH (*black circles*) from serum. Unbound METH is either excreted unchanged by the kidney or metabolized to Phase I (*open circle*) and Phase II METH metabolites (*open circles with attached triangle*). These in vivo METH elimination processes (e.g., metabolic and renal excretion) allow the long-acting mAb to become quickly available for more METH binding, which regenerates its capacity

This ability to restore METH binding capacity allows each molecule of anti-METH mAb to block or reduce the effects of many molecules of METH during its prolonged biological half-life. This mechanism of regeneration likely has major impact on the functional capacity of the mAb to neutralize METH effects, especially when METH is administered in excess of available mAb binding sites.

A clear understanding of how the antibodies function in vivo came through years of studying several prototype mAb medications. We will now discuss the discovery process and testing of these anti-METH mAb.

9.6 Selection of Anti-METH mAb Medications and Preclinical Testing

Our initial goal was to discover a METH-specific mAb with a K_d value of ≤10 nM. We set this criteria based on success with the preclinical testing of an anti-phencyclidine mAb medication with a K_d value of 1 nM for phencyclidine binding (Hardin et al. 2002). The first anti-METH mAb to achieve this criterion was mAb6H4. The lessons learned from the testing of this mAb (both good and bad) helped us establish many of the selection criteria needed to discover an optimized clinical candidate mAb.

The general methods and experimental strategies for selection and large-scale production of mAb are reported in previous publications (Peterson et al. 2007;

Carroll et al. 2009). In this section, a brief overview of the process will be described. To produce anti-METH mAb, we start by immunizing female BALB/c mice with a METH-conjugate vaccine (MCV). This MCV is composed of a carefully designed METH-like hapten and antigenic carrier protein such as ovalbumin or bovine serum albumin. After several months of booster immunizations to maximize anti-METH titers and affinity, we select a single mouse for use in generating high-affinity mAb. The selection of the optimal mouse is based on immunochemical characteristics of the anti-METH polyclonal antibodies in their serum.

The initial immunochemical criterion for selection of a candidate mouse includes high-affinity METH binding of the mouse antiserum (as measured by the dissociation constant [K_d] for METH), specificity for METH-like chemicals and drugs, and lack of significant cross-reactivity with other small-molecule ligands. Radioimmunoassays using a [^{3}H]-METH radioligand are used for these immunochemical studies (Owens et al. 1988; Peterson et al. 2007).

Initially, the affinity of mAb6H4 for METH was determined to be $K_d = 11$ nM (Byrnes-Blake et al. 2003), but with improvements in the radioimmunoassay determination, the K_d value was found to actually be 4 nM (Owens et al. 2011). MAb6H4 was highly specific for METH with <0.1 % cross-reactivity with a wide range of test drugs and compounds, which included chemicals that were structurally related and structurally unrelated to METH. The only exception was methylenedioxymethamphetamine (MDMA, commonly known as ecstasy). MAb6H4 bound (+)-MDMA (a drug of abuse administered as a racemic mixture) with a marginally higher affinity than METH. Besides (+)-MDMA, mAb6H4 showed negligible affinity for drugs like amphetamine or pseudoephedrine and no affinity for endogenous monoamines like dopamine or norepinephrine.

MAb6H4 was designed to have specificity for the (+)-METH enantiomer. This enantiomeric specificity was created by connecting the carrier protein to the para-position on the phenyl ring of METH distal to the chiral portion of the (+)-METH molecule (Peterson et al. 2007). Much of the illicit METH currently being produced contains both (+)-METH and (−)-METH, because it is synthesized using the phenyl-2-propenone production method (Maxwell and Brecht 2011). While the (−)-enantiomer of METH has some stimulant effects, it has a shorter duration of action and is less desirable to users than (+)-METH (Mendelson et al. 2006). Therefore, development of an anti-(+)-METH-specific mAb is the best strategy since production of antibodies against a racemic form of METH would lead to mAb binding of the less active, less addicting (−)-METH enantiomer. Binding to both enantiomers with high affinity could have a negative impact on the capacity of the mAb to bind the more active and highly addictive (+)-METH isomer.

Extensive preclinical testing of anti-METH mAb6H4 in rat models of METH abuse demonstrated efficacy in acute treatment scenarios. For example, in a METH overdose model, mAb6H4 (367 mg/kg) was administered 30 min after a 0.3, 1, or 3 mg/kg iv METH dose (0.3, 1, or 3 METH molecules per mAb binding site) followed by measurements of changes in METH-induced rearing events and distance traveled (Byrnes-Blake et al. 2003). In the 0.3 and 1 mg/kg METH groups, the number of rearing events and total distance traveled were both significantly reduced when compared to the baseline level of each METH dose before mAb treatment. Surprisingly, the two behavioral activity measurements were significantly increased in the mAb6H4-treated animals following a 3 mg/kg METH dose. This was initially a major concern since it suggested an additive or synergistic effect of high METH doses in the presence of antibody or that the antibody binding was perhaps serving as a sustained-release formulation for the METH. While these findings were difficult to understand at the time of the studies, it made us seek better direct measures and criteria for screening of sustained in vivo mAb function. It was also an early indication that anti-METH mAb6H4 had problems binding METH in vivo.

On the positive side, these data showed the mAb was capable of substantially increasing serum METH concentrations and immediately decreasing brain METH concentrations for at least 2.5 h. In a model of acute METH overdose, high-affinity mAb6H4 administration (367 mg/kg) was then compared to a very high dose (1000 mg/kg) of a lower-affinity mAb6H8 (METH K_d=250 nM). The mAb dosing occurred 30 min after a 1 mg/kg METH dose (Byrnes-Blake et al. 2005). Despite the substantially larger mAb6H8 dose, the mAb6H4 treatment resulted in significantly greater reduction in both METH-induced rearing (78 % vs. 27 %) and distance traveled (74 % vs. 35 %). These experiments provided evidence of the anti-METH mAb mechanism of action, the immediate anti-METH effects upon mAb administration, and the importance of high anti-METH mAb affinity for the attainment of anti-METH effects.

In other studies, mAb6H4 was administered prior to METH administration in an attempt to understand mAb effects on METH when given as a pretreatment. This pretreatment model was intended to simulate the use of the antibody for the clinical treatment of relapse to METH use in addicted patients.

In a pharmacokinetic study, mAb6H4 (503 mg/kg) was administered 17 h before a 1 mg/kg iv METH dose. This mAb6H4 dose was calculated to be equimolar in available mAb binding sites to the total body burden of METH administered (Laurenzana et al. 2003). This treatment dramatically increased area under the serum METH concentration-time curve (AUC) from 0 to 4.5 h. When compared to the AUC of vehicle control-treated rats after a 1 mg/kg METH dose, the AUC was 6600 % greater in the mAb6H4-treated rats. Importantly, brain METH AUC values in mAb6H4-treated rats were decreased by more than 60 %. Additionally, mAb6H4 significantly reduced METH concentrations in the kidney. It also showed that anti-METH mAb can reduce tissue concentrations, even though the mAb treatment did not decrease free METH concentrations in the serum compared to vehicle control. This lack of substantive changes in serum-free drug concentrations is a consistent finding in all of our studies of mAb treatment of METH and phencyclidine in rats, even though brain concentrations (and pharmacological effects) of the drugs of abuse are significantly lowered. We now know this high free drug concentration allows for the antibody binding capacity to be regenerated, as discussed earlier.

The next study was in a mAb pretreatment model designed to test the ability of high- and low-affinity anti-METH mAb to both protect against METH-induced effects and constantly reduce these METH effects over time. In these behavioral studies, rats were first preconditioned to repeated METH dosing until stable baseline values of locomotor activity were achieved (Byrnes-Blake et al. 2005). MAb6H4 (503 mg/kg) was then administered, followed by three 1 mg/kg METH challenges 1, 4, and 7 days later. Measurements of distance traveled and rearing behavior were determined immediately after each METH challenge dose. The much lower-affinity mAb6H8 (K_d for METH = 250 nM) was also tested in an identical manner. The dose of mAb6H8 (1000 mg/kg) was greater than the mAb6H4 dose in an attempt to partially compensate for its lower affinity. MAb6H4 treatment produced a significant reduction in METH-induced distance traveled on the first day after the first mAb administration, but it ceased to have a significant effect on post-mAb days 4 and 7. The mAb6H4 reduction in rearing was significant on all 3 days, but it slowly decreased over the course of the three METH administrations. As expected, the low-affinity mAb6H8 was less effective than mAb6H4, even though it was administered at a higher dose.

In a broader study of mAb6H4 efficacy, METH-induced locomotor activity and rearing were measured along with hemodynamics in a model of chronic METH use. The doses of mAb6H4 were 175, 300, or 525 mg/kg. The challenge dose of 1 mg/kg METH was administered 1 and 4 days after mAb6H4 (Gentry et al. 2006). The doses of mAb6H4 were equivalent to 0.32, 0.56, or 1 mol of mAb binding sites for each METH molecule, respectively. The highest mAb6H4 dose produced significant reductions in the duration of locomotor activity, blood pressure, and heart rate effects from 2 to 3 h to about 1 h, and there were significant reductions in locomotor activity and the heart rate and blood pressure area under the hemodynamic effect vs. time curves. In addition, the time to peak locomotor activity was decreased after the 1 mol-eq. mAb6H4 dose compared to the lower mAb6H4 doses. MAb6H4's protective effects only lasted for one METH challenge.

While extensive early pharmacokinetics, behavioral, and hemodynamic studies of mAb6H4 demonstrated the importance of mAb affinity as a prerequisite for therapeutic success in acute situations (McMillan et al. 2004; Byrnes-Blake et al. 2005), this series of studies also demonstrated the need for an antibody with a long-acting (e.g., weeks not days) METH binding function in vivo.

There are many potential reasons for why mAb6H4 appeared to lose function in vivo faster than expected (Byrnes-Blake et al. 2003, 2005; Gentry et al. 2006), but we eventually narrowed the cause down to two possibilities: increased clearance of the mAb protein (as indicated by a short half-life) or in vivo inactivation resulting in changes in K_d or B_{max}. To test these hypotheses, we devised in vivo tests (Laurenzana et al. 2009). First we measured the pharmacokinetic properties of several mAb in rats and determined there were no substantive differences in the clearance, volume of distribution, or half-life between any of the mAb. These pharmacokinetic studies indicated the mAb were long lasting in the vasculature, with an average half-life of about 1 week.

To test for long term in vivo changes in binding function (i.e., K_d and B_{max}), groups of rats were implanted with sc osmotic minipumps set to infuse 5.6 mg/kg/day of METH for 2 weeks. The rats were administered a 180 mg/kg dose of one of several candidate anti-METH mAb, including mAb6H4. A control group of rats without mAb treatment was used to determine baseline METH steady-state serum concentrations. Blood samples were collected over 2 weeks and the serum concentrations of METH were determined. We reasoned that the longest acting mAb would show the highest METH serum concentrations over time and that if some of the mAb were losing METH binding function (e.g., a decrease in B_{max}), they would show much lower METH concentrations over time.

During the first two hours after mAb6H4 dosing, METH serum concentrations were elevated compared to pre-mAb control values. However, relative to the METH concentration values in the longest acting mAb, there was a considerable loss of binding function before the 24 h time point and therefore a much shorter duration of binding action. MAb6H4 was one of several antibodies (e.g., mAb10D1 and mAb6H7) that quickly showed a substantial loss of METH binding (Fig. 9.3). However, other antibodies did not show this loss of METH binding over time (i.e., mAb9C10, mAb7F9, and mAb4G9). From this group, mAb7F9 and mAb4G9 became our lead candidates for development of a therapeutic anti-METH mAb.

All three of the longer acting mAb presented in Fig. 9.3 were originally discovered from mice immunized with a hapten containing a 10 molecule spacer group between the METH backbone structure of the hapten and the site of conjugation on the protein carrier. This hapten is designated as MO10. All of the inactivated mAb resulted from immunization of mice with an antigenic carrier protein coupled to a METH-like hapten containing a 4- or 6-molecule spacer group. Because of this observation, we realized the use of haptens with longer spacer arms could prevent inactivation of the mAb.

We concluded that loss of the mAb function over time was not the result of increased clearance of the protein. Measurements of K_d values before and after in vivo administration of mAb6H4 suggested the affinity was not changing over

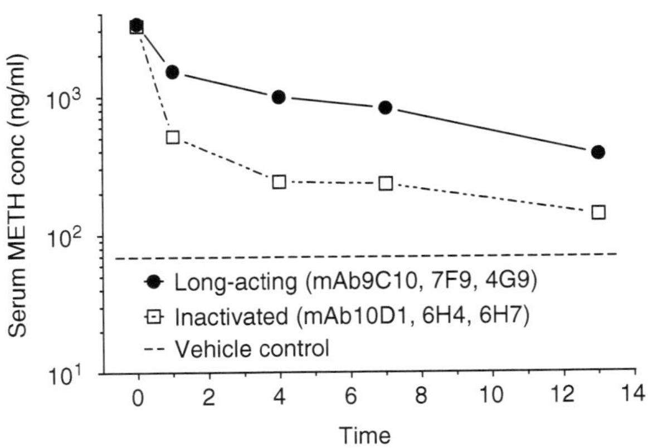

Fig. 9.3 Composite graph of average serum concentrations resulting from a 5.6 mg/kg/day sc METH dose to separate groups of male Sprague-Dawley rats after administration of long-acting mAb (*circles*) and inactivated mAb (*squares*). The horizontal dashed line shows the average METH steady-state concentration value resulting from the steady-state infusion of METH without mAb treatment. Data are summarized from previous publications (Laurenzana et al. 2009; Owens et al. 2011)

time. However the binding capacity (B_{max}) was changing. Results of more extensive testing of the mechanism for the loss of mAb6H4 activity in vivo will be reported in a future manuscript.

The production of mAb that are susceptible to inactivation in vivo could be an issue for other mAb targets (including non-drug abuse applications) and for polyclonal antibodies produced by active immunizations. For in vivo use of antibodies, we think it is very important to screen for long-term antibody function, before undertaking more extensive preclinical studies.

The hapten used to generate our best monoclonal antibodies (MO10) has other important structural features. It is linked to the aromatic group of METH at a distal site to the chiral center of the METH molecule. This allows (+)-METH stereospecificity for the resulting antibodies. It also has the 10-molecule linker group attached to the meta-site of METH's aromatic ring (Carroll et al. 2009, 2011). The previously used shorter linker group haptens were attached either at the meta- or para-positions of METH's aromatic ring. As stated earlier, these changes led to the production of high-affinity, long-acting mAb4G9 and mAb7F9 (Laurenzana et al. 2009). The cross-reactivity of these mAb for non-amphetamine-like stimulant drugs of abuse and for (−)-isomers is clinically insignificant (Peterson et al. 2007; Carroll et al. 2009). MAb4G9 is a murine IgG2b isotype antibody with a κ light chain that has a METH $K_d = 16$ nM and AMP $K_d = 110$ nM. MAb7F9 is a murine IgG1 isotype antibody with a κ light chain that has a METH $K_d = 8$ nM and an AMP $K_d = 270$ nM (Carroll et al. 2009; Stevens et al. 2014b; Laurenzana et al. 2014).

9.7 Comparisons of mAb7F9 and mAb4G9 as Possible Lead Candidates for Clinical Testing

Based on data from immunochemical studies (affinity, specificity), pharmacokinetic studies with and without METH, behavioral studies in rat models of METH abuse, and results of testing for long-term function, mAb7F9 and mAb4G9 were considered the lead candidates for conversion to a chimeric mouse/human form for use in clinical trials. Their affinity for METH was not substantially different (8 nM vs. 16 nM, respectively), and the relatively low affinity for AMP (270 nM vs. 110 nM, respectively) was not considered an important difference. Therefore, we considered other strengths and weaknesses of each antibody, including studies in which they were directly compared for efficacy against METH pharmacological effects.

Studies in male Sprague-Dawley rats by Laurenzana et al. (2014) tested four doses (from 36.2 to 362 mg/kg) of each mAb for their capacity to attenuate METH-induced locomotor activity following a 1 mg/kg METH dose. The mAb doses were calculated to result in 1:10 to 1:1 molar ratios of mAb binding sites to METH molecules at the time of mAb administration 30 min after METH dosing. METH pharmacokinetics in the presence of 362 mg/kg and 116 mg/kg mAb doses were determined in a separate group of rats. This study was useful for lead candidate selection because it was a direct comparison of the antibodies with a relatively simple study design, a range of mAb doses, and both behavioral and pharmacokinetic measures. By starting the behavioral comparisons at 30 min after METH dosing, we avoided much of the early stereotypic, horizontal motion inhibiting effects produced by amphetamine-like stimulants (Segal and Mandell 1974). We also reasoned that administration of mAb near the peak of horizontal motion activity (typically around 30 min at this METH dose) would be very useful in assessing the capacity of an anti-METH mAb to immediately reduce METH behavioral effects.

Both mAb7F9 and mAb4G9 treatment of the rats resulted in significant reduction of METH-induced distance traveled at mAb doses of ≥116 mg/kg. Only the 362 mg/kg mAb7F9 dose resulted in decreased total rearing or a decreased duration in locomotor activity. In the pharmacokinetic studies, both doses of each mAb substantially reduced the METH volume of distribution. Both doses of mAb7F9 and the higher dose of mAb4G9 significantly increased the METH AUC (34–360 min) compared to vehicle control. The higher mAb7F9 dose significantly increased METH serum AUC values relative to the same dose of mAb4G9. In contrast, both doses of mAb4G9 and the highest dose of mAb7F9 resulted in significantly elevated amphetamine (AMP) metabolite AUC (34–360 min) values compared to control values produced by METH administration alone. This AMP AUC value was significantly elevated in both mAb4G9 dose groups relative to their corresponding mAb7F9 groups.

MAb7F9, in addition to having better anti-METH dispositional and behavioral effects than mAb4G9, was more easily formulated for dosing in the preclinical studies. Considering that mAb7F9 had a higher affinity for METH than mAb4G9, it was not a surprise that it proved the better of the two antibodies.

Based on the overall in vitro and in vivo results and other preclinical data from testing of mAb4G9 and mAb7F9 in a rodent model of relapse to METH use (to be published), mAb7F9 was chosen as the best prototype medication. An additional study of chronic treatment with anti-METH mAb7F9 was then conducted to determine the long-term function of the antibody during repeated METH challenges.

9.8 Repeated METH Challenges of mAb7F9 Capacity over a Month Period

Considering the known executive control impairment, withdrawal, and craving in METH-addicted individuals (Koob and Volkow 2010), it is likely that METH-addicted patients will attempt to use METH during mAb treatment and poorly comply with the treatment regimen (Hillhouse et al. 2007). Thus an effective METH addiction treatment needs to provide constant protection against METH effects (i.e., at all times during the treatment regimen regardless of proximity to the time of administration). For patient safety, the mAb treatment must not result in additive or synergistic effects in the presence of METH, because addicted patients could decide to self-administer very high METH doses in an attempt to overwhelm the anti-METH mAb effects.

The doses of mAb7F9 used in these and other preclinical studies in rats are much higher than are currently feasible in humans. However, we made the assumption that these were proof of principle studies and that only human clinical trials can accurately determine the dose of mAb needed to produce efficacy in addicted patients. Anti-METH mAb therapy would not likely be a standalone medicine for chronic addiction. The antibody would be used to aid in prevention of adverse effects resulting from relapse to METH use. We also envision METH addiction therapy would include cognitive behavioral therapy to help patients learn better ways for coping with day-to-day life, dealing with craving, and the self-motivation needed to overcome their addiction. Behavioral treatments like these are not possible to include in rat models of addiction therapy.

Since previously described preclinical experiments showed that anti-METH mAb can acutely decrease the effects of METH, we wanted to test mAb7F9 in a chronic treatment scenario using male Sprague-Dawley rats (Hambuchen et al. 2014). The first dose of anti-METH mAb7F9 was administered as a 282 mg/kg loading dose followed by two weekly 141 mg/kg maintenance doses. The loading dose of mAb7F9 was used to rapidly bring the mAb to steady-state serum concentrations, which is a clinically relevant treatment strategy. MAb7F9 was dosed weekly since the half-life of the proteins was presumed to be about 1 week (Laurenzana et al. 2009).

To test the ability of mAb7F9 to continuously inhibit the effects of METH administration during the treatment regimen, vehicle- or mAb-treated male Sprague-Dawley rats were challenged with a total of seven 0.56 mg/kg METH doses. These METH challenge doses were administered every 3 or 4 days from day 0 until day 21. The mAb7F9 maintenance dose was sufficient to bind one-half of each METH challenge dose. Behavioral measures of horizontal movement and rearing were assessed for 4 h after each METH dose. METH and AMP serum concentrations were determined at 5 h after each METH dose.

To test the safety of mAb7F9 at METH doses beyond its binding capacity, a 1.68 mg/kg METH dose was given 10 and 14 days after the final dose of mAb7F9 (on experimental days 24 and 28, respectively). This produced METH serum concentrations that were 8- and 12-fold, respectively, greater than the number of mAb binding sites. This part of the study was designed to model the consequences of a patient missing a dose of antibody and then attempting to surmount the antibody protective effects with a significantly higher dose of METH. Behavioral measures of horizontal movement and rearing were again assessed. Five hours after the end of the last studies on day 28, rat blood and brain were removed for use in determining brain and serum METH and AMP concentration measurements after METH dosing on day 28 of the experiment.

MAb7F9 treatment resulted in significantly elevated METH concentrations after METH administration on days 0–21. It reduced total METH-induced locomotor activity (measured as distance traveled, 0–240 min post METH) after three of seven METH challenges and rearing after four of seven METH challenges. Our first analysis of these data suggested the effectiveness of the mAb7F9 treatment appeared to be decreasing with the repeated METH doses despite the continued function of mAb7F9 seen as elevations of total serum METH on each experimental day. We then considered that prior to mAb7F9 administration, the 0.56 mg/kg METH dose produced locomotor activity of about a 2 h duration. In the mAb7F9-treated animals, the behavioral measurements during the second hour of horizontal locomotor activity were significantly lower than those of the vehicle-treated animals after each challenge from days 0 to 21. These data showed mAb7F9 was substantially shortening the METH duration of action. Indeed the duration of locomotor activity was significantly reduced after five of the seven METH challenges doses on these days. Rearing events during the second hour of locomotor activity were also significantly reduced after six of the seven METH challenge doses administered (days 0–17).

In the second part of the study, after the 3-fold greater 1.68 mg/kg METH challenge dose on days 24 and 28 (10 and 14 days after the final mAb dose), the mAb7F9 treatment still increased METH serum concentrations, decreased METH brain concentrations on day 28, and reduced the duration of METH horizontal motion and rearing events. There were no signs of loss of in vivo function. While the results supporting the safety and efficacy of mAb7F9 treatment were promising, we did not study the effects on other critical organs like the heart. We concluded from these studies that mAb7F9 could continuously bind METH and reduce METH-induced stimulant effects even if mAb treatment is discontinued and the animals receive substantially higher doses of METH.

9.9 Design and Development of Chimeric mAb7F9

Once mouse anti-METH mAb7F9 was chosen as the lead candidate, it was converted to a form suitable for safe use in humans. Acceptable choices for possible FDA approval included a mouse/human chimeric monoclonal antibody, a humanized monoclonal antibody, or a fully human monoclonal antibody. The best choice for us was the production of a chimeric antibody because of the lower cost for conversion to an acceptable human dosage form and the desire to maintain critical features of the mouse anti-METH binding site.

The variable region from the mouse mAb7F9 was used as the starting template to create the new mouse/human chimeric anti-METH mAb called ch-mAb7F9. RNA was extracted from the hybridoma cell line that produced mAb7F9. Reverse transcription of the RNA was used to obtain the light- and heavy-chain cDNA sequences of the variable regions. These two sequences were joined to the coding sequences of the constant domains of a human IgG_{2K} antibody. This set of sequences was inserted into a Chinese hamster ovary cell line to establish a new cell line for production of ch-mAb7F9 (Stevens et al. 2014b).

Characterization of ch-mAb7F9 showed that it maintains high affinity for METH (K_d=6.9 nM vs. 7.7 nM for murine mAb7F9) (Stevens et al. 2014b). It also shows high affinity for the (+)-isomer of MDMA (K_I=6.7 nM). There was only negligible cross-reactivity with other structural analogues of METH (e.g., K_I for (+)-AMP=370 nM). There is no substantive cross-reactivity with other drugs, over-the-counter medications, neurotransmitters, or drugs of abuse. This precise specificity is important for both the efficacy and the safety of ch-mAb7F9. If the mAb had high affinity for a readily available legal drug like phenylephrine, an addicted individual could administer a large dose of the non-METH drug to saturate antibody binding sites and negate its effect. Additionally, any adverse effects resulting from patients consuming large doses of structurally related drugs could be a serious safety concern. Fortunately with ch-mAb7F9, this is not a likely issue.

As part of the strategy for improving the safety of the ch-mAb7F9 in humans, the murine mAb7F9 was changed from a mouse IgG_1 isotype to a human IgG_2 isotype. Unlike other human IgG isotypes like IgG_1, the human IgG_2 constant domain lacks significant complement-dependent activity. This reduces the possibility of activating constant region effector functions such as the ability to stimulate complement-dependent cytotoxicity. C1q binding is a requirement for this activity and the lack of C1q binding by ch-mAb7F9 suggested it did not have this function (Stevens et al. 2014b).

Male Sprague-Dawley rats administered ch-mAb7F9 in vivo remained healthy (Stevens et al. 2014b). This included stable weight and hematocrit values over time, and all rats appeared healthy at the end of the study. As with murine mAb7F9, ch-mAb7F9 has a long elimination half-life in rats. It is slightly longer than mAb7F9 with an approximate value of 11 days (Table 9.3). Importantly, the ch-mAb7F9 version of mAb7F9 has a long duration of METH binding function like the murine form. After pretreating rats with a 150 mg/kg dose of ch-mAb7F9, a 1 mg/kg METH dose is detectable in the serum well beyond 24 h. In contrast, early antibody prototypes like murine mAb6H4 are known to become inactive before this time point. Like murine mAb7F9, the half-life of METH is extended in the presence of ch-mAb7F9 (6.5 h rather than 1.1 h in absence of ch-mAb7F9), but this half-life is considerably shorter than the ~11 day half-life of the ch-mAb7F9. As discussed earlier in this review, this means METH can be eliminated in the presence of the mAb allowing regeneration of METH binding sites and allowing renewed protection against repeated METH administration.

Considered together, these preclinical data, along with many other forms of FDA required supporting documentation and testing, showed that ch-mAb7F9 was ready for clinical trials.

9.10 Clinical Trial of Anti-METH Chimeric mAb7F9

Ch-mAb7F9 has been tested in a first-in-human Phase 1a, double-blind, randomized, placebo-controlled, single iv dose study of safety and pharmacokinetics in healthy volunteers with no history of stimulant abuse (Stevens et al. 2014a). For the studies, subjects were assigned randomly into five ch-mAb7F9 dosing groups (0.2, 0.6, 2, 6, 20 mg/kg) with two of eight subjects in each group receiving placebo control. During the 3 weeks prior to dosing, subjects were screened, and then vehicle control or ch-mAb7F9 was infused over two hrs. After administration, each subject was observed for 48 h as an inpatient and then as an outpatient until day 147. The outpatient appointments were on a weekly basis for 6 weeks, followed by observations every 3 weeks for the remainder of the study. Blood samples were collected prior to ch-mAb7F9 administration and several blood samples were collected during the 48 h inpatient period. Less frequent blood sampling continued until the end of the study. An ELISA was used to determine serum ch-mAb7F9 concentrations. Pharmacokinetic parameters were determined by non-compartmental analysis. In addition, the serum samples were screened for human anti-chimeric antibodies (HACA) and tested by standard blood chemistry assays. Vital signs were observed and electrocardiograms (ECG) and physical examinations were performed.

Overall, ch-mAb7F9 was found to be safe at all doses tested. In vehicle- compared to ch-mAb7F9-treated subjects and with increasing dose, there did not appear to be any trends in occurrence, relatedness, or intensity of adverse events. The presence of HACA occurred in four of the 32 treated subjects in a non-dose-dependent manner. Also, the laboratory serum analysis, vital signs, and ECG measurements showed no important trends or changes.

The ch-mAb7F9 was also found to have favorable pharmacokinetic properties in humans. In the 2 to 20 mg/kg administered groups, there was an approximately 18-day half-life, an 8.5 ml/h clearance, and a 5.4 L volume of distribution, and in the two low-dose groups, there was an approximately 15-day half-life, a 10 ml/h clearance, and an approximately 5.2 L volume of distribution. As discussed previously, slow elimination and limited volume of distribution are both beneficial properties for a monoclonal antibody expected to both restrict entry to METH active sites as well as continuously maintain this activity for a substantial time period.

While ch-mAb7F9 shows clinical safety and useful pharmacokinetic properties and murine mAb7F9 shows acute and chronic anti-METH effects, the true efficacy of this medication will need to be tested in further clinical trials. The preclinical trials used doses of anti-METH mAb7F9 that are relatively high for humans (i.e., >20 mg/kg). We calculate that a 20 mg/kg dose of ch-mAb7F9 provides sufficient mAb binding sites to bind serum METH concentrations resulting from a 30 mg dose (Stevens et al. 2014a). This METH dose produces an ~110 ng/ml serum concentration which could be fully bound by the greater than 50 μg/ml ch-mAb7F9 concentrations which were maintained for greater than 5 weeks after a 20 mg/kg mAb dose. While these mAb concentrations are only accounting for METH in the serum, in the Martell et al. (2009) active vaccination study for cocaine abuse, patients who achieved anti-cocaine antibody titers of ≥43 μg/ml had a significant reduction in cocaine use. This concentration is similar to the aforementioned 50 μg/ml target value. That these relatively low antibody concentrations resulted in an observable beneficial therapeutic effect is encouraging, but not entirely surprising considering the effects of mAb on METH doses in substantial excess of available binding sites (Laurenzana et al. 2014; Hambuchen et al. 2014). Further, each ch-mAb7F9 molecule administered has the same high affinity for METH while the anti-cocaine vaccine generates polyclonal antibodies of a variety of affinities.

Because of the unique physiological recycling of mAb (Lobo et al. 2004; Wang et al. 2008), they are expected to have long half-lives and a likely long duration of action. As discussed earlier in this review, mAb frequency of dosing will likely be based on ch-mAb half-life. This means treatment once every 3 weeks. To achieve maximal steady-state effects, ch-mAb7F9 would have to be administered for at least four half-lives (i.e., about 8–12 weeks). A loading dose given over the first week or two of treatment is a possible option to more rapidly achieve steady-state conditions. Examples of predicted concentrations achieved after four different maintenance doses are shown in Table 9.4. The frequency of dosing in each case is once every 3 weeks.

Figure 9.4 shows the predicted serum mAb concentrations after administering 5 mg/kg ch-mAb7F9 every 3 weeks with and without a loading dose of 8.8 mg/kg. Note that without the initial 8.8 mg/kg loading dose, approximately four half-lives are required to achieve steady-state concentrations (C_{ss}, C_{max}, and C_{min}) and several administrations are required to achieve serum mAb concentrations above the previ-

Table 9.4 Predicted steady-state (C_{ss}), minimum (C_{min}), and maximum (C_{max}) plasma concentrations of ch-mAb7F9 in human subjects after four different dosing regimens of ch-mAb7F9 administered once every 3 weeks (ch-mAb7F9 $t_{1/2}$ = 18 days)

Maintenance dose (mg/kg)[a]	3	5	10	20
C_{ss} (µg/ml)	53	88	176	319
C_{min} (µg/ml)	34	57	113	215
C_{max} (µg/ml)	78	131	261	460

[a]The 20 mg/kg treatment values for ch-mAb7F9 are based on pharmacokinetic parameters from a 20 mg/kg experimental group with an average body weight of 72 kg in the studies of Stevens et al. (2014a). The concentration calculated for the other dose groups is based on pharmacokinetic parameters from a 6 mg/kg experimental group with an average body weight of 76 kg.

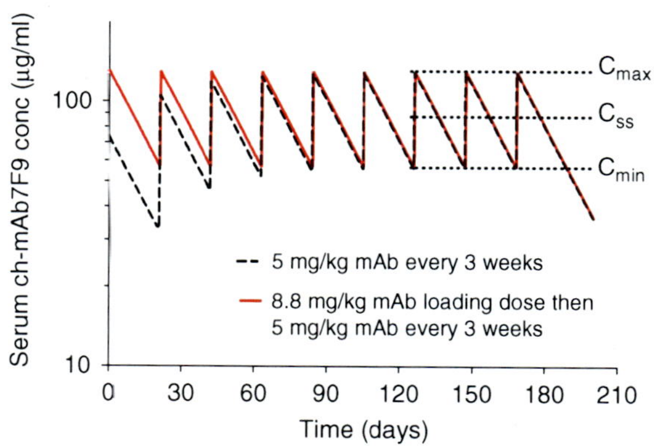

Fig. 9.4 Example predicted serum ch-mAb7F9 concentrations over a >6 month time period. The chronic administration included 5 mg/kg dose every 3 weeks with an 8.8 mg/kg loading dose (*solid line*) starting at time zero or without a loading dose (*small dashed line*). The dotted lines in the top right depict final values for C_{max}, C_{ss}, and C_{min} (see Table 9.4 for actual values after a 5 mg/kg dose). The lower bolder horizontal dashed line depicts an example 50 µg/ml target value for mAb serum concentrations. Pharmacokinetic parameters used to calculate these predicted values were reported by Stevens et al. (2014a)

ously mentioned example target value of 50 μg/ml of ch-mAb7F9. As with small-molecule medications, the mAb loading dose can result in drug concentrations within the desired range at the start of therapy.

Importantly, even patients who are immune compromised can be dosed so that they have high anti-METH antibody serum concentrations. Assuming the antibody does not become antigenic in the patient, the major limitation is cost. However, like most medications, cost can be decreased with improvements in mAb production. Due to its specific anti-METH action, this mAb therapy could likely be administered with any concurrent medication, other future small molecules for treating METH addiction, or even a carefully designed MCV (Carrera et al. 2000; Roiko et al. 2008; Cornish et al. 2011).

9.11 Future Directions and Conclusions

Our preclinical study of chronic mAb7F9 treatment (Hambuchen et al. 2014) showed that the mAb7F9 can maintain anti-METH activity for an extended period of time and in the presence of large doses of METH in a rat model of a patient attempting to overwhelm the binding capacity of METH. However, this only showed the inhibition of a METH-induced CNS effect. Safety data is still needed concerning peripheral toxicities including cardiovascular toxicity (Stevens et al. 2014a). The safety of METH in the presence of ch-mAb7F9 will be determined in a series of planned rat studies (Stevens et al. 2014a). Assuming safety of the combination of METH and ch-mAb7F9 is demonstrated in rats, ch-mAb7F9 can then be tested in Phase 1b human trials, in which the in vivo safety of combined use of METH and ch-mAb7F9 will be ascertained. While safety is the primary concern with the Phase 1b study, this study will also allow the collection of some early efficacy data. Though the planned METH challenge regimen will not test the ability of ch-mAb7F9 treatment to decrease use, it will allow for evaluation of the treatment's capabilities to alter the subjective (e.g., euphoria, energy, dollar value of METH dose) and physiological (e.g., blood pressure) effects of METH.

The results of clinical testing of this first-generation anti-METH ch-mAb should help to define the criteria for testing of antibody-based medications for the treatment of drug abuse. If needed, it is also possible to make improvements in the protein sequence that could improve the affinity for the target drug of abuse, extend the half-life of the protein, or reduce antigenicity. In addition to improving efficacy, these changes could also lower the doses and reduce cost.

In conclusion, developing specific medications for the treatment of METH addiction is challenging. A major hurdle is the inability to protect patients from impulsive, sporadic relapse to METH use, especially during the early stages of therapy. Protecting patients from the powerful rewarding effects of a relapse to METH use during their most vulnerable periods could be accomplished by treatment with a long-lasting anti-METH mAb medication.

Funding Sources Research funding was provided by the National Institutes of Health; the National Institute on Drug Abuse Grants DA11560, DA028915, and DA031944; the National Center for Advancing Translational Sciences (Grant ULITR000039); and the Arkansas Biosciences Institute (the major research component of the Arkansas Tobacco Settlement Proceeds Act of 2000).

Notes S. Michael Owens and W. Brooks Gentry are Chief Scientific Officer and Chief Medical Officer, respectively, and have financial interests in InterveXion Therapeutics, LLC, a pharmaceutical biotech company, whose main interest is the development of antibody medications for the treatment of human diseases, including drug abuse.

References

Abreu ME, Bigelow GE, Fleisher L, Walsh SL. Effect of intravenous injection speed on responses to cocaine and hydromorphone in humans. Psychopharmacology (Berl). 2001;154:76–84.

Brensilver M, Heinzerling KG, Shoptaw S. Pharmacotherapy of amphetamine-type stimulant dependence: an update. Drug Alcohol Rev. 2013;32:449–60. doi:10.1111/dar.12048.

Byrnes-Blake KA, Laurenzana EM, Carroll FI, et al. Pharmacodynamic mechanisms of monoclonal antibody-based antagonism of (+)-methamphetamine in rats. Eur J Pharmacol. 2003;461:119–28.

Byrnes-Blake KA, Laurenzana EM, Landes RD, et al. Monoclonal IgG affinity and treatment time alters antagonism of (+)-methamphetamine effects in rats. Eur J Pharmacol. 2005;521:86–94.

Carrera MR, Ashley JA, Zhou B, et al. Cocaine vaccines: antibody protection against relapse in a rat model. Proc Natl Acad Sci U S A. 2000;97:6202–6.

Carroll FI, Abraham P, Gong PK, et al. The synthesis of haptens and their use for the development of monoclonal antibodies for treating methamphetamine abuse. J Med Chem. 2009;52:7301–9. doi:10.1021/jm901134w.

Carroll FI, Blough BE, Pidaparthi RR, et al. Synthesis of mercapto-(+)-methamphetamine haptens and their use for obtaining improved epitope density on (+)-methamphetamine conjugate vaccines. J Med Chem. 2011;54:5221–8.

Cook CE, Jeffcoat AR, Hill JM, et al. Pharmacokinetics of methamphetamine self-administered to human subjects by smoking S-(+)-methamphetamine hydrochloride. Drug Metab Dispos. 1993;21:717–23.

Cornish KE, Harris AC, LeSage MG, et al. Combined active and passive immunization against nicotine: minimizing monoclonal antibody requirements using a target antibody concentration strategy. Int Immunopharmacol. 2011;11:1809–15. doi:10.1016/j.intimp.2011.07.009.

Cruickshank CC, Dyer KR. A review of the clinical pharmacology of methamphetamine. Addiction. 2009;104:1085–99. doi:10.1111/j.1360-0443.2009.02564.x.

Diagnostics Q. Quest Diagnostics Drug Testing Index ™. 2012. In: www.questdiagnostics.com. http://www.questdiagnostics.com/home/physicians/health-trends/drug-testing. Accessed 24 Mar 2015.

Gentry WB, Laurenzana EM, Williams DK, et al. Safety and efficiency of an anti-(+)-methamphetamine monoclonal antibody in the protection against cardiovascular and central nervous system effects of (+)-methamphetamine in rats. Int Immunopharmacol. 2006;6:968–77.

Gentry WB, Rüedi-Bettschen D, Owens SM. Development of active and passive human vaccines to treat methamphetamine addiction. Hum Vaccin. 2009;5:206–13.

Hambuchen MD, Rüedi-Bettschen D, Williams DK, et al. Treatment of rats with an anti-(+)-methamphetamine monoclonal antibody shortens the duration of action of repeated (+)-methamphetamine challenges over a one month period. Vaccine. 2014. doi:10.1016/j.vaccine.2014.09.025.

Hardin JS, Wessinger WD, Wenger GR, et al. A single dose of monoclonal anti-phencyclidine IgG offers long-term reductions in phencyclidine behavioral effects in rats. J Pharmacol Exp Ther. 2002;302:119–26.

Hillhouse MP, Marinelli-Casey P, Gonzales R, et al. Predicting in-treatment performance and post-treatment outcomes in methamphetamine users. Addiction. 2007;102 Suppl 1:84–95. doi:10.1111/j.1360-0443.2007.01768.x.

Koob GF, Volkow ND. Neurocircuitry of addiction. Neuropsychopharmacology. 2010;35:217–38. doi:10.1038/npp.2009.110.

Kresina TF, Normand J, Khalsa J, et al. Addressing the need for treatment paradigms for drug-abusing patients with multiple morbidities. Clin Infect Dis. 2004;38 Suppl 5:S398–401. doi:10.1086/421403.

Laurenzana EM, Byrnes-Blake KA, Milesi-Hallé A, et al. Use of anti-(+)-methamphetamine monoclonal antibody to significantly alter (+)-methamphetamine and (+)-amphetamine disposition in rats. Drug Metab Dispos. 2003;31:1320–6. doi:10.1124/dmd.31.11.1320.

Laurenzana EM, Hendrickson HP, Carpenter D, et al. Functional and biological determinants affecting the duration of action and efficacy of anti-(+)-methamphetamine monoclonal antibodies in rats. Vaccine. 2009;27:7011–20. doi:10.1016/j.vaccine.2009.09.072.

Laurenzana EM, Stevens MW, Frank JC, et al. Pharmacological effects of two anti-methamphetamine monoclonal antibodies: supporting data for lead candidate selection for clinical development. Hum Vaccin Immunother. 2014. doi:10.4161/hv.29707.

Lobo ED, Hansen RJ, Balthasar JP. Antibody pharmacokinetics and pharmacodynamics. J Pharm Sci. 2004;93:2645–68.

Martell B, Orson F, Poling J, et al. Cocaine vaccine for the treatment of cocaine dependence in methadone-maintained patients: a randomized, double-blind, placebo-controlled efficacy trial. Arch Gen Psychiatry. 2009;66:1116.

Maxwell JC, Brecht M-L. Methamphetamine: here we go again? Addict Behav. 2011;36:1168–73. doi:10.1016/j.addbeh.2011.07.017.

McMillan DE, Hardwick WC, Li M, et al. Effects of murine-derived anti-methamphetamine monoclonal antibodies on (+)-methamphetamine self-administration in the rat. J Pharmacol Exp Ther. 2004;309:1248–55. doi:10.1124/jpet.103.061762.

Mendelson J, Jones RT, Upton R, Jacob P. Methamphetamine and ethanol interactions in humans. Clin Pharmacol Ther. 1995;57:559–68. doi:10.1016/0009-9236(95)90041-1.

Mendelson J, Uemura N, Harris D, et al. Human pharmacology of the methamphetamine stereoisomers. Clin Pharmacol Ther. 2006;80:403–20. doi:10.1016/j.clpt.2006.06.013.

Newton TF, De La Garza R, Kalechstein AD, et al. Theories of addiction: methamphetamine users' explanations for continuing drug use and relapse. Am J Addict. 2009;18:294–300. doi:10.1080/10550490902925920.

Nicosia N, Pacula RL, Kilmer B, et al. The economic cost of methamphetamine use in the United States, 2005. Santa Monica: Rand Corporation; 2009.

Owens SM, Atchley WT, Hambuchen MD, et al. Monoclonal antibodies as pharmacokinetic antagonists for the treatment of (+)-methamphetamine addiction. CNS Neurol Disord Drug Targets. 2011;10:892–8.

Owens SM, Zorbas M, Lattin DL, et al. Antibodies against arylcyclohexylamines and their similarities in binding specificity with the phencyclidine receptor. J Pharmacol Exp Ther. 1988;246:472–8.

Peterson EC, Gunnell M, Che Y, et al. Using hapten design to discover therapeutic monoclonal antibodies for treating methamphetamine abuse. J Pharmacol Exp Ther. 2007;322:30–9. doi:10.1124/jpet.106.117150.

Rivière GJ, Byrnes KA, Gentry WB, Owens SM. Spontaneous locomotor activity and pharmacokinetics of intravenous methamphetamine and its metabolite amphetamine in the rat. J Pharmacol Exp Ther. 1999;291:1220–6.

Roiko SA, Harris AC, Keyler DE, et al. Combined active and passive immunization enhances the efficacy of immunotherapy against nicotine in rats. J Pharmacol Exp Ther. 2008;325:985–93. doi:10.1124/jpet.107.135111.

Rowland M, Tozer TN. Clinical pharmacokinetics. 3rd ed. Baltimore: Williams & Wilkins; 1995.

Rüedi-Bettschen D, Wood SL, Gunnell MG, et al. Vaccination protects rats from methamphetamine-induced impairment of behavioral responding for food. Vaccine. 2013;31:4596–602. doi:10.1016/j.vaccine.2013.07.038.

Schiorring E. Amphetamine induced selective stimulation of certain behaviour items with concurrent inhibition of others in an open-field test with rats. Behaviour. 1971;39:1–17.

Segal DS, Mandell AJ. Long-term administration of d-amphetamine: progressive augmentation of motor activity and stereotypy. Pharmacol Biochem Behav. 1974;2:249–55.

Sellings LHL, Clarke PBS. Segregation of amphetamine reward and locomotor stimulation between nucleus accumbens medial shell and core. J Neurosci. 2003;23:6295–303.

Shoptaw S, Huber A, Peck J, et al. Randomized, placebo-controlled trial of sertraline and contingency management for the treatment of methamphetamine dependence. Drug Alcohol Depend. 2006;85:12–8. doi:10.1016/j.drugalcdep.2006.03.005.

State Summaries of Client Admissions Data: Treatment Episode Data Set (TEDS). Substance abuse and mental health services administration. Rockville; 2012. http://wwwdasis.samhsa.gov/webt/newmapv1.htm. Accessed 16 Mar 2015.

Stevens MW, Henry RL, Owens SM, et al. First human study of a chimeric anti-methamphetamine monoclonal antibody in healthy volunteers. MAbs. 2014a;6:1649–56. doi:10.4161/19420862.2014.976431.

Stevens MW, Tawney RL, West CM, et al. Preclinical characterization of an anti-methamphetamine monoclonal antibody for human use. MAbs. 2014b;6:547–55. doi:10.4161/mabs.27620.

Sulzer D, Sonders MS, Poulsen NW, Galli A. Mechanisms of neurotransmitter release by amphetamines: a review. Prog Neurobiol. 2005;75:406–33. doi:10.1016/j.pneurobio.2005.04.003.

Tiihonen J, Kuoppasalmi K, Föhr J, et al. A comparison of aripiprazole, methylphenidate, and placebo for amphetamine dependence. Am J Psychiatry. 2007;164:160–2. doi:10.1176/ajp.2007.164.1.160.

Wang W, Wang EQ, Balthasar JP. Monoclonal antibody pharmacokinetics and pharmacodynamics. Clin Pharmacol Ther. 2008;84:548–58. doi:10.1038/clpt.2008.170.

White SJ, Hendrickson HP, Atchley WT, et al. Treatment with a monoclonal antibody against methamphetamine and amphetamine reduces maternal and fetal rat brain concentrations in late pregnancy. Drug Metab Dispos. 2014;42:1285–91. doi:10.1124/dmd.114.056879.

Part III
Enzymes

Chapter 10
Enzyme-Based Cocaine Pharmacotherapies: Current Status and Projections for the Future

James H. Woods and Chang-Guo Zhan

Abbreviations

Albu-CocH	Albumin-tagged cocaine hydrolase
CocE	Cocaine esterase
CocH	Cocaine hydrolase
PBS	Phosphate-buffered saline
DM CocE	Double mutant cocaine esterase
PEG CCRQ CocE	Pegylated CocE with the dimer tightly bound
MDMA	Methylenedioxymethamphetamine

Cocaine is an alkaloid, present in the leaves of the coca plant that grows in the mountainous portions of South America. The coca leaf has been used for centuries by the human populace in these locations as an orally consumed or buccally absorbed substance. Other routes of cocaine salt or cocaine base administration, e.g., intranasal, smoked, or intravenous, became more common among North and South American as well as European recreational users once cocaine was isolated from the coca leaf and could be easily transported worldwide. Administration of concentrated cocaine in any form is far more dangerous, in terms of both acute toxicity and risk of addiction.

J.H. Woods (✉)
Department of Pharmacology and Psychology, University of Michigan, Ann Arbor, MI, USA
e-mail: jhwoods@umich.edu

C.-G. Zhan
Department of Pharmaceutical Sciences, College of Pharmacy, University of Kentucky, Lexington, KY, USA

I.D. Montoya (ed.), *Biologics to Treat Substance Use Disorders: Vaccines, Monoclonal Antibodies, and Enzymes*, DOI 10.1007/978-3-319-23150-1_10

10.1 Toxic Effects

Patients with cocaine overdose usually present to the emergency department with chest pain; have increased blood pressure, heart rate, and body temperature; and are in an agitated state. If the bout of cocaine use has been long, evidence of paranoia and delirium may be present. These symptoms are difficult to separate from amphetamine intoxication, and discussions with the patient himself, friends that accompanied him to the emergency department, and a urine assay for benzoylecgonine, a cocaine metabolite, may be necessary for a differential diagnosis.

Cocaine achieves its effects in the body and brain through several mechanisms. It blocks the reuptake of three biogenic monoamine neurotransmitters (norepinephrine, dopamine, and serotonin) in the synaptic cleft upon their release – thus enhancing the intensity and duration of action of each of these neurotransmitters. In addition, and at higher concentrations, it can produce local anesthesia by blocking neuronal voltage-gated sodium channels. These combined actions produce a large number of toxic effects throughout the body and brain. Vasoconstrictive and sympathomimetic effects predominate: blood pressure and heart rate are increased – usually in a dose-related manner. Cocaine can also enhance aspects of inflammation and blood clotting factors (Zimmerman 2012). Hemorrhagic or ischemic stroke is a potential outcome of cocaine intoxication, the first due to elevated blood pressure and the second from the vasoconstrictive effects of the stimulant. Hyperthermia can result from disruption of central temperature regulation, compounded by increased motor activity. The possibility of myocardial infarction is the primary concern in case of cocaine overdose. Increases in heart rate, blood pressure, and blood clotting tendency are major contributing factors to the risk of heart attack. Other cardiac-related problems include atrial and ventricular arrhythmias as well as the potential for aortic dissection. Cocaine can also have deleterious effects on the pulmonary, renal, musculoskeletal, and gastrointestinal systems (Zimmerman 2012). When overdose patients present in emergency rooms with chest pain, lives are seldom lost with appropriate care (McCord et al. 2008). Nevertheless, symptoms of cocaine overdose, including convulsions and delirium, require extensive supportive therapy and cannot be treated simply. Unfortunately, the treatment of cocaine overdose is entirely symptomatic. The recommended treatment of the agitated mental state is administration of benzodiazepines. These drugs also reduce the likelihood of cocaine-induced seizures. Treatment of increased blood pressure and body temperature proceeds as they would for these symptoms in the absence of cocaine overdose.

Although many of the issues that can result from cocaine overdose are not amenable to pharmacotherapy (e.g., aortic dissection, myocardial infarction), if it was possible to remove cocaine quickly from the body, a majority of the signs of cocaine toxicity (agitation, increased heart rate, blood pressure, and body temperature) would resolve. This in turn would reduce the likelihood that more serious problems would develop and would permit treatment, surgical or otherwise, of remaining symptoms in the absence of high cocaine blood levels. Both of the enzyme therapies discussed in this presentation have the potential for dramatically increasing the rate of cocaine metabolism, effectively terminating its action, and permitting a careful evaluation of the patient in the absence of the instigating substance. These therapies would also be helpful in diagnosis of the nature of the ingested toxin. Only people suffering from cocaine intoxication would be helped by the enzyme therapy, establishing whether or not cocaine is the culprit or whether ingestion of other drugs such as amphetamine or MDMA or an acute psychotic episode is responsible for presenting symptoms. Being able to reduce the amount of cocaine present in plasma rapidly would be extremely useful, and simple, relative to dealing with each presenting symptom individually. In these circumstances, time can be of the essence for therapeutic usefulness.

10.2 Abuse Liability

Cocaine has presented complex problems of abuse for a long time, essentially, since it was introduced into medicine in the late nineteenth century. The number of people who are abusing cocaine at any one time tends to fluctuate with a variety of environmental factors. The levels of abuse in the United States were much larger in the 1980s, for example, than they are now and have retreated dramatically in the last several years. However, cocaine use is on the upswing in Europe where there may be many more users than currently in North America (Zimmerman 2012). In addition, as long as the drug remains available and inexpensive, its reinforcing properties are such that its abuse will remain a problem for a substantial number of people. With cocaine abuse comes the likelihood of potentially fatal cocaine overdose. There are no currently available FDA-approved pharmacotherapies for either acute cocaine intoxication or chronic cocaine abuse.

Although the enhanced effect of all biogenic amines through reuptake blockade is likely the strongest contributor to both the peripheral and central toxic effects of cocaine, it is the enhanced effect of dopamine alone that is thought to contribute most to cocaine's central stimulus effects. This includes the strong reinforcing effect that is the basis of cocaine's abuse liability. Although this suggests that dopamine antagonists should be very effective and quite selective in reducing the effects of dopamine and treating both abuse and toxicity, this seems not to be the case. A great many studies of a wide variety of general and selective dopamine antagonists have yielded mostly negative results in behavioral models of cocaine abuse (Pierce et al. 2012). Although we are continuing to learn more about the nature of dopamine's actions, and scientists are developing more selective dopamine antagonists (e.g., Newman et al. 2012), it seems unlikely at this point that treatment of cocaine abuse will come from compounds that act at the dopamine transporter or receptors.

Although the chronic abuse of cocaine has not been described definitively in nearly the detail as have the effects of acute intoxication, it seems clear that the pattern is one of long periods of intense use (binges or runs) that lead to sustained periods of intoxication, sometimes on the order of days. These episodes may be interrupted by variable periods of time when cocaine is not used, typically followed by a relapse to another run of cocaine intoxication.

For appropriate pharmacotherapy of cocaine abuse, it is likely that intoxication will have to be prevented whenever it might occur – either from the continuation of a binge or from a relapse to cocaine use. This requires a sustained capacity to interrupt and prevent the actions of cocaine for weeks, if not months, on a continuous basis. This is a far more complex problem of pharmacotherapy compared with that of acute intoxication. In both acute intoxication and prolonged cocaine abuse, a pharmacokinetic approach to removing cocaine has distinct advantages over pharmacodynamic approaches. A compound that attaches strongly to cocaine in the periphery, is too large to cross the blood-brain barrier, and thus serves as a sink for central cocaine could quickly reverse the central effects of the drug. If such a compound also metabolizes the cocaine and thereby frees itself to bind to another cocaine molecule, the advantages are even more striking. This is the profile of action of both the bacteria-based and cholinesterase-based enzymes being developed for these anti-cocaine indications.

10.3 In Vivo Evaluation of Pharmacotherapies

There are procedures designed to measure the ability of compounds to modify the toxic effects of cocaine, as well as procedures to measure the ability of compounds to modify the abuse-related effects of cocaine. Toxic effects are typically evaluated in rats or mice, although some studies of the effects of CocE on cocaine-induced blood pressure and heart rate measures have also been done in rhesus monkeys (Collins et al. 2012). Evaluations in rodents can involve measures of cocaine-induced death, which usually follows a pattern of increased heart rate and blood pressure, hypermobility, seizure, and death. These develop over a period of about 5 min following intraperitoneal administration of a lethal dose (180 mg/kg) of cocaine (Wood et al. 2010). The ability to interrupt this pattern of toxic effects can be measured by giving the rodent a pretreatment with an anti-cocaine enzyme and observing the number of animals that proceed to die. The duration of action of the enzyme can be established by lengthening the time between enzyme administration and cocaine administration. Since treatment of cocaine overdose is going to occur following the onset of signs of toxicity, this model of cocaine overdose can also involve administration of the enzyme once signs of cocaine toxicity have developed (Wood et al 2010).

10.4 Behavioral Measures of Cocaine's Abuse Liability and Its Treatment

Two measures of how anti-cocaine enzymes can reduce cocaine's abuse liability are particularly popular. Both evaluate the ability of the enzymes to reduce the stimulus effects of cocaine. One, used primarily to evaluate CocE, is simply to establish cocaine as a reinforcing stimulus in self-administration assays. Rats or monkeys are given several hours each day during which they can respond on a lever and receive response-contingent intravenous injections of small doses of cocaine. The availability of cocaine is typically signaled by the illumination of a light in the animals' working environment. The number of responses required to earn each cocaine injection can be varied, as can the amount of time between the opportunities to respond for the drug. Under these conditions, experienced animals show short latencies to respond when the stimulus light is illuminated and earn substantial amounts of cocaine. Rates of responding typically decrease as the dose per injection of cocaine is increased, reflecting the feedback effects of accumulated cocaine on the animals' behavior. When saline replaces cocaine, rates of responding may increase briefly, and then decline, indicating "extinction" of responding in the absence of cocaine delivery. The ability of presession administration of anti-cocaine enzymes to change rates of responding maintained by cocaine to those that are more like saline-maintained responding will reflect the potential of these enzymes to block the stimulus effects of cocaine that lead to its abuse. Dose-related and time-course-related effects of the enzymes can be established in both rats and rhesus monkeys using these self-administration procedures. Control procedures involve the use of food or drugs other than cocaine to maintain responding. If the enzymes do not modify non-cocaine-maintained responding, it is an indication that general motivational and behavioral processes are not affected by the enzyme, and the blocking effect is directed specifically at cocaine.

The other measure is a model of cocaine-induced reinstatement of previously established cocaine self-administration. This has been used extensively to evaluate the potential therapeutic effects of CocH. Rats are given the opportunity to self-administer cocaine, much as described above. The cocaine is then removed from the situation, saline replaces the cocaine, and behavior gradually declines. Passive, experimenter-delivered administration of i.p. cocaine or other drugs with stimulus properties in common with cocaine (e.g., amphetamine, methylphenidate) elicit increased responding, even when cocaine is not returned to the situation as a response consequence. The rates of responding following stimulant administration are related to the dose of stimulant given. Saline does not elicit responding. This means that anti-cocaine enzymes that make cocaine's stimulus effects resemble those of saline will markedly reduce the ability of cocaine to reinstate behavior. The duration of action of the enzymes can be evaluated by testing the effects of cocaine on a regular basis over time. This is possible because cocaine continues to reinstate responding even if long periods of time (months) occur between injections of the stimulant.

10.5 Characterization of Enzymatic Therapy for Acute Toxicity

Cocaine's chemical structure is shown in Fig. 10.1a. In the body of humans and other animals, cocaine is attacked at the ester bridge (shown by the arrow) by endogenous butyrylcholinesterase which reduces cocaine to virtually inactive metabolites. Native butyrylcholinesterase activity is too inefficient, even at large doses, to be of therapeutic value, but this endogenous enzyme has been modified to much more active hydrolases by the Zhan group (Pan et al. 2005, 2007; Zheng et al. 2008; Xue et al. 2011) and these form the basis for much promise in pharmacotherapy of

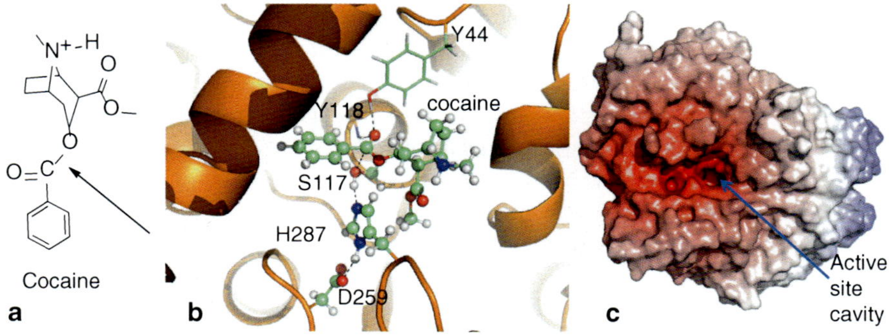

Fig. 10.1 (**a**) Molecular structure of cocaine in which the arrow points to the ester bond to be broken during butyrylcholinesterase-catalyzed hydrolysis of cocaine. (**b**) CocE-cocaine binding structure modeled by Liu et al. (2009). (**c**) Space-filled model of CocE

acute cocaine toxicity and abuse, as discussed below. A problem with the development of mammalian enzymes for therapeutics is that it is extremely difficult to produce these enzymes in the large quantities required for evaluation, let alone therapy. This issue has been largely overcome by recent developments (Xue et al. 2013; Larrimore et al. 2013). The advantage of mammalian enzymes such as butyrylcholinesterase is that they can be generated from the particular mammal that is under study and avoid the potential hazards of immunological reactions that can cause allergic responses or can simply remove the protein quickly from the circulation. Bacterial enzymes, on the other hand, have the advantage of being easy to produce in large quantities using bacterium such as *E. coli*, but either additional processing of the enzyme is necessary to remove any bacterial endotoxins or a form of *E. coli* that does not make endotoxins (Meredith et al. 2007) must be used; the possibility of immune responses to a bacterial enzyme continues to carry risk.

10.5.1 Bacterial Cocaine Esterase

An inventive group of British investigators (Bresler et al. 2000) found a form of esterase in a strain of the *Rhodococcus* bacterium growing in the soil around the roots of the coca plant. They isolated and purified this esterase, named it cocaine esterase (CocE), and proceeded to characterize its enzymatic activity. They found that it converts cocaine to ecgonine methyl ester and benzoate, providing an eventual source of nitrogen and carbon as food for the bacterium. The enzyme was highly efficient, much more so than any other naturally occurring enzyme that breaks down cocaine. They sequenced and crystallized the esterase and found that it is composed of 574 amino acids arranged in three domains (Larsen et al. 2002). The active site is located at the intersection of the three domains. Figure 10.1b depicts cocaine located in the active site of the enzyme, and Fig. 10.1c shows a space-filling drawing of the CocE enzyme.

Turner et al. (2002) added significantly to the cellular characterization of CocE by finding that a naturally occurring combination (transesterification) of ethanol and cocaine, called cocaethylene, is also destroyed by CocE; indeed, it did so with almost the same efficiency as it used cocaine as a substrate. Modifications of the structure of cocaine esterase by simple manipulations of single amino acids within the active site completely destroyed its ability to act as an esterase (Turner et al. 2002). This is an enzymatically common fact, but a highly important one, since it illustrates the remarkable selectivity of the enzymes. These investigators also found cocaine esterase to be similarly efficient as did the original discovers of CocE; it is approximately 500 times more efficient than native butyrylcholinesterase in breaking down cocaine. Turner et al. (2002) made a number of important observations regarding the biochemical properties of cocaine esterase. For example, although many enzymes are slowed in efficiency by feedback factors associated with their metabolites, this is not true of cocaine esterase.

Native CocE and modified CocE have been studied extensively in animal models of cocaine toxicity. Native CocE prevents the convulsant and lethal effect of cocaine in mice and rats (Cooper et al. 2006; Ko et al. 2007, 2009). It also reverses the cardiovascular and seizurogenic effects of cocaine in rats (Jutkiewicz et al. 2009; Wood et al. 2010). In addition, Zheng and Zhan (2012) computationally modeled cocaine pharmacokinetics in the presence of a constant concentration of CocE in comparison with native human BChE and CocHs by using available human positron emission tomography (PET) data (Fowler et al. 1989). However, native cocaine esterase is active for only minutes when heated to body temperature (Cooper et al. 2006); presumably, the enzyme evolved to be most efficient at soil temperatures. The short half-life of the wild-type cocaine esterase, considerably less than the half-life of cocaine, may limit its therapeutic usefulness. Gao et al. (2009) and Huang et al. (2012) carried out molecular dynamics (MD) simulations to examine areas of the enzyme that were sensitive to heating and determined amino acid modifications that would enhance its thermostability. These MD simulations were validated by in vivo assessments of esteratic protection against cocaine toxicity in mice (Gao et al. 2009). Slight, critical changes in the structure of the esterase led to durations of action that extended beyond the half-life of cocaine. There were excellent predictions from the model to in vivo function suggesting that thermostability was a major determinant of the enzyme's half-life in plasma of the mouse (Brim et al. 2010). Interestingly, the single or double exchanges in amino acids that increased thermostability occurred at residues that were far from the active site of the enzyme and therefore did not modify the efficiency of the enzyme (Narasimhan et al. 2010). Because some of these changes in structure extended the enzymatic half-life beyond the normal residence time of cocaine, a single administration of the mutant enzyme was sufficient, in principle, to destroy an intoxicating amount of cocaine.

The mutant, more thermostable, esterase has two amino acids modified (CocE T172R/G173Q; referred to in subsequent descriptions as double mutant or DM CocE). DM CocE is active for 4.5 h in rats; increasing the enzyme's duration of action does not appear dramatically to slow its onset of action. Collins, Zaks, Cunningham, St Clair, Nichols, Narasimhan et al. (2011) demonstrated that increasing doses of DM CocE reduced the potency of cocaine in producing convulsions and subsequent death in rats.

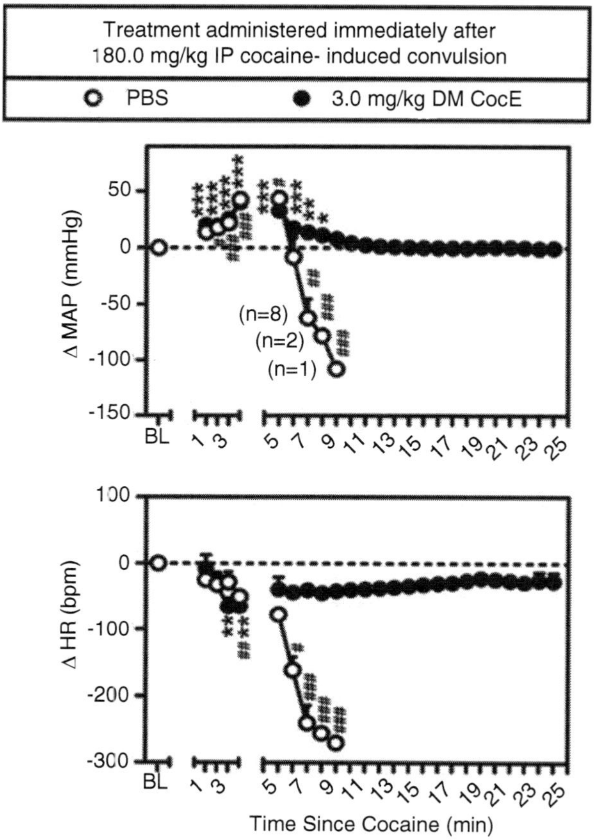

Fig. 10.2 Capacity of DM CocE to rescue rats from the cardiovascular effects of 180.0 mg/kg; IP cocaine. Baseline measures of mean arterial pressure (MAP; mmHg) and heart rate (HR; bpm) were collected for 30 min prior to the IP administration of 180.0 mg/kg cocaine. PBS or 3 mg/kg DM CocE was administered i.v., immediately after the onset of cocaine-induced convulsion, with cardiovascular measures collected for at least 20 min thereafter. Data are expressed as the mean ± SEM ($n = 10$/group) change in MAP or HR from baseline (1-min bin immediately prior to cocaine administration). Numbers in parentheses represent the number of rats remaining in the group at each time point following the first incidence of lethality. * $p < 0.05$, ** $p < 0.01$, *** $p < 0.001$, # $p < 0.05$, ## $p < 0.01$, ### $p < 0.001$. Significant differences from baseline for the DM CocE (*) and PBS (#) groups were determined using one-way ANOVA with post hoc Dunnett's tests (Taken with permission from Collins et al. (2011))

The magnitude of change in potency was on the order of tenfold. A pretreatment dose of 10 mg/kg of DM CocE continued to produce a protective effect against a lethal cocaine dose for 4 h. If DM CocE was administered intravenously *after* a lethal dose of intraperitoneal cocaine, it could reverse the cardiovascular effects of cocaine as shown in Fig. 10.2, as well as death; it was not determined how close to cocaine-induced death a rat might be and still be rescued by administration of DM CocE. Also of interest, but not studied, was the plasma concentrations of DM CocE and cocaine during the time course of the experiment illustrated in Fig. 10.2.

DM CocE has been given to rhesus monkeys following the administration of radiolabeled cocaine. PET scans demonstrated that the egress of the labeled cocaine was much faster following DM CocE administration, presumably due to the creation of a strong concentration gradient by CocE-enhanced plasma cocaine elimination. This effect was not obtained with a cocaine analogue without the ester bridge attack point (Howell et al. 2013).

Brim et al. (2011a) reported that DM CocE, given subsequent to cocaine administration, would hydrolyze norcocaine and cocaethylene somewhat less efficiently than it hydrolyzed cocaine, but it did not hydrolyze benzoylecgonine. The latter is a relatively unimportant metabolite, having far weaker capacity to induce cocaine-like effects. This is an important confirmation of an earlier finding with cocaethylene by Turner et al. (2002), and both reports suggest that the enzyme will clear the most active metabolites quickly.

Brim et al. (2011b) determined that DM CocE hydrolytic capacity was not interfered with significantly by a number of commonly abused substances that may be coadministered with cocaine, including alcohol, nicotine, morphine, phencyclidine, ketamine, methamphetamine, naltrexone, naloxone, and midazolam. Diazepam interfered with the enzyme somewhat, but this effect may be unreliable (S. Schwartz, personal communication).

In virtually all cases, the biological fate of the enzymes that utilize cocaine as a substrate has been inadequately studied. An exception is the work of Brim et al. (2012) who found that a labeled form of DM CocE had a half-life of 2.1 h in rats. The primary mechanism of its termination of action was proteolysis, though some was eliminated in urine as well. This suggests the possibility of effective multiple administrations of the enzyme as a potential therapeutic for repeated episodes of toxicity in the same individual.

There may be another advantage to a therapy that works through the elimination of substrate. There may be less species variation relative to, for example, a receptor-based antagonism. This is highly speculative at present given the small number of examples to use as a basis of comparison. Regardless, we are impressed by the lack of differences in effect across species. For example, the effects of DM CocE in rhesus monkey were similar to the rodent examples described above. Collins et al. (2011) showed that in non-human primates, cocaine would produce increases in blood pressure and heart rate that were reduced by the mutant CocE in a dose-dependent fashion over a range of 0.03–3.2 mg/kg i.v. without evoking cardiovascular change on its own. The speed and magnitude of effect were dose dependent. Over the course of studying the enzyme, it was given repeatedly to the monkeys. There were small increases in antibody production to the DM CocE, but they were short-lived and failed to produce a marked change in sensitivity to the hydrolytic activity of the enzyme. Collins et al. (2012) made a more exacting study of repeated dosing to alter cardiovascular effects of cocaine. As shown in Fig. 10.3, repeated administration of 0.32 mg/kg of DM CocE failed to produce a striking change in the hydrolytic capacity of the enzyme rapidly to reduce cocaine blood levels. There were commensurate changes in cardiovascular effects of intravenous cocaine as shown in Fig. 10.4. By the fourth administration of DM CocE, there was a tenfold increase in anti-CocE antibodies. These increases were transient and dissipated

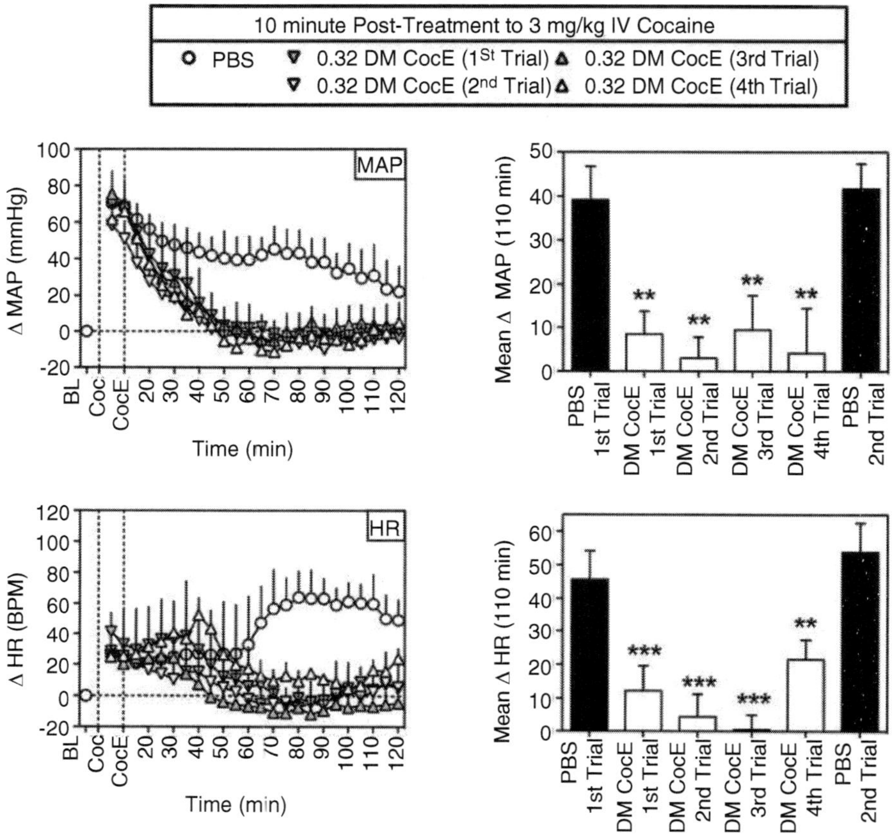

Fig. 10.3 Effects of repeated doses of DM CocE (0.32 mg/kg i.v.) or PBS on the cocaine-induced changes in MAP (*top*) and HR (*bottom*) when administered 10 min after an intravenous dose of 3 mg/kg cocaine ($n=3$) during six biweekly trials. *Left*, data points represent the mean ± S.E.M. change from baseline for MAP or HR over successive 5-min blocks of time during sessions in which 3 mg/kg cocaine was followed by PBS (○) or 0.32 mg/kg DM CocE (*triangles*). *Right*, data represent the mean ± S.E.M. change from baseline for MAP or HR over the entire 110 min after the administration of PBS (*filled bars*) or 0.32 mg/kg DM CocE (*open bars*). **, $p<0.001$; ***, $p<0.001$. Significant differences in mean change in MAP or HR among conditions were determined by one-way ANOVA with repeated measures with post hoc Bonferroni's tests (Taken with permission from Collins et al. (2012))

within 8 weeks. Both of these studies suggest the possibility that DM CocE might be administered with impunity on more than one occasion to humans for the treatment of intoxication.

Although a 4 h duration of action is quite satisfactory for the treatment of cocaine toxicity, it is far from satisfactory for the treatment of cocaine abuse. Our group found that DM CocE is active as a dimer in plasma, which is a duplicate and connected version of the enzyme molecule shown in Fig. 10.1 (Narasimhan et al. 2010).

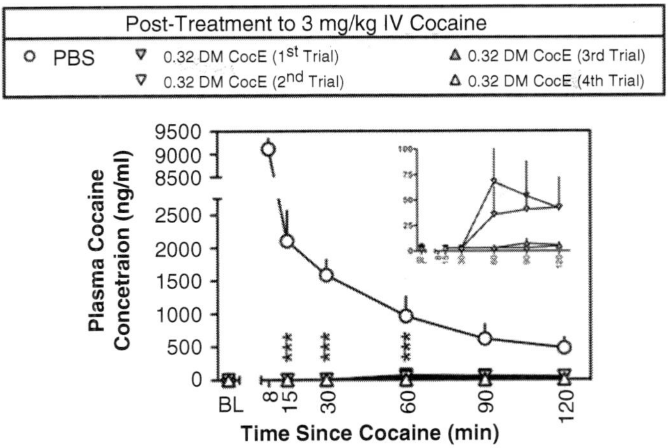

Fig. 10.4 Plasma concentrations of cocaine produced by intravenous doses of 3 mg/kg cocaine during five biweekly trials in two rhesus monkeys. Plasma cocaine concentrations were assessed by mass spectrometry ~ 2 min before cocaine (baseline; BL) and at 8, 15, 30, 60, 90, and 120 min after the administration of cocaine. ○ represent the mean ± S.E.M. plasma concentrations of cocaine when PBS was administered 10 min after 3 mg/kg cocaine. Plasma concentrations of cocaine during the first (▾), second (▿), third (▴), and fourth (▵) trials in which 0.32 mg/kg DM CocE was administered as a posttreatment to 3 mg/kg cocaine are shown. Data from the 8-min time point were excluded because of differences in the posttreatment times (UR, 10-min posttreatment; BE, 1-min posttreatment). Inset shows plasma cocaine concentrations during the four DM CocE conditions plotted on a *y*-axis with a smaller range of concentrations. *** $p < 0.001$. Significant differences in plasma cocaine concentrations were determined by two-way ANOVA with repeated measures and post hoc Bonferroni's tests (Taken with permission from Collins et al. (2012))

Increases in the strength of the linkage between the individual monomers of the pair produced complete thermostability at body temperatures (Narasimhan et al. 2011). The enzyme, however, remained susceptible to peptide degradation in the body. Potential ways to protect against enzyme degradation include additions of polyethylene glycol polymers to the enzymes and/or further enhancement or alteration of the linkage between the monomers. Current research is also being devoted to approaches that provide sustained release of the longer acting versions of the esterases (Sunahara and colleagues, unpublished observations).

10.5.2 *Modified Human Butyrylcholinesterase (BChE)*

The human endogenous esterase, BChE, has an inefficient capacity to attack cocaine as a substrate. It is by far more efficient at breaking down acetylcholine and the biologically inactive cocaine isomer, (+) cocaine. An early modification of native BChE resulted in a mutant form that had increased capacity to metabolize cocaine (Sun et al. 2002; Table 10.1). Through a series of state-of-the-art molecular dynamic simulations based on the structure of BChE as well as on comparisons of the

Table 10.1 Kinetic parameters of human BChE and its mutants against cocaine

Enzyme (BChE or mutant)	k_{cat} (min^{-1})	K_M (μM)	k_{cat}/K_M (min^{-1} M^{-1})	RCE[a]
Wild-type BChE[b]	4.1	4.5	9.1×10^{-5}	1
A328W/Y332A[b]	154	18	8.6×10^{6}	9.4
A328W/Y332G[c]	240	17	1.4×10^{7}	15
F227A/S287G/A328W/Y332M (AME359)[d]	620	20	3.1×10^{7}	34
A199S/A328W/Y332G[e]	389	5.4	7.2×10^{7}	79
A199S/S287G/A328W/Y332G (CocH1)[f]	3060	3.1	9.9×10^{-8}	1080
A199S/F227A/S287G/A328W/E441D (CocH2)[g]	1730	1.1	1.6×10^{-9}	1730
A199S/F227A/S287G/A328W/Y332G (CocH3)[h]	5700	3.1	1.8×10^{-9}	2020

[a]RCE – relative catalytic efficiency (k_{cat}/K_M) value (relative to wild-type human BChE) against (−)-cocaine
[b]Sun et al. (2002)
[c]Hamza et al. (2005)
[d]Gao et al. (2005)
[e]Pan et al. (2007)
[f]Pan et al. (2005) and Yang et al. (2010)
[g]Yang et al. (2009) and Xue et al. (2011)
[h]Zheng et al. (2008)

dynamics of the BChE-(−)-cocaine complex with the BChE-(+)-cocaine complex, modifications of butytylcholinesterase were made that resulted in quadruple and quintuple mutant forms of human BChE that were at least 1000 times more efficient in degrading (−)-cocaine (Pan et al. 2005; Zheng et al. 2008; Zheng and Zhan 2008a, b, 2012; Yang et al. 2010; Xue et al. 2011). Molecular modifications of BChE, in contrast to those made in CocE, were in the active site of the enzyme, far from its surface. Several different forms of mutant BChE, generically termed cocaine hydrolases (CocH), have been described in the literature, as listed and characterized in Table 10.1, and modifications continue to be made to enhance the activity and the duration of action of compounds. The most recently published set of changes resulted in a modified butyrylcholinesterase that surpassed the efficiency of cocaine esterase on a molar basis. Direct comparisons in vivo among the various forms of enzyme would be very interesting, but have not been described. Nevertheless, the altered forms of butyrylcholinesterase are a remarkable improvement in efficiency. The design and implementation of the chemical modifications required to produce these highly efficient anti-cocaine cholinesterases required a number of in silico as well as actual chemical iterations (e.g., Zhan et al. 2003; Zhan and Gao 2005; Zheng et al. 2008; Zheng and Zhan 2009; Zheng et al. 2010).

The Zhan group (Pan et al. 2005) advanced a form of CocH, referred to as CocH1 in Table 10.1. This compound has been fused with human albumin in attempts to increase its in vivo residence time (Gao et al. 2008). At a dose of 10 mg/kg with cocaine delivered 10 min later, CocH1 reduced cocaine toxicity by approximately tenfold. It was effective in both male and female rats. At a dose of 3 mg/kg, it reduced cocaine-induced changes in blood pressure. At the same dose, it reduced cocaine levels in the plasma, heart, and brain of the rat assayed 10 min after cocaine administration (3.5 mg/kg) (Brimijoin et al. 2008).

10.6 Addiction Pharmacotherapy

As noted earlier, the problems of cocaine abuse require a therapy that lasts much, much longer than does therapy for a single episode of intoxication. Although there is no agreement regarding the shortest duration that is necessary and sufficient for treating abuse, the possibility that synthesis of anti-cocaine enzymes can be produced through gene expression raises the possibility of lifetime exposure to the enzyme – certainly an upper limit on duration of protective effect. Although no one is, at present, advocating the possibility of therapy through virally mediated alterations in gene expression, it is at least feasible to entertain this possibility as an eventual therapeutic intervention.

It is clear from the success of long-acting esterases (e.g., DM CocE and CocH1), in reversing or preventing the toxic effects of cocaine, that it might be possible to study the effect of cancellation of cocaine's stimulus effect in animals. Various assessments have been carried out in rodents that indicate that the reinforcing effects of cocaine can be significantly attenuated with these compounds. It is important to appreciate that there is no way "to erase" the cocaine exposure completely with these pharmacotherapies, but they represent remarkably effective ways of reducing the likelihood that reexposure to cocaine will increase the probability of relapse as long as compliance with therapy administration is maintained.

As described earlier, studies of the reinforcing effects of cocaine are very popular in assessing potential antagonists of cocaine abuse, and these were among the first approaches to be used with anti-cocaine enzymes. When an animal has been trained to administer cocaine and cocaine delivery is then removed by substituting a null substance (e.g., saline), the animal gradually reduces (extinguishes) responding. Not surprisingly, the speed and pattern of decrease in responding depend upon the past history of reinforced responding (e.g., Johanson and Fischman 1989).

10.6.1 CocE

There are two excellent examples of the effects of anti-cocaine enzymes that illustrate the principles of reinforcement theory applied to cocaine. One demonstrates that, as the dose of cocaine esterase is increased, it can produce a partial elimination of cocaine's reinforcing effect, mimicking a reduction in cocaine dose. If the dose of the enzyme is increased further, it cancels completely the reinforcing effect of cocaine, converting the pattern of cocaine self-administration to one like saline self-administration. These experiments used rats with intravenous catheters that were

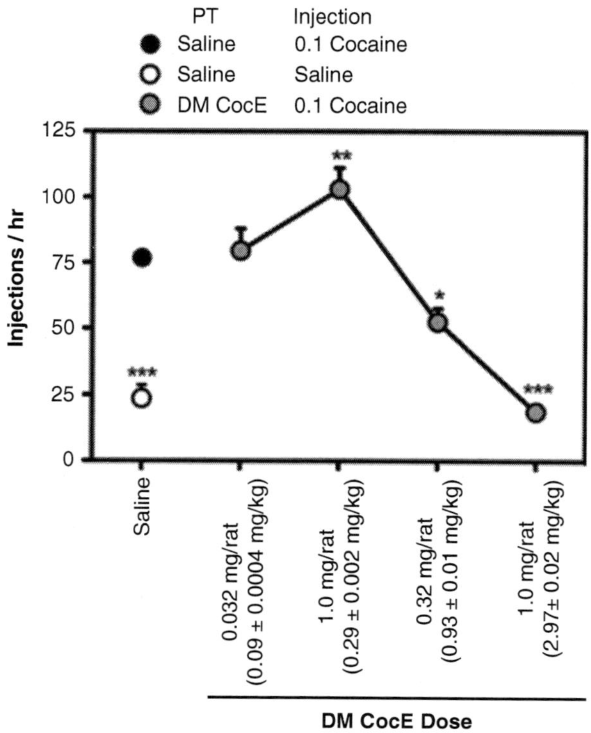

Fig. 10.5 Dose-response analysis of the capacity of CocE T172R/G173Q (DM CocE) to alter responding reinforced by 0.1 mg/kg/injection cocaine. Rats were maintained on 0.1 mg/kg/injection cocaine during daily 60-min sessions in which responding was reinforced under a FR5TO5 schedule of reinforcement. Data represent the mean (±S.E.M.) number of injections earned during 60-min sessions. • responding under baseline conditions, ○ responding during a single-session saline substitution, • responding during sessions in which rats were pretreated on a milligram per rat basis with 0.032, 0.1, 0.32, or 1.0 mg i.v. DM CocE and allowed to respond for 0.1 mg/kg/injection cocaine. * $p<0.05$, ** $p<0.01$, *** $p<0.001$. Significant differences in responding compared with baseline conditions were determined by one-way ANOVA with post hoc Bonferroni's tests (Taken with permission from Collins et al. (2009))

taught to respond on a lever to deliver i.v. injections of cocaine. Figure 10.5 illustrates the effects of increasing doses of DM CocE on the reinforcing effects of 0.1 mg/kg/inj of cocaine. In the left margin of the figure, the effects of saline substitution for cocaine are shown for comparative purposes. The first active dose of DM CocE (0.3 mg/rat) increased cocaine-maintained responding, just as substituting a smaller dose of cocaine would do. A larger dose of the enzyme (1 mg/rat) reduced cocaine-maintained responding to levels equal to those obtained when saline was substituted for cocaine. If the native, short-acting version of CocE was given prior to a 1-h session of cocaine self-administration, there was a small change in behavior, but only for the period that the cocaine esterase was active (15 min or so). DM CocE failed to change the reinforcing effect of a cocaine analogue without an ester bridge, nor did it change the speed of collecting food reinforcers. The enzyme was therefore acting specifically against cocaine and not acting to suppress behavior in general (Collins et al. 2009).

Cocaine esterase has been further modified to link the monomers more tightly (CCRQ CocE) and to add polyethylene glycol groups to the enzyme (PEG CCRQ CocE); both approaches extend the residence time of the enzyme without altering the efficiency of the enzyme (Narasimhan et al. 2011). Collins et al. (2012) showed that this form of cocaine esterase, delivered intravenously, was maximally active in reducing the potency of cocaine as a reinforcer immediately after administration. The effect of the esterase was reduced over the course of 3–4 days. At its maximum, the reinforcing potency of cocaine was reduced by more than 30-fold, the reinforcing potency of methylphenidate was unchanged, and rates of food-reinforced responding were unchanged. The discriminative stimulus effects of cocaine were also markedly attenuated by PEG CCRQ CocE; the most effective dose (32 mg/kg) completely eliminated the discriminative stimulus effect of a lethal dose of cocaine (180 mg/kg). A tenfold rightward shift in the potency of cocaine remained 72 h after administration of this dose of PEG CCRQ CocE. The Michigan group is attempting to provide this form of CocE in a sustained-release formulation to gain still further increases in functional, residence time.

10.6.2 CocH

Brimijoin et al. (2008) reported that albumin-conjugated CocH1 (denoted as Albu-CocH) blocked completely the ability of cocaine to reinstate cocaine-maintained responding that had been extinguished. However, amphetamine's capacity to produce reinstatement of cocaine self-administration was unchanged, illustrating the selectivity of the effects of CocH1. Neither locomotor behavior nor rates of food-reinforced responding were altered by the dose of CocH1 that eliminated cocaine's capacity to reinstate cocaine-reinforced responding. Carroll et al. (2011) reported that Albu-CocH was mildly effective in reducing cocaine self-administration in rats responding under a progressive ratio schedule. The effect was not maintained beyond the session immediately following administration of the enzyme. Schindler and colleagues (Schindler et al. 2013) studied the effect of Albu-CocH on the reinforcing and discriminative stimulus effects of cocaine and on the ability of cocaine to reinstate extinguished responding in squirrel monkeys. They reported that the enzyme (5 mg/kg, i.m.) had a half-life of between 45.5 and 65.5 h in the squirrel monkey. At this dose, Albu-CocH had the capacity to reduce the reinforcing effect of a large but not a smaller dose of cocaine significantly for three days, with rates of cocaine-maintained responding increasing toward baseline levels over those four sessions. Albu-CocH was effective at blocking cocaine reinstatement and cocaine discrimination at 2 h but not at 48 h following enzyme administration. Some of the monkeys developed antibodies to this human form of CocH, something that would not be expected in humans, but needs yet to be evaluated. This form of the modified enzyme has recently been registered for cocaine abuse trials in humans by Teva Pharmaceuticals (see below for details).

The Brimijoin group has been employing different CocH gene delivery devices to produce high levels of the butyrylcholinesterase mutants (including AME359 and CocH1 to CocH3 in Table 10.1) in rats for a long period of time, and the advances have been very impressive. Early approaches utilized adenoviral vectors driven by a cytomegalovirus promoter (CMV-AV). Four days after being given directly into the caudate nucleus, this vector provided local protection against cocaine administration (Gao et al. 2005). They then turned to delivery of helper-dependent adenoviral expression (ApoE-hdAV), designed to produce a weaker immune response and maintain longer transduction. This also protected the brain from cocaine following intracerebral administration. Given systemically (i.v.), ApoE-hdAV produced a 25,000-fold increase in plasma cocaine hydrolase activity and also provided protection against cocaine's effects in the brain. Levels of expression of cocaine hydrolase remained near 80 % after 2 months and at 10–20 % after a year (Gao and Brimijoin 2009). It was important in these experiments to build the animal-selective forms of helper-dependent adenoviral vectors; when such species-selective agents were used, an impressive, long-term effect was obtained. Anker et al. (2012) demonstrated this type of effect. These investigators first conditioned rats to self-administer cocaine intravenously. Then, the rats were given a single injection of the ApoE-hdAV vector or a vector that was absent in the enzyme. Cocaine self-administration behavior was extinguished for 2 weeks by substituting saline for cocaine; rates of responding decreased over this period. The rats were then given one of three doses of cocaine (5, 10, or 15 mg/kg) over a period of 6 months to evaluate the ability of these doses to reinstate responding that was previously reinforced with cocaine (drug-primed reinstatement). Across this entire time period, the hydrolase vector continued to suppress the capacity of cocaine to reinstate responding, although the control vector animals responded robustly. At the end of the 6-month period of evaluation, amphetamine (2 mg/kg) was administered to both groups, and both responded vigorously and non-differentially. This is an interesting result because it indicates that the animals treated with the CocH vector, and receiving no effect from cocaine for 6 months, continued to be responsive to amphetamine. Overall, the data suggest not only that CocH generated from the CocH gene transfer may have a duration of action that satisfies the unspecified requirements for treatment of cocaine abuse but also that successful treatment of cocaine abuse requires pharmacotherapy that lasts a very long time or is renewed on an appropriate time frame.

Another major advance in the field of gene-related therapies takes into account differences in the genomes of the subjects of the experiments. The human form of BChE has been the model enzyme to work from since the eventual target is human cocaine abusers. Nevertheless, it is important to examine the possibility of improvement by employing a rodent form of BChE for gene transfer for evaluation in rodents. The implication of the concept is that conspecies are more important for assessment of "true" effect than are cross-species evaluations. An experiment utilizing the mouse genome has recently been reported. Geng et al. (2013) utilized the mouse form (mCocH) of CocH3 (see Table 10.1 for details of the amino acid changes) for gene transfer in the mouse (AAV-CMV-mCocH). There were vector-amount increases in functioning hydrolase activity with no changes related to obvious toxicity in the mouse, for example, in general cholinergic functions nor evident toxicity related to amount of hydrolase expressed in the mice. The mouse mutant BChE (mCocH) continued to enhance cocaine hydrolysis over the animals' lifetime. Human mutant BChE (CocH3), on the other hand, was effective for only 2 months. Nevertheless, the expressed hydrolase was capable of reducing the effects of cocaine in the mouse. This result generally suggests that wide variations in hydrolases, expressed within the same species, can be accomplished with reduced concern for immune effects. The effectiveness of repeated or long-term exposure to esterases can be evaluated only in human studies; this makes the variety of modeling in animals less important than it might be under other circumstances. The predictability across species is uncharted water.

Under these proof-of-concept studies, DM CocE altered cocaine-reinforced responding directly and CocH1 altered cocaine's capacity to reinstate responding previously reinforced by cocaine, arguing more directly for its ability to prevent relapse in humans. Neither enzyme changed ongoing behavior reinforced by non-drug reinforcers or normal locomotor behavior. It is no longer a question as to whether these enzymes are capable of intercepting cocaine fast enough to totally remove the effects of small doses of cocaine delivered repeatedly intravenously in rodents or primates. The question remains as to whether sufficiently long-acting enzymes can be designed and rendered appropriate for human trials.

10.7 Summary and Projections

The general issues associated with developing pharmacotherapies of cocaine toxicity and abuse should be clearer to the reader, and it should also be clearer that we might be on the brink of delivery of viable compounds for both therapeutic goals within the next decade. Active and passive immunization against cocaine (see Kosten's contribution to this volume) were the first approaches using selective cocaine-binding proteins to sequester cocaine in the periphery. In contrast to the anti-cocaine enzymes, cocaine antibodies have been evaluated in humans and have provided proof of the concept that cocaine sequestration, when it is achieved, can reduce cocaine's effects and cocaine abuse. Generally, active immunization takes a long time (weeks) whereas passive immunization simply administers a developed antibody. Early forms of vaccines were not quite adequate in terms of capacity and there were considerable individual differences in antibody development. In addition, the vaccines simply bind to cocaine in a saturable interaction, as compared with the esterases and hydrolases that are released once they have metabolized cocaine and can continue to react with cocaine as long as the stimulant is present in the blood.

Landry and colleagues (Landry et al. 1993) provided a conceptual jump forward by combining for the first time an enzyme with a cocaine antibody in the molecule, a cocaine-directed, catalytic antibody. Although it was active in vivo, it suffered from a lack of efficiency (Mets et al. 1998). Catalytic antibodies have lanquished in attention although they should not be ruled out for future ventures if there are unforeseen problems with current approaches.

The enzymes described in this review represent the next step forward in the use of anti-cocaine proteins to treat clinical pathologies related to cocaine use. It has taken two decades to get this far toward enzyme therapy of either cocaine toxicity or abuse, but the progress has been substantial, involving heroic molecular biological techniques. Many questions remain to be answered: how much cocaine needs to be guarded against (i.e., prevented completely from having any effect) and how long will the therapy need to be given to be effective in preventing relapse. The discovery and implementation of anti-cocaine esterases and hydrolases allow these questions to be posed for the first time. The first form of human hydrolase has been registered for human evaluation for cocaine abuse. Teva Pharmaceuticals has registered a 12-week trial for recombinant human serum albumin-fused CocH1 (known as Albu-CocH or TV-1380 or AlbuBChE) for the facilitation of abstinence in cocaine abusers (NCT01887366, ClinicalTrials.gov). Likewise, the first clinical trials using DM CocE for the treatment of cocaine overdose are also currently ongoing (NCT01846481, ClinicalTrials.gov). It will be very exciting to see how these enzymes interact with cocaine in humans.

Most experts believe that no single therapy will prevail, but approaches that combine different therapies will be the model of the future. For example, the Kosten and Brimijoin groups are exploring the combination of vaccine and gene transfer-assisted hydrolase. They find that they act more effectively when combined (Gao et al. 2013). Carroll et al. (2012) studied the effects of cocaine on locomotor behavior with small amounts of either hydrolase, vaccine, or their combination and found the combination of approaches was more effective in either mice or rats in different experiments. Brimijoin et al. (2013) have provided similar findings in mice. One could easily see combinations of approaches in which an esterase-based effect might have the capacity to exert most effect early and could be followed by a vaccine that would be the longer acting therapeutic for cocaine abuse. For example, a long-acting form of enzymatic monotherapy might work for a month or so, giving the vaccine time to develop greater activity.

There is another significant advantage of pharmacokinetic approaches to cocaine pharmacotherapies. Still other forms of therapy can easily be combined with either of these pharmacokinetic approaches. There may be small-molecule antagonists that act at dopamine receptors (D3 is a favorite type, at the moment; Newman et al. 2012; Heidbreder 2013) that will reduce the relapse proclivity even further. Still other types of compounds, e.g., buspirone or phendimetrazine (Banks et al. 2013), may be helpful as well. In short, there are a variety of other approaches that are conceptually compatible with pharmacokinetic-based approaches to cocaine abuse.

Behavioral therapies are much more successful than many acknowledge. With some types of approach, 80 % of patients remain totally abstinent without any pharmacological support (e.g., Secades-Villa et al. 2011; Kirby et al. 2013). The implementation of sustained-release forms of narcotic antagonists for the treatment of opioid abuse is similar conceptually to approaches that take an enzymatic, pharmacokinetic approach to cocaine abuse. These types of approach need to be studied intensively to learn what is most effective so that they can be transferred across drugs of abuse and can be used in conjunction with other approaches.

Drug abuse is a chronic, relapsing disorder. Compliance with whatever therapy is provided is essential, but not easy to ensure. We think that treatment approaches that have very long durations of action are an appropriate way to approach problems of compliance but that remains to be determined. A long-lasting, depot preparation of an opioid antagonist (Vivitrol) is available for the treatment of opioid abuse, but it is sufficiently new to providers that its success cannot yet be evaluated. The several approaches at increasing the duration of action of the cocaine esterases and hydrolases have been sufficiently successful to suggest that these approaches may overcome even the relative intractable compliance issues.

The near future in the treatment of cocaine-related problems could be very exciting. It has taken many years to come this far, but we have come quite a distance. Continued progress will require vigilance and attention by all interested parties: the pharmaceutical industry, academic researchers, and vital governmental support. All are experiencing enormous changes in scientific and administrative disposition. It is vital that all keep their eyes on the prize. Each delay costs time, human investments, and battered objectives.

Conflict of Interest Statement Both authors hold patents related to some of the enzymes described in this paper.

References

Anker JJ, Brimijoin S, Gao Y, Geng L, Zlebnik NE, Parks RJ, Carroll ME. Cocaine hydrolase encoded in viral vector blocks the reinstatement of cocaine seeking in rats for 6 months. Biol Psychiatry. 2012;71:700–5.

Banks ML, Blough BE, Fennell TR, Snyder RW, Negus SS. Effects of phendimetrazine treatment on cocaine vs food choice and extended-access cocaine consumption in rhesus monkeys. Neuropsychopharmacology. 2013;38(13):2698–707.

Bresler MM, Rosser SJ, Basran A, Bruce NC. Gene cloning and nucleotide sequencing and properties of a cocaine esterase from Rhodococcus sp. strain MB1. Appl Environ Microbiol. 2000;66:904–8.

Brim RL, Noon KR, Collins GT, Nichols J, Narasimhan D, Sunahara RK, Woods JH. The ability of bacterial cocaine esterase to hydrolyze cocaine metabolites and their simultaneous quantification using high-performance liquid chromatography-tandem mass spectrometry. Mol Pharmacol. 2011a;80:1119–27.

Brim RL, Noon KR, Nichols J, Narasimhan D, Woods JH, Sunahara RK. Evaluation of the hydrolytic activity of a long-acting mutant bacterial cocaine in the presence of commonly co-administered drugs. Drug Alcohol Depend. 2011b;119:224–8.

Brim RL, Noon KR, Collins GT, Stein A, Nichols J, Narasimhan D, Ko M-C, Woods JH, Sunahara RK. The fate of bacterial cocaine esterase (CocE), an in vivo study of CocE-mediated cocaine hydrolysis, CocE pharmacokinetics, and CocE elimination. J Pharmacol Exp Ther. 2012;340:83–95.

Brim RL, Nance MR, Youngstrom DW, Narasimhan D, Zhan CG, Tesmer JJ, Sunahara RK, Woods JH. A thermally stable form of bacterial cocaine esterase: a potential therapeutic agent for treatment of cocaine abuse. Mol Pharmacol. 2010;77:593–600.

Brimijoin S, Gao Y, Anker JJ, Gliddon LA, Lafleur D, Shah R, Zhao Q, Singh M, Carroll ME. A cocaine hydrolase engineered from human butyrylcholinesterase selectively blocks cocaine toxicity and reinstatement of drug seeking in rats. Neuropsychopharmacology. 2008;33:2715–25.

Brimijoin S, Orson F, Kosten TR, Kinsey B, Shen XY, White SJ, Gao Y. Anti-cocaine antibody and butyrylcholinesterase-derived cocaine hydrolase exert cooperative effects on cocaine pharmacokinetics and cocaine-induced locomotor activity in mice. Chem Biol Interact. 2013;203:212–6.

Carroll ME, Gao Y, Brimijoin S, Anker JJ. Effects of cocaine hydrolase on cocaine self-administration under a PR schedule and during extended access (escalation) in rats. Psychopharmacology (Berl). 2011;213:817–29.

Carroll ME, Zlebnik NE, Anker JJ, Kosten TR, Orson FM, Shen X, Kinsey B, Parks RJ, Gao Y, Brimijoin S. Combined cocaine hydrolase gene transfer and anti-cocaine vaccine synergistically block cocaine-induced locomotion. PLoS One. 2012;7(8):e43536. doi:10.1371/journal.pone.0043536.

Collins GT, Zaks ME, Cunningham AR, St Clair C, Nichols J, Narasimhan D, Ko M-C, Sunahara RK, Woods JH. Effects of a long-acting mutant bacterial cocaine esterase on acute cocaine toxicity in rats. Drug Alcohol Depend. 2011;118:158–65.

Collins GT, Brim RL, Noon KR, Narasimhan D, Lukacs NW, Sunahara RK, Woods JH, Ko M-C. Repeated administration of a mutant cocaine esterase, effects on plasma cocaine levels, cocaine-induced cardiovascular activity, and immune responses in rhesus monkeys. J Pharmacol Exp Ther. 2012;342:205–13.

Collins GT, Brim RL, Narasimhan D, Ko MC, Sunahara RK, Zhan CG, Woods JH. Cocaine esterase prevents cocaine-induced toxicity and the ongoing intravenous self-administration of cocaine in rats. J Pharmacol Exp Ther. 2009;331:445–55.

Cooper ZD, Narasimhan D, Sunahara RK, Mierzejewski P, Jutkiewicz EM, Larsen NA, Wilson IA, Landry DW, Woods JH. Rapid and robust protection against cocaine-induced lethality in rats by the bacterial cocaine esterase. Mol Pharmacol. 2006;70:1885–91.

Fowler JS, Volkow ND, Wolf AP, Dewey SL, Schlyer DJ, MacGregor RR, Hitzemann R, Logan J, Bendriem B, Gatley SJ, Christman D. Mapping cocaine binding sites in human and baboon brain in vivo. Synapse. 1989;4:371–7.

Gao Y, Atanasova E, Sui N, Pancook JD, Watkins JD, Brimijoin S. Gene transfer of cocaine hydrolase suppresses cardiovascular responses to cocaine in rats. Mol Pharmacol. 2005;67:204–11.

Gao Y, Brimijoin S. Lasting reduction of cocaine action in neostriatum – a hydrolase gene therapy approach. J Pharmacol Exp Ther. 2009;330:449–57.

Gao Y, Geng L, Orson F, Kinsey B, Kosten TR, Shen X, Brimijoin S. Effects of anti-cocaine vaccine and viral gene transfer of cocaine hydrolase in mice on cocaine toxicity including motor strength and liver damage. Chem Biol Interact. 2013;20:208–11.

Gao Y, LaFleur D, Shah R, Zhao Q, Singh M, Brimijoin S. An albumin-butyrylcholinesterase for cocaine toxicity and addiction: catalytic and pharmacokinetic properties. Chem Biol Interact. 2008;175:83–7.

Gao D, Narasimhan DL, Macdonald J, Brim R, Ko M-C, Landry DW, Woods JH, Sunahara RK, Zhan CG. Thermostable variants of cocaine esterase for long-time protection against cocaine toxicity. Mol Pharmacol. 2009;75:318–23.

Geng L, Gao Y, Chen X, Hou S, Zhan C-G, Radic Z, Parks RJ, Russell SJ, Pham L, Brimijoin S. Gene transfer of mutant mouse cholinesterase provides high lifetime expression and reduced cocaine responses with no evident toxicity. PLoS One. 2013;8(6):e67446. doi:10.1371/journal.pone.0067446.

Hamza A, Cho H, Tai H-H, Zhan C-G. Molecular dynamics simulation of cocaine binding with human butyrylcholinesterase and its mutants. J Phys Chem B. 2005;109:4776–82.

Heidbreder C. Rationale in support of the use of selective dopamine D_3 receptor antagonists for the pharmacotherapeutic management of substance use disorders. Naunyn Schmiedebergs Arch Pharmacol. 2013;386:167–76.

Howell L, Nye J, Stehouwer J, Voll R, Mun J, Narasimhan D, Nichols J, Sunahara R, Goodman M, Carroll I, Woods JH. A mutant bacterial cocaine esterase rapidly eliminates cocaine from brain in nonhuman primates. 2013.

Huang X, Zhao X, Zheng F, Zhan C-G. Cocaine esterase-cocaine binding process and the free energy profiles by molecular dynamics and potential of mean force simulations. J Phys Chem B. 2012;116:3361–8.

Johanson CE, Fischman MW. The pharmacology of cocaine related to its abuse. Pharmacol Rev. 1989;41:3–52.

Jutkiewicz EM, Baladi MG, Cooper ZD, Narasimhan D, Sunahara RK, Woods JH. A bacterial cocaine esterase protects against cocaine-induced epileptogenic activity and lethality. Ann Emerg Med. 2009;54:409–20.

Kirby KC, Carpenedo CM, Dugosh KL, Rosenwasser BJ, Benishek LA, Janik A, Keashen R, Bresani E, Silverman K. Randomized clinical trial examining duration of voucher-based reinforcement therapy for cocaine abstinence. Drug Alcohol Depend. 2013;132(3):639–45.

Ko M-C, Narasimhan D, Berlin AA, Lukacs NW, Sunahara RK, Woods JH. Effects of cocaine esterase following its repeated administration with cocaine in mice. Drug Alcohol Depend. 2009;101:202–9.

Ko M-C, Bowen LD, Narasimhan D, Berlin AA, Lukacs NW, Sunahara RK, Cooper ZD, Woods JH. Cocaine esterase: interactions with cocaine and immune responses in mice. J Pharmacol Exp Ther. 2007;320:926–33.

Landry DW, Zhao K, Yang GX, Glickman M, Georgiadis TM. Antibody-catalyzed degradation of cocaine. Science. 1993;259:1899–901.

Larrimore KE, Barcus M, Kannan L, Gao Y, Zhan C-G, Brimijoin S, Mor T. Gene transfer of mutant mouse cholinesterase provides high lifetime expression and reduced cocaine responses with no evident toxicity. PLoS One. 2013;8(6):e67446. doi:10.1371/journal.pone.0067446.

Larsen NA, Turner JM, Stevens J, Rosser SJ, Basran A, Lerner RA, Bruce NC, Wilson IA. Crystal structure of a bacterial cocaine esterase. Nat Struct Biol. 2002;9:17–21.

Liu J, Hamza A, Zhan C-G. Fundamental reaction mechanism and free energy profile for (−)-cocaine hydrolysis catalyzed by cocaine esterase. J Am Chem Soc. 2009;131:11964–75.

McCord J, Jneid H, Hollander JE, de Lemos JA, Cercek B, Hsue P, Gibler WB, Ohman EM, Drew B, Philippides G, Newby LK. Management of cocaine-associated chest pain and myocardial infarction: a scientific statement from the American Heart Association Acute Cardiac Care Committee of the Council on Clinical Cardiology. Circulation. 2008;117:1897–907.

Meredith TC, Mamat U, Kaczynski Z, Lindner B, Holst O, Woodard RW. Modification of lipopolysaccharide with colanic acid (M-antigen) repeats in Escherichia coli. J Biol Chem. 2007;282:7790–8.

Mets B, Winger G, Cabrera C, Seo S, Jamdar S, Yang G, Zhao K, Briscoe RJ, Almonte R, Woods JH, Landry DW. A catalytic antibody against cocaine prevents cocaine's reinforcing and toxic effects in rats. Proc Natl Acad Sci U S A. 1998;95:10176–81.

Narasimhan D, Nance MR, Gao D, Ko M-C, Macdonald J, Tamburi P, Yoon D, Landry DM, Woods JH, Zhan CG, Tesmer JJ, Sunahara RK. Structural analysis of thermostabilizing mutations of cocaine esterase. Protein Eng Des Sel. 2010;23:537–47.

Narasimhan D, Collins GT, Nance MR, Nichols J, Edwald E, Chan J, Ko M-C, Woods JH, Tesmer JJ, Sunahara RK. Subunit stabilization and polyethylene glycolation of cocaine esterase improves in vivo residence time. Mol Pharmacol. 2011;80:1056–65.

Newman AH, Blaylock BL, Nader MA, Bergman J, Sibley DR, Skolnick P. Medication discovery for addiction: translating the dopamine D3 receptor hypothesis. Biochem Pharmacol. 2012;84:882–90.

Pan Y, Gao D, Yang W, Cho H, Yang G, Tai HH, Zhan C-G. Computational redesign of human butyrylcholinesterase for anticocaine medication. Proc Natl Acad Sci U S A. 2005;102: 16656–61.

Pan Y, Gao D, Yang W, Cho H, Zhan C-G. Free energy perturbation (FEP) simulation on the transition-states of cocaine hydrolysis catalyzed by human butyrylcholinesterase and its mutants. J Am Chem Soc. 2007;129:13537–43.

Pierce RC, O'Brien CP, Kenny PJ, Vanderschuren LJ. Rational development of addiction pharmacotherapies: successes, failures, and prospects. Cold Spring Harb Perspect Med. 2012;2(6): a012880.

Schindler CW, Justinova Z, Lafleur D, Woods D, Roschke V, Hallak H, Sklair-Tavron L, Redhi GH, Yasar S, Bergman J, Goldberg SR. Modification of pharmacokinetic and abuse-related effects of cocaine by human-derived cocaine hydrolase in monkeys. Addict Biol. 2013;18:30–9.

Secades-Villa R, García-Rodríguez O, García-Fernández G, Sánchez-Hervás E, Fernandez-Hermida JR, Higgins ST. Community reinforcement approach plus vouchers among cocaine-dependent outpatients: twelve-month outcomes. Psychol Addict Behav. 2011;25:174–9.

Sun H, Shen ML, Pang YP, Lockridge O, Brimijoin S. Cocaine metabolism accelerated by a re-engineered human butyrylcholinesterase. J Pharmacol Exp Ther. 2002;302:710–6.

Turner JM, Larsen NA, Basran A, Barbas 3rd CF, Bruce NC, Wilson IA, Lerner RA. Biochemical characterization and structural analysis of a highly proficient cocaine esterase. Biochemistry. 2002;41:12297–307.

Wood SK, Narasimhan D, Cooper Z, Sunahara RK, Woods JH. Prevention and reversal by cocaine esterase of cocaine-induced cardiovascular effects in rats. Drug Alcohol Depend. 2010;106:219–29.

Xue L, Hou S, Tong M, Fang L, Chen X, Jin Z, Tai HH, Zheng F, Zhan C-G. Preparation and in vivo characterization of a cocaine hydrolase engineered from human butyrylcholinesterase for metabolizing cocaine. Biochem J. 2013;453:447–54.

Xue L, Ko M-C, Tong M, Yang W, Hou S, Fang L, Liu J, Zheng F, Woods JH, Tai HH, Zhan C-G. Design, preparation, and characterization of high-activity mutants of human butyrylcholinesterase specific for detoxification of cocaine. Mol Pharmacol. 2011;79:290–7.

Yang W, Xue L, Fang L, Chen X, Zhan C-G. Characterization of a high-activity mutant of human butyrylcholinesterase against (−)-cocaine. Chem Biol Interact. 2010;187:148–52.

Yang W, Pan Y, Zheng F, Cho H, Tai H-H, Zhan C-G. Free-energy perturbation simulation on transition states and redesign of butyrylcholinesterase. Biophys J. 2009;96:1931–8.

Zhan C-G, Gao D. Catalytic mechanism and energy barriers for butyrylcholinesterase-catalyzed hydrolysis of cocaine. Biophys J. 2005;89:3863–72.

Zhan C-G, Zheng F, Landry DW. Fundamental reaction mechanism for cocaine hydrolysis in human butyrylcholinesterase. J Am Chem Soc. 2003;125:2462–74.

Zheng F, Yang W, Xue L, Hou S, Liu J, Zhan CG. Design of high-activity mutants of human butyrylcholinesterase against (−)-cocaine: structural and energetic factors affecting the catalytic efficiency. Biochemistry. 2010;49:9113–9.

Zheng F, Yang W, Ko M-C, Liu J, Cho H, Gao D, Tong M, Tai H-H, Woods JH, Zhan C-G. Most efficient cocaine hydrolase designed by virtual screening of transition states. J Am Chem Soc. 2008;130:12148–55.

Zheng F, Zhan C-G. Recent progress in protein drug design and discovery with a focus on novel approaches to the development of anti-cocaine medications. Future Med Chem. 2009;1:515–28.

Zheng F, Zhan C-G. Rational design of an enzyme mutant for anti-cocaine therapeutics. J Comput Aided Mol Des. 2008a;22:661–71.

Zheng F, Zhan C-G. Structure-and-mechanism-based design and discovery of therapeutics for cocaine overdose. Org Biomol Chem. 2008b;6:836–43.

Zheng F, Zhan C-G. Modeling of pharmacokinetics of cocaine in human reveals the feasibility for development of enzyme therapies for drugs of abuse. PLoS Comput Biol. 2012;8(7):e1002610. doi:10.1371/journal.pcbi. 1002610.

Zimmerman JL. Cocaine intoxication. Crit Care Clin. 2012;28:517–26.

Chapter 11
Viral Gene Transfer of Enzymes

W. Stephen Brimijoin

11.1 Introduction

11.1.1 Delivering Anti-drug Proteins by Gene Transfer

Among the agents recently showing potential as future treatments for drug abuse are drug-targeting antibodies and enzymes. Antibodies are commonly induced by vaccines, which can be regarded as an indirect mechanism for long-term delivery of a therapeutic protein. Elsewhere in this volume are chapters that offer extensive discussions of antidrug vaccines directed against cocaine, amphetamine, nicotine, heroin, novel stimulants, and other important agents of abuse. Some of these vaccines, in particular those for nicotine, appear to be on the verge of generating antibodies of very high avidity in titers that should have a substantial impact on the abuse potential of the targeted drug. In principle it is also possible to provide antidrug antibodies by means of gene transfer, as demonstrated in recent animal studies of monoclonal anti-nicotine antibodies. Given the growing efficacy of modern vaccine technologies, however, it seems unlikely that such an approach will soon be adapted for clinical use.

In contrast to immunoglobulins, enzymes cannot be elicited indirectly. They must either be delivered as purified proteins or generated within the body by some type of expression vector, typically a virus. As the half-life of a free protein in the body is likely several days at most, direct enzyme delivery must be repeated at frequent intervals. A need for recurring treatments thus becomes a drawback that can impose severe practical limitations of cost and effectiveness over the long term. As for cost, de novo protein synthesis, or protein harvest followed by purification, is an expensive

W.S. Brimijoin, PhD
Department of Molecular Pharmacology and Experimental Therapeutics, Mayo Clinic,
200 First Street SW, #W4, Rochester, MN 55905, USA
e-mail: brimijoi@mayo.edu

I.D. Montoya (ed.), *Biologics to Treat Substance Use Disorders: Vaccines, Monoclonal Antibodies, and Enzymes*, DOI 10.1007/978-3-319-23150-1_11

undertaking. Although mass production may lead to economies of scale, costs of each episode of treatment for a single patient may run into tens of thousands of dollars, mounting to hundreds of thousands over the course of a year. As for the issue of effectiveness, over the long term the treated individual will need to make repeated positive decisions to continue therapy. Since an addiction therapy is unlikely to deliver immediate benefit in terms of general well-being and might even be mildly aversive, the patient who is battling an addiction will be at risk of prematurely abandoning treatment. These two issues should *not* be fatal to strategies based on direct administration of a therapeutic protein, because there are promising solutions to the problem. In particular, new developments such as slow-release nanoparticle depots are making it possible to sustain therapeutic levels of desired proteins for several weeks at a time. Further consideration of such possibilities, especially with regard to cocaine hydrolyzing enzymes, will be touched upon later in this article and in greater detail elsewhere in this volume (see Chap. 12 by Chang-Guo Zhan).

Here we will survey a strategy for treating cocaine addiction by gene transfer of an enzyme known as butyrylcholinesterase (BChE), which after multiple active-site mutations for breakdown and elimination of cocaine has gained high efficiency against that target and can rightly be described as a cocaine hydrolase (CocH). This strategy can be taken as an example of an alternative or complementary approach for delivering proteins that reduce or eliminate access of addictive substances to brain reward centers and, therefore, accomplish two major goals: (1) aiding a treatment-seeking drug user to avoid relapse into drug taking in the early stages of recovery and (2) sustaining that effect long enough for robust drug resistance and better habits to take hold.

In principle, gene transfer can be accomplished in any of several ways, but by far the most durable and effective approach in terms of sustained protein levels is currently based on use of viral vectors. Accumulated data have established that, with some viral vectors, one can attain extremely high levels of a desired protein in the general circulation or the liver, or brain, for essentially as long as desired. Even a permanent expression window is possible in principle though it may not be desirable. Later on this chapter will consider specific examples in terms of expression levels, duration, and locus. We will also take up the issue of intrinsic toxicity, acute and chronic, arising directly from the vector itself (i.e., adverse responses to the presence of the vehicle administered to drive the expression of a therapeutic protein).

Before launching into these matters, it is worth looking at alternative approaches to gene transfer that involve no virus and might ultimately prove intrinsically safe. One such alternative is based on a liposomal nanoparticle or "nanocomplex" that has been designed to encapsulate plasmid DNA encoding a therapeutic protein. Investigators have had some success in using liposomal nanoparticles encapsulating DNA to drive the expression of peptides, proteins, or other "molecular medicines" for cancer chemotherapy (Freedman et al. 2009). An interesting variation on this technology involves incorporation of a single-chain antibody fragment recognizing the transferrin receptor, which enables i.v.-injected nanoparticles to cross the blood–brain barrier and drive protein expression in the brain. The author is aware of unpublished research indicating that this approach is suitable for use with cDNA of enzymes that hydrolyze cocaine. It remains to be seen whether it will be capable of bringing the payload protein to levels that impact drug reward. It is also not yet clear how long the elevated expression will last and what sort of decay curve it will follow. Although this novel and proprietary technology has not been available to other investigators in a way that allows full evaluation of its potential, it appears likely to be intrinsically safe and it might sustain expression of a desired transgene product much longer than would a direct injection of "naked" protein. Furthermore, there could be added therapeutic impact from favorable actions in the periphery and within the central nervous system. At present, however, available information does not allow firm predictions about the ultimate impact of nanoparticle technology in addiction therapy.

11.2 General Overview of Viral Gene Transfer

11.2.1 Historical Background

More than two decades ago, viral gene transfer began to demonstrate its potential for generating and sustaining levels of protein and peptides that are crucial to normal physiology but, for genetic reasons, were deficient or entirely lacking in certain patients. Initially the therapeutic impact of viral vectors on such life-threatening conditions aroused widespread enthusiasm. One early application for such agents was to reverse inherited and life-threatening disorders stemming from congenital inability to express one or more peptides or proteins involved in the essential process of clot formation. What initially appeared to be a powerful means of curing such crippling diseases soon proved riskier than investigators had imagined. A tragic sentinel event at the University of Pennsylvania was the acute anaphylactic reaction of a young patient who received a large dose of "classical adenoviral vector" (AD) intended to overcome his life-threatening problems with a genetically based clotting deficiency disorder. This treatment evoked an intense "cytokine storm," probably triggered by the adenoviral coat proteins, which led to the subject's death 4 days later. Not surprisingly, the outcome led to a complete and immediate hiatus of viral vector trials. During this moratorium there was a widespread search for vectors with far lower acute toxicity.

For a brief period it was believed that retroviruses were well suited to serve that role. In fact the *acute* toxicity of such agents did appear to be significantly lower than that of AD vectors. Several patients were treated successfully for inherited combined immunodeficiency disorder (SCID) and showed an excellent response. Approximately 3 years later, however, a presumably treatment-related leukemia arose in several recipients. This effect was eventually tied to disruption of oncogenes during the process of inserting vector DNA into host chromosomes. Again viral gene transfer for clinical application came under intense scrutiny. Eventually, cautious studies of gene transfer resumed, but under stricter guidelines. By the year 2005, approximately 1000 trials had been launched or scheduled worldwide, virtually all of them falling into the FDA category of "phase one," that is, aimed at testing risk/safety issues rather than actual clinical effectiveness. As this chapter was being written, an online website, "Gene Therapy Net," was reporting trials initiated or updated at a rate of more than one per day. This statistic is one clear indication that clinical applications of gene transfer are now being actively pursued despite prior missteps and regulatory hurdles.

11.2.2 Classes of Vector

Viral gene transfer vectors fall into two general categories: integrating and non-integrating. The former are specifically designed to incorporate into chromosomal DNA and therefore have a potential to remain active for the life of the recipient, unless gene silencing occurs. In contrast, the latter may persist in the cytoplasm or in the nucleus as "episomal concatemers," which are typically lost when host cells undergo mitosis. Thus, expression of a non-integrating vector may also last indefinitely in tissues composed of nondividing cells, such as skeletal muscle, and neurons in both the brain and the peripheral nervous system. These cells are in fact potential targets for vectors of certain specific serotypes. In comparison, vector persistence in the liver is limited by the lifetime of hepatocytes, which is 2–3 years in humans and rodents as well. Of course, at any given moment, the hepatic population consists of old cells in the process of dying and new ones that will last for years. Thus the time course of "vector load" in that tissue will follow an exponential decay curve with a half-life of ~2 years. This feature holds particularly important implications for therapeutic gene transfer of proteins intended for addiction treatment, because the liver is the key organ for surveillance and metabolism of biologically active substances of all kinds, including drugs of abuse.

Two important examples of the integrating vectors are lentiviruses and onco-retroviruses. Those two classes will not be discussed further in this article beyond stating that they pose a risk of oncogenesis. If that problem is ever definitively resolved, integrating vectors might indeed prove useful in achieving lifelong transduction of a transgene. Such a result would not only present a means of curing single-gene deficits but might also offer meaningful assistance to patients with major neuropsychiatric disorders that are also essentially permanent and unresponsive to medication. Meanwhile, however, it is not clear that permanent gene transduction is needed to treat drug addiction, and recent work discussed below indicates that less problematic, non-integrating vectors may well be able to serve such purposes with considerably less risk.

Examples of *non-integrating* vectors, which are the primary focus of this chapter, are as follows: (1) AD, the classic adenovirus vectors of various serotypes, especially type 5 (involved in the Pennsylvania incident); (2) hdAD, the so-called "helper-dependent adenoviruses" of the same serotypes; and (3) AAV, the adeno-associated virus vectors. Each of these vector types is inherently capable of generating high levels of transgene product by co-opting host systems to transcribe cDNA encoding the protein of therapeutic interest.

Broadly speaking, recent research indicates that the two safest and generally effective non-integrating viral vectors are hdAD and AAV. The former has been artificially deprived of coding information for proteins essential for viral replication, which requires a helper virus to package therapeutic DNA into preformed adenovirus coat proteins of the chosen serotype. Recent work has demonstrated that gene transfer of CocH with a liver-directed hdAD vector can sustain very high levels of circulating enzyme in rodents. Specifically, we obtained 1000-fold increases of cocaine hydrolyzing activity for at least six months in rats (Anker et al. 2012). In separate and ongoing studies, mice have shown substantial hydrolase transduction for 24 months or more after initial treatment [unpublished results]. Therefore continued testing is focused on hepatotropic viral vectors incorporating liver-specific promoters. Signs of toxicity have been absent at the doses used (up to 10^{13} particles per mouse, delivered through the tail vein), which elevated circulating cocaine hydrolase activity by a factor of approximately 1,000,000 (Geng et al. 2013). In particular, blood monitoring for liver enzymes detected no elevation of markers that serve as signals of damage to hepatocytes. Furthermore, liver tissue has appeared entirely normal in postmortem histological sections. Treated mice show normal behavior patterns, normal levels of spontaneous activity, and weight gain, and when challenged with doses of cocaine that are hepatotoxic or lethal in unprotected animals, they show dramatically reduced toxicity or none at all.

The second vector to consider, AAV, is naturally replication incompetent and also requires packaging help. One important limitation of AAV vectors is their relatively small "cloning capacity" or "packaging capacity." This is measured by the length, in kilobases (kb), of the extrinsic sequences that a vector can accommodate to drive high-level expression of an encoded therapeutic protein (i.e., the DNA "payload"). In AAV, the packaging capacity is strictly limited to 4.7 kb including the full coding sequence, the promoter and enhancer elements, and the inverted terminal repeats (ITRs). Thus, AAV vectors are much more readily suited to deliver cDNA for peptides or small proteins than, for example, large proteins like G-protein-coupled receptors. Nevertheless, a fully formed BChE monomer is only about 68 kilo-daltons in mass, and its coding sequence is relatively small at approximately 1.8 kb. This leaves room to incorporate multiple promoter and enhancer elements without exceeding the AAV cloning capacity. In most of our recent experiments with BChE expression vectors, we have relied on a so-called VIP system developed in Professor David Baltimore's lab at Caltech. This system incorporates a CMV enhancer, a chicken beta-actin promoter, and a UBC enhancer upstream of the cDNA insert. Also included, downstream of the insert, is an SV40 late poly-A signal and a WPRE sequence (woodchuck hepatitis posttranscriptional regulatory element). Altogether, these components bring the inserted DNA up to a total length of 2.6 kb. Such a vector in our hands has recently proved capable of generating high-level expression of native BChE and, more importantly, of alternate BChE versions incorporating mutations that confer high efficiency in metabolizing cocaine.

Metrics for choosing between AAV and hdAD as candidates for an enzyme gene transfer to treat cocaine addiction are not fully developed. Both of these vectors will support long-sustained transduction in mice. There is a general perception that AAV poses less risk of acute toxicity than hdAD. Our experience in rodents is in line with that perception when equivalent viral doses are compared. However, recent test results indicate that the yield-to-dose ratio is much higher with type 5 hdAD than with an AAV vector that had been designed to express the identical coding sequence for our therapeutic enzyme candidate. Specifically, regardless of species tested, it appears that a roughly 10-fold higher dose of AAV vector (measured by viral genome copies) is required to match the transduction effect achieved by hdAD encoding the same enzyme DNA. Transduction by either vector in mice is similarly long lasting (i.e., the time course of enzyme levels in the circulation is approximately the same, with significant expression still persisting 2 years after treatment). In rats, for reasons not known to us, this vector generates much less BChE expression. Expression levels driven by AAV are higher in rhesus monkeys, and moderately long lasting, but still not equal to what can be achieved with hdAD vector encoding the same cDNA (Brimijoin, Carroll, 2015).

The issue of transduction durability and choice of vector platform is complicated by regulatory concerns. Naively, our initial concept was that an optimal gene therapy approach to addiction would be the one that led to the longest window of enzyme expression. Instead, recent experience with the US FDA revealed that this agency regards gene transfer of enzymes for drug dependency as a very different issue than gene transfer to remedy a genetically based deficiency of clotting factors or proteins critically involved in the immune response to pathogens. Instead it is seen as a treatment that, in most cases, should *not* continue indefinitely. Official comments from an FDA "pre-IND meeting" suggested that, in their view, an expression window on the order of 2–3 years in duration would be optimal. Fortunately such an interval might be able to bridge the period of maximum risk for relapse.

This process of protein expression is termed "viral gene transduction." Studies from our laboratory, based on such vectors in mice and rats, demonstrated the feasibility of using this technology to raise plasma levels of a natural enzyme by more than 1000-fold, making it the second most abundant protein in the bloodstream. These levels were also long sustained and were not associated with overt toxicity.

11.3 Long-Term Delivery of Cocaine Hydrolase by Viral Gene Transfer

11.3.1 Initial Studies

Most of the author's research into treatments for cocaine addiction has involved the ubiquitous plasma enzyme formerly known as pseudocholinesterase and currently as "butyrylcholinesterase" (BChE). Now, in a pentamutant version that seems close to being optimally mutated for cocaine hydrolysis, it can legitimately be called "cocaine hydrolase" (CocH). Positive results of recent behavioral experiments with enzyme-treated rats suggest that therapies based on CocH might indeed be effective if comparable levels of enzyme can be delivered and sustained in human beings. In rats the direct effects of enzyme injection last only a few hours, limited by the protein half-life (8 h for the tested mutant versus 40 h for native rat BChE). We realized that it might be possible to extend the duration of enzyme treatments with various protein modifications to increase in vivo half-life, such as PEGylation (covalent modification of peptide or protein by conjugation with polyethylene glycol), or with slow-release depot preparations. However, with a view toward truly long-sustained therapeutic effects after a single treatment, and in view of the huge costs associated with treatments requiring gram quantities of pure protein, we began investigating gene transfer approaches. Initial experiments with this technology involved early-stage, E-1 deleted adenoviral vectors with mutant hBChE cDNA sequences driven by a CMV promoter. This type of construct was known for ability to transduce substantial levels of various transgenes in the liver but also to arouse immune responses that limited the duration of such a response. Overall our results were in line with previous data on gene transfer of other proteins. In that sense they provided little new information but they did serve to demonstrate basic feasibility. At peak expression, 5–7 days after treatment with 2.2×10^9 plaque-forming units (active viral particles) of vector encoding a double-mutant human BChE (A328W, Y332A), cocaine hydrolase activity in rat plasma had risen 3000 times above its initial level (Gao et al. 2005). At these levels the mutated BChE accelerated cocaine breakdown to a point at which locomotor responses to i.p. cocaine injection were sharply curtailed.

Further studies on the efficiency of BChE transduction were carried out with a helper-dependent adenoviral vector (hdAD) incorporating a liver-specific human ApoE promoter. This advanced vector lacks DNA for all viral proteins and is much less prone than a first-generation AD vector to provoke immunological reactions (Parks et al. 1996). Our results showed that transduction of a cocaine hydrolase, based on the quadruple mutant referred to above, was sustained at high levels for long periods of time. Peak activity was reached approximately 2 weeks after vector injection, leveling off in the range of 1000–2000 mU/ml. One year later, the longest interval tested up to that point, plasma cocaine hydrolase activity in the recipient rats was still more than 20 % of the initial peak levels (Gao and Brimijoin 2009). To investigate the in vivo turnover of transduced enzyme 9 months after vector delivery, we used iso-OMPA, an organophosphate known for selective and irreversible inactivation of BChE. This agent was given in a dose that inactivated BChE by 98–99 %% but largely spared AChE (<5 % inactivation). From the quasi-exponential recovery of cocaine hydrolase activity in these animals, we deduced a plasma half-life of 60 h for the expressed transgene. That value actually exceeded the half-life estimated for native BChE in rats that had received no vector. In other words the mutated BChE was as stable as the unmodified enzyme, even though, as a human protein given to mice, it elicited trace amounts of anti-BChE antibody in the plasma samples that were screened.

11.3.2 Locus of Expression

The locus of transgene expression is highly relevant in terms of efficacy and even more so, looking ahead to possible clinical trials, in terms of safety. After delivery of a viral vector encoding appropriate cDNA, the extent of enzyme expression in different tissues is determined by two key factors. First is the tissue tropism of the vector itself, i.e., relative preferences for specific organs of the body and for specific cell types within these organs. Second is the promoter sequence incorporated into the vector that must drive transgene expression. To impact a behavioral problem like drug addiction, there seem to be two logical sites for expressing an antidrug agent. One would be the central nervous system itself, where drugs of abuse exert their primary actions. The other would be a peripheral tissue that is naturally involved in surveillance of foreign substances entering the bloodstream and, for this reason, is adapted to produce and release enzymes into plasma where they can intercept or destroy drug before it reaches CNS targets. The liver fits both of these requirements. Among the viral vectors that are plausible candidates for a "drug interception therapy," none of them are likely to cross the blood–brain barrier and drive gene expression in the brain unless they are administered directly into brain tissue (i.e., by stereotaxic surgery). Such a highly invasive approach might be considered for treatment of a fatal illness like malignant glioblastoma or a progressive and irreversible condition like Parkinson's disease, but it appears to be radically inappropriate for treatment of a behavioral disorder. Fortunately, our animal data indicated that systemic transduction of cocaine hydrolase is at least as effective as transduction in neostriatal reward nuclei (Gao and Brimijoin 2009).

As targets for systemic delivery, there are few choices. Muscle is an accessible, large-mass tissue with the advantage that minor dysfunction is unlikely to pose extreme risks. This tissue site may be desirable when attempting to replace a deficient protein such as a clotting factor that is not required in large quantities. However muscle is a poor choice if there is need for high levels of expression, e.g., to intercept large drug doses entering the circulation. A focus on circulation and blood flow led us toward the one tissue that has evolved specifically for eliminating or neutralizing toxic xenobiotics, namely, the liver. The liver receives a large fraction of the total cardiac output, and over a period of not more than one or two circulation times (i.e., a few minutes at most), it has the opportunity to interact with essentially all blood-borne substances. The liver is also the natural location for synthesis and release of butyrylcholinesterase, which, after appropriate protein engineering, has shown great promise as a means of degrading cocaine en route to the brain. Acceleration of cocaine metabolism by a liver-transduced cocaine hydrolase is likely to be an efficient means of reducing blood levels of this stimulant. The metabolic effect has been demonstrated to include two components: (1) a diminished peak level of circulating cocaine and (2) drastically increased rate of clearance from the bloodstream. These effects can be attributed partially to the fact that any blood-borne chemical must pass repeatedly through the liver and, if it crosses cell membranes, will be in direct contact with metabolic enzymes in the hepatocytes. In addition, as directed by the signaling sequences in the BChE gene, a large fraction of the newly synthesized enzyme is secreted into the circulation, where it remains with a half-life of many days and has the ability to destroy cocaine on contact.

11.3.3 Impact of Optimal BChE Vector on Cocaine Metabolism

As noted earlier in this essay, accelerated drug metabolism has been developing as an alternative to vaccines as a way of reducing cocaine's brain access, which is a key step in the reward process that generates and maintains addictive behaviors. This approach is tenable for two main reasons. First, native BChE converts cocaine directly into two metabolites, benzoic acid and ecgonine methyl ester. Based on the older literature, these compounds were expected to have little or no reward properties. We have now confirmed that expectation in a recent study utilizing a "conditioned place preference" paradigm, which assesses drug reward by determining the relative time spent in a chamber where drug was repeatedly given, versus a chamber associated with saline (Murthy et al. 2015). Second, CocH, a BChE with 5 active-site mutations, drives the same reaction with greatly increased activity (see below). It is unfortunate that this strategy does not readily generalize to the metabolism of other addictive substances such as amphetamines, nicotine, "bath salts," and many other stimulant drugs whose metabolism requires cytochrome-p450-dependent pathways in the liver (Howard et al. 2002; Sellers et al. 2000). These pathways require intact electron transport chains that only operate in an intracellular environment and cannot readily be enhanced by an exogenous enzyme. Therefore, if a BChE-based therapy is ever approved for clinical use in treating drug addiction, cocaine might be the only drug that can be effectively targeted.

As a potential therapeutic agent, BChE and its key mutant CocH both appear very safe. Unlike acetylcholinesterase (AChE), BChE has no major impact on cholinergic neurotransmission that would be disturbed by increased levels of enzyme. Although it does hydrolyze acetylcholine, BChE accompanies every transfusion without ill effect. In view of these facts, Gorelick in 1997 proposed using human BChE to treat cocaine overdose (Gorelick 1997). Natural BChE is not highly efficient with cocaine. In an attempt to increase its ability to metabolize that drug, Lockridge and collaborators used site-directed mutagenesis to obtain a BChE with fourfold improved catalytic activity (Xie et al. 1999). This process, aided by computer-based modeling of cocaine docking and catalysis, continued in our laboratory and that of C.-G. Zhan in Kentucky, leading to a series of "rationally designed" BChE mutants with increasing catalytic activity against cocaine (Pan et al. 2005; Sun et al. 2002; Sun and Lau 2001; Yang et al. 2010; Zheng et al. 2008). The key enzyme yardstick is "catalytic efficiency," defined as the ratio between "k_{cat}" (molecules of substrate hydrolyzed per min, per active site) and "K_m" (substrate concentration at half-maximal velocity). Unless drug saturates the binding site (an improbable or very transient condition), an efficient enzyme will outperform others with higher catalytic "power" (larger k_{cat}) but disproportionately higher K_m. Compared with natural BChE, the optimal mutant cocaine hydrolase, "CocH," has lost catalytic efficiency with acetylcholine but has gained 1500-fold greater efficiency with cocaine (Chen et al. 2015).

The advent of a near optimal CocH led to observations that an efficient cocaine-metabolizing enzyme not merely prevents cocaine toxicity in animal models but will also *reverse* it. In our hands CocH protein proved able to abort lethal cocaine-induced seizures in rats and reliably rescue them even when delivered after major convulsions had already begun (Brimijoin et al. 2008). Still more interesting with regard to addictive behaviors were a series of findings with instrumented rats trained on lever pressing for i.v. cocaine reward. Collaborating with Marilyn Carroll and her students at University of Minnesota, we were able to demonstrate that i.p. injection of purified CocH enzyme delivered immediately before a behavioral session reliably prevents "reinstatement" behavior (Brimijoin et al. 2008). The reinstatement paradigm is a model of addiction relapse. Briefly described, the procedure allows subjects to establish a pattern of robust responding for drug delivered directly into the vena cava, inducing a virtually immediate reward as the cocaine bolus passes into the brain. When this behavioral pattern is well established, the reward link is canceled and, over time, lever-pressing behavior extinguishes. But later on, when these same animals receive "free cocaine" just before entering the behavioral apparatus, they show a brief burst of activity on the lever formerly associated with drug reward. This behavior is termed "reinstatement responding" and it was completely suppressed by an injection of purified CocH given shortly before the test. As could be expected, however, the protective effect of CocH protein was brief (1 or 2 days). In contrast, when an efficient hdAD-CocH vector became available, an equally powerful blockade of cocaine-stimulated reinstatement behavior was achieved, and the effect persisted for months (Fig. 11.1). To confirm that this outcome was entirely due to enhanced cocaine metabolism, a final experiment was performed with amphetamine as the "priming stimulus." Not surprisingly, since CocH does not hydrolyze amphetamine, this drug provoked a strong reinstatement response in vector-treated rats as well as in the control rats.

The sustained and specific blockade of reinstatement was an encouraging sign that CocH gene transfer might eventually prove useful in protecting a treatment-seeking human from experiencing a major relapse into cocaine abuse triggered by a single re-encounter with that drug. A weakness in the simple reinstatement model, however, was that the "priming exposure" involved a relatively slow route of drug delivery (i.e., subcutaneous or intraperitoneal injection). Since the intensity of reward typically increases with the speed of drug delivery to the brain, more realistic experiments based on rapid drug delivery were clearly needed. The most rigorous test we could construct was to assess the effect of gene transfer upon ongoing responding for i.v. cocaine reward delivered through a cannula permanently implanted in the vena cava. Such experiments, carried out in Dr. Carroll's laboratory, used two groups of rats fully trained on lever pressing for cocaine reward and maintaining a steady level of responding. These groups were given different doses

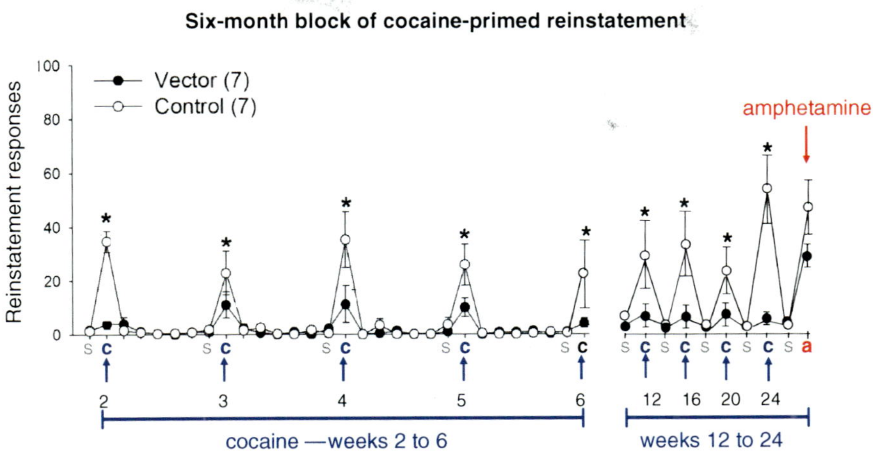

Fig. 11.1 Long-term blockade of cocaine-primed reinstatement responding. CocH vector-treated rats ($N=14$) made significantly fewer responses (# $p<0.05$) on the lever previously paired with cocaine than control rats ($N=26$) following a 10 mg/kg cocaine i.p. priming injection during reinstatement testing sessions up to 24 weeks after vector or control injections. This effect was specific to cocaine, as 2 mg/kg d-amphetamine i.p. priming injections administered at 24 weeks post-vector injection elicited a similar number of responses in CocH vector-treated and control rats

of hdAD vector encoding CocH (10^{11} and 10^{12} viral genomes per rat). The results were clear cut (Fig. 11.2). With either dose there was a lag of several days during which ongoing responding continued at the same stable level as before treatment. Then at about 5 days, the lever-pressing behavior began to *increase*. This outcome occurred in both experimental groups. It was interpreted as an attempt to compensate for a loss of reward derived from the drug delivery, which was unchanged in the amount of cocaine. This compensatory behavior was apparently successful for the rats that received low-dose vector, which continued with their increased lever pressing indefinitely. In sharp contrast, the rats that received high-dose vector abandoned lever pressing altogether and for the entire remainder of the 2-month study.

11.4 Avoiding Vector Toxicity

Despite these encouraging results, there are serious challenges to the clinical application of hdAD vectors. The greatest of these is the demonstrated risk of short term toxicity, particularly in the liver, induced by transient exposure to the capsid proteins in the viral vector. These proteins are required for initial interaction with hepatocytes, our preferred cell type for enzyme transduction, but they evoke a dose-related response from the innate host immune system, which can be rapid and severe (Brunetti-Pierri et al. 2004; Muruve 2004). Hepatocytes are particularly vulnerable during the process of vector uptake. This reaction is equivalent to the one provoked by early-generation E-1 deleted AD vectors, which is suspected as the primary

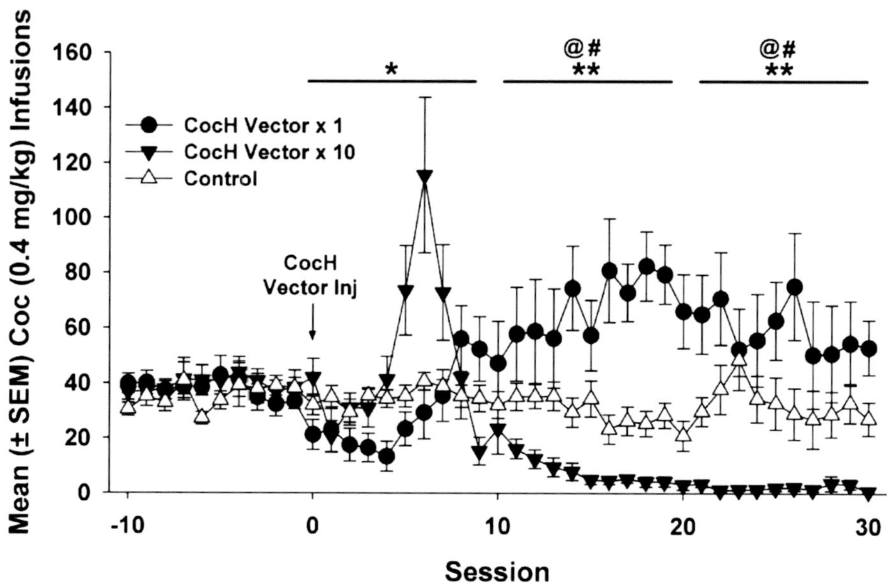

Fig. 11.2 Long-term blockade of ongoing responding for cocaine reward. Mean (± SEM) cocaine infusions before and after delivery of CocH vector or vehicle. CocH vector × 1 rats notably increased their infusions relative to controls (** $p<0.01$) and baseline (at $p<0.01$) following hdAD-CocH vector injection. While the CocH vector × 10 rats increased their infusions for 10 days following vector delivery, their infusions subsequently decreased to near-zero levels and were significantly lower than their infusions at baseline (at $p<0.01$) and lower than that of CocH vector × 1 rats (** $p<0.01$)

cause of the fatal outcome in one of the earliest clinical trials of AD gene therapy (Raper et al. 2003). Since the immune response is transient and limited to the period during which viral capsid proteins remain in situ, the problem can be mitigated to an extent by temporary immune suppression. In fact, although multiple factors come into play, it has been reported that pretreatment with the anti-inflammatory steroid, dexamethasone (Seregin et al. 2009), reduces the innate toxicity of adenoviral coat proteins. We used this approach in studies with rhesus monkeys given relatively high doses of hdAD under thiofluorane anesthesia: up to 10^{12} viral particles per animal. None of the treated animals exhibited signs of discomfort or distress after recovering from the anesthesia or later on. Nonetheless, it would be premature to conclude that clinical application of such vectors is completely safe.

The principal alternative to hdAD in gene therapy for cocaine abuse is AAV. AAV vectors have seen limited applications because of the tight restrictions on packaging capacity, i.e., the length of DNA sequences that can be introduced as transgene payload is less than 5 kB as noted earlier. A second problem is that infections with wild type AAV are prevalent in the human population and the resulting immunity prevents effective use of vectors with the same serotype. On the positive side, AAV has never been associated with human illness, and it has proved relatively benign in animal studies. As a result, and despite the drawbacks just noted, several clinical trials have been completed with AAV vectors and more are ongoing or pending. In our early mouse experiments, however, AAV-8 vector loaded with cocaine hydrolase generated only 20 % as much plasma cocaine hydrolase activity as the equivalent hdAD vector. If this problem can be overcome, the stage will be set for a fair comparison between two promising vector platforms, in which the primary standard will be delivery of the greatest drug-metabolizing power with the risk of adverse effect.

11.4.1 Probable Duration of Expression in Humans

It should not be necessary to provide permanent gene transduction in order to treat addiction effectively. However, at least 6 months of effective drug interception is needed, and a period of 2 or 3 years may be desirable to aid in cessation of drug intake and avoidance of relapse. This time frame would not require a vector that incorporates into genomic DNA (with attendant risk of disrupting oncogenes), but can be achieved with a vector that persists as a quasi-stable episomal element (e.g., helper-dependent "gutted" adenoviral vector or adeno-associated viral vector). The latter two vectors show long persistence even though they do not propagate from cell to cell and are diluted or lost as a result of mitosis. Even in rats and mice, whose hepatocytes turn over with a half-life of a year or less, effective levels of transgene remain for many months after initial vector treatment. Life spans for hepatocytes in adult human liver are estimated to lie between 300 and 500 days (Spalding et al. 2005). Therefore, if cell turnover is actually the primary mechanism for loss of vector DNA, one could expect a therapeutic window on the order of a year or two at most.

11.4.2 Drawbacks and Obstacles to Gene Transfer

One major present drawback is a persistent concern for safety, which may be well founded and certainly deserves attention. A key risk factor appears to be the brief but intense innate immune response to viral capsid proteins (Muruve 2004). Much research has concentrated on this issue and how to minimize or avoid it (Brunetti-Pierri and Ng 2008, 2011). Deletion of multiple viral genes while preserving transduction capability is one important step, as in the engineered helper-dependent adenoviral vectors (Morral et al. 1999) or the vectors based on naturally helper-dependent adeno-associated virus (Brantly et al. 2009; Manno et al. 2006). These modified agents typically have no ability to express viral proteins in vivo and thus, longer term, may remain "hidden" from immune surveillance (Vetrini and Ng 2011). On the other hand, to deliver an engineered DNA payload, viral particles must first attach to the plasma membranes of host cells that can translate the genetic information into a protein product. This function requires packaging of the functional DNA within a coat that (a) protects it from dispersal and metabolic attack in body fluids, (b) selectively binds surface targets characteristic of the host cells chosen for transgene product, and (c) stimulates endocytosis of the delivered DNA. At the present state of vector technology, the most efficient means of accomplishing this objective uses artificial protein coats derived from the shell of a relatively benign "helper virus." The immune system still recognizes these coats, which remain able to trigger a seriously adverse response. Such responses are typically short lived, however. They are also dose related and can be minimized by delivering a smaller load of vector, albeit at the price of obtaining less transgene product.

Fortunately, transient immunosuppression with anti-inflammatory steroids, such as dexamethasone, will reduce host immune responses to viral vector and lessen subsequent toxicity (Seregin et al. 2009) while also prolonging transgene expression (Kumahara et al. 2005). In some of our animal studies, immunosuppression was also required for adequate levels of therapeutic protein because the subjects had undergone prior procedures that established a state of chronic inflammation. This happened in animals subjected to procedures creating sustained inflammatory stress (e.g., implantation of multiple cannulas), which can impair subsequent virally mediated transgene expression (Gao, Brimijoin, 2015). In higher organisms, especially nonhuman primates and humans, the acute immune response to vector is very strong, associated with a sharp rise in cytokines such as interleukin 6, while immunosuppression is more difficult and less effective (Brunetti-Pierri et al. 2004). Progress in this arena is critical to future success.

11.5 Long-Term Safety Issues

In view of the high bar that must eventually be cleared if BChE/CocH gene transfer can be tested in clinical trial, our research group has carried out numerous studies to evaluate safety issues. These studies were carried out largely in mice but also to an extent in rats and in a few rhesus monkeys. These studies involved delivery of viral vector in doses up to 3×10^4 genomes per kg body weight in rodents and 3×10^{12} genomes per kg in rhesus (several times larger than would likely be given to a human patient). Multiple issues were examined, many of them selected in light of the fact that BChE gene transfer necessarily increases the capacity for hydrolysis of acetylcholine, the cholinergic neurotransmitter. For example, grip strength and maximum treadmill effort were evaluated in mice (Murthy et al. 2014a). Also, even though systemic gene transfer should not affect CNS function and our prior studies showed no viral particles in the brains of treated rodents, cognitive function was tested with mice in a structured water maze. No deficits were observed. Liver function appeared normal and there was no elevation of sentinel enzymes such as alanine aminotransferase in plasma. Resting mouse blood pressure was normal as measured by semiautomatic plethysmography. EKG telemetry with indwelling sensors revealed no alteration of resting heart rate or QT interval (unpublished data). Spontaneous locomotor activity was not affected, nor was body temperature, O_2–CO_2 exchanger, or overall metabolic rate as assessed from 24-h sessions in a metabolic chamber (Murthy et al. 2014a, b). And finally, no differences between treated and untreated mice were detected in a pathology analysis of multiple tissues including the liver, kidney, heart, lung, brain, muscle, stomach, and small intestine, in professional harvests at 1 week, 3 weeks, 3 months, and 22 months after vector delivery.

11.6 FDA Concerns

When it comes to protein-based therapeutics, the US FDA appears to have several general concerns focusing on duration of action, immunological responses, and amount of protein delivery over time, among other issues. A gene therapy approach necessarily complicates the process of seeking approval for an investigational therapy of this nature. There are two key reasons. First, the vector is seen as a potential risk in itself, regardless of the nature of encoded protein, and second, the magnitude and time course of the vector-transduced protein is more difficult to predict and control as compared with direct administration of a highly purified final product (enzyme). In fact, after a recent pre-IND conference with the FDA, the agency explicitly stated concerns about the duration, level, and enhanced affinity of our proposed transgene expression product (i.e., cocaine hydrolase) which could persist for years in subjects receiving this investigational treatment (viral vector). Based on those concerns, the FDA asked for extensive new data demonstrating vector biodistribution and persistence, as well as transgene expression levels over time. The agency also expressed a need for supporting data addressing the potential that overexpression of this enzyme and its resulting effect on endogenous biochemical pathways (e.g., cholinergic synapses) and clinical medications (e.g., pharmacological muscle relaxants, morphine-based pain medication, antibiotics, etc.) that might be administered to these subjects over the course of their lifetime. Proponents of a gene therapy for cocaine addiction must take all possible steps to address such issues. What the FDA did *not* pose as a precondition for eventual clinical trial was to duplicate all preclinical testing on vector transduction with essentially identical tests based upon purified CocH. In short, the focus is upon the candidate therapeutic (i.e., viral vector) and not the downstream enzyme product. Our attempts to allay all concerns expressed in regard to BChE gene transfer are extensive and ongoing. They are briefly summarized below in the interests of guiding other investigators with similar goals and issues.

11.6.1 Addressing FDA Concerns

The general literature on cholinergic pharmacology and physiology provides no reason to expect serious toxicity from high levels of BChE per se. Nonetheless any potential harm deserves close attention. As noted previously, BChE is largely viewed as a metabolic enzyme that hydrolyzes bioactive esters in the diet and also, under certain circumstances, may play an auxiliary role in cholinergic neurotransmission by virtue of its capacity to hydrolyze acetylcholine. In fact BChE is about 20 % as efficient in hydrolyzing acetylcholine as is acetylcholinesterase (AChE), which is the key enzyme for clearing that transmitter from the neuromuscular junction and other cholinergic synapses. This catalytic property raises the possibility that elevated BChE levels would shorten or weaken synaptic potentials evoked by acetylcholine at the neuromuscular junction and at sympathetic and parasympathetic ganglia in the heart, blood vessels, glands, and intestinal smooth muscle. Nonetheless, there are good reasons to think that systemic BChE gene transfer will not disturb cholinergic function by reducing synaptic acetylcholine concentration either in the periphery or in the central nervous system. First, all tested BChE-based hydrolases for cocaine have shown *reduced* activity with acetylcholine as a substrate. In particular, if gene transfer of highly efficient CocH resulted in twice-normal plasma BChE levels, one could expect a nearly 2000-fold increase in hydrolysis of cocaine but less than a twofold increase in hydrolysis of acetylcholine. Such an effect should be trivial since transgene expression is largely confined to the liver and plasma while AChE is concentrated in cholinergic synapses where it reaches levels hundreds of times greater than those that could be achieved by transduced BChE. This theoretical picture is in line with the outcome of our own as yet unreported studies with large nonhuman primates (rhesus macaques). It is also in line with unpublished data from the US Department of Defense (personal communication, B.P. Doctor), which recently conducted experiments that involved delivery of BChE to human subjects for evaluating its potential to protect against chemical warfare agents. Unpublished results from the preclinical studies carried out at Walter Reed and USAMRICD the US Army Medical Research Institute of Chemical Defense (personal communications from B.P. Doctor and D. Cerasoli) revealed no physiologic disturbances of any sort from doses of highly purified human enzyme that raised the plasma BChE activity to levels several-fold above normal.

11.6.2 Species Selection for Preclinical Studies

We take note of FDA's statement that, for preclinical studies, in order to generate relevant data to guide clinical trial design, the selected animal species should demonstrate a biological response to the intended clinical product similar to that expected in humans. Some factors to consider include (a) comparability of physiology and anatomy to that of humans, (b) similar susceptibility to infection by the vector, (c) immune tolerance to the expressed human transgene, and (d) preexisting immunity to your clinical vector/transgene (e.g., neutralizing antibodies). In fact there is no ideal species but in our view a reasonable plan can be based primarily on mice.

FDA's guidance summary also recognizes that, due to the species-specific nature of the final clinical product (e.g., human versus mouse CocH, species-specific immunogenicity, etc.), testing the exact product intended for clinical administration in animals may not be informative. Therefore we intend to evaluate murine CocH as an analogous product, which we have already found not to evoke antibodies in mice. We will also test clinical grade human CocH under conditions where a moderate immune response to that protein should not confound the results.

11.7 What Remains Before CocH Vector Can Undergo Clinical Trial?

It is now clear that the remaining obstacles to a so-called "first-in-human" clinical trial of CocH viral vector are quite substantial but not insuperable if adequate funding can be secured. Funding for a trial itself is an obvious requirement. Unfortunately, it will also be expensive to complete the investigations that FDA will regard as "definitive preclinical studies." Such studies must be carried out either with clinical grade vector produced under good manufacturing process (GMP) standards or with a comparable vector generated by "essentially similar" production methods. Initial quotes from not-for-profit, university-associated manufacturers are in the range of \$1.5 million for a single batch of 10^{15} genomes of AAV 2/8 vector encoding human CocH. Our task will now be to obtain "comparable vectors" encoding mouse and rhesus CocH (mimicking our lab-generated vectors). We will use them to compile the remaining data needed for the IND application, making sure that each of the most important studies will be validated by quality assurance personnel with strict regard to explicit protocols for each intervention and observation.

References

Anker JJ, Brimijoin S, Gao Y, Geng L, Zlebnik NE, Parks RJ, Carroll ME. Cocaine hydrolase encoded in viral vector blocks the reinstatement of cocaine seeking in rats for 6 months. Biol Psychiatry. 2012;71:700–5.

Brantly ML, Chulay JD, Wang L, Mueller C, Humphries M, Spencer LT, Rouhani F, Conlon TJ, Calcedo R, Betts MR, et al. Sustained transgene expression despite T lymphocyte responses in a clinical trial of rAAV1-AAT gene therapy. Proc Natl Acad Sci U S A. 2009;106:16363–8.

Brimijoin S, Gao Y, Anker JJ, Gliddon LA, Lafleur D, Shah R, Zhao Q, Singh M, Carroll ME. A cocaine hydrolase engineered from human butyrylcholinesterase selectively blocks cocaine toxicity and reinstatement of drug seeking in rats. Neuropsychopharmacology. 2008;33: 2715–25.

Brunetti-Pierri N, Ng P. Progress and prospects: gene therapy for genetic diseases with helper-dependent adenoviral vectors. Gene Ther. 2008;15:553–60.

Brunetti-Pierri N, Ng P. Helper-dependent adenoviral vectors for liver-directed gene therapy. Hum Mol Genet. 2011;20:R7–13.

Brunetti-Pierri N, Palmer DJ, Beaudet AL, Carey KD, Finegold M, Ng P. Acute toxicity after high-dose systemic injection of helper-dependent adenoviral vectors into nonhuman primates. Hum Gene Ther. 2004;15:35–46.

Chen X, Huang X, Geng L, Xue L, Hou S, Zheng X, Brimijoin S, Zheng F, Zhan CG. Kinetic characterization of a cocaine hydrolase engineered from mouse butyrylcholinesterase. Biochem J. 2015;466:243–51.

Freedman M, Chang EH, Zhou Q, Pirollo KF. Nanodelivery of MRI contrast agent enhances sensitivity of detection of lung cancer metastases. Acad Radiol. 2009;16:627–37.

Gao Y, Atanasova E, Sui N, Pancook JD, Watkins JD, Brimijoin S. Gene transfer of cocaine hydrolase suppresses cardiovascular responses to cocaine in rats. Mol Pharmacol. 2005;67:204–11.

Gao Y, Brimijoin S. Lasting reduction of cocaine action in neostriatum – a hydrolase gene therapy approach. J Pharmacol Exp Ther. 2009;330:449–57.

Geng L, Gao Y, Chen X, Hou S, Zhan CG, Radic Z, Parks RJ, Russell SJ, Pham L, Brimijoin S. Gene transfer of mutant mouse cholinesterase provides high lifetime expression and reduced cocaine responses with no evident toxicity. PLoS One. 2013;8, e67446.

Gorelick D. Enhancing cocaine metabolism with butyrylcholinesterase as a treatment strategy. Drug Alcohol Depend. 1997;48:159–65.

Howard LA, Sellers EM, Tyndale RF. The role of pharmacogenetically-variable cytochrome P450 enzymes in drug abuse and dependence. Pharmacogenomics. 2002;3:185–99.

Kumahara K, Nagata H, Watanabe K, Shimizu N, Arimoto Y, Isoyama K, Okamoto Y, Shirasawa H. Suppression of inflammation by dexamethasone prolongs adenoviral vector-mediated transgene expression in murine nasal mucosa. Acta Otolaryngol. 2005;125:1301–6.

Manno CS, Pierce GF, Arruda VR, Glader B, Ragni M, Rasko JJ, Ozelo MC, Hoots K, Blatt P, Konkle B, et al. Successful transduction of liver in hemophilia by AAV-Factor IX and limitations imposed by the host immune response. Nat Med. 2006;12:342–7.

Morral N, O'Neal W, Rice K, Leland M, Kaplan J, Piedra PA, Zhou H, Parks RJ, Velji R, Aguilar-Cordova E, et al. Administration of helper-dependent adenoviral vectors and sequential delivery of different vector serotype for long-term liver-directed gene transfer in baboons. Proc Natl Acad Sci U S A. 1999;96:12816–21.

Murthy V, Gao Y, Geng L, LeBrasseur N, White T, Brimijoin S. Preclinical studies on neurobehavioral and neuromuscular effects of cocaine hydrolase gene therapy in mice. J Mol Neurosci. 2014a;53:409–16.

Murthy V, Gao Y, Geng L, LeBrasseur NK, White TA, Parks RJ, Brimijoin S. Physiologic and metabolic safety of butyrylcholinesterase gene therapy in mice. Vaccine. 2014b;32:4155–62.

Murthy V, Geng L, Gao Y, Zhang B, Miller JD, Reyes S, Brimijoin S. Reward and toxicity of cocaine metabolites generated by cocaine hydrolase. Cell Mol Neurobiol. 2015;35:819–826.

Muruve DA. The innate immune response to adenovirus vectors. Hum Gene Ther. 2004;15:1157–66.

Pan Y, Gao D, Yang W, Cho H, Yang G, Tai HH, Zhan CG. Computational redesign of human butyrylcholinesterase for anticocaine medication. Proc Natl Acad Sci U S A. 2005;102:16656–61.

Parks RJ, Chen L, Anton M, Sankar U, Rudnicki MA, Graham FL. A helper-dependent adenovirus vector system: removal of helper virus by Cre-mediated excision of the viral packaging signal. Proc Natl Acad Sci U S A. 1996;93:13565–70.

Raper SE, Chirmule N, Lee FS, Wivel NA, Bagg A, Gao GP, Wilson JM, Batshaw ML. Fatal systemic inflammatory response syndrome in a ornithine transcarbamylase deficient patient following adenoviral gene transfer. Mol Genet Metab. 2003;80:148–58.

Sellers EM, Kaplan HL, Tyndale RF. Inhibition of cytochrome P450 2A6 increases nicotine's oral bioavailability and decreases smoking. Clin Pharmacol Ther. 2000;68:35–43.

Seregin SS, Appledorn DM, McBride AJ, Schuldt NJ, Aldhamen YA, Voss T, Wei J, Bujold M, Nance W, Godbehere S, et al. Transient pretreatment with glucocorticoid ablates innate toxicity of systemically delivered adenoviral vectors without reducing efficacy. Mol Ther. 2009;17:685–96.

Spalding KL, Bhardwaj RD, Buchholz BA, Druid H, Frisen J. Retrospective birth dating of cells in humans. Cell. 2005;122:133–43.

Sun H, Pang YP, Lockridge O, Brimijoin S. Re-engineering butyrylcholinesterase as a cocaine hydrolase. Mol Pharmacol. 2002;62:220–4.

Sun L, Lau CE. Simultaneous pharmacokinetic modeling of cocaine and its metabolites, norcocaine and benzoylecgonine, after intravenous and oral administration in rats. Drug Metab Dispos. 2001;29:1183–9.

Vetrini F, Ng P. Liver-directed gene therapy with helper-dependent adenoviral vectors: current state of the art and future challenges. Curr Pharm Des. 2011;17:1886–1917.

Xie W, Altamirano CV, Bartels CF, Speirs RJ, Cashman JR, Lockridge O. An improved cocaine hydrolase: the A328Y mutant of human butyrylcholinesterase is 4-fold more efficient. Mol Pharmacol. 1999;55:83–91.

Yang W, Xue L, Fang L, Chen X, Zhan CG. Characterization of a high-activity mutant of human butyrylcholinesterase against (−)-cocaine. Chem Biol Interact. 2010;187:148–52.

Zheng F, Yang W, Ko MC, Liu J, Cho H, Gao D, Tong M, Tai HH, Woods JH, Zhan CG. Most efficient cocaine hydrolase designed by virtual screening of transition states. J Am Chem Soc. 2008;130:12148–55.

Chapter 12
Cocaine Hydrolases Designed from Butyrylcholinesterase

Fang Zheng and Chang-Guo Zhan

12.1 Butyrylcholinesterase as a Promising Protein Scaffold to Design Cocaine Hydrolases

As discussed in the above chapters, the inherent difficulties in antagonizing cocaine in the central nervous system (CNS) have led to the development of alternative approaches to alter the pharmacokinetics of cocaine. In particular, an ideal anti-cocaine medication would accelerate cocaine metabolism producing biological inactive metabolites (Gorelick 1997, 2008; Zheng and Zhan 2012a, b).

The primary pathway for the metabolism of cocaine in primates is hydrolysis at the benzoyl ester or methyl ester group (Meijler et al. 2005; Carrera et al. 2004; Landry et al. 1993; Zhan et al. 2005; Kamendulis et al. 1996; Gorelick 2008). Benzoyl ester hydrolysis generates ecgonine methyl ester (EME), whereas the methyl ester hydrolysis yields benzoylecgonine (BE). The major cocaine-metabolizing enzymes in humans are butyrylcholinesterase (BChE) which catalyzes benzoyl ester hydrolysis and two liver carboxylesterases (denoted by hCE-1 and hCE-2) that catalyze hydrolysis at the methyl ester and the benzoyl ester, respectively. Among the three, BChE is the principal cocaine-metabolizing enzyme in human serum. Hydrolysis accounts for most of cocaine metabolism in humans. The remaining cocaine is metabolized through oxidation by the liver microsomal cytochrome P450 (CYP) 3A4 to produce norcocaine.

EME appears the least pharmacologically active of the cocaine metabolites and may even cause vasodilation, whereas both BE and norcocaine appear to cause

F. Zheng • C.-G. Zhan, PhD (✉)
Molecular Modeling and Biopharmaceutical Center, College of Pharmacy, University of Kentucky, 789 South Limestone Street, Lexington, KY 40536, USA

Department of Pharmaceutical Sciences, College of Pharmacy, University of Kentucky, 789 South Limestone Street, Lexington, KY 40536, USA
e-mail: zhan@uky.edu

I.D. Montoya (ed.), *Biologics to Treat Substance Use Disorders: Vaccines, Monoclonal Antibodies, and Enzymes*, DOI 10.1007/978-3-319-23150-1_12

vasoconstriction and lower the seizure threshold, similar to cocaine itself (Gorelick 1997, 2008). In fact, norcocaine was found to be more toxic than cocaine (Zhan et al. 2014), but the lethality of BE has not been noted. In addition, the known hepatotoxic activity of cocaine is associated with further oxidative reactions of norcocaine (Pellinen et al. 2000). Thus, hydrolysis of cocaine at the benzoyl ester by an enzyme is the pathway most suitable for amplification.

Ignoring hCE-2, so far, two types of known native enzymes may be used to catalyze the hydrolysis of cocaine at the benzoyl ester: human BChE and bacterial cocaine esterase (CocE) (Larsen et al. 2002). Both enzymes have their own advantages and disadvantages. BChE from human source can be tolerated perfectly in human body. In fact, BChE has a long history of successful clinical use, and no adverse effects have been noted with increased BChE plasma activity (Gorelick 2008). In addition, at least 65 naturally occurring mutants of human BChE have been identified (Lockridge 2015), and there is no evidence that these mutants are antigenic. So BChE might be an ideal protein scaffold for rational design of a cocaine hydrolase, if a highly efficient mutant of human BChE can be designed and discovered (Zheng and Zhan 2012a). Compared to wild-type BChE, the bacterial CocE has a significantly higher catalytic efficiency against (−)-cocaine but thermally instable (Gao et al. 2009). In order to develop CocE into a therapeutic enzyme, one must significantly improve its thermal stability. Encouraging progress has been made on both types of enzymes. We will focus on mutants of human BChE in this chapter, whereas the development of thermostable mutants of CocE (Gao et al. 2009; Brim et al. 2010; Collins et al. 2009; Narasimhan et al. 2010, 2011; Fang et al. 2014a) is discussed in another chapter.

BChE, known in older literature as pseudocholinesterase or plasma cholinesterase to distinguish it from its close cousin acetylcholinesterase (AChE), is synthesized in the liver and widely distributed in the body, including the plasma, brain, and lung (Gorelick 1997). Studies in animals and humans demonstrated that enhancement of BChE activity by the administration of exogenous enzyme substantially decreased cocaine half-life (Gorelick 1997, 2008). So enhancement of cocaine metabolism by the administration of BChE was considered a promising pharmacokinetic approach for the treatment of cocaine abuse and dependence (Gorelick 1997). Unfortunately, wild-type BChE has a too low catalytic activity against naturally occurring (−)-cocaine ($k_{cat}=4.1\ \text{min}^{-1}$ and $K_M=4.5\ \mu\text{M}$) (Sun et al. 2002a; Hamza et al. 2005; Gatley 1991; Darvesh et al. 2003; Giacobini 2003) to be used therapeutically. Interestingly, the catalytic activity of wild-type human BChE is three orders of magnitude lower against the naturally occurring (−)-cocaine than that against the unnatural, biologically inactive (+)-cocaine enantiomer (Gatley 1991). (+)-Cocaine can be cleared from plasma in seconds and prior to partitioning into the central nervous system (CNS). Thus, positron emission tomography (PET) applied to mapping of the binding of (−)-cocaine and (+)-cocaine in baboon CNS showed marked uptake corresponding to (−)-cocaine in the striatum along with other areas of low uptake, whereas no CNS uptake corresponding to (+)-cocaine was observed (Gately et al. 1990). (+)-Cocaine was hydrolyzed by BChE so rapidly that it never reached the CNS for PET visualization. One may expect a great progress in the pharmacological treatment for cocaine if a BChE mutant capable of hydrolyzing (−)-cocaine with the rate of (+)-cocaine hydrolysis by wild-type BChE can be developed. Hence, human BChE may serve as a promising protein scaffold to rationally design a cocaine hydrolase (CocH), i.e., a BChE mutant with a considerably improved catalytic activity against (−)-cocaine. On the other hand, it is always very challenging to design an enzyme mutant with a considerably improved catalytic activity for a given substrate.

Recently developed computational enzyme redesign strategies and protocols (Pan et al. 2005, 2007, 2008; Zheng et al. 2008, 2010, 2014; Yang et al. 2009; Xue et al. 2011), to be discussed in Sect. 12.3, have allowed to rationally design highly efficient enzyme mutants. The computational enzyme redesign is based on the detailed understanding of the three-dimensional (3D) protein structure and catalytic mechanism. As discussed in the following sections, the structure- and mechanism-based computational design has led to the discovery of highly efficient mutants of human BChE suitable for clinical development of pharmacological treatment of cocaine abuse.

For convenience, in the following sections, we will always refer cocaine to (−)-cocaine unless stated otherwise explicitly.

12.2 Structure and Catalytic Mechanism of BChE

12.2.1 BChE Structure

Generally speaking, for the purpose of rational enzyme redesign, one first needs to know the detailed 3D structure of the enzyme and uncover the catalytic mechanism. Human BChE (with a common accession number in the UniProtKB and NCBI databases: P06276) is a secreted protein including 28 residues in the signal peptide and 574 residues in the mature secreted protein. With the 574 amino-acid residues, the native human BChE exists in tetramer. Recombinant BChE may exist in the forms of monomer, dimer, and tetramer. The first crystal structure of BChE was solved for a recombinant form of a truncated BChE in which the tetramerization domain (i.e., the last 40 residues on the C-terminus) had been deleted (Nicolet et al. 2003). So the first X-ray crystal structure was determined for the BChE monomer. Before the X-ray crystal structure was available, a homology model of human BChE (based on the use of an X-ray crystal structure of AChE) had been used to study detailed BChE-substrate complex structures and catalytic mechanisms concerning how human BChE catalyzes the hydrolysis of (−)-cocaine and (+)-cocaine (Zhan et al. 2003). Notably, the reported X-ray crystal structure (Nicolet et al. 2003) of the BChE monomer confirmed the previously modeled human BChE structure, as discussed in literature (Nicolet et al. 2003; Hamza et al. 2005). The main difference between the X-ray crystal structure and the homology model was found at the acyl loop (Nicolet et al. 2003) which does not significantly affect the enzyme interacting with a substrate. Comparing the simulated protein backbone structures to the X-ray crystal structure, the root-mean-square deviation (RMSD) values were all smaller than 1.3 Å for the overall protein structures (Hamza et al. 2005); an RMSD value of 1.3 Å is within the resolution of the X-ray crystal structure. Both the homology model and X-ray crystal structure of BChE consistently revealed that BChE has a catalytic triad consisting of residues S198, H438, and E325 and a three-pronged oxyanion hole consisting of residues G116, G117, and A199.

Native BChE tetramer has not been crystallized to date, but a 3D model (depicted in Fig. 12.1) was built by the team at the University of Kentucky (Pan et al. 2009). The model of BChE tetramer complexed with a proline-rich attachment domain (PRAD) was constructed by carrying out homology modeling followed by molecular dynamics (MD) simulation of the explicit water-solvated protein system. The 3D structural model enabled to clearly identify the orientation of the BChE subunits in the tetramer and to study how the tetramerization domain of BChE binds with the proline-rich peptide to form a stable tetramer of human BChE. According to the 3D model, the four helices of tryptophan amphiphilic tetramerization (WAT) domain of BChE form a left-hand superhelix wrapping around the proline-rich peptide in the middle. Six conserved hydrophobic residues located on the C-terminus of BChE are responsible for the key interaction between the tetramerization domain and PRAD. Three equally spaced tryptophan residues on adjacent WAT chains have a dynamic hydrogen-bond network with consecutive residues of PRAD to form 12 hydrogen bonds; there are hydrophobic interactions between the side chain of tryptophans and the proline rings located on the PRAD. The simulated model structures suggested that mutation of three residues, i.e., Phe547, Met554, and Phe561, to other hydrophobic residues could be beneficial for increasing the binding between the tetramerization domain of BChE and the proline-rich peptide.

12.2.2 Doors and Dynamics of the Active Site

MD simulations have also been performed to understand how a substrate molecule can enter the active site of BChE in comparison with AChE in their monomer and tetramer structures (Fang et al. 2011). BChE and AChE are highly homologous proteins with distinct substrate preferences. The MD simulations revealed some similarities but also some differences between the AChE and BChE monomers. BChE has a larger main entrance than AChE, which seems reasonable as BChE can bind substrates as large as cocaine. Two previously proposed alternative doors (side door and back door in BChE) are larger in size than those in AChE. The acyl loop back doors in both enzymes are too small to be significant channels leading to the active sites. Based on these results, the back door and the side door are more likely and more important alternative doors than the acyl loop back door, as the former ones have larger radii and can exist for longer time. As discussed in a previous study (Tara et al. 1999a), there was no direct experimental evidence to prove the function of these alternative doors. However, multiple simulations performed by different groups using different forms of enzymes and different force fields all predicted the existence of these doors (Tai et al. 2001, 2002; Tara et al. 1999a, b; Suarez and Field 2005). Regardless,

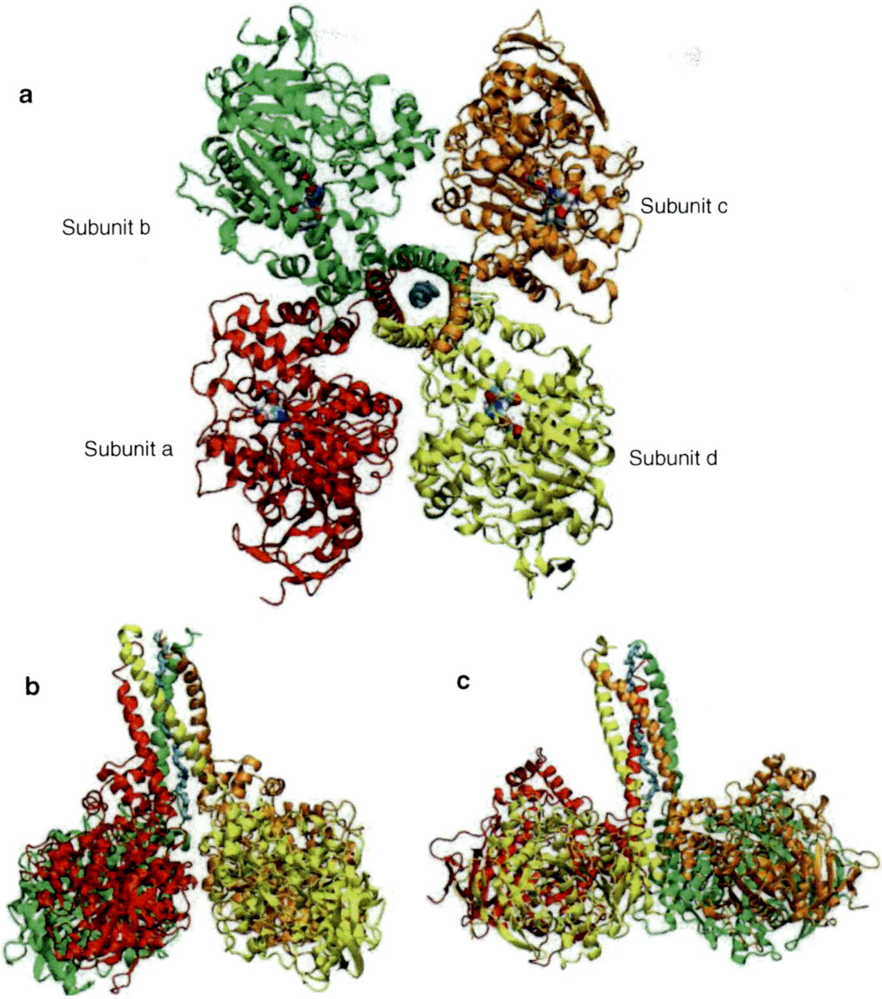

Fig. 12.1 Overall structural of the $[BChE]_4$-PRAD complex derived from MD simulation (Pan et al. 2009). The ribbons in color *red*, *green*, *orange*, and *yellow* represent chains a, b, c, and d of the BChE subunits, and the cyan tube represents chain e or the PRAD chain. (**a**) Viewed from the top of tetramerization domain of BChE. The multicolored regions refer to the active sites of the tetramer. Two of active sites in subunits indicated by chains a and c are exposed to outside solvent, while the other two face the central cavity of the BChE tetramer. (**b**) Viewed from the side of the twofold axis of BChE tetramer. This picture has 90° rotation from figure (**a**). (**c**) This picture has 90° clockwise rotation from figure (**b**) around the twofold symmetry axis

for a substrate as large as cocaine, the substrate can only enter the active site of BChE through the main door (Fang et al. 2011). In light of the MD simulations (Fang et al. 2011), the main door of BChE is significantly larger than that of AChE, which explains why BChE can have a variety of large substrates including cocaine, ghrelin, and prodrug CPT-11, whereas AChE is specific for small substrates like acetylcholine (ACh).

Further, according to the MD simulations (Fang et al. 2011), the overall structures of AChE and BChE tetramers are similar, and the gating mechanisms of the main doors of AChE and BChE are responsible for their different substrate specificities. It has also been demonstrated that both AChE and BChE tetramers could have two dysfunctional active sites due to their restricted accessibility to substrates.

12.2.3 Catalytic Mechanism for Cocaine Hydrolysis

12.2.3.1 Prechemical Reaction Process

In order to rationally design an enzyme mutant with improved catalytic activity for a given substrate, one first needs to understand the detailed catalytic mechanism including how the substrate binds with the enzyme and the subsequent chemical transformation process. Modern computational modeling and simulations can provide this detailed information. It was demonstrated that for both (−)-cocaine and (+)-cocaine, the BChE-substrate binding involves two different types of complexes: non-prereactive and prereactive BChE-substrate complexes (Zhan et al. 2003; Hamza et al. 2005). Specifically, (−)/(+)-cocaine first slides down the substrate-binding gorge to bind to W82 and stands vertically in the gorge between D70 and W82 (non-prereactive complex) and then rotates to a position in the catalytic site within a favorable distance for nucleophilic attack and hydrolysis by S198 (prereactive complex). In the prereactive complex, cocaine lies horizontally at the bottom of the gorge. The main structural difference between the BChE–(−)-cocaine and BChE–(+)-cocaine complexes exists in the relative position of the cocaine methyl ester group (Zhan et al. 2003; Hamza et al. 2005).

The MD simulations (Hamza et al. 2005) have further revealed that the (−)-cocaine rotation in the active site of wild-type BChE from the non-prereactive complex to the prereactive complex is hindered by some residues including Y332, A328, and F329 residues in the non-prereactive complex that are significantly different from those in the prereactive complex. Compared to (−)-cocaine binding with wild-type BChE, (−)-cocaine can more strongly bind with the A328W/Y332A and A328W/Y332G mutants in the prereactive complexes. More importantly, the (−)-cocaine rotation in the active site of the A328W/Y332A and A328W/Y332G mutants from the non-prereactive complex to the prereactive complex did not cause considerable changes of the positions of A332 or G332, W328, and F329 residues. These results suggest that the A328W/Y332A and A328W/Y332G mutants should be associated with lower energy barriers than wild-type BChE for the (−)-cocaine rotation from the non-prereactive complex to the prereactive complex. Further, (−)-cocaine binding with the A328W/Y332G mutant is very similar to the binding with the A328W/Y332A mutant, but the position change of F329 residue caused by the (−)-cocaine rotation was significant only in the A328W/Y332A mutant, thus suggesting that the energy barrier for (−)-cocaine rotation in the A328W/Y332G mutant should be slightly lower than that in the A328W/Y332A mutant. It has also been demonstrated that (−)-cocaine binds with the A328W/Y332A/Y419S mutant in a way that is not suitable for the catalysis (Hamza et al. 2005).

Based on the computational results, both the A328W/Y332A and A328W/Y332G mutants were expected to have catalytic activity for (−)-cocaine hydrolysis higher than that of wild-type BChE, and the catalytic activity of the A328W/Y332G mutant should be slightly higher than that of the A328W/Y332A mutant, whereas the A328W/Y332A/Y419S mutant was expected to lose the catalytic activity. The computational analysis on the A328W/Y332A mutant is consistent with the known experimental data (Sun et al. 2002a), and the computational predictions concerning the A328W/Y332G and A328W/Y332A/Y419S mutants were confirmed by the experimental kinetic analysis (Hamza et al. 2005).

Further MD and potential of mean force (PMF) simulations were performed to determine the detailed enzyme-substrate (ES) binding pathway and the corresponding free energy profiles for wild-type BChE binding with (−)/(+)-cocaine and for the A328W/Y332G mutant binding with (−)-cocaine (Huang et al. 2010, 2011). It was revealed that the non-prereactive binding pathway for (+)-cocaine binding with wild-type BChE is similar to that for (−)-cocaine binding with wild-type BChE and the A328W/Y332G mutant. For each ES binding system, the simulated PMF free energy profile revealed a local minimum on the free energy surface corresponding to the formation of an ES1-like complex (in which the substrate binds with the enzyme at the presumed peripheral anionic site around the entrance of the active-site gorge) prior to the formation of the non-prereactive ES complex during the enzyme-substrate-binding process; the ES1 complex was proposed for BChE binding with smaller substrates/reactants (Masson et al. 1997, 1999). However, further evolution from the ES1-like complex to the non-prereactive ES complex is nearly barrierless, with a free energy barrier being lower than 1.0 kcal/mol (Huang et al. 2010, 2011). So the non-prereactive ES binding process should be very fast. The rate-determining step of the entire ES binding process is the further evolution from the non-prereactive ES complex to the prereactive ES complex. The combined MD and PMF simulations also demonstrated that all of the three simulated non-prereactive complexes have similar free energy profiles for the binding processes, and the calculated binding free energies are close to each other. Further accounting for the PMF-simulated free energy change from the non-prereactive ES complex to the prereactive ES complex allowed to estimate the binding free energy for the entire ES binding process. Depicted in Fig. 12.2 are obtained PMF free energy profiles for the entire ES binding process in which the right side represents the pre-ES binding state and the local minimum on the left site refers to the final state of the ES binding (i.e., the prereactive ES complex). The PMF simulations qualitatively reproduced the relative order of the experimentally derived binding free energies, i.e., ΔG_{bind}(wild-type BChE–(−)-cocaine) < ΔG_{bind}(wild-type BChE–(+)-cocaine) < ΔG_{bind}(A328W/Y332G BChE–(−)-cocaine), although the simulations systematically overestimated the magnitude of the binding affinity and systematically underestimated the differences between the ΔG_{bind} values (Huang et al. 2010, 2011).

The structural transformation from the non-prereactive ES complex to the prereactive complex was simulated through a combined use of targeted molecular dynamics (TMD) and PMF methods (Huang et al. 2010). The combined TMD and PMF

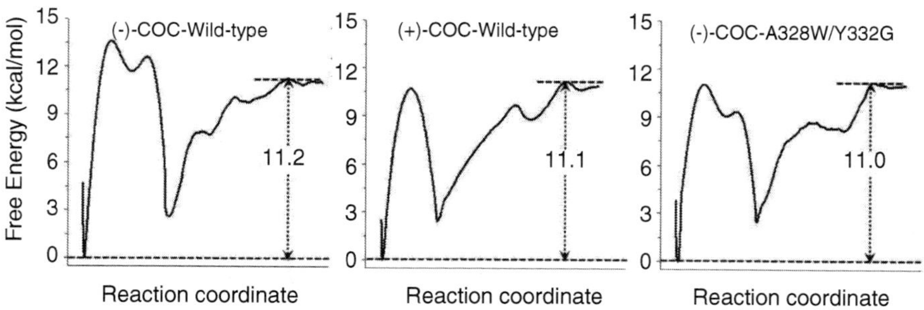

Fig. 12.2 Free energy profiles for the formation of prereactive ES complex for wild-type BChE binding with (−)-cocaine (*left*), wild-type BChE binding with (+)-cocaine (*middle*), and the A328W/Y332G mutant binding with (−)-cocaine (*right*)

simulations revealed that the structural transformation involves two transition states, denoted as $TS1_{rot}$ and $TS2_{rot}$. The transition-state $TS1_{rot}$ is mainly associated with the deformation of the non-prereactive complex in which the benzoyl ester group of (−)-cocaine moves toward the catalytic residue S198 of BChE. The transition-state $TS2_{rot}$ is mainly associated with the formation of the prereactive complex in which the methyl ester group of (−)-cocaine rotates and the carbonyl oxygen at the benzoyl ester group of (−)-cocaine moves into the oxyanion hole of BChE. The combined TMD and PMF simulations also demonstrated that the A328W/Y332G mutations do not change the fundamental pathway for the structural transformation from the non-prereactive binding to the prereactive binding. However, the A328W/Y332G mutations significantly reduce the steric hindrance for (−)-cocaine rotation in the binding pocket of BChE and, thus, decrease the free energy barrier for the structural transformation from the non-prereactive binding to the prereactive binding. The calculated relative free energy barriers are all consistent with the experimental kinetic data (Huang et al. 2010; Hamza et al. 2005), suggesting that the computational insights are reasonable. The general computational strategy and approach (Huang et al. 2010, 2011) based on the combined TMD and PMF simulations may be also valuable in computational studies of detailed pathways and free energy profiles for other similar mechanistic problems involving ligand rotation or another type of structural transformation in the binding pocket of a protein.

12.2.3.2 Chemical Reaction Pathway

Starting from the prereactive ES complex, one may explore the detailed reaction pathway for the chemical reaction process through reaction-coordinate calculations. The first reaction-coordinate calculations on BChE-catalyzed hydrolysis of cocaine (Zhan et al. 2003) were based on the use of *ab initio* quantum mechanical (QM) approach and an active-site model of the enzyme. Subsequent reaction-coordinate calculations on BChE (or BChE mutant)-catalyzed hydrolysis reactions were based on hybrid quantum mechanical/molecular mechanical (QM/MM) calculations or

QM/MM-free energy (QM/MM-FE) calculations (Zhan and Gao 2005; Zheng et al. 2008, 2014; Liu and Zhan 2012; Chen et al. 2011, 2012). Based on the reaction-coordinate calculations, the fundamental pathway for the chemical reaction process of BChE-catalyzed hydrolysis of (−)-cocaine (see Fig. 12.3) is essentially the same as that for BChE-catalyzed hydrolysis of other esters such as ACh, acetylthiocholine (ATC), and (+)-cocaine in terms of the covalent bond breaking and formation.

As seen in Fig. 12.3 (Zhan et al. 2003), the chemical reaction process includes both the acylation and deacylation stages. The acylation is initialized by the hydroxyl oxygen (O^{γ}) of S198 side chain attacking at the carbonyl carbon of the cocaine benzoyl ester to form the first tetrahedral intermediate (INT1) through the first transition state (TS1). During the formation of INT1, the C–O bond between the carbonyl carbon and S198 O^{γ} gradually forms, while the proton at S198 O^{γ} gradually transfers to the imidazole N atom of H438 side chain which acts as a general base. The second step of the acylation is the decomposition of INT1 to the metabolite ecgonine methyl ester and acyl-BChE (INT2a) through the second transition state (TS2). During the change from INT1 to INT2a, the proton gradually transfers to the benzoyl ester oxygen, while the C–O bond between the carbonyl carbon and the ester oxygen gradually breaks. Also, during the first step of acylation, the carbonyl oxygen may potentially form up to three hydrogen bonds with the NH groups of G116, G117, and A199. Note that these potential hydrogen bonds do not necessarily exist in the prereactive complex (ES) and in other structures, even though they are, for convenience, indicated throughout the reaction process in Fig. 12.3 (Zhan et al. 2003). The potential hydrogen bonds of the carbonyl oxygen of the substrate with the NH groups of G116, G117, and A199 are expected to play a key role in stabilizing the transition states during the reaction process.

It should be noted in Fig. 12.3 that there is no proton transfer between H438 and E325 throughout the reaction process. So the role of E325 is to stabilize the positively charged H438 during the reaction process, according to the aforementioned QM/MM-FE calculations at high levels. This reaction pathway is remarkably different from the double-proton transfer mechanism known for other serine hydrolases with a similar catalytic triad (Ser-His-Glu or Ser-His-Asp).

12.3 Transition-State Modeling and Simulation for Computational Enzyme Redesign

It has been well known that computational design of high-activity mutants of an enzyme is extremely challenging, particularly when the chemical reaction process is rate determining for the enzymatic reaction (Gao and Zhan 2005, 2006; Gao et al. 2006; Zheng et al. 2014). Generally speaking, for computational design of a mutant enzyme with an improved catalytic activity for a given substrate, one needs to design possible amino-acid mutations that can accelerate the rate-determining step of the catalytic reaction process (Zhan et al. 2003; Hamza et al. 2005; Zhan and Gao 2005), while other steps of the reaction are not slowed down by the mutations. It has been known (Zhan et al. 2003; Zhan and Gao 2005; Hamza et al. 2005; Gao and Zhan

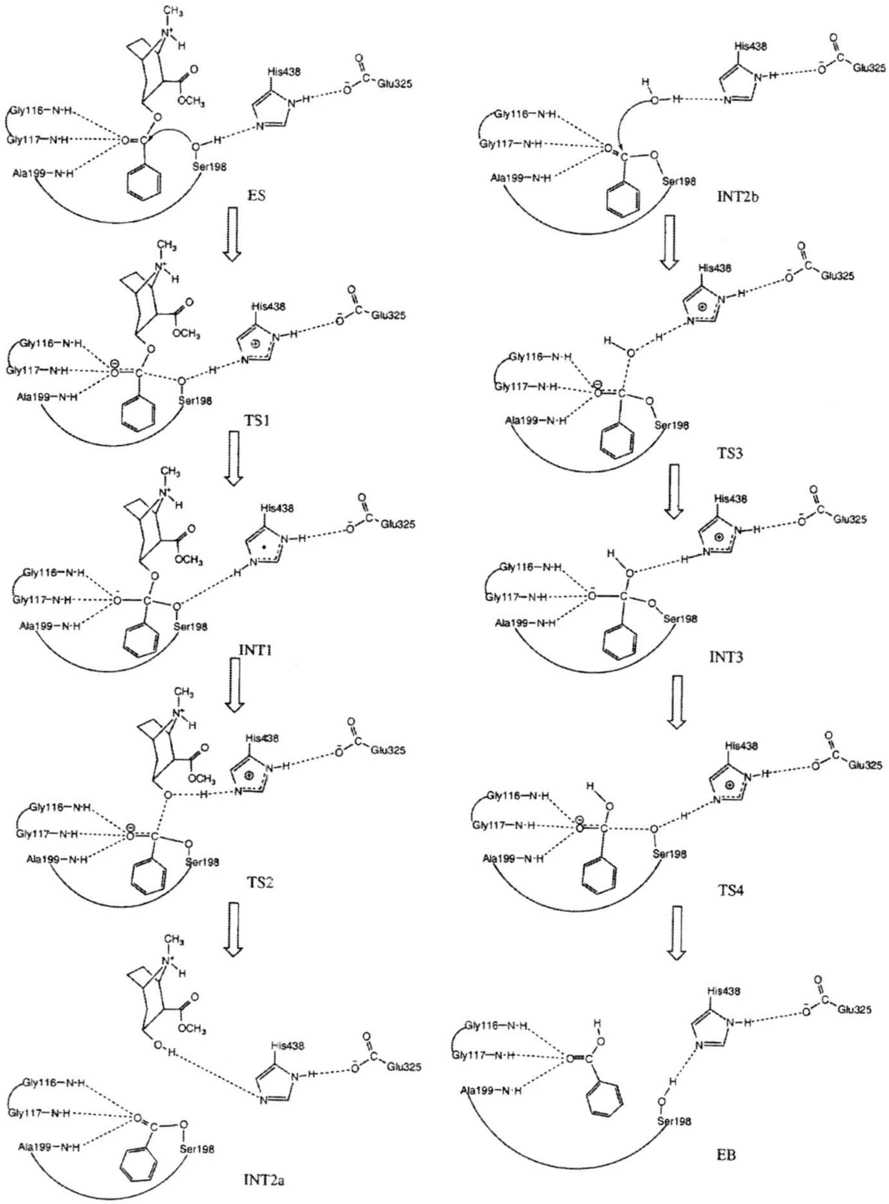

Fig. 12.3 Schematic representation of the chemical reaction pathway (Zhan et al. 2003) for BChE-catalyzed hydrolysis of (−)-cocaine at the benzoyl ester. The *dash lines* between the carbonyl oxygen of (−)-cocaine and backbone NH groups of residues G116, G117, and A199 refer to the potential hydrogen bonding (HB) interactions that may exist during the catalytic reaction process. However, these desirable HB interactions do not always exist for (−)-cocaine hydrolysis catalyzed by wild-type BChE

2006; Pan et al. 2005) that the rate-determining step of (−)-cocaine hydrolysis catalyzed by the A328W/Y332A and A328W/Y332G mutants of BChE is the first step of the chemical reaction process. Therefore, starting from the A328W/Y332A or A328W/Y332G mutant, rational design of BChE mutants against (−)-cocaine should focus on decreasing the energy barrier for the first reaction step without significantly affecting other steps of the reaction. Thus, to computationally design a mutant with a significantly improved catalytic activity, one needs to model the possible transition-state structures associated with a variety of possible mutants of the enzyme. When a mutant of the enzyme is predicted to have a more stable transition state for the rate-determining step and, thus, is expected to have a significantly lower free energy barrier for the enzymatic reaction, the mutant will be recommended for wet experimental tests for their actual catalytic activity against (−)-cocaine (Pan et al. 2005).

12.3.1 QM/MM and QM/MM-FE Calculations

In principle, a reliable QM/MM approach may be used to evaluate the transition-state structures associated with a variety of possible mutants and predict the corresponding free energy barriers. Generally speaking, a QM/MM approach allows us to describe reaction center of an enzymatic reaction system (including the substrate atoms and key atoms in the active site of the enzyme) quantum mechanically (QM) while dealing with the remaining part of enzyme molecular mechanically (MM) and appropriately accounting for the interactions between the QM-treated atoms and the MM-treated atoms (QM/MM interactions). Different QM/MM methods differ mainly in the treatment of the QM/MM boundary atoms. A pseudobond first-principles QM/MM method has actually been used to successfully design high-activity mutants of human BChE (Zheng et al. 2008, 2014).

The pseudobond QM/MM method was initially implemented in revised Gaussian and Tinker programs (Zhang et al. 2000; Zhang 2005, 2006). The revised Gaussian and Tinker programs can be used to carry out the QM and MM parts of the QM/MM calculation iteratively until the full self-consistency is achieved. The pseudobond QM/MM method uses a seven-valence-electron atom with an effective core potential constructed to replace the boundary atom of the environment part and to form a pseudobond with the boundary atom of the active part. The main idea of the pseudobond approach is as follows: one considers that a large molecule is partitioned into two parts, an active part and an environment part, by cutting a covalent σ-bond Y–X. Y and X refer to boundary atoms of the environment part and the active part, respectively. Instead of using a hydrogen atom to cap the free valence of X atom as in the conventional link-atom approach, a pseudobond Y_{ps}–X is formed by replacing the Y atom with a one-free-valence boundary Y atom (Y_{ps}). The Y_{ps} atom is parametrized to make the Y_{ps}–X pseudobond mimic the original Y–X bond with similar bond length and strength and also to have similar effects on the rest of the active part. In the pseudobond approach, the Y_{ps} atom and all atoms in the active part form a well-defined QM subsystem which can be treated by a QM method. Excluding Y atom, the remaining atoms in the environment part form the MM subsystem treated by an MM method. The pseudobond *ab initio* QM/MM approach has been demonstrated to be powerful in studies of enzymatic reactions.

The Kentucky team developed a revised version (Zheng et al. 2008; Liu and Zhan 2012) of the Gaussian and Amber programs that allow users to use the more popularly used Amber force field in the QM/MM calculations. Compared to the original version of the revised Gaussian and Tinker programs (Zhang et al. 2000; Zhang 2005, 2006), the development of the revised version of the Gaussian and Amber programs enabled to perform parallel computing for the pseudobond QM/MM method for the first time (Zheng et al. 2008).

Using the QM/MM method, one may perform reaction-coordinate calculations to uncover a detail reaction pathway (the minimum-energy path), including the structures of all transition states, and the corresponding free energy barriers. To more accurately determine the free energy barriers for an enzymatic reaction, the QM/MM calculations can be followed by an appropriately planned free energy perturbation (FEP) calculations – the QM/MM-FE approach. In general, FEP calculations can be performed to evaluate free energy change caused by a small structural change (Kollman 1993; Beveridge and DiCapua 1989; Acevedo and Jorgensen 2010). Specifically, after the minimum-energy path is determined by the QM/MM calculations, the free energy changes associated with the QM/MM interactions can be determined by using the FEP method (Zhang et al. 2000). In the FEP calculations, sampling of the MM subsystem is carried out with the QM subsystem frozen at each state along the reaction path. The point charges on the frozen QM atoms used in the FEP calculations are determined by fitting the electrostatic potential (ESP) in the QM part of the QM/MM single-point calculations. The FEP calculations enable us to more reasonably determine the relative free energy changes due to the QM/MM interactions. Technically, the final (relative) free energy determined by the QM/MM-FE calculations is the QM part of the QM/MM energy (excluding the Coulombic interaction energy between the point charges of the MM atoms and the ESP charges of the QM atoms) plus the relative free energy change determined by the FEP calculations.

The QM/MM-FE calculations on the entire enzymatic reaction system allow the evaluation of the free energy barriers for each forward and reverse reaction step. The first-principles QM/MM-FE approach has been proven reliable in predicting the free energy barriers for enzymatic reactions (Hu and Zhang 2006; Zhang et al. 2002; Zheng et al. 2008, 2014; Liu et al. 2009a, b, 2011; Chen et al. 2011; Liu and Zhan 2012).

12.3.2 Transition-State Modeling and Simulation Using Classical Force Field

As noted above, the QM/MM-FE calculations have been proven reliable in predicting the free energy barriers for enzymatic reactions. On the other hand, the calculations using a truly reliable QM/MM approach (in which the QM calculation is performed at a high level of first-principles theory) are very time-consuming and, hence, are not suitable for virtual screening of a large number of possible mutants. It is highly desired to have a more efficient computational strategy which allows rapid modeling and simulation of the transition states associated with a variety of mutants.

For practical computational enzyme redesign, the Kentucky team developed a strategy to efficiently model and simulate the transition-state modeling using a classical force field (molecular mechanics) (Pan et al. 2005, 2007; Gao et al. 2006; Zheng et al. 2008, 2010, 2014; Yang et al. 2009; Xue et al. 2011). It should be pointed out that, in theory, computational modeling, such as energy minimization or MD simulation, using a classical force field can only simulate a stable structure corresponding to a local minimum on the potential energy surface, whereas a transition state during a reaction process is always associated with a first-order saddle point on the potential energy surface. Hence, energy minimization (or MD simulation) using a classical force field cannot directly simulate a transition state without any restraint on the geometry of the transition state. Nevertheless, if we can technically remove the freedom of imaginary vibration in the transition-state structure, then the number of the degrees of vibrational freedom (normal vibration modes) for a nonlinear molecule will decrease from $3N$-6 to $3N$-5 or less represents the number of atoms of the reaction system. The transition-state structure is associated with a local minimum on the potential energy surface within a subspace of the reduced degrees of vibrational freedom, although it is associated with a first-order saddle point on the potential energy surface with all of the $3N - 6$ degrees of vibrational freedom. Theoretically, the degree of vibrational freedom associated with the imaginary vibrational frequency in the transition-state structure can be removed by appropriately freezing the reaction coordinate. The reaction coordinate corresponding to the imaginary vibration of the transition state is generally characterized by a combination of some key geometric parameters (Pan et al. 2005). These key geometric parameters are bond lengths of the transition bonds, i.e., the forming and breaking covalent bonds during this reaction step of the enzymatic reaction. Thus, we just need to maintain the lengths of the transition bonds during the modeling of a transition state. Technically, we can maintain the lengths of the transition bonds by simply fixing all atoms within the reaction center, by using some constraints on the transition bonds, or by redefining the transition bonds. It should be pointed out that the purpose of performing such type of computational modeling on a transition state is only to examine the change of the protein environment surrounding the reaction center and the interaction between the reaction center and the protein environment (Pan et al. 2005).

The computational strategy for using a classical force field to efficiently model and simulate transition states in large-scale has opened doors to develop various practically useful approaches for computational enzyme redesign as noted below.

12.3.3 Free Energy Perturbation on the Rate-Determining Transition State (FEP-TS)

On the basis of the general strategy for the transition-state modeling and simulation mentioned above, a novel computational approach (Pan et al. 2007) was developed to carry out FEP simulations on the mutation-caused changes of the rate-determining

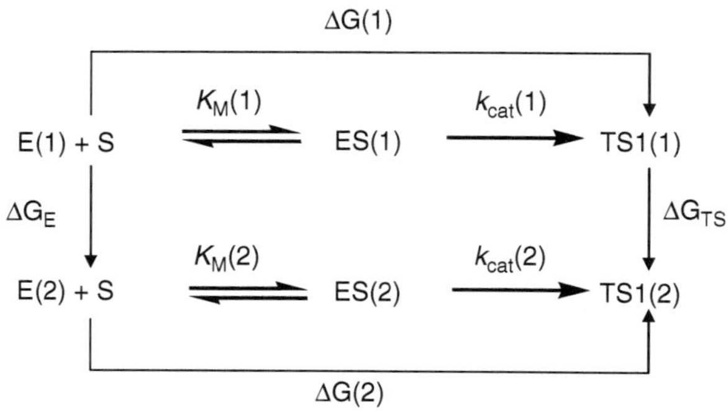

Fig. 12.4 The relationship between different free energy changes for the enzymatic reactions catalyzed by two enzymes. E(i) is the free enzyme, ES(i) represents the enzyme–substrate complex, and TS1(i) refers to the transition state (Pan et al. 2007)

transition states and directly estimate the mutation-caused shifts of the catalytic efficiency of an enzyme for a given substrate. This type of FEP approach for transition state (TS) is denoted as FEP-TS for convenience.

Depicted in Fig. 12.4 are the free energy changes associated with two reaction systems: one is the enzymatic reaction catalyzed by a reference mutant of the enzyme (or the wild-type), denoted by Enzyme 1 or E(1); the other is the enzymatic reaction catalyzed by another mutant, denoted by Enzyme 2 or E(2). As seen in Fig. 12.4, the catalytic efficiency, i.e., $k_{cat}(i)/K_M(i)$, for the enzymatic reaction catalyzed by enzyme E(i) is determined by the Gibbs free energy change $\Delta G(i)$ of the reaction system from E(i) plus substrate S to the corresponding rate-determining transition state TS1(i). $\Delta G(i)$ is the sum of the enzyme-substrate-binding free energy $\Delta G_{ES}(i)$ and the activation free energy $\Delta G_{av}(i)$:

$$\Delta G(i) = \Delta G_{ES}(i) + \Delta G_{av}(i), \quad i = 1 \text{and} 2. \tag{12.1}$$

Assuming that a mutation on an amino-acid residue can change the enzyme from E(1) to E(2), we want to know the corresponding free energy change from $\Delta G(1)$ to $\Delta G(2)$ for the computational design of the high-activity mutants of the enzyme. There are two possible paths to determine the free energy change $\Delta\Delta G(1\rightarrow 2)\equiv\Delta G(2) - \Delta G(1)$. One path is to directly calculate $\Delta G_{ES}(i)$ and $\Delta G_{av}(i)$ associated with E(1) and E(2), which is very computationally demanding in terms of the level of theory. For an alternative path, the relatively less-demanding FEP simulations allow us to estimate $\Delta\Delta G(1\rightarrow 2)$ by determining the free energy changes ΔG_E and ΔG_{TS1} from E(1) to E(2):

$$\Delta\Delta G(1 \rightarrow 2) = \Delta G_{TS1} - \Delta G_E \tag{12.2}$$

where ΔG_E and ΔG_{TS1} are the free energy changes from E(1) to E(2) for the free enzyme and TS1, respectively. ΔG_E and ΔG_{TS1} can be estimated by performing the FEP simulations. By using the calculated $\Delta\Delta G(1\rightarrow 2)$, the ratio of the catalytic efficiency associated with E(2) to that associated with E(1) can be evaluated *via*

$$\Delta\Delta G(1 \rightarrow 2) = -RT \ln \frac{k_{cat}(2)/K_M(2)}{k_{cat}(1)/K_M(1)}. \tag{12.3}$$

According to Eq. (12.3), one can predict the catalytic efficiency (k_{cat}/K_M) associated with E(2) from the calculated $\Delta\Delta G(1 \rightarrow 2)$ value and the known catalytic efficiency (k_{cat}/K_M) associated with E(1) (Pan et al. 2007). Equation (12.3) can also be used to derive the experimental $\Delta\Delta G(1 \rightarrow 2)$ value from the experimental ratio of the catalytic efficiency (k_{cat}/K_M) associated with E(2) to that associated with E(1).

The FEP-TS approach has been proven reliable in practical prediction of the mutation-caused shifts of the free energy barriers for the purpose of BChE mutant design (Pan et al. 2007; Yang et al. 2009, 2010a).

12.3.4 Systematic Virtual Screening of the Transition States

The basic computational strategies and methods mentioned above have been used to virtually screen a variety of hypothetical mutants of human BChE in an automated way (Pan et al. 2005, 2007; Gao et al. 2006; Zheng et al. 2008, 2010, 2014; Yang et al. 2009; Xue et al. 2011). Depicted in Fig. 12.5 is a general representation of the integrated computational–experimental effort for rational design and discovery of the enzyme mutants with an improved catalytic efficiency for a given substrate. The integrated computational–experimental effort includes the automated virtual screening of transition states, followed by wet experimental studies.

Using the general approach depicted in Fig. 12.5 for human BChE mutants against (−)-cocaine, the entire virtual screening process may consist of multiple steps (up to five steps depicted in Fig. 12.5). Steps #1 and #2 are for the preparation. For the preparation, step #1 is based on the detailed reaction coordinates and free energy profile determined by the QM/MM-FE calculations for the reference mutant, i.e., the most active one of the known BChE mutants against (−)-cocaine. The transition state for the rate-determining step (i.e., the step associated with the highest free energy barrier) may be used as the starting transition state for virtual screening. Starting from the rate-determining transition-state structure optimized for (−)-cocaine hydrolysis catalyzed by the reference mutant, one can conveniently build the initial structures of the transition state to be modeled for various hypothetical BChE mutants by only changing the side chains of the mutated residues.

Step #2 is to generate an appropriately designed library of hypothetical BChE mutants for practical virtual screening according to two basic requirements. The first requirement is that the library will be made sure to include BChE mutants with possibly higher catalytic efficiency against (−)-cocaine compared to the reference mutant. Certainly, this requirement can be satisfied most likely by building a complete library of all combinations of the possible mutations. Unfortunately, such a complete library would be too large to screen practically with any meaningful molecular modeling/simulation approach. Hence, the second requirement is that the library should be sufficiently small (say, $<$ 1,000,000 or 100,000 mutants) so that the virtual screening with this library can be done practically. To satisfy both of these two necessary requirements, one must appropriately consider possible mutations on the residues that could directly or indirectly influence the reaction center based on

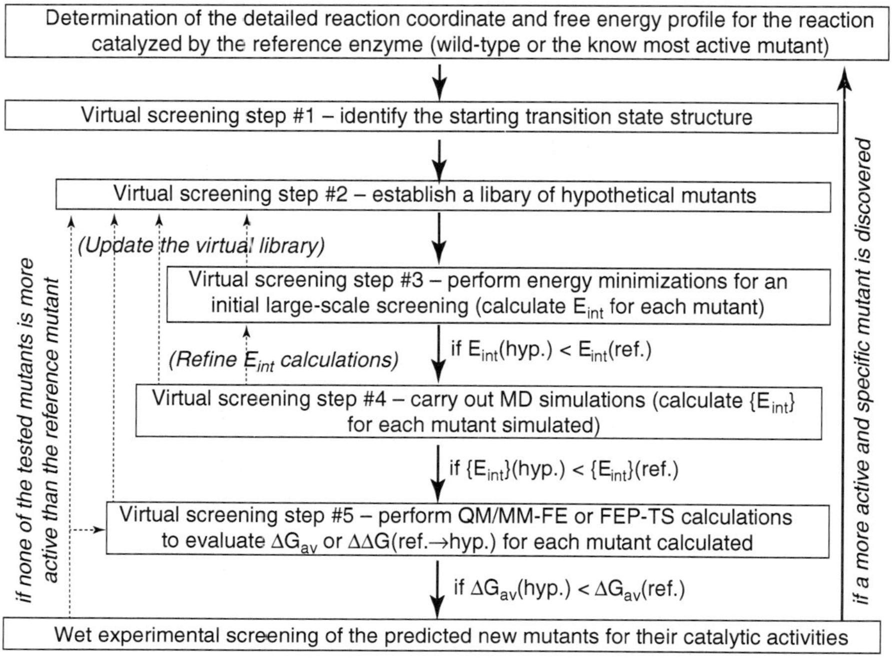

Fig. 12.5 Integrated computational-experimental effort for rational design and discovery of the enzyme mutants with an improved catalytic efficiency against a given substrate, such as (−)-cocaine. The *dash lines with arrows* represent the optional refinement process whenever necessary. For example, in case there is no mutant passing step #3, one may go back to step #2, updating the virtual library (with new hypothetical mutants). E_{int} is the overall interaction energy (or another indicator for the interaction energy) between the substrate atoms and the protein environment for the hypothetical (hyp.) or the reference (ref.) mutant. $\{E_{int}\}$ (Zheng et al. 2008) refers to the dynamically averaged overall interaction energy between the substrate atoms and the protein environment for a given mutant. ΔG_{av} is the free energy barrier for the rate-determining step of the reaction catalyzed by the hypothetical (hyp.) or reference (ref.) mutant

the structural and mechanistic insights obtained from the detailed computational studies on the catalytic mechanism.

Steps #3 to #5 are for the practical computational screening at various levels. It should be noted that the ultimate criterion used in the virtual screening should be the free energy barrier (ΔG_{av}) for the rate-determining step of the reaction process. A conceptually simple, but practically very time-consuming, way is to directly evaluate the ΔG_{av} values associated with all of the hypothetical BChE mutants and select only a few mutants corresponding to the lowest ΔG_{av} values for wet experimental tests. In order to speed up the virtual screening process, during the initial virtual screening steps (prior to step #5), one may first focus on the major factor affecting the free energy barrier, e.g., the interaction energy (E_{int}) between all atoms of (−)-cocaine and the protein environment in the rate-determining transition state, without directly calculating the free energy barrier. It has been demonstrated that the lower the interaction energy, the more stable the transition state structure (Pan et al. 2005; Zheng et al. 2008).

The more stable transition-state structure means the lower energy barrier for the catalytic reaction process and, therefore, the higher catalytic efficiency. The virtual screening based on the calculation of the overall interaction energy, i.e., E_{int} (in step #3) or $\{E_{int}\}$ (in step #4) shown in Fig. 12.5, without directly evaluating the ΔG_{av} values, is computationally efficient and makes the large-scale virtual screening possible. It has also been known that a major factor affecting the overall interaction energy E_{int} or $\{E_{int}\}$ for a BChE mutant is the overall hydrogen bonding (HB) interactions between the carbonyl oxygen of (−)-cocaine benzoyl ester and the oxyanion hole of the enzyme. The overall HB interactions may be represented by the total hydrogen bonding energy (tHBE). For this reason, some of the successfully accomplished virtual screening of the transition states actually evaluated tHBE, instead of E_{int} or $\{E_{int}\}$ (Pan et al. 2005; Gao et al. 2006; Zheng et al. 2010, 2014).

As discussed below, the systematic virtual screening of transition states has led to successful design and discovery of human BChE mutants with considerably improved catalytic efficiency against (−)-cocaine.

12.4 Highly Efficient Cocaine Hydrolases (CocHs) Designed from Human BChE

The early rational BChE mutant design efforts were focused on the prereactive BChE–(−)-cocaine complex (ES) formation process (Sun et al. 2001, 2002a; Gao et al. 2005; Hamza et al. 2005). This strategy was reasonable because the formation of the prereactive ES complex is the rate-determining step of (−)-cocaine hydrolysis catalyzed by wild-type BChE (Zhan et al. 2003; Hamza et al. 2005; Huang et al. 2010, 2011), as noted above. Indeed, the use of this strategy led to the discovery of several mutants of human BChE with a ~9- to 34-fold improved catalytic efficiency (k_{cat}/K_M) against (−)-cocaine (Sun et al. 2002a; Hamza et al. 2005; Gao et al. 2005). In particular, cocaine rotation in the BChE active site from the non-prereactive ES complex to the prereactive ES complex is hindered mainly by the bulky side chain of Y332 residue in wild-type BChE, but the hindering can be removed by the Y332A mutation and the Y332G mutation can produce a more significant improvement (Zhan et al. 2003; Hamza et al. 2005). However, extensive computational modeling and simulations including the detailed reaction-coordinate calculations (Zhan et al. 2003; Pan et al. 2005; Zhan and Gao 2005) revealed that the rate-determining step of (−)-cocaine hydrolysis catalyzed by the A328W/Y332A mutant (Sun et al. 2002a) or A328W/Y332G mutant (Hamza et al. 2005) is the first step of the chemical reaction process. Therefore, starting from the A328W/Y332A or A328W/Y332G mutant, further efforts (Pan et al. 2005, 2007; Gao et al. 2006; Zheng et al. 2008, 2010, 2014; Xue et al. 2011) in improving the catalytic efficiency of human BChE against (−)-cocaine aimed to stabilize the transition state (TS1) for the first step of the chemical reaction process and, thus, decrease the energy barrier without significantly affecting the prechemical process and the other steps of the chemical reaction process. In these efforts, the aforementioned computational strategies and methods were used to virtually screen the transition-state structures associated with a variety of hypothetical mutants of human BChE, followed by in vitro activity assays on the actual catalytic efficiency of computationally selected mutants. The integrated computational–experimental efforts based on virtual screening of transition-state structures led to successful design and discovery of human BChE mutants (including those summarized in Table 12.1) with considerably improved catalytic efficiency against (−)-cocaine, as discussed below, without significantly changing the catalytic efficiencies against other substrates (Hou et al. 2013).

12.4.1 *First* True *CocH (CocH1): The A199S/S287G/A328W/Y332G Mutant*

The first integrated computational–experimental effort based on virtual screening of transition-state structures, reported by the Kentucky team (Pan et al. 2005), identified that the A199S/S287G/A328W/Y332G mutant of human BChE has a significantly improved catalytic efficiency against (−)-cocaine. Based on the virtual screening of the TS1 structures, the initial in vitro activity assay was based on the measurement of the time-dependent radiometric data associated with a low concentration of [^{3}H](−)-cocaine and fitting of the data to the kinetic equation. Such a kinetic assay was designed to quickly estimate the relative k_{cat}/K_M values of various BChE mutants without determining the individual k_{cat} and K_M values. Based on this simple assay, the A199S/S287G/A328W/Y332G mutant was estimated to have a ~456-fold improved catalytic efficiency compared to wild-type human BChE against (−)-cocaine (Pan et al. 2005). Subsequent, standard Michaelis–Menten kinetic analysis (Yang et al. 2010b) determining the individual k_{cat} and K_M values revealed that the A199S/S287G/A328W/Y332G mutant ($k_{cat}=3,060$ min^{-1}, $K_M=3.1$ μM, and $k_{cat}/K_M=9.9\times10^8$ min^{-1} M^{-1}) has ~1,080-fold improved catalytic efficiency compared to wild-type human BChE ($k_{cat}=4.1$ min^{-1}, $K_M=4.5$ μM, and $k_{cat}/K_M=9.1\times10^5$ min^{-1} M^{-1}) against (−)-cocaine without improving the catalytic efficiency against neurotransmitter ACh. Pretreatment with the mutant (i.e., 1 min prior to cocaine administration) dose dependently protected mice against the acute toxicity of a lethal dose (180 mg/kg, i.p.) of cocaine (LD_{100}) (Xue et al. 2011). The A199S/S287G/A328W/Y332G mutant of human BChE at the dose of 0.03 mg/mouse (i.v.) (or ~0.9 mg/kg) produced full protection in mice after receiving 180 mg/kg of cocaine.

The original report of the A199S/S287G/A328W/Y332G mutant (Pan et al. 2005) has stimulated extensive preclinical and clinical studies on this mutant by multiple research labs (Brimijoin et al. 2008, 2013; Gao et al. 2008, 2010; Schindler et al. 2013; Schindler and Goldberg 2012; Carroll et al. 2011; Cohen-Barak et al. 2015). Through in vitro activity validation, Brimijoin et al. (Brimijoin et al. 2008) concluded that this BChE mutant is "a true CocH with a catalytic efficiency that is 1,000-fold greater than wild-type BChE." If a *true* CocH can be defined as a BChE mutant with a catalytic efficiency that is at least 1,000-fold greater than wild-type

Table 12.1 Kinetic parameters determined for (−)-cocaine, (+)-cocaine, acetylcholine (ACh), acetylthiocholine (ATC), and butyrylthiocholine (BTC) hydrolyses catalyzed by wild-type human BChE and the representative mutants designed by the Kentucky team

Substrate	Enzyme[a]	K_M (μM)	k_{cat} (min^{-1})	k_{cat}/K_M (min^{-1} M^{-1})	RCE[b]
(−)-Cocaine	Wild-type BChE[c]	4.5	4.1	9.1×10^5	1
	A199S/A328W/Y332G	5.1	560	1.1×10^8	121
	A199S/F227A/A328W/Y332G	4.4	1,560	3.6×10^8	396
	A199S/S287G/A328W/Y332G	3.1	3,060	9.9×10^8	1,080
	A199S/F227A/S287G/A328W/E441D	1.1	1,730	1.6×10^9	1,730
	A199S/F227A/S287G/A328W/Y332G	3.1	5,700	1.8×10^9	2,020
(+)-Cocaine	Wild-type BChE	4.7	6,420	1.4×10^9	1
	A199S/A328W/Y332G	5.0	2,820	5.6×10^8	0.40
	A199S/F227A/A328W/Y332G	4.4	6,060	1.4×10^9	1.01
	A199S/S287G/A328W/Y332G	6.3	5,620	8.9×10^8	0.65
	A199S/F227A/S287G/A328W/E441D	4.7	10,800	2.3×10^9	1.68
	A199S/F227A/S287G/A328W/Y332G	4.6	8,990	2.0×10^9	1.43
ACh	Wild-type BChE[d]	148	61,200	4.1×10^8	1
	A199S/A328W/Y332G	156	4,190	2.7×10^7	0.066
	A199S/F227A/A328W/Y332G	189	7,430	3.9×10^7	0.095
	A199S/S287G/A328W/Y332G	36	5,320	1.5×10^8	0.37
	A199S/F227A/S287G/A328W/E441D	27	10,400	3.9×10^8	0.95
	A199S/F227A/S287G/A328W/Y332G	37	11,900	3.2×10^8	0.78
ATC	Wild-type BChE[e]	33	20,200	6.1×10^8	1
	A199S/A328W/Y332G	31	3,410	1.1×10^8	0.18
	A199S/F227A/A328W/Y332G	41	6,870	1.6×10^8	0.26
	A199S/S287G/A328W/Y332G	21	7,880	3.7×10^8	0.60
	A199S/F227A/S287G/A328W/E441D	12	14,000	1.2×10^9	1.99
	A199S/F227A/S287G/A328W/Y332G	20	14,800	7.2×10^8	1.19
BTC	Wild-type BChE[f]	17	29,500	1.7×10^9	1
	A199S/A328W/Y332G	8.9	6,100	6.8×10^8	0.39
	A199S/F227A/A328W/Y332G	11	74,700	6.8×10^9	3.91
	A199S/S287G/A328W/Y332G	5.3	14,400	2.7×10^9	1.57
	A199S/F227A/S287G/A328W/E441D	8.9	17,800	2.0×10^9	1.15
	A199S/F227A/S287G/A328W/Y332G	13	28,000	2.2×10^9	1.24

[a]Unless indicated otherwise, all kinetic parameters listed in this table came from reference Hou et al. (2013)
[b]RCE refers to the relative catalytic efficiency (k_{cat}/K_M), i.e., the ratio of the k_{cat}/K_M value of the mutant to that of wild-type BChE against the same substrate
[c]Data for wild-type BChE from reference Sun et al. (2002a)
[d]The k_{cat} value for wild-type BChE was reported in reference Brimijoin et al. (2008)
[e]The k_{cat} value for wild-type BChE from reference Sun et al. (2001)
[f]The k_{cat} value for wild-type BChE was reported in reference Gao et al. (2008)

BChE, then one may say that the A199S/S287G/A328W/Y332G mutant of human BChE (Pan et al. 2005) is the first *true* CocH. The A199S/S287G/A328W/Y332G mutant of human BChE is also known as CocH1 or E14-3 in literature (Gao et al. 2010; Xue et al. 2011; Zhan et al. 2014; Hou et al. 2013, 2014; Brimijoin et al. 2013). Through in vivo studies, Brimijoin et al. (Brimijoin et al. 2008) demonstrated that this BChE mutant (A199S/S287G/A328W/Y332G), fused with human serum albumin (HSA) to extend the in vivo half-life, selectively blocked the cocaine-induced toxicity and reinstatement of drug seeking in rats that had previously self-administered cocaine. In this HSA-fused BChE mutant (with a biological half-life of ~8 h in rats (Brimijoin et al. 2008)), the C-terminus tetramerization domain of the BChE mutant (Pan et al. 2005) was removed to express the protein using a mammalian expression system as a monomer, and the truncated BChE mutant (residues #1 to #529) was fused to the N-terminus of HSA in order to express the recombinant protein as a single, continuous polypeptide to increase its stability and residence time in vivo (Brimijoin et al. 2008). This HSA-fused form of the A199S/S287G/A328W/Y332G mutant (Pan et al. 2005) is known as Albu-CocH, Albu-CocH1, AlbuBChE, or TV-1380 in literature (Brimijoin et al. 2008, 2013; Gao et al. 2008, 2010; Schindler and Goldberg 2012; Schindler et al. 2013; Cohen-Barak et al. 2015; Carroll et al. 2011). The in vivo efficacy of the HSA-fused A199S/S287G/A328W/Y332G mutant in monkeys was demonstrated in self-administration and drug discrimination studies (Schindler and Goldberg 2012; Schindler et al. 2013).

Besides testing the abovementioned A199S/S287G/A328W/Y332G mutant (CocH1) as a potential therapeutic enzyme for the treatment of cocaine abuse, additional in vivo studies were carried out to examine the feasibility of CocH1-based gene therapy approach for cocaine addiction treatment using viral gene transfer vectors (Gao and Brimijoin 2009; Anker et al. 2012; Carroll et al. 2012; Gao et al. 2013), demonstrating that CocH1 may also be used *via* gene therapy for the treatment of cocaine addiction using a viral gene transfer vector encoding CocH1.

In light of the promising outcomes of the preclinical studies, Teva Pharmaceutical Industries Ltd went ahead to conduct double-blind, placebo-controlled studies on TV-1380 or Albu-CocH or Albu-CocH1 or AlbuBChE (i.e., the HSA-fused form of the A199S/S287G/A328W/Y332G mutant (Pan et al. 2005)) in humans for cocaine addiction treatment (Cohen-Barak et al. 2015). Two randomized, blinded phase I studies, conducted to evaluate the safety, pharmacokinetics, and pharmacodynamics of TV-1380 following single and multiple administration in healthy subjects, revealed that TV-1380 (at the 50–300 mg dose range, i.m.) was safe and well tolerated with a half-life of 43–77 h (Cohen-Barak et al. 2015). It was shown that TV-1380 can rapidly eliminate cocaine in the plasma, thus forestalling entry of cocaine into the brain and heart. TV-1380 activity clearly increased upon treatment in a dose-dependent manner, which is consistent with preclinical results. Overall, the enzyme offers a safe once-weekly therapy to increase cocaine hydrolysis in humans (Cohen-Barak et al. 2015). TV-1380 is currently under phase II clinical trial (NCT01887366) for cocaine addiction treatment; see https://clinicaltrials.gov/ct2/show/NCT01887366.

In addition to the clinical application in cocaine addiction treatment, TV-1380 was also tested for its efficacy as a stoichiometric bioscavenger of organophosphorus

(OP) nerve agents including tabun (GA), sarin (GB), soman (GD), cyclosarin (GF), VX, Russian VX (VR), and VM (Seavey et al. 2014). The measured inhibition rate constants ($\times 10^5$ min^{-1} M^{-1}) for TV-1380 were 6.12 (GA), 10.3 (GB), 109 (GD), 203 (GF), 0.398 (VX), 0.339 (VR), and 17.8 (VM). Protection studies on TV-1380 in guinea pigs showed 100 % survival against GB, GD, GF, and VR and 50 % survival against GA for 50 mg/kg pretreatment of TV-1380 (i.v.). 50 mg/kg of TV-1380 had no protection against VX, but a higher dose (267 mg/kg) of TV-1380 showed 100 % survival against VX. The protection studies suggested that TV-1380 may also act as a promising stoichiometric nerve agent bioscavenger by binding various OP agents in circulation and preventing them from interacting with AChE (Seavey et al. 2014).

All of the preclinical and clinical studies discussed above have demonstrated that the first *true* CocH, i.e., the A199S/S287G/A328W/Y332G mutant of human BChE designed and discovered by the Kentucky team (Pan et al. 2005), in an HSA-fused form (known as TV-1380 or Albu-CocH or Albu-CocH1 or AlbuBChE) is promising for the treatment of both cocaine addiction and pharmacological prophylaxis against OP nerve agent poisoning.

12.4.2 CocH2 and CocH3 with Further Improved Catalytic Efficiency

Through further integrated computational–experimental efforts (Zheng et al. 2008, 2014; Yang et al. 2009; Xue et al. 2011) based on virtual screening of transition-state structures, the Kentucky team also successfully designed and discovered other BChE mutants with further improved catalytic efficiency against (−)-cocaine. For example, the A199S/F227A/S287G/A328W/E441D mutant (Yang et al. 2009; Xue et al. 2011; Hou et al. 2013) is known as E12-4 or CocH2 ($k_{cat}=1{,}730$ min^{-1}, $K_M=1.1$ μM, and $k_{cat}/K_M=1.6\times10^9$ min^{-1} M^{-1}) with ~1,730-fold improved catalytic efficiency, and the A199S/F227A/S287G/A328W/Y332G mutant is known as E12-7 or CocH3 ($k_{cat}=5{,}700$ min^{-1}, $K_M=3.1$ μM, and $k_{cat}/K_M=1.8\times10^9$ min^{-1} M^{-1}) with ~2,020-fold improved catalytic efficiency, compared to wild-type human BChE against (−)-cocaine, as seen in Table 12.1. In order to characterize these CocHs more extensively, a lentiviral vector (pCSC-SP-PW) encoding a CocH (CocH3 or CocH2 or another BChE mutant) was used to develop stable HEK 293 F cell lines (Xue et al. 2011) and stable CHO-S cells lines (Xue et al. 2013a) for scale-up production of the CocHs. In particular, the stable CHO-S cell line developed by using a lentivirus-based repeated-transduction method can be used to more efficiently produce CocH3 (Xue et al. 2013a).

Notably, both computational modeling and kinetic analysis (Hou et al. 2013) have consistently revealed that all of the amino-acid mutations leading to the BChE mutants (including CocH1 to 3) listed in Table 12.1 only considerably improve the catalytic efficiency of human BChE against (−)-cocaine, without significantly improving the catalytic efficiency of the enzyme against anyone of the other substrates examined (Xue et al. 2013b; Hou et al. 2013). In particular, all of the BChE mutants listed in Table 12.1 have an even slightly lower catalytic efficiency against neurotransmitter ACh compared to the wild-type BChE. The observed substrate selectivity of these mutations may be used to address a potential question concerning whether the enzyme therapy using a high-activity mutant of human BChE would significantly affect the cholinergic transmission and, thus, produce adverse effects. In fact, reported studies evaluating wide-type human BChE as a prophylaxis against chemical warfare nerve agents found no autonomic or motor impairment in rats, guinea pigs, or primates, even with the high doses raising the plasma enzyme levels from 50- to 100-fold (Myers et al. 2012; Saxena et al. 2005, 2011; Rosenberg et al. 2010; Genovese et al. 2010; Weber et al. 2011). This is not surprising due to several factors. First, the molar concentrations of AChE and BChE in blood are roughly similar (Li et al. 2000), and BChE has a lower catalytic efficiency against ACh compared to AChE. Second, cholinergic synapses in the brain are insulated from plasma enzymes by the blood–brain barrier, and, thus, the exogenous enzymes in plasma would not reach the brain. In addition, peripheral cholinergic synapses are densely packed with AChE. It has been known that mouse neuromuscular junction has 5×10^{19} catalytic AChE subunits per cc, i.e., ~0.1 mM (Anglister et al. 1998), whereas mouse plasma BChE levels are below 0.1 μM (Li et al. 2000). For these reasons, even high levels of plasma BChE activity are unlikely to affect motor transmission. The observation that none of these high-activity mutants of human BChE had an improved catalytic efficiency against ACh compared to the wild-type BChE gave us additional confidence in the development of a more efficient enzyme therapy using one of the highly efficient CocHs.

In fact, CocH2 and CocH3 have been tested extensively in animals. The first in vivo study on CocH3 (Zheng et al. 2008) revealed that pretreatment with CocH3 (i.e., 1 min prior to cocaine administration) dose dependently protected mice against cocaine-induced convulsions and lethality. In fact, CocH3 can rapidly hydrolyze cocaine in vivo and effectively block cocaine-induced hyperactivity (Xue et al. 2013a). With pretreatment of 2 mg/kg CocH3 (i.v.), 25 mg/kg cocaine (i.p.) did not induce any notable hyperactivity in mice. So 2 mg/kg CocH3 completely blocked the hyperactivity induced by 25 mg/kg cocaine (Xue et al. 2013a).

CocH2 also effectively protected mice from the acute toxicity of a lethal dose (180 mg/kg, i.p.) of cocaine (Xue et al. 2011). The minimum (i.v.) dose of enzyme required to protect all of the mice from the acute toxicity of 180 mg/kg cocaine was determined to be 0.03 mg/mouse (or ~0.9 mg/kg) for CocH1, 0.02 mg/mouse (or ~0.6 mg/kg) for CocH2, and 0.01 mg/mouse (or ~0.3 mg/kg) for CocH3. So compared to CocH1, both CocH2 and CocH3 are more effective in the protection experiments. The relative in vivo potency of CocH1 to 3 in the protection assays was consistent with the relative catalytic efficiency of the enzymes against (−)-cocaine determined in vitro (Zheng et al. 2008; Xue et al. 2011). The higher the catalytic efficiency (k_{cat}/K_M) observed in vitro, the lower the minimum dose of the enzyme required to protect all of the animals from the acute toxicity of 180 mg/kg cocaine. Compared to CocH1 and CocH2, CocH3 is more active in vitro and, thus, more effective in vivo.

In addition to the above in vitro and in vivo testing of CocH2 and CocH3 as potential therapeutic enzymes for the treatment of cocaine abuse, the gene therapy approach was also used to test CocH2 and CocH3 for their effectiveness and safety using viral gene transfer vectors encoding CocH2 or CocH3 (Geng et al. 2013; Murthy et al. 2014a, b; Zlebnik et al. 2014). The CocHs tested using the viral gene transfer vectors also included mouse BChE (mBChE)-based CocHs (mCocHs) with equivalent mutations in mBChE. For example, human BChE (hBChE)-based CocH3 (hCocH3) is the A199S/F227A/S287G/A328W/Y332G mutant of hBChE, whereas mCocH3 is the A199S/S227A/S287G/A328W/Y332G mutant of mBChE (Chen et al. 2015b).

According to the in vitro activity assays (Chen et al. 2015b), mCocH3 had an improved catalytic efficiency compared to mBChE but had a significantly lower catalytic efficiency compared to hCocH3, against (−)-cocaine. On the other hand, mCocH3 was accommodated perfectly in mice such that a viral gene transfer vector (AAV-CMV-mCocH) encoding mCocH3 was able to increase the plasma cocaine hydrolase activity for over one year with no observed immune response (Geng et al. 2013). A more advanced viral gene transfer vector (AAV-VIP-mCocH) encoding mCocH3 generated a dose-dependent increase in plasma cocaine hydrolase activity from 20-fold to 20,000-fold, and another viral vector (hdAD-ApoE-mCocH) encoding mCocH3 produced a 300,000-fold increase in the plasma cocaine hydrolase activity (Geng et al. 2013). These viral gene transfer vectors encoding mCocH3 did not generate adverse reactions such as motor weakness, elevated liver enzymes, or disturbance in spontaneous activity (Geng et al. 2013). It has been demonstrated that the gene transfer using a viral vector encoding a CocH (CocH3 or CocH2) can yield plasma CocH levels that effectively detoxify cocaine, block cocaine-induced physiological effects, and diminish long-term cocaine intake for lengthy periods without immune reactions or cholinergic dysfunction (Geng et al. 2013; Murthy et al. 2014a, b; Zlebnik et al. 2014).

Most recently, during mouse studies of the CocH-based gene therapy for cocaine abuse, it was noted (Chen et al. 2015a) that the viral gene transfer of mouse/human CocH3 or CocH2 or wild-type BChE exhibited sharply reduced plasma ghrelin in mice *via* the enzymatic hydrolysis of ghrelin and, thus, helped to control aggression. With increased plasma enzyme activity for ghrelin hydrolysis, the animals fought less, both spontaneously and in a resident/intruder provocation model (Chen et al. 2015a). Meanwhile, ongoing animal studies of the CocH-based enzyme therapy for cocaine abuse by the Kentucky team revealed that the administration of a purified CocH enzyme significantly decreased the body weight gain of the animals (mice and rats) that were given high-fat diet, compared to the corresponding control animals without the CocH enzyme administration. More extensive efforts will be needed to thoroughly evaluate its therapeutic potential in obesity treatment. All of these findings suggest that the cocaine hydrolases may also have valuable anti-aggression and anti-obesity effects due to their catalytic activity for ghrelin hydrolysis.

Collectively, it has been demonstrated that CocH3 and CocH2 (Zheng et al. 2008; Yang et al. 2009; Xue et al. 2011) designed and discovered by the Kentucky team are promising for treating not only cocaine overdose and addiction but also aggression and obesity.

12.4.3 Catalytic Activities Against Cocaethylene and Norcocaine

As discussed above, the *true* CocHs (including CocH1 to 3) are promising for therapeutic treatment of both cocaine addiction and overdose. For cocaine addiction treatment, one may use either the enzyme therapy or gene therapy approach to keep an effective CocH level in the plasma. In the presence of an effective CocH level in plasma, whenever the patients take cocaine again, cocaine will be hydrolyzed rapidly by the CocH in plasma to produce biologically inactive metabolites EME and benzoic acid such that the patients could not feel the "high" of cocaine. So for the cocaine addiction treatment, the contributions from the other metabolic reactions to the overall cocaine metabolism may be negligible.

However, for cocaine overdose treatment, a cocaine user has already taken a high dose of cocaine prior to the administration of an exogenous enzyme (CocH *via* enzyme therapy). Prior to the enzyme administration, certain amount of cocaine has already been metabolized *via* multiple metabolic pathways. So an effective treatment of cocaine overdose should account for not only cocaine itself but also its potentially toxic metabolites, particularly norcocaine (Zhan et al. 2014).

As an additional challenge to cocaine abuse treatment, statistical data revealed that the majority of cocaine users (e.g., 92 % as of August 2013) (Gorelick et al. 2013) also consume alcohol (ethanol or EtOH depicted in Fig. 12.6). Alcohol can react with cocaine under hCE-1 catalysis to produce a significantly more cytotoxic compound, cocaethylene, through transesterification. With alcohol coadministration, ~24 % (intravenous), ~34 % (oral), or ~18 % (smoked) of cocaine is converted to cocaethylene through transesterification (Herbst et al. 2011). Hence, a truly valuable mutant of human BChE for anti-cocaine enzyme therapy development should be efficient for not only cocaine but also norcocaine and cocaethylene depicted in Fig. 12.6 (Hou et al. 2014).

The catalytic parameters (k_{cat} and K_M) of human BChE and representative mutants (including CocH1 and CocH3 discussed above) for cocaethylene and norcocaine were characterized by the Kentucky team, for the first time, in comparison with those for cocaine (Zhan et al. 2014; Hou et al. 2014). Based on the obtained kinetic data summarized in Table 12.2, wild-type human BChE has a lower catalytic activity for cocaethylene/norcocaine compared to its catalytic activity for (−)-cocaine. The CocHs have a considerably improved catalytic activity against cocaethylene and norcocaine compared to the wild-type BChE. In particular, CocH3 has a 1,080-fold improved catalytic efficiency for norcocaine ($k_{cat} = 2{,}610$ min^{-1}, $K_M = 13$ μM, and $k_{cat}/K_M = 2.01 \times 10^8$ min^{-1} M^{-1}) and an 861-fold improved catalytic efficiency for cocaethylene ($k_{cat} = 3{,}600$ min^{-1}, $K_M = 9.5$ μM, and $k_{cat}/K_M = 3.79 \times 10^8$ min^{-1} M^{-1}). It has been demonstrated that CocH3 as an exogenous enzyme can indeed rapidly metabolize norcocaine and cocaethylene, in addition to (−)-cocaine, in rats (Zhan et al. 2014; Hou et al. 2014). Further kinetic modeling suggested that CocH3 with an identical concentration as that of the endogenous BChE in human plasma can effectively eliminate

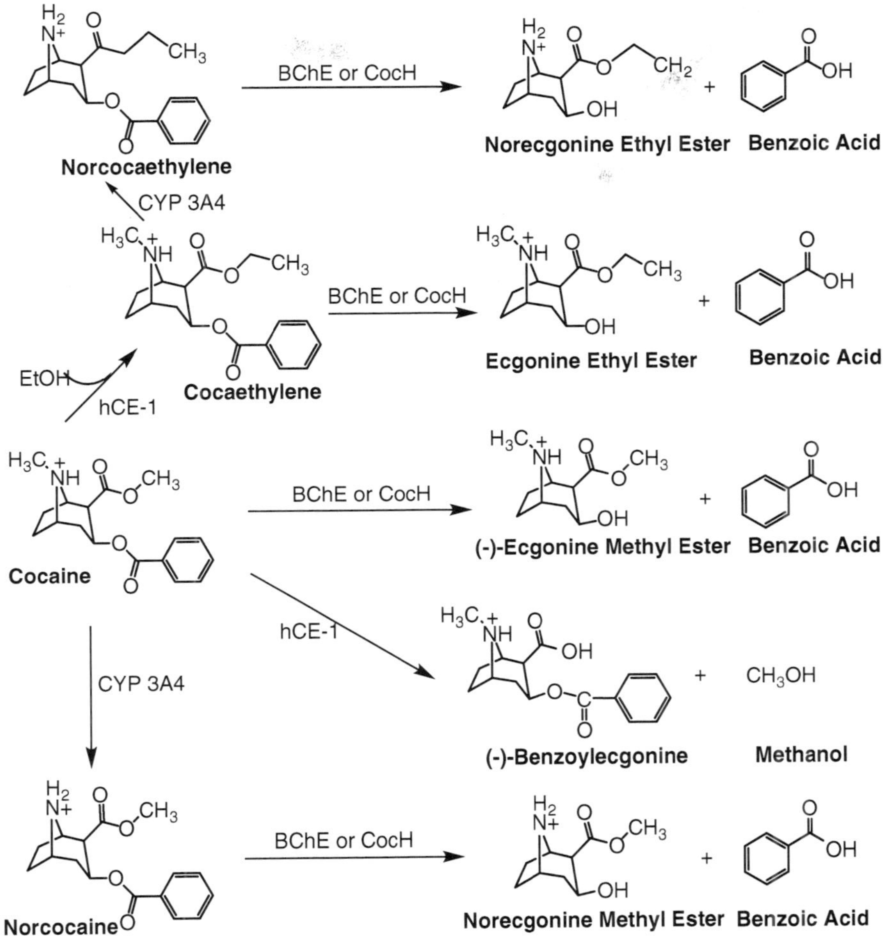

Fig. 12.6 Cocaine metabolites produced in humans through hydrolysis catalyzed by CocH and/or BChE, oxidation by CYP 3A4, and reaction of cocaine with alcohol (catalyzed by liver hCE-1)

(−)-cocaine, cocaethylene, and norcocaine in simplified kinetic models of cocaine abuse and overdose associated with the concurrent use of cocaine and alcohol (Hou et al. 2014).

12.4.4 Computational Prediction of the Effectiveness of CocHs in Human

To predict how effective a cocaine-metabolizing enzyme can actually prevent cocaine from entering brain and producing physiological effects, the Kentucky team (Zheng and Zhan 2012b) developed a two-compartment pharmacokinetic model of

Table 12.2 Kinetic parameters determined in vitro for (−)-cocaine, norcocaine, and cocaethylene hydrolyses catalyzed by wild-type human BChE and its representative mutants

Substrate	Enzyme[a]	K_M (μM)	k_{cat} (min^{-1})	k_{cat}/K_M (M^{-1} min^{-1})	RCE[b]
(−)-Cocaine[c]	WT BChE	4.5	4.1	9.11×10^5	1
	CocH1	3.1	3,060	9.87×10^8	1,080
	CocH3	3.1	5,700	1.84×10^9	2,020
Norcocaine[c]	WT BChE	15	2.8	1.87×10^5	1
	CocH1	12	766	6.38×10^7	343
	CocH3	13	2,610	2.01×10^8	1,080
Cocaethylene[d]	WT BChE	7.5	3.3	4.40×10^5	1
	CocH1	8.0	1,820	2.28×10^8	517
	CocH3	9.5	3,600	3.79×10^8	861

[a]The enzyme under the studies (Hou et al. 2014; Zhan et al. 2014) was wild-type human BChE (WT BChE), A199S/S287G/A328W/Y332G mutant (CocH1 or E14-3), or A199S/F227A/S287G/A328W/Y332G mutant (CocH3 or E12-7)

[b]RCE refers to the relative catalytic efficiency (k_{cat}/K_M), i.e., the ratio of the k_{cat}/K_M value of the mutant to that of wild-type BChE against the same substrate

[c]Data for wild-type human BChE against (−)-cocaine came from Sun et al. (2002a), data for CocH1 against (−)-cocaine came from reference Xue et al. (2011), data for CocH3 against (−)-cocaine came from Zheng et al. (2008), and data for all enzymes against norcocaine came from Zhan et al. (2014)

[d]All of the kinetic data for cocaethylene came from Hou et al. (2014)

cocaine through a combined use of in vitro kinetic parameters and positron emission tomography (PET) data (Fowler et al. 1989) in human to examine the effects of a cocaine-metabolizing enzyme in plasma on the time course of cocaine in plasma and brain of human. The model has one compartment representing brain (striatum) tissue, which exchanges cocaine with plasma compartment where cocaine molecules experience enzymatic Michaelis–Menten elimination. According to the modeling, without an exogenous enzyme, cocaine half-lives in both brain and plasma are almost linearly dependent on the initial cocaine concentration in plasma. For a given exogenous cocaine-metabolizing enzyme, a sufficiently high concentration of the enzyme in plasma can completely block physiological effects of cocaine. The computational prediction was supported by subsequent observations in various animal models. For example, the nearly constant concentration of mCocH3 generated *via* viral gene transfer effectively diminished long-term cocaine intake in rats (Zlebnik et al. 2014), and the administration of hCocH3 completely blocked cocaine-induced hyperactivity in mice (Xue et al. 2013a).

Further, based on the modeling (Zheng and Zhan 2012b), the threshold concentration of cocaine in the brain required to produce physiological effects was estimated to be 0.22 ± 0.07 μM, and the threshold area under the cocaine concentration versus time curve (AUC) value in the brain (denoted by $AUC2_\infty$) required to produce physiological effects was estimated to be 7.9 ± 2.7 μM · min. The modeling (Zheng and Zhan 2012b) also predicted that the administration of a CocH or cocaine esterase (CocE) can considerably decrease the cocaine half-lives in both brain and plasma, the peak cocaine concentration in the brain, and

Table 12.3 Kinetic parameters for enzymatic hydrolysis of (−)-cocaine and ACh

Enzyme	Substrate	K_M (μM)	k_{cat} (min^{-1})	k_{cat}/K_M (min^{-1} M^{-1})
E30-6 (CocH4)[a]	(−)-Cocaine	3.65	14,600	4.0×10^9
E30-6 (CocH4)[a]	ACh	54.7	8,710	1.6×10^8
BChE[b]	ACh	150	61,200	4.1×10^8
AChE[c]	ACh	90	702,000	7.8×10^9

[a]Data for E30-6 or CocH4 (which is the A199S/F227A/P285A/S287G/A328W/Y332G mutant of human BChE) came from Zheng et al. (2014). The kinetic analysis for (−)-cocaine hydrolysis was carried out at 37 °C and pH 8

[b]Data for wild-type BChE came from Gao et al. (2008)

[c]Data for wild-type AChE came from Wolfenden and Yuan (2011)

the $AUC2_\infty$. The estimated maximum cocaine plasma concentration which a given concentration of drug-metabolizing enzyme can effectively prevent from entering the brain and producing physiological effects may be used to guide preclinical and clinical studies on cocaine-metabolizing enzymes. In fact, this pharmacokinetic model (Zheng and Zhan 2012b) was used in combination with the time-dependent enzyme concentration to guide phase IIa clinical trial (Nasser et al. 2014) on a thermally stable CocE mutant (T172R/G173Q) (Gao et al. 2009) which is also known as RBP-8000. As understanding of drug-metabolizing enzymes is key to the science of pharmacokinetics, the general insights (Zheng and Zhan 2012b) into the effects of a drug-metabolizing enzyme on drug kinetics in human should be valuable also in future development of enzyme therapies for other drugs of abuse.

12.4.5 Novel, More Efficient CocHs Under Investigation

In addition to the well-characterized CocHs discussed above, further integrated computational–experimental studies (Zheng et al. 2014) led to successful design and discovery of additional BChE mutants with further improved catalytic efficiency against (−)-cocaine, including the A199S/F227A/P285A/S287G/A328W/Y332G mutant of human BChE (E30-6 or CocH4) in Table 12.3. As seen in Table 12.3, E30-6 has much higher catalytic efficiency for cocaine conversion than for conversion of the natural BChE substrate, ACh. It is interesting to note that the catalytic efficiency of E30-6 for cocaine hydrolysis is comparable to that of the most efficient naturally occurring hydrolytic enzyme, AChE, the catalytic activity of which against ACh approaches the diffusion limit.

Further, E30-6 can protect mice from a subsequently administered lethal dose of cocaine, suggesting the enzyme may have therapeutic potential in the setting of cocaine detoxification or cocaine abuse (Zheng et al. 2014). The minimum dose of E30-6 required to fully protect mice from the acute toxicity of a lethal dose of cocaine (180 mg/kg, i.p.) was 0.15 mg/kg (i.v.). This highly efficient mutant of human BChE is currently under further studies by the Kentucky team.

12.5 Further Rational Design of Protein Engineering to Prolong the Biological Half-Life

In order to effectively suppress cocaine reward for a long period of time after the administration of an exogenous CocH, the therapeutic enzyme (CocH) should have not only a high catalytic efficiency against cocaine but also a sufficiently long circulation time (biological half-life). It should be pointed out that the observed time-dependent concentrations of an active CocH usually follow a well-known double exponential equation ($[E]_t = Ae^{-k_1 t} + Be^{-k_2 t}$) which accounts for both the enzyme distribution process (the fast phase, associated with k_1) and elimination process (the slow phase, associated with k_2). The half-life associated with the enzyme elimination rate constant k_2 is called the biological half-life (the usually referred in vivo half-life).

Particularly for cocaine addiction treatment using a cocaine-metabolizing enzyme, it is desired to have a highly efficient cocaine-metabolizing enzyme circulating in the body for a long time. With a highly efficient cocaine-metabolizing enzyme circulating in the body, whenever a cocaine user takes cocaine again, the enzyme will metabolize cocaine rapidly such that the user will not feel the reward effects of the drug. In addition to the aforementioned efforts to improve catalytic activities of the BChE mutants, further rational design of protein engineering was carried out to prolong the in vivo half-lives of the enzymes, as discussed below.

All strategies discussed below may be used separately to prolong the biological half-lives of CocHs, but a combined use of multiple strategies could be more effective.

12.5.1 *Posttranslational Modifications and PEGylation*

Native human BChE has a biological half-life of ~24 h in mice and ~7 to 12 days in humans (Sun et al. 2002b). However, recombinant forms of wild-type human BChE and the known BChE mutants have a much shorter biological half-life compared to the native human BChE (Duysen et al. 2002), due to the difference in the posttranslational modifications such as subunit oligomerization, *N*-glycosylation, and sialylation. In particular, human BChE is a glycosylated, tetrameric serum protein (with highly sialylated *N*-glycans) (Schneider et al. 2014). Native BChE is fully glycosylated with whole nine N-linked oligosaccharides, whereas recombinant BChE is either not fully glycosylated or glycosylated differently (Lockridge et al. 1987b; Geyer et al. 2010; Huang et al. 2007; Saxena et al. 1998). So recombinant BChE (or a mutant) proteins expressed in different systems differ in the glycosylation and oligomerization and, thus, have different pharmacokinetic (PK) profiles. For example, CocH3 expressed in Chinese hamster ovary (CHO) cells had a significantly longer biological half-life (7.3 h in rats) compared to that expressed in human embryonic kidney (HEK) 293 cells (2.8 h in rats) (Xue et al. 2013a). Recombinant

BChE expressed in transgenic goats or plants usually had a very short biological half-life (Huang et al. 2007; Larrimore et al. 2012; Schneider et al. 2014). Nevertheless, recombinant cholinesterases (including BChE and its mutants) decorated with sialylated *N*-glycans are expected to have significantly prolonged biological half-lives (Kronman et al. 1995), and it is possible to decorate BChE (or its mutant) with sialylated *N*-glycans during protein expression. In fact, recombinant BChE decorated with sialylated *N*-glycans was generated by the coexpression of BChE with a gene-stacking vector encoding six mammalian genes necessary for *in planta* protein sialylation (Schneider et al. 2014).

Further, for a given recombinant BChE (or mutant) produced in an expression system, one may also try to extend its biological half-life by PEGylation, i.e., covalent attachment of polyethylene glycol (PEG) polymer chains. PEGylation is a well-known approach to improvement of the PK profile of a therapeutic protein. For example, PEGylation of recombinant BChE produced in transgenic goats significantly prolonged the biological half-life (Huang et al. 2007), and PEGylation of bacterial CocE mutants also significantly extended the biological half-life (Fang et al. 2014a; Narasimhan et al. 2011). To assist rational design of PEGylation of BChE and its highly efficient mutants in the future, a detailed 3D structural model of glycosylated human BChE (Fang et al. 2014c) was developed. The developed 3D model allows the investigation of the influence of glycans on the PEGylation modification. According to 3D model and MD simulations, glycans did not change the overall stability of the BChE structure, but could increase the flexibility of some local structures. Some lysine residues are expected to have a significant decrease in solvent accessible surface area (SASA) due to the direct or indirect influence of their surrounding glycans. The computational results also revealed that PEGylation reaction agents with smaller functional groups could have a better chance to react with lysine residues (Fang et al. 2014c).

12.5.2 Design of Amino-Acid Mutations to Stabilize the Oligomer Structure

Native and recombinant human BChE proteins are also different in the distribution of the oligomeric forms. Native BChE consists of more than 95 % of tetramer, whereas predominant forms of a recombinant BChE are monomer and dimer (Duysen et al. 2002; Blong et al. 1997). Oligomerization status could influence subcellular deposition and glycosylation of recombinant BChE (Schneider et al. 2014) and, thus, affect the biological half-life of the recombinant BChE (Xue et al. 2013a; Fang et al. 2014b).

Lockridge et al. (Altamirano and Lockridge 1999; Duysen et al. 2002; Altamirano et al. 2000; Biberoglu et al. 2012; Parikh et al. 2011; Li et al. 2008) demonstrated that coexpression of a proline-rich peptide with recombinant human BChE can form a complex between the proline-rich peptide and BChE tetramer, and the complex has a longer biological half-life. The same approach may be used to extend the biological half-life of a cocaine hydrolase (BChE mutant).

For the purpose of practical protein drug development, it might also be interesting to extend the biological half-life of a CocH through an alternative method without coexpression of another peptide. Specifically, one might want to rationally design further mutations on its amino-acid residues that are not available for intermolecular interactions with any other proteins in the body; such type of amino-acid mutations are not expected to produce immune response (Fang et al. 2014b).

On the other hand, it is a challenge to design amino-acid mutations that can extend the biological half-life of a protein, although rational or computational design has been used to successfully identify thermostable mutants of proteins (Korkegian et al. 2005; Gao et al. 2009; Fei et al. 2013; Joo et al. 2011; Kim et al. 2010). This is because the biological half-life of a protein is determined by many factors, in addition to the thermal stability. For a protein to have a desirably long biological half-life, the protein must be thermostable enough at the body temperature (37 °C) to have an in vitro half-life at 37 °C which is at least not shorter than the desired biological half-life. So when a protein has a short biological half-life because the protein is thermally unstable, one may design a thermostable mutant of the protein to extend the biological half-life (Gao et al. 2009). However, for most proteins, their short biological half-lives are due to factors other than the thermal stability. In particular, BChE (wild-type or the mutant) is very thermostable at 37 °C. But the recombinant form of the thermostable protein is quickly eliminated from the body. So further improving the protein thermal stability is not expected to extend its biological half-life. One must account for other factors affecting the biological half-life (Fang et al. 2014b).

A recently reported study (Fang et al. 2014b) aimed to extend the biological half-life of cocaine hydrolase CocH3 through further amino-acid mutations on CocH3 without changing its high catalytic activity against cocaine. The strategy (Fang et al. 2014b) was to design possible amino-acid mutations that can introduce cross subunit disulfide bond(s) and, thus, stabilize the multimeric forms and decrease the concentration of the monomer. This rational design strategy was based on the observation that the multimeric forms of BChE have a longer biological half-life compared to the monomer and that the formation of the multimeric forms of wild-type human BChE relies on an interchain disulfide bond (C571a-C571b) that, once formed, can covalently link two subunits (Lockridge et al. 1987a).

For rational design of cross subunit disulfide bonds (Fang et al. 2014b), MD simulation was carried out on the CocH3 structure using an initial structure built from the previously modeled BChE tetramer structure (Pan et al. 2009). According to the tetramer structure, a tetramer consists of two equivalent dimers, and the rational design was focused on the amino-acid residues on the intersubunit interface within a dimer. For this reason, one only needed to model a BChE dimer, instead of a tetramer, for the practical rational design. A detailed analysis of the MD trajectory predicted that mutations F364C/M532C, V377C/A516C, and N535C may introduce the desirable cross subunit disulfide bond(s) (Fang et al. 2014b). For example, F364C/M532C mutations were predicted to have a more stable dimer structure with the desirable cross subunit disulfide bonds: one between C364 of subunit a (C364a) and C532 of subunit b (C532b), and the other between C532 of subunit a (C532a) and C364 of subunit b (C364b). The rational design was followed by experimental tests in vitro and in vivo, confirming that the rationally designed new BChE mutants (with additional mutations like F364C/M532C, V377C/A516C, or N535C) indeed had a remarkably different distribution of the oligomeric forms and prolonged biological half-life in rats from ~7 h to ~13 h without significantly changing the catalytic activity against (−)-cocaine. The similar strategy using computational simulations was also used to successfully design cross subunit disulfide bonds in a thermally stable bacterial CocE, and the designed cross subunit disulfide bonds (confirmed by the X-ray structural analysis) have not only considerably extended the in vitro half-life at 37 °C to >100 days but also significantly improved the catalytic efficiency against cocaine (Fang et al. 2014a).

12.5.3 Fusion Proteins

It has been known that pharmacokinetic profile of a therapeutic protein may be improved by genetically fusing the protein to another peptide, such as albumin or Fc portion of human immunoglobulin G (IgG). In fact, both Fc and albumin have widely been used as carrier proteins in the development of fusion protein drugs with a prolonged half-life (Dumont et al. 2006; Schulte 2008), and various albumin-fused and Fc-fused protein drugs have been approved by FDA for use in humans. The idea for development of an Fc (or albumin)-fused protein for the in vivo half-life extension is based on the fact that IgG has a very long biological half-life. IgG is a class of antibody predominantly present in the normal human serum, and additional amount of IgG could be generated from the secondary response under continuous stimulation of an external pathogen. The Fc portion of IgG can bind with neonatal Fc receptor (FcRn) in the acidic environment of endosome and is later transported to the cell surface where upon exposure to a neutral pH IgG is released back to the main bloodstream. The primary function of FcRn is to maintain the long half-life of IgG in the serum through binding with the Fc portion of IgG. For this reason, the Fc portion of an Fc-fused protein may also bind with FcRn to extend in vivo half-life of an Fc-fused protein. Similarly, albumin can also bind with FcRn, and, thus, an albumin-fused protein may also have a prolonged in vivo half-life.

In fact, TV-1380 (or Albu-CocH, Albu-CocH1, or AlbuBChE in literature) is an albumin-fused protein of CocH1 (an BChE mutant designed, discovered, and patented by the Kentucky team (Pan et al. 2005), as noted above), and the fusion with albumin has indeed improved the PK profile of CocH1 (Cohen-Barak et al. 2015). The biological half-life of the albumin-fused CocH1 was ~8 h in rats (Brimijoin et al. 2008) and 43–77 h in humans (Cohen-Barak et al. 2015). In ongoing research, the Kentucky team genetically fused Fc (wild-type or rationally designed mutant) of IgG1 to various CocHs and demonstrated that some Fc-fused CocHs have considerably prolonged half-lives (>100 h) in mice and rats. Through computational modeling and simulations on FcRn binding with the possible fusion proteins (Huang et al. 2013), the team has been designing and testing various mutants of the Fc-fused and albumin-fused CocHs in order to further extend the biological half-lives of the fused CocH proteins.

12.6 Summary and Perspectives

Accelerating metabolism of cocaine and its toxic metabolites by using a highly efficient cocaine hydrolase (CocH) catalyzing cocaine hydrolysis at cocaine benzoyl ester is recognized as an ideal approach to the treatment of cocaine overdose and addiction. As the principal endogenous cocaine-metabolizing enzyme in human plasma, butyrylcholinesterase (BChE) can catalyze cocaine hydrolysis at cocaine benzoyl ester, producing biologically inactive metabolites. But the catalytic activity of the wild-type BChE against the naturally occurring, biologically active (−)-cocaine is too low. It is highly desired to develop a much more active mutant of human BChE with considerably improved catalytic efficiency against (−)-cocaine. It has been well known that computational design of a highly efficient enzyme is extremely challenging, particularly when the chemical reaction process is rate determining for the enzymatic reaction. To solve the problem, the Kentucky team developed unique computational enzyme redesign strategies and approaches and employed the computational approaches to rationally design and discover a variety of BChE mutants with at least ~1,000-fold improved catalytic efficiency compared to the wild-type BChE against (−)-cocaine. These highly efficient mutants are recognized the *true* CocHs, such as CocH1 (which is the A199S/S287G/A328W/Y332G mutant or enzyme E14-3), CocH2 (which is the A199S/F227A/S287G/A328W/E441D mutant or enzyme E12-4), CocH3 (which is the A199S/F227A/S287G/A328W/Y332G mutant or enzyme E12-7), and CocH4 (which is the A199S/F227A/P285A/S287G/A328W/Y332G mutant or enzyme E30-6).

Of the *true* CocHs, CocH1 to 4 have been tested in vivo and demonstrated to be potent for accelerating cocaine metabolism, detoxifying cocaine, and eliminating abuse-related physiological effects of cocaine. Hence, these CocHs are promising therapeutic candidates for the treatment of cocaine overdose and addiction and may be used *via* either enzyme therapy (suitable for the treatment of both cocaine overdose and addiction) or gene therapy (suitable for the treatment of cocaine addiction only). In addition to their therapeutic potential for cocaine abuse treatment, these CocHs could also be used as therapeutic agents for the treatment of aggression and obesity as well as promising bioscavengers for organophosphorus nerve agents.

The first *true* CocH (i.e., CocH1) is currently under clinical development (phase II with weekly dosing) for cocaine addiction treatment by Teva Pharmaceutical Industries Ltd. The CocH1-based enzyme formulation used in the clinical trials is the HSA-fused form of CocH1 (i.e., the A199S/S287G/A328W/Y332G mutant or enzyme E14-3 designed and discovered by the Kentucky team), known as TV-1380 or Albu-CocH or Albu-CocH1 or AlbuBChE. The clinical data reported so far are encouraging.

Compared to CocH1 or CocH1-based TV-1380 formulation, the more recently reported CocHs (including CocH2 to 4) have further improved catalytic efficiency against (−)-cocaine, and the latest CocH forms developed by the Kentucky team are expected to have significantly longer biological half-lives. The newly developed long-lasting enzyme forms of the more active CocHs are expected to be much more effective. One may expect to see the development of a much improved CocH formulation with not only significantly higher catalytic efficiency against (−)-cocaine but also a significantly longer biological half-life, suitable for a monthly dosing in cocaine addiction treatment.

Acknowledgment This work was supported by the National Institute on Drug Abuse of the National Institutes of Health (grants R01 DA035552, R01 DA032910, R01 DA013930, and R01 DA025100) and the National Science Foundation (grant CHE-1111761). We also acknowledge the Computer Center at the University of Kentucky for a large amount of supercomputing time over the years.

References

Acevedo O, Jorgensen WL. advances in quantum and molecular mechanical (QM/MM) simulations for organic and enzymatic reactions. Acc Chem Res. 2010;43:142–51.

Altamirano CV, Lockridge O. Conserved aromatic residues of the C-terminus of human butyrylcholinesterase mediate the association of tetramers†. Biochemistry. 1999;38:13414–22.

Altamirano CV, Bartels CF, Lockridge O. The butyrylcholinesterase K-variant shows similar cellular protein turnover and quaternary interaction to the wild-type enzyme. J Neurochem. 2000;74:869–77.

Anglister L, Eichler J, Szabo M, Haesaert B, Salpeter MM. 125i-labeled fasciculin 2: a new tool for quantitation of acetylcholinesterase densities at synaptic sites by EM-autoradiography. J Neurosci Methods. 1998;81:63–71.

Anker JJ, Brimijoin S, Gao Y, Geng L, Zlebnik NE, Parks RJ, Carroll ME. Cocaine hydrolase encoded in viral vector blocks the reinstatement of cocaine seeking in rats for 6 months. Biol Psychiatry. 2012;71:700–5.

Beveridge DL, Dicapua FM. Free energy via molecular simulation: applications to chemical and biomolecular systems. Annu Rev Biophys Biophys Chem. 1989;18:431–92.

Biberoglu K, Schopfer LM, Tacal O, Lockridge O. The proline-rich tetramerization peptides in equine serum butyrylcholinesterase. FEBS J. 2012;279:3844–58.

Blong RM, Bedows E, Lockridge O. Tetramerization domain of human butyrylcholinesterase is at the C-terminus. Biochem J. 1997;327:747–57.

Brim RL, Nance MR, Youngstrom DW, Narasimhan D, Zhan C-G, Tesmer JJ, Sunahara RK, Woods JH. A thermally stable form of bacterial cocaine esterase: a potential therapeutic agent for treatment of cocaine abuse. Mol Pharmacol. 2010;77:593–600.

Brimijoin S, Gao Y, Anker JJ, Gliddon LA, Lafleur D, Shah R, Zhao Q, Singh M, Carroll ME. A cocaine hydrolase engineered from human butyrylcholinesterase selectively blocks cocaine toxicity and reinstatement of drug seeking in rats. Neuropsychopharmacology. 2008;33:2715–25.

Brimijoin S, Orson F, Kosten TR, Kinsey B, Shen XY, White SJ, Gao Y. Anti-cocaine antibody and butyrylcholinesterase-derived cocaine hydrolase exert cooperative effects on cocaine pharmacokinetics and cocaine-induced locomotor activity in mice. Chem Biol Interact. 2013;203:212–6.

Carrera MRA, Kaufmann GF, Mee JM, Meijler MM, Koob GF, Janda KD. Treating cocaine addiction with viruses. Proc Natl Acad Sci U S A. 2004;101:10416–21.

Carroll ME, Gao Y, Brimijoin S, Anker JJ. Effects of cocaine hydrolase on cocaine self-administration under a PR schedule and during extended access (escalation) in rats. Psychopharmacology (Berl). 2011;213:817–29.

Carroll ME, Zlebnik NE, Anker JJ, Kosten TR, Orson FM, Shen X, Kinsey B, Parks RJ, Gao Y, Brimijoin S. Combined cocaine hydrolase gene transfer and anti-cocaine vaccine synergistically block cocaine-induced locomotion. PLoS One. 2012;7, E43536.

Chen X, Fang L, Liu J, Zhan C-G. Reaction pathway and free energy profile for butyrylcholinesterase-catalyzed hydrolysis of acetylcholine. J Phys Chem B. 2011;115:1315–22.

Chen X, Fang L, Liu J, Zhan C-G. Reaction pathway and free energy profiles for butyrylcholinesterase-catalyzed hydrolysis of acetylthiocholine. Biochemistry. 2012;51:1297–305.

Chen VP, Gao Y, Geng L, Parks RJ, Pang YP, Brimijoin S (2015a) Plasma butyrylcholinesterase regulates ghrelin to control aggression. Proc Natl Acad Sci USA. pii: 201421536 [Epub ahead of print 2015, 112:2251–6].

Chen X, Huang X, Geng L, Xue L, Hou S, Zheng X, Brimijoin S, Zheng F, Zhan C-G. Kinetic characterization of a cocaine hydrolase engineered from mouse butyrylcholinesterase. Biochem J. 2015b;466:243–51.

Cohen-Barak O, Wildeman J, Van De Wetering J, Hettinga J, Schuilenga-Hut P, Gross A, Clark S, Bassan M, Gilgun-Sherki Y, Mendzelevski B, Spiegelstein O. Safety, pharmacokinetics, and pharmacodynamics of TV-1380, a novel mutated butyrylcholinesterase treatment for cocaine addiction, after single and multiple intramuscular injections in healthy subjects. J Clin Pharmacol. 2015. doi:10.1002/Jcph.450. [Epub ahead of print 2014 Dec 18].

Collins GT, Brim RL, Narasimhan D, Ko M-C, Sunahara RK, Zhan C-G, Woods JH. Cocaine esterase prevents cocaine-induced toxicity and the ongoing intravenous self-administration of cocaine in rats. J Pharmacol Exp Ther. 2009;331:445–55.

Darvesh S, Hopkins DA, Geula C. Neurobiology of butyrylcholinesterase. Nat Rev Neurosci. 2003;4:131–8.

Dumont JA, Low SC, Peters RT, Bitonti AJ. Monomeric Fc fusions: impact on pharmacokinetic and biological activity of protein therapeutics. BioDrugs. 2006;20:151–60.

Duysen EG, Bartels CF, Lockridge O. Wild-type and A328W mutant human butyrylcholinesterase tetramers expressed in Chinese hamster ovary cells have a 16-hour half-life in the circulation and protect mice from cocaine toxicity. J Pharmacol Exp Therap. 2002;302:751–8.

Fang L, Pan Y, Muzyka J, Zhan C-G. Active site gating and substrate specificity of butyrylcholinesterase and acetylcholinesterase: insights from molecular dynamics simulations. J Phys Chem B. 2011;115:8797–805.

Fang L, Chow KM, Hou S, Xue L, Rodgers DW, Zheng F, Zhan C-G. Rational design, preparation, and characterization of a therapeutic enzyme mutant with improved stability and function for cocaine detoxification. ACS Chem Biol. 2014a;9:1764–72.

Fang L, Hou S, Xue L, Zheng F, Zhan C-G. Amino-acid mutations to extend the biological half-life of a therapeutically valuable mutant of human butyrylcholinesterase. Chem Biol Interact. 2014b;214:18–25.

Fang L, Zheng F, Zhan C-G. A model of glycosylated human butyrylcholinesterase. Mol Biosyst. 2014c;10:348–54.

Fei B, Xu H, Cao Y, Ma S, Guo H, Song T, Qiao D, Cao Y. A multi-factors rational design strategy for enhancing the thermostability of Escherichia coli appa phytase. J Ind Microbiol Biotechnol. 2013;40:457–64.

Fowler JS, Volkow ND, Wolf AP, Dewey SL, Schlyer DJ, Macgregor RR, Hitzemann R, Logan J, Bendriem B, Gatley SJ, et al. Mapping cocaine binding sites in human and baboon brain in vivo. Synapse. 1989;4:371–7.

Gao Y, Brimijoin S. Lasting reduction of cocaine action in neostriatum – a hydrolase gene therapy approach. J Pharmacol Exp Ther. 2009;330:449–57.

Gao D, Zhan C-G. Modeling effects of oxyanion hole on the ester hydrolysis catalyzed by human cholinesterases. J Phys Chem B. 2005;109:23070–6.

Gao D, Zhan C-G. Modeling evolution of hydrogen bonding and stabilization of transition states in the process of cocaine hydrolysis catalyzed by human butyrylcholinesterase. Proteins Struct Funct Bioinf. 2006;62:99–110.

Gao Y, Atanasova E, Sui N, Pancook JD, Watkins JD, Brimijoin S. Gene transfer of cocaine hydrolase suppresses cardiovascular responses to cocaine in rats. Mol Pharmacol. 2005;67:204–11.

Gao D, Cho H, Yang W, Pan Y, Yang G, Tai HH, Zhan C-G. Computational design of a human butyrylcholinesterase mutant for accelerating cocaine hydrolysis based on the transition-state simulation. Angew Chem Int Ed. 2006;45:653–7.

Gao Y, Lafleur D, Shah R, Zhao Q, Singh M, Brimijoin S. An albumin-butyrylcholinesterase for cocaine toxicity and addiction: catalytic and pharmacokinetic properties. Chem Biol Interact. 2008;175:83–7.

Gao D, Narasimhan DL, Macdonald J, Ko M-C, Landry DW, Woods JH, Sunahara RK, Zhan C-G. Thermostable variants of cocaine esterase for long-time protection against cocaine toxicity. Mol Pharmacol. 2009;75:318–23.

Gao Y, Orson FM, Kinsey B, Kosten T, Brimijoin S. The concept of pharmacologic cocaine interception as a treatment for drug abuse. Chem Biol Interact. 2010;187:421–4.

Gao Y, Geng L, Orson F, Kinsey B, Kosten TR, Shen X, Brimijoin S. Effects of anti-cocaine vaccine and viral gene transfer of cocaine hydrolase in mice on cocaine toxicity including motor strength and liver damage. Chem Biol Interact. 2013;203:208–11.

Gately SJ, Macgregor RR, Fowler JS, Wolf AP, Dewey SL, Schlyer DJ. Rapid stereoselective hydrolysis of (+)-cocaine in baboon plasma prevents its uptake in the brain: implications for behavioral studies. J Neurochem. 1990;54:720–3.

Gatley SJ. Activities of the enantiomers of cocaine and some related compounds as substrates and inhibitors of plasma butyrylcholinesterase. Biochem Pharmacol. 1991;41:1249–54.

Geng L, Gao Y, Chen X, Hou S, Zhan C-G, Radic Z, Parks R, Russell SJ, Pham L, Brimijoin S. Gene transfer of mutant mouse cholinesterase provides high lifetime expression and reduced cocaine responses with no evident toxicity. PLoS One. 2013;8, E67446.

Genovese RF, Sun W, Johnson CC, Ditargiani RC, Doctor BP, Saxena A. Safety of administration of human butyrylcholinesterase and its conjugates with soman or VX in rats. Basic Clin Pharmacol Toxicol. 2010;106:428–34.

Geyer BC, Kannan L, Garnaud P-E, Broomfield CA, Cadieux CL, Cherni I, Hodgins SM, Kasten SA, Kelley K, Kilbourne J, Oliver ZP, Otto TC, Puffenberger I, Reeves TE, Robbins N, Woods RR, Soreq H, Lenz DE, Cerasoli DM, Mor TS. Plant-derived human butyrylcholinesterase, but not an organophosphorous-compound hydrolyzing variant thereof, protects rodents against nerve agents. Proc Natl Acad Sci. 2010;107:20251–6.

Giacobini E. Butyrylcholinesterase: its function and inhibitors. London: Martin Dunitz, An Imprint of the Taylor and Francis Group plc; 2003.

Gorelick DA. Enhancing cocaine metabolism with butyrylcholinesterase as a treatment strategy. Drug Alcohol Depend. 1997;48:159–65.

Gorelick DA. Pharmacokinetic approaches to treatment of drug addiction. Exp Rev Clin Pharmacol. 2008;1:277–90.

Gorelick DA, Saxon AJ, Hermann R. Cocaine use disorder in adults: epidemiology, pharmacology, clinical manifestations, medical consequences, and diagnosis. 2013. http://www.uptodate.com/contents/cocaine-use-disorder-in-adults-epidemiology-pharmacology-clinical-manifestations-medical-consequences-and-diagnosis. Updated: 15 Aug 2013.

Hamza A, Cho H, Tai H-H, Zhan C-G. Molecular dynamics simulation of cocaine binding with human butyrylcholinesterase and its mutants. J Phys Chem B. 2005;109:4776–82.

Herbst ED, Harris DS, Everhart ET, Mendelson J, Jacob P, Jones RT. Cocaethylene formation following ethanol and cocaine administration by different routes. Exp Clin Psychopharmacol. 2011;19:95–104.

Hou S, Xue L, Yang W, Fang L, Zheng F, Zhan C-G. Substrate selectivity of high-activity mutants of human butyrylcholinesterase. Org Biomol Chem. 2013;11:7477–85.

Hou S, Zhan M, Zheng X, Zhan C-G, Zheng F. Kinetic characterization of human butyrylcholinesterase mutants for hydrolysis of cocaethylene. Biochem J. 2014;460:447–57.

Hu P, Zhang YK. Catalytic mechanism and product specificity of the histone lysine methyltransferase SET7/9: an ab initio QM/MM-FE study with multiple initial structures. J Am Chem Soc. 2006;128:1272–8.

Huang Y-J, Huang Y, Baldassarre H, Wang B, Lazaris A, Leduc M, Bilodeau AS, Bellemare A, Côté M, Herskovits P, Touati M, Turcotte C, Valeanu L, Lemée N, Wilgus H, Bégin I, Bhatia B, Rao K, Neveu N, Brochu E, Pierson J, Hockley DK, Cerasoli DM, Lenz DE, Karatzas CN, Langermann S. Recombinant human butyrylcholinesterase from milk of transgenic animals to protect against organophosphate poisoning. Proc Natl Acad Sci. 2007;104:13603–8.

Huang X, Pan Y, Zheng F, Zhan C-G. Reaction pathway and free energy profile for pre-chemical reaction step of human butyrylcholinesterase-catalyzed hydrolysis of (–)-cocaine by combined targeted molecular dynamics and potential of mean force simulations. J Phys Chem B. 2010;114:13545–54.

Huang X, Zheng F, Zhan C-G. Human butyrylcholinesterase-cocaine binding pathway and free energy profiles by molecular dynamics and potential of mean force simulations. J Phys Chem B. 2011;115:11254–60.

Huang X, Zheng F, Zhan C-G. Binding structures and energies of human neonatal Fc receptor with human Fc and its mutants by molecular modeling and dynamics simulations. Mol Biosyst. 2013;9:3047–58.

Joo JC, Pack SP, Kim YH, Yoo YJ. Thermostabilization of Bacillus circulans xylanase: computational optimization of unstable residues based on thermal fluctuation analysis. J Biotechnol. 2011;151:56–65.

Kamendulis LM, Brzezinski MR, Pindel EV, Bosron WF, Dean RA. Metabolism of cocaine and heroin is catalyzed by the same human liver carboxylesterases. J Pharmacol Exp Therap. 1996;279:713–7.

Kim SJ, Lee JA, Joo JC, Yoo YJ, Kim YH, Song BK. The development of a thermostable CiP (coprinus cinereus peroxidase) through in silico design. Biotechnol Prog. 2010;26:1038–46.

Kollman P. Free-energy calculations – applications to chemical and biochemical phenomena. Chem Rev. 1993;93:2395–417.

Korkegian A, Black ME, Baker D, Stoddard BL. Computational thermostabilization of an enzyme. Science. 2005;308:857–60.

Kronman C, Velan B, Marcus D, Ordentlich A, Reuveny S, Shafferman A. Involvement of oligomerization, N-glycosylation and sialylation in the clearance of cholinesterases from the circulation. Biochem J. 1995;311:959–67.

Landry DW, Zhao K, Yang GX, Glickman M, Georgiadis TM. Antibody-catalyzed degradation of cocaine. Science. 1993;259:1899–901.

Larrimore KE, Barcus M, Kannan L, Gao Y, Zhan C-G, Brimijoin S, Mor T. Plants as a source of butyrylcholinesterase variants designed for enhanced cocaine hydrolase activity. Chem Biol Interact. 2012;203:217–20.

Larsen NA, Turner JM, Stevens J, Rosser SJ, Basran A, Lerner RA, Bruce NC, Wilson IA. Crystal structure of a bacterial cocaine esterase. Nat Struct Mol Biol. 2002;9:17–21.

Li B, Stribley JA, Ticu A, Xie W, Schopfer LM, Hammond P, Brimijoin S, Hinrichs SH, Lockridge O. Abundant tissue butyrylcholinesterase and its possible function in the acetylcholinesterase knockout mouse. J Neurochem. 2000;75:1320–31.

Li H, Schopfer LM, Masson P, Lockridge O. Lamellipodin proline rich peptides associated with native plasma butyrylcholinesterase tetramers. Biochem J. 2008;411:425–32.

Liu J, Zhan C-G. Reaction pathway and free energy profile for cocaine hydrolase-catalyzed hydrolysis of (–)-cocaine. J Chem Theory Comput. 2012;8:1426–35.

Liu JJ, Hamza A, Zhan C-G. Fundamental reaction mechanism and free energy profile for (–)-cocaine hydrolysis catalyzed by cocaine esterase. J Am Chem Soc. 2009a;131:11964–75.

Liu JJ, Zhang YK, Zhan C-G. Reaction pathway and free-energy barrier for reactivation of dimethylphosphoryl-inhibited human acetylcholinesterase. J Phys Chem B. 2009b;113:16226–36.

Liu JJ, Zhao XY, Yang WC, Zhan C-G. Reaction mechanism for cocaine esterase-catalyzed hydrolyses of (+)- and (–)-cocaine: unexpected common rate-determining step. J Phys Chem B. 2011;115:5017–25.

Lockridge O. Review of human butyrylcholinesterase structure, function, genetic variants, history of use in the clinic, and potential therapeutic uses. Pharmacol Ther. 2015;148c:34–46.

Lockridge O, Adkins S, La Du BN. Location of disulfide bonds within the sequence of human serum cholinesterase. J Biol Chem. 1987a;262:12945–52.

Lockridge O, Bartels CF, Vaughan TA, Wong CK, Norton SE, Johnson LL. Complete amino acid sequence of human serum cholinesterase. J Biol Chem. 1987b;262:549–57.

Masson P, Legrand P, Bartels CF, Froment M-T, Schopfer LM, Lockridge O. Role of aspartate 70 and tryptophan 82 in binding of succinyldithiocholine to human butyrylcholinesterase. Biochemistry. 1997;36:2266–77.

Masson P, Xie W, Froment M-T, Levitsky V, Fortier P-L, Albaret C, Lockridge O. Interaction between the peripheral site residues of human butyrylcholinesterase, D70 and Y332, in binding and hydrolysis of substrates. Biochim Biophys Acta. 1999;1433:281–93.

Meijler MM, Kaufmann GF, Qi L, Mee JM, Coyle AR, Moss JA, Wirsching P, Matsushita M, Janda KD. Fluorescent cocaine probes: a tool for the selection and engineering of therapeutic antibodies. J Am Chem Soc. 2005;127:2477–84.

Murthy V, Gao Y, Geng L, Lebrasseur N, White T, Brimijoin S. Preclinical studies on neurobehavioral and neuromuscular effects of cocaine hydrolase gene therapy in mice. J Mol Neurosci. 2014a;53:409–16.

Murthy V, Gao Y, Geng L, Lebrasseur NK, White TA, Parks RJ, Brimijoin S. Physiologic and metabolic safety of butyrylcholinesterase gene therapy in mice. Vaccine. 2014b;32:4155–62.

Myers TM, Sun W, Naik RS, Clark MG, Doctor BP, Saxena A. Characterization of human serum butyrylcholinesterase in rhesus monkeys: behavioral and physiological effects. Neurotoxicol Teratol. 2012;34:323–30.

Narasimhan D, Nance MR, Gao D, Ko M-C, Macdonald J, Tamburi P, Yoon D, Landry DM, Woods JH, Zhan C-G, Tesmer JJG, Sunahara RK. Structural analysis of thermostabilizing mutations of cocaine esterase. Protein Eng Des Sel. 2010;23:537–47.

Narasimhan D, Collins GT, Nance MR, Nichols J, Edwald E, Chan J, Ko M-C, Woods JH, Tesmer JJG, Sunahara RK. Subunit stabilization and polyethylene glycolation of cocaine esterase improves in vivo residence time. Mol Pharmacol. 2011;80:1056–65.

Nasser AF, Fudala PJ, Zheng B, Liu Y, Heidbreder C. A randomized, double-blind, placebo-controlled trial of Rbp-8000 in cocaine abusers: pharmacokinetic profile of Rbp-8000 and cocaine and effects of Rbp-8000 on cocaine-induced physiological effects. J Addict Dis. 2014;33:289–302.

Nicolet Y, Lockridge O, Masson P, Fontecilla-Camps JC, Nachon F. Crystal structure of human butyrylcholinesterase and of its complexes with substrate and products. J Biol Chem. 2003; 278:41141–7.

Pan Y, Gao D, Yang W, Cho H, Yang G, Tai H-H, Zhan C-G. Computational redesign of human butyrylcholinesterase for anticocaine medication. Proc Natl Acad Sci U S A. 2005;102:16656–61.

Pan Y, Gao D, Yang W, Cho H, Zhan C-G. Free energy perturbation (FEP) simulation on the transition states of cocaine hydrolysis catalyzed by human butyrylcholinesterase and its mutants. J Am Chem Soc. 2007;129:13537–43.

Pan Y, Gao D, Zhan C-G. Modeling the catalysis of anti-cocaine catalytic antibody: competing reaction pathways and free energy barriers. J Am Chem Soc. 2008;130:5140–9.

Pan Y, Muzyka J, Zhan C-G. Model of human butyrylcholinesterase tetramer by homology modeling and dynamics simulation. J Phys Chem B. 2009;113:6543–52.

Parikh K, Duysen EG, Snow B, Jensen NS, Manne V, Lockridge O, Chilukuri N. Gene-delivered butyrylcholinesterase is prophylactic against the toxicity of chemical warfare nerve agents and organophosphorus compounds. J Pharmacol Exp Therap. 2011;337:92–101.

Pellinen P, Kulmala L, Konttila J, Auriola S, Pasanen M, Juvonen R. Kinetic characterization of norcocaine N-hydroxylation in mouse and human liver microsomes: involvement of CYP enzymes. Arch Toxicol. 2000;74:511–20.

Rosenberg YJ, Saxena A, Sun W, Jiang X, Chilukuri N, Luo C, Doctor BP, Lee KD. Demonstration of in vivo stability and lack of immunogenicity of a polyethyleneglycol-conjugated recombinant CHO-derived butyrylcholinesterase bioscavenger using a homologous macaque model. Chem Biol Interact. 2010;187:279–86.

Saxena A, Ashani Y, Raveh L, Stevenson D, Patel T, Doctor BP. Role of oligosaccharides in the pharmacokinetics of tissue-derived and genetically engineered cholinesterases. Mol Pharmacol. 1998;53:112–22.

Saxena A, Sun W, Luo C, Doctor BP. Human serum butyrylcholinesterase: in vitro and in vivo stability, pharmacokinetics, and safety in mice. Chem Biol Interact. 2005;157–158:199–203.

Saxena A, Sun W, Fedorko JM, Koplovitz I, Doctor BP. Prophylaxis with human serum butyrylcholinesterase protects guinea pigs exposed to multiple lethal doses of soman or VX. Biochem Pharmacol. 2011;81:164–9.

Schindler CW, Goldberg SR. Accelerating cocaine metabolism as an approach to the treatment of cocaine abuse and toxicity. Future Med Chem. 2012;4:163–75.

Schindler CW, Justinova Z, Lafleur D, Woods D, Roschke V, Hallak H, Sklair-Tavron L, Redhi GH, Yasar S, Bergman J, Goldberg SR. Modification of pharmacokinetic and abuse-related effects of cocaine by human-derived cocaine hydrolase in monkeys. Addict Biol. 2013;18:30–9.

Schneider JD, Marillonnet S, Castilho A, Gruber C, Werner S, Mach L, Klimyuk V, Mor TS, Steinkellner H. Oligomerization status influences subcellular deposition and glycosylation of recombinant butyrylcholinesterase in Nicotiana benthamiana. Plant Biotechnol J. 2014;12: 832–9.

Schulte S. Use of albumin fusion technology to prolong the half-life of recombinant factor viia. Thromb Res. 2008;122:S14–9.

Seavey MM, Cerasoli DM, Cadieux CL, Boeri MV, Hodgins SM, Hofstetter CA, Kasten SA, Otto TC, Hallak H, Darvish L, Gross A, Clark S, Singh M, Bock J, Shaw J, Bassan M, Eliaz R, Orbach A. Recombinant human serum albumin fused with human butyrylcholinesterase (TV-1380) as a bioscavenger of organophosphorus nerve agents. Neuroscience. 2014. Presentation Abstract 713.01/Aa12.

Suarez D, Field MJ. Molecular dynamics simulations of human butyrylcholinesterase. Proteins. 2005;59:104–17.

Sun H, El Yazal J, Lockridge O, Schopfer LM, Brimijoin S, Pang Y-P. Predicted michaelis-menten complexes of cocaine-butyrylcholinesterase: engineering effective butyrylcholinesterase mutants for cocaine detoxification. J Biol Chem. 2001;276:9330–6.

Sun H, Pang Y-P, Lockridge O, Brimijoin S. Re-engineering butyrylcholinesterase as a cocaine hydrolase. Mol Pharmacol. 2002a;62:220–4.

Sun H, Shen ML, Pang Y-P, Lockridge O, Brimijoin S. Cocaine metabolism accelerated by a re-engineered human butyrylcholinesterase. J Pharmacol Exp Therap. 2002b;302:710–6.

Tai K, Shen T, Börjesson U, Philippopoulos M, Mccammon JA. Analysis of a 10-ns molecular dynamics simulation of mouse acetylcholinesterase. Biophys J. 2001;81:715–24.

Tai K, Shen T, Henchman RH, Bourne Y, Marchot P, Mccammon JA. Mechanism of acetylcholinesterase inhibition by fasciculin: a 5-ns molecular dynamics simulation. J Am Chem Soc. 2002;124:6153–61.

Tara S, Helms V, Straatsma TP, Mccammon JA. Molecular dynamics of mouse acetylcholinesterase complexed with huperzine A. Biopolymers. 1999a;50:347–59.

Tara S, Straatsma TP, Mccammon JA. Mouse acetylcholinesterase unliganded and in complex with huperzine a: a comparison of molecular dynamics simulations. Biopolymers. 1999b;50: 35–43.

Weber A, Butterweck H, Mais-Paul U, Teschner W, Lei L, Muchitsch EM, Kolarich D, Altmann F, Ehrlich HJ, Schwarz HP. Biochemical, molecular and preclinical characterization of a double-virus-reduced human butyrylcholinesterase preparation designed for clinical use. Vox Sang. 2011;100:285–97.

Wolfenden R, Yuan Y. The "neutral" hydrolysis of simple carboxylic esters in water and the rate enhancements produced by acetylcholinesterase and other carboxylic acid esterases. J Am Chem Soc. 2011;133:13821–3.

Xue L, Ko M-C, Tong M, Yang W, Hou S, Fang L, Liu J, Zheng F, Woods JH, Tai H-H, Zhan C-G. Design, preparation, and characterization of high-activity mutants of human butyrylcholinesterase specific for detoxification of cocaine. Mol Pharmacol. 2011;79:290–7.

Xue L, Hou S, Tong M, Fang L, Chen X, Jin Z, Tai H-H, Zheng F, Zhan C-G. Preparation and in vivo characterization of a cocaine hydrolase engineered from human butyrylcholinesterase for metabolizing cocaine. Biochem J. 2013a;453:447–54.

Xue L, Hou S, Yang W, Fang L, Zheng F, Zhan C-G. Catalytic activities of a cocaine hydrolase engineered from human butyrylcholinesterase against (+)- and (−)-cocaine. Chem Biol Interact. 2013b;203:57–62.

Yang W, Pan Y, Zheng F, Cho H, Tai H-H, Zhan C-G. Free-energy perturbation simulation on transition states and redesign of butyrylcholinesterase. Biophys J. 2009;96:1931–8.

Yang W, Pan Y, Fang L, Gao D, Zheng F, Zhan C-G. Free-energy perturbation simulation on transition states and high-activity mutants of human butyrylcholinesterase for (−)-cocaine hydrolysis. J Phys Chem B. 2010a;114:10889–96.

Yang W, Xue L, Fang L, Chen X, Zhan C-G. Characterization of a high-activity mutant of human butyrylcholinesterase against (−)-cocaine. Chem Biol Interact. 2010b;187:148–52.

Zhan C-G, Gao D. Catalytic mechanism and energy barriers for butyrylcholinesterase-catalyzed hydrolysis of cocaine. Biophys J. 2005;89:3863–72.

Zhan C-G, Zheng F, Landry DW. Fundamental reaction mechanism for cocaine hydrolysis in human butyrylcholinesterase. J Am Chem Soc. 2003;125:2462–74.

Zhan C-G, Deng SX, Skiba JG, Hayes BA, Tschampel SM, Shields GC, Landry DW. First-principle studies of intermolecular and intramolecular catalysis of protonated cocaine. J Comput Chem. 2005;26:980–6.

Zhan M, Hou S, Zhan C-G, Zheng F. Kinetic characterization of high-activity mutants of human butyrylcholinesterase for the cocaine metabolite norcocaine. Biochem J. 2014;457:197–206.

Zhang YK. Improved pseudobonds for combined ab initio quantum mechanical/molecular mechanical methods. J Chem Phys. 2005;122:024114.

Zhang YK. Pseudobond ab initio QM/MM approach and its applications to enzyme reactions. Theor Chem Acc. 2006;116:43–50.

Zhang YK, Liu HY, Yang WT. Free energy calculation on enzyme reactions with an efficient iterative procedure to determine minimum energy paths on a combined ab initio QM/MM potential energy surface. J Chem Phys. 2000;112:3483–92.

Zhang YK, Kua J, Mccammon JA. Role of the catalytic triad and oxyanion hole in acetylcholinesterase catalysis: an ab initio QM/MM study. J Am Chem Soc. 2002;124:10572–7.

Zheng F, Zhan C-G. Are pharmacokinetic approaches feasible for treatment of cocaine addiction and overdose? Future Med Chem. 2012a;4:125–8.

Zheng F, Zhan C-G. Modeling of pharmacokinetics of cocaine in human reveals the feasibility for development of enzyme therapies for drugs of abuse. PLoS Comput Biol. 2012b;8, E1002610.

Zheng F, Yang WC, Ko MC, Liu JJ, Cho H, Gao DQ, Tong M, Tai HH, Woods JH, Zhan C-G. Most efficient cocaine hydrolase designed by virtual screening of transition states. J Am Chem Soc. 2008;130:12148–55.

Zheng F, Yang W, Xue L, Hou S, Liu J, Zhan C-G. Design of high-activity mutants of human butyrylcholinesterase against (−)-cocaine: structural and energetic factors affecting the catalytic efficiency. Biochemistry. 2010;49:9113–9.

Zheng F, Xue L, Hou S, Liu J, Zhan M, Yang W, Zhan C-G. A highly efficient cocaine detoxifying enzyme obtained by computational design. Nat Commun. 2014;5:3457. doi:10.1388/Ncomms4457.

Zlebnik NE, Brimijoin S, Gao Y, Saykao AT, Parks RJ, Carroll ME. Long-term reduction of cocaine self-administration in rats treated with adenoviral vector-delivered cocaine hydrolase: evidence for enzymatic activity. Neuropsychopharmacology. 2014;39:1538–46.

Part IV
Strategies to Optimize the Development of Biologics to Treat Addictions

Chapter 13
Adenovirus-Based Vaccines for the Treatment of Substance Use Disorders

David F. Havlicek, Jonathan B. Rosenberg, Dolan Sondhi, Ronald G. Crystal, and Stephen M. Kaminsky

13.1 Introduction

Addiction to small-molecule drugs including opiates, nicotine, and cocaine is a major, worldwide problem, and few effective therapies exist (Degenhardt et al. 2008; Kinsey et al. 2009; Ross and Peselow 2009). One strategy to reduce the use of addictive drugs utilizes vaccines to stimulate the production of circulating drug-specific antibodies, which bind to the addictive molecules, creating antibody–drug complexes incapable of crossing the blood–brain barrier (Brimijoin et al. 2013; Jupp and Lawrence 2010; Kinsey 2014; Leshner 1996; Orson et al. 2009; Shen et al. 2012; Spector et al. 1973; Yahyavi-Firouz-Abadi and See 2009). Effective vaccination in the context of addictive drug use would prevent the drug from reaching cognate receptors in the central nervous system (CNS), thereby preventing the drug from activating the reinforcing effects of a drug-induced "high" that underlie addiction (Brimijoin et al. 2013; Kinsey 2014; Leshner 1996; Orson et al. 2009; Shen et al. 2012; Spector et al. 1973).

Unlike vaccines to infectious agents that seek to protect individuals from inadvertent exposure, vaccines for substance use disorders must protect against intentional exposure, where the number of target molecules is orders of magnitude larger than that typically seen during involuntary infection. While vaccines utilizing drug analogs conjugated to immunogenic macromolecules such as cholera toxin and tetanus toxoid have been evaluated in clinical trials, none have generated antidrug titers robust enough to abrogate the large number of addictive molecules administered by drug users (Kinsey et al. 2009; Shen et al. 2012; Cornuz et al. 2008; Fahim et al. 2013; Haney et al. 2010; Hatsukami et al. 2011; Kosten et al. 2002, 2014; Martell

D.F. Havlicek • J.B. Rosenberg • D. Sondhi • R.G. Crystal (✉) • S.M. Kaminsky
Department of Genetic Medicine, Weill Medical College of Cornell University, 1300 York Avenue, Box 164, New York, NY 10065, USA
e-mail: geneticmedicine@med.cornell.edu

I.D. Montoya (ed.), *Biologics to Treat Substance Use Disorders: Vaccines, Monoclonal Antibodies, and Enzymes*, DOI 10.1007/978-3-319-23150-1_13

et al. 2005, 2009; Maurer et al. 2005; Orson et al. 2013). The challenge, therefore, is to develop more immunogenic carrier proteins, drug analog haptens with greater specificity, and more potent adjuvants, in hopes that these improved vaccines will evoke potent antidrug immunity with the capacity to achieve widespread efficacy.

Our group has developed a novel platform strategy for the development of immunity to addictive drugs based on the knowledge that adenovirus (Ad) gene transfer vectors act as potent immunogens (Chirmule et al. 1999; De et al. 2013; Harvey et al. 1999; Hicks et al. 2011, 2014; Maoz et al. 2013; Rosenberg et al. 2013; Wee et al. 2012). We hypothesized that a vaccine made by covalently linking the addictive drugs or their analogs to Ad capsid proteins would elicit high-titer antidrug antibodies sufficient to sequester systemically administered drugs in the blood and restrict their access to the brain. To achieve this, we chemically conjugated an addictive drug analog to the capsid proteins of a disrupted, noninfectious, replication-incompetent, E1^{-}E3^{-}, serotype 5 Ad gene transfer vector, which has an extensive safety record in clinical studies, creating adenovirus-based vaccines for the treatment of substance use disorders.

13.2 Adenovirus-Based Therapeutics

The adenovirus, first isolated from the human adenoids in 1953, is an 80 to 100 nm non-enveloped, icosahedral double-stranded DNA virus that commonly causes respiratory tract infections (Ginsberg 1984). Since the discovery of adenovirus, its full viral genome has been sequenced, over 50 serotypes have been identified, and the biology of viral replication and assembly has been well characterized (Ginsberg 1984; Hackett and Crystal 2008; Russell 2009; Wilson 1996). By the early 1990s a foundational understanding of adenovirus biology presented the opportunity to engineer recombinant adenovirus particles to deliver therapeutic genetic sequences to somatic cells. It is this attained knowledge that enabled the use of an adenovirus as the first effective in vivo gene delivery vector in 1991 (Crystal et al. 1994; Rosenfeld et al. 1992; Zabner et al. 1993; Zuckerman et al. 1999; Crystal 2014). Since that time, the field of gene therapy has grown considerably, adenovirus-based gene therapy vectors have been used safely and effectively in clinical trials, and increasingly more has been revealed about adenovirus biology.

Most current adenovirus-based treatments are genetic therapies, which employ the adenovirus to deliver therapeutic genetic sequences to target organs. Classic adenovirus-based gene therapies have sought to treat individuals by delivering a functional gene to those with disease caused inherently by the mutation or absence of that gene. These therapies typically use the common human adenovirus serotype 5 deleted in the E1 genes (the adenovirus genes that control replication of the virus) and the E3 genes (genes protecting the virus from the host immune system). The first example was adenovirus-based gene therapy for the pulmonary manifestations of cystic fibrosis, where an E1^{-}E3^{-} adenovirus gene transfer vector was used to transfer the human cystic fibrosis transmembrane conductance regulator (CFTR) coding sequences to the airway epithelium of individuals with cystic fibrosis (Wilson 1996;

Crystal et al. 1994; Zabner et al. 1993; Zuckerman et al. 1999). While successful in transferring the CFTR coding sequences (Wilson 1996; Crystal et al. 1994; Zabner et al. 1993; Zuckerman et al. 1999), the expression of the normal CFTR gene was short-lived because the host immune system recognized the adenovirus as foreign and mounted a response that suppressed expression directed by the transferred CFTR expression cassette (Chirmule et al. 1999; Harvey et al. 1999; Hackett and Crystal 2008; Hackett et al. 2000; Hartman et al. 2008; Jooss and Chirmule 2003; Nemerow 2009; Shayakhmetov 2010; Thaci et al. 2011; Worgall et al. 1997; Yang et al. 1994, 1996; Zaiss et al. 2009). This and many experimental animal and human studies with adenovirus gene transfer vectors led to the conclusion that the adenovirus capsid proteins are highly immunogenic, and thus, adenovirus vector-mediated gene transfer is limited to applications where the duration of expression of the gene is about 2–3 weeks (Crystal 2014; Jooss and Chirmule 2003). Taking advantage of this short duration of expression, examples of the successful use of adenovirus as a gene transfer vector include expressing genes that build new biologic structures (e.g., angiogenesis) or evoke destruction of cells (e.g., cancer therapy) (Aguilar et al. 2011; Aurisicchio and Ciliberto 2012; Crystal et al. 2012; Deisseroth et al. 2013; Duarte et al. 2012; Fukazawa et al. 2010; Mack et al. 1998; Matthews et al. 2009; Patel et al. 1999; Rosengart et al. 1999a, b; Tagawa et al. 2008; Wu et al. 2005).

13.3 Adenovirus as a Basis for Vaccines

While the highly immunogenic properties of the adenovirus capsid are a disadvantage for gene therapy applications requiring long-term gene expression, its immunogenic properties are an advantage for the development of vaccines. The first example of this was a development by the US military in the 1960s, a vaccine against adenovirus using an oral formulation of live serotypes 4 and 7 to evoke immunity against acute febrile respiratory tract illness (Hoke and Snyder 2013). We, and others, expanded this concept by using $E1^{-}E3^{-}$ adenovirus to express protein antigens that would evoke immunity against infectious agents or cancer (Barouch and Picker 2014; Boyer et al. 2005; Chiuchiolo et al. 2006; Hashimoto et al. 2005; Krause and Worgall 2011; Rein et al. 2006; Song et al. 1997; Tan et al. 2003). Another strategy, used to evoke immunity against cancer, is to use adenovirus vectors designed to replicate only in cancer cells, both destroying the target cells and evoking immunity against the neoplasm (Choi et al. 2012; Short and Curiel 2009; Zeyaullah et al. 2012).

Based on the highly immunogenic properties of the adenovirus capsid, we hypothesized that if we could covalently link an addictive molecule (or analogs of addictive molecules) to the adenovirus capsid, it might be possible to evoke high titers of antibodies against the addictive molecule, by tricking the immune system to see the addictive molecule as a component of the adenovirus capsid (De et al. 2013; Hicks et al. 2011, 2014; Maoz et al. 2013; Rosenberg et al. 2013; Wee et al. 2012). If correct, these antibodies would bind to the addictive molecule entering the circulation, restricting access of the addictive molecule to the central nervous system (CNS).

13.4 Hapten-Carrier Addictive Molecule Vaccines

The idea of conjugating an addictive molecule to an immunogenic protein was first developed over 40 years ago. In 1972, a vaccine was developed based on a morphine hapten conjugated to bovine serum albumin (BSA). This vaccine evoked anti-morphine antibodies which reduced the amount of free morphine in the serum of rats following drug administration (Berkowitz and Spector 1972). Two years later the principle was applied to a similar vaccine which decreased heroin self-administration behavior in non-human primates (Bonese et al. 1974). Since that time, several other opiate vaccines have been developed using this same concept. These include a morphine–tetanus toxoid vaccine that demonstrated the capacity to reduce the acquisition of heroin self-administration in rats (Anton and Leff 2006); a heroin-like hapten conjugated to keyhole limpet hemocyanin (KLH), which prevented heroin self-administration and the analgesic effects of heroin in rodents (Stowe et al. 2011); and a morphine hapten conjugated to KLH that significantly inhibited morphine-induced pain relief and the reinforcing effects of the drug as measured by conditioned place preference studies (Shen et al. 2012). Hapten-based vaccines to addictive molecules have also been developed for the treatment of methamphetamine addiction with hapten analogs conjugated to KLH, BSA, or the outer membrane protein complex of *Neisseria meningitidis* group B (Shen et al. 2012, 2013; Byrnes-Blake et al. 2001). All of these strategies generate anti-methamphetamine antibody titers sufficient to inhibit methamphetamine-induced locomotor activity in vaccinated animals.

Several addictive molecule hapten-carrier vaccines for cocaine addiction have been developed with carriers including BSA, KLH, and cholera toxin B (Carrera et al. 1995; Fox et al. 1996; Fox 1997; Kantak et al. 2000). One TA-CD, a cocaine hapten conjugated to the cholera toxin B subunit, has progressed to clinical trials (Haney et al. 2010; Kosten et al. 2002, 2014; Martell et al. 2005, 2009; Orson et al. 2013). This vaccine stimulates anti-cocaine immunity and blocks the addictive effects of cocaine in animal models (Kantak et al. 2000, 2001). In humans, the vaccine had few side effects (Kosten et al. 2002, 2014; Martell et al. 2005). In a phase IIb clinical trial, the subset of subjects with anti-cocaine antibody titers >43 μg/ml showed significant reductions in cocaine use, demonstrating the potential for anti-cocaine vaccines as a therapy for cocaine addiction (Martell et al. 2009). However, only 38 % of vaccinated subjects produced anti-cocaine antibody titers >43 μg/ml and those who did not showed no significant reduction in cocaine use when compared with placebo controls (Martell et al. 2009). While phase III clinical trials revealed anti-cocaine antibody titers >43 μg/ml in two-thirds of vaccinated patients and demonstrated some trends for efficacy, there was no statistically significant attenuation of cocaine use (Kosten et al. 2014). The disappointing results may reflect the lack of potency (insufficient anti-cocaine antibody titers), efforts by the trial participants to overwhelm the anti-cocaine immune response through higher cocaine doses, and/or a clinical trial design that tested the vaccine in a population with too many confounding factors (Kosten et al. 2014).

Hapten-carrier vaccines to treat nicotine addiction have also been tested in clinical trials (Shen et al. 2012; Fahim et al. 2013): Nic002 (Cornuz et al. 2008; Maurer et al. 2005); NicVax (Hatsukami et al. 2005, 2011; Wagena et al. 2008); SCL-0068 (Pittet et al. 2012); Niccine (de Villiers et al. 2002, 2010; Lindblom et al. 2002); TA-NIC (St.Clair Roberts J et al. 2003). A phase II clinical trial evaluated the virus-like particle-based vaccine, Nic002, consisting of a nicotine analog linked to the coat protein from the bacteriophage Qβ demonstrated higher rates of nicotine abstinence in patients with the highest anti-nicotine antibody titers (Cornuz et al. 2008). However, the drug produced frequent side effects consisting of flu-like symptoms, and subjects with lower anti-nicotine titers showed nicotine use similar to that of subjects receiving a placebo (Cornuz et al. 2008). While another phase II trial with a reformulation of Nic002 showed fewer side effects, insufficient anti-nicotine antibody titers limited the success of the vaccine (Shen et al. 2012; Cytos Biotechnology ZS 2006).

Another strategy was to link a nicotine analog to the *Pseudomonas aeruginosa* recombinant exoprotein (Hatsukami et al. 2005). This vaccine (NicVax) did not reduce smoking in subjects with low titers, but demonstrated significantly higher rates of abstinence among individuals with the highest anti-nicotine titers (Hatsukami et al. 2011). However, phase III clinical trials with NicVax did not demonstrate efficacy, presumably because the drug failed to provoke sufficient immunity (Fahim et al. 2013; Nabi.com. 2011; Nicotine Conjugate Vaccine 2015). Other hapten-carrier anti-nicotine vaccines have been evaluated in clinical trials, including SCL-068, based on nanoparticle technology; Niccine, which employs a tetanus toxoid carrier; and TA-NIC, which uses a recombinant cholera toxin carrier, but clinical results with these vaccines have not yet been reported (Fahim et al. 2013).

In summary, active vaccines have been shown to stimulate immunity against an array of addictive molecules and have demonstrated a capacity to reduce substance use in animal models and in humans that respond with the highest titer antidrug immunity. If successful, an advantage of vaccines for addiction is the reduced reliance on patient compliance due to the reduced number and frequency of required interventions compared to traditional pharmaceutical-based therapy. However, most of these vaccine strategies have been limited by a failure to achieve a breadth of coverage with a sufficient level of immunity to meet expectations of efficacy. In this context, the effort to improve antidrug vaccines has focused on improving hapten design, adjuvants, and carrier molecules.

13.5 Adenovirus-Based Therapies for Substance Use Disorders

Vaccines for substance use have been designed to present the addictive molecule (or an analog) in the context of potent immunogenic carrier proteins. Given that the limits of efficacy have been tied to a lack of adequate immunopotency, the identification of the most immunogenic carrier is paramount to the success of this therapeutic strategy. While carriers such as BSA, KLH, tetanus toxoid, *Pseudomonas*, and cholera toxins have been shown to elicit antidrug immunity in animal models, none have been able to evoke immunity that ensures widespread efficacy in the clinic. Based on our experience with adenovirus as a vector for gene therapy in vivo, we hypothesized that an adenovirus-based carrier, which employs the capsid proteins of adenovirus known to be highly immunogenic in humans, would be an effective immunogenic carrier for addictive molecule haptens (Hicks et al. 2011).

Our first design of an adenovirus-based vaccine against an addictive drug utilized chemical conjugation of the cocaine analog GNC [6-(2R,3S)-3-(benzoyloxy)-8-methyl-8-azabicyclo [3.2.1] octane-2-carbonyloxy-hexanoic acid] to the capsid proteins of a replication-incompetent $E1^{-}E3^{-}$ serotype 5 adenovirus (Hicks et al. 2011). Early studies with this approach demonstrated high-titer (~10^5) anti-cocaine antibodies. However, we quickly realized that if the adenovirus capsid was disrupted prior to conjugation to GNC, the result was a vaccine with superior potency (titers $>5\times10^5$). This disrupted adenovirus, dAd5GNC, demonstrated the potential of a therapeutic vaccine for substance use disorders by blocking administered cocaine from reaching the CNS of vaccinated mice and suppressing cocaine-induced hyperactivity (Hicks et al. 2011). A greater immune response was next obtained with an improved design for the cocaine analog GNE [6-(2R,3S)-3-(benzoyloxy)-8-methyl-8-azabicyclo [3.2.1] octane-2-carboxoamido-hexanoic acid] (Fig. 13.1). dAd5GNE has been evaluated for efficacy in numerous preclinical studies, formal safety and toxicology studies are complete, and human studies will be initiated shortly (De et al. 2013; Hicks et al. 2014; Maoz et al. 2013; Wee et al. 2012).

13.6 dAd5GNE Design

The adenovirus-based vaccine platform was derived from the concept that the carrier protein provides the signaling to the immune system to overcome the lack of response to the small addictive molecules. Of the many serotypes of adenovirus, serotype 5 (Ad5) has the best-characterized immune profile as a gene therapy vector and an excellent safety record in the clinic (Crystal et al. 2002; Harvey et al. 2002). Rather than using a wild-type Ad5, the E1 genes of the vector genome were removed, creating a replication-incompetent starting material, minimizing potential safety concerns associated with residual vector DNA (Wold et al. 1999). Although the intact adenovirus evokes potent humoral immunity, there are several additional advantages of disrupting the $E1^{-}E3^{-}$ adenovirus. First, the disrupted capsid vaccine circumvents the minor risk associated with infectious adenovirus vectors, which already have a well-documented and clinically acceptable safety profile (Crystal et al. 2002; Harvey et al. 2002). Second, the disrupted proteins of the adenovirus circumvent preexisting anti-adenovirus immunity (De et al. 2013). Third, the disrupted capsid likely exposes additional sites for the conjugation of GNE haptens,

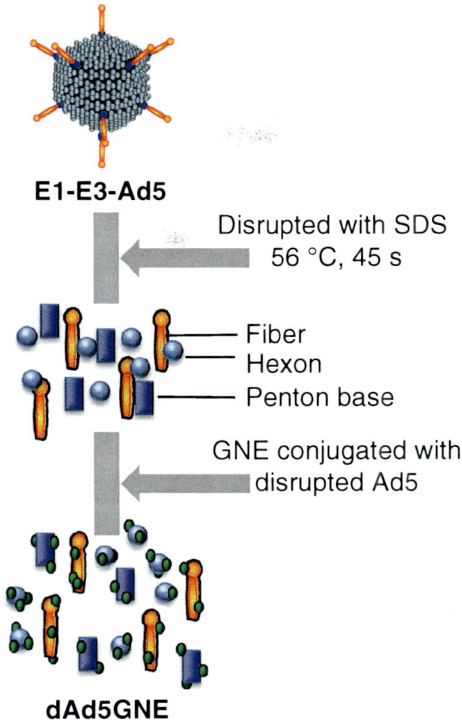

Fig. 13.1 The production of the disrupted adenovirus vaccine dAd5GNE. Recombinant, $E1^{-}E3^{-}$ replication-incompetent adenovirus serotype 5 is disrupted by detergent and heat, and the disassociated capsid proteins (fiber, hexon, and penton base) are chemically coupled to the cocaine analog GNE

increasing the effective dose of the antigen. Finally, the inclusion of the beta-galactosidase transgene in the vector's expression cassette provides a sensitive assay used for in-process quality control and detection of residual infectious Ad5 after the disruption process.

Hapten design is very important for small-molecule-targeted vaccines. The first-generation cocaine hapten, GNC, was designed based on the need for it to be relatively easy to manufacture, safe to administer, and linkable to the carrier protein without disruption of the cocaine-like antigenic character (Hicks et al. 2011; Carrera et al. 1995). While GNC demonstrated efficacy, a new hapten, GNE, provided greater chemical stability and thus more sustained presentation to the host immune system. The carboxyl groups on the cocaine analogs GNE and GNC are activated with 1-ethyl-3-[3-dimethylaminopropyl] carbodiimide and N-hydroxysulfosuccinimide for coupling to the primary amines of lysines on the adenovirus capsid, forming the covalently linked protein–hapten conjugates that serve as the key components of the vaccine. Optimization of several parameters was required to maximize the density of haptens. For example, the conjugation ratios of hapten to capsid protein differed for each hapten. The hapten GNC/carrier ratio of 100:1 was sufficient to saturate the binding to adenovirus capsid proteins, whereas for GNE that ratio was 300:1. A formulation had to be defined that provided stability to the dAd5GNE, was compatible with the adjuvant, and would not impact the safety profile, particularly at the site of injection. Lastly, the purification and formulation must remove conjugation residuals to avoid adverse effects on potency and safety. The formulation buffer for dAd5GNE enabled stable −80 °C storage for at least 1 year. Head-to-head comparison of several adjuvants with dAd5GNE demonstrated that Adjuplex® (Advanced BioAdjuvants LLC, Omaha NE) provided the greatest immunostimulatory boost, providing the optimal balance of potency and risk analysis for adjuvant components and potential safety concerns.

13.7 dAd5GNE-Evoked Immune Response

Studies with dAd5GNC in mice demonstrated classic vaccine immunity with early response anti-cocaine IgM antibody levels that dropped below the limit of detection by week 5, inversely related to rising anti-cocaine IgG titers (Hicks et al. 2011). An evaluation of IgG subtypes demonstrated that IgG1 levels were highest, followed by IgG2a and IgG2b. Additionally, the polyclonal response had similar avidities for cocaine and for the conjugated cocaine analog, suggesting excellent hapten/cocaine characteristics (Hicks et al. 2011). Although the most desired immunoglobulin isotype in mice is not clear, it is important to note that IgG1 is not the most potent of the immunoglobulin isotypes to activate complement, a process not needed for a response to addictive drugs (Schroeder and Cavacini 2010).

Subsequent experiments with dAd5GNE confirmed the capacity of the vaccine to stimulate robust anti-cocaine IgG immunity in mice, rats, and non-human primates (De et al. 2013; Hicks et al. 2014; Maoz et al. 2013; Wee et al. 2012). Evaluation of the serum from dAd5GNE-vaccinated non-human primates revealed antibodies with high specificity not only for cocaine but also for the active cocaine metabolite cocaethylene and lower, but measureable, specificity for the active cocaine metabolite norcocaine (Hicks et al. 2014). Further, reduced affinity for the non-active metabolites benzoylecgonine and ethyl methyl ester suggests that the anti-cocaine immunity to the hapten recognized the essence of the cocaine molecule that embodies the functional action of the drug.

Many studies evaluating vaccines for the treatment of substance use disorders have demonstrated that vaccines with the highest antibody titers tend to demonstrate some measure of efficacy (Cornuz et al. 2008; Haney et al. 2010; Hatsukami et al. 2011; Martell et al. 2009). Similarly in preclinical studies, dAd5GNE mediated CNS protection following cocaine administration in non-human primates with anti-cocaine antibody titers $>4\times10^5$, whereas animals with anti-cocaine antibody titers $<4\times10^5$ had only mildly reduced cocaine levels in the brain. Cocaine administration at the weight-adjusted typical human dose showed significant reduction in cocaine binding at the site of the dopamine transporter in high-titer non-human primates relative to non-immunized animals and animals with titers $<4\times10^5$ (Maoz et al. 2013). Similarly, a study in mice demonstrated that following cocaine challenge, there was no significant reduction of cocaine levels in the brain when anti-cocaine antibody titers were $<5\times10^5$. However, when anti-cocaine antibody titers were $>5\times10^5$, cocaine levels in the brain were reduced significantly.

Vaccination regimen and dAd5GNE dose were evaluated with the goal of achieving the high, persistent anti-cocaine antibody titers required for efficacy. Long-term sustained titers are necessary for the vaccine to provide coverage in the context of unpredictable instances of addictive drug use. Dose escalation results from mice, rats, and non-human primates were neither consistent nor predictable by body weight or surface area, and therefore, the definitive extrapolation to humans will require clinical study. However, the evaluation of anti-cocaine antibody titers over time in two studies of vaccinated non-human primates demonstrated that the anti-cocaine antibody titer half-life was approximately 4 weeks. Consistent with this, monthly vaccinations of non-human primates yielded sustained, high anti-cocaine antibody titers, which remained stable for 6 months, the duration of the study, suggesting that the optimal dosing regimen for humans will be monthly.

13.8 dAd5GNE Efficacy in the Context of Preexisting Anti-adenovirus Immunity

The translation of a vaccine to widespread use requires that it is broadly effective in the target population. Vaccines against infectious agents have different criteria for success that include sufficient coverage to provide herd protection, limiting propagation of the target through a population. While this is not an important characteristic for a therapeutic vaccine for drug use, there is a shared need for efficacy in the context of a target population with preexisting immunity to the vaccine vector, as vaccines based on adenovirus have suffered from widespread seroprevalence in human populations (D'Ambrosio et al. 1982; Mast et al. 2010; Nwanegbo et al. 2004; Piedra et al. 1998). The possibility that preexisting anti-adenovirus immunity may limit the potency of dAd5GNE is therefore an important concern to address. However, in mice treated to evoke potent neutralizing anti-adenovirus immunity, subsequent vaccination with dAd5 did not significantly affect total or isotype-specific anti-cocaine antibody levels and did not affect the vaccine-mediated abrogation of cocaine access to the CNS (De et al. 2013).

13.9 dAd5GNE-Induced CNS Protection and Redistribution of Cocaine

Evaluation of the capacity of dAd5GNE to evoke high-titer anti-cocaine antibodies is necessary, but not sufficient for an efficacious and safe anti-cocaine vaccine. Assessment of the vaccine must include an evaluation of vaccine function in the context of cocaine use. As such, the distribution of a sequestered bolus of the drug throughout the body was evaluated, with assessment of local toxicity to organs that can be adversely affected by cocaine, such as the heart (Benowitz 1993; Brody et al. 1990; Derlet and Albertson 1989; Hollander et al. 1995; Kloss et al. 1984; Lange and Hillis 2001; Lipton et al. 2000; Muscholl 1961; Restrepo et al. 2007; Rump et al. 1995; Silva et al. 1991).

The biodistribution of ^{3}H-cocaine was evaluated in naive and dAd5GNE-vaccinated rodents. In both mice and rats, dAd5GNE vaccination significantly increased the amount of ^{3}H-cocaine maintained in the serum of vaccinated animals, most of which was IgG bound (De et al. 2013; Wee et al. 2012). Vaccination significantly reduced cocaine access to the brain in mice by 63 % ($p<0.003$) and in rats by 61 % ($p<0.009$) (De et al. 2013; Wee et al. 2012). Positron emission tomography (PET) was used to evaluate access of administered cocaine to the brains of naive and dAd5GNE-vaccinated non-human primates (Maoz et al. 2013). A high-affinity, dopamine transporter (DAT)-specific ligand ^{11}C-PE2I was displaced by cocaine and the loss of the PET signal correlated with cocaine access. When naive animals were challenged with cocaine, there was a 62 % loss of ^{11}C-PE2I-labeled DAT in the caudate and putamen, a level significantly greater than the 47 % threshold needed to evoke a subjective "high" in humans (Maoz et al. 2013; Volkow et al. 1997). In contrast, dAd5GNE-vaccinated animals showed less than 20 % cocaine-occupied DAT when anti-cocaine titers were $>4\times10^5$.

Systemic distribution of administered cocaine and cocaine metabolites was assessed in vaccinated and naive non-human primates. As expected, dAd5GNE vaccination significantly reduced cocaine and cocaine metabolite levels in the brain, but despite increased levels in the serum, levels of cocaine and cocaine metabolites were reduced in peripheral organs (adrenal gland, spleen, lung, heart, kidney, and liver), suggesting that antibody-bound cocaine restricts access to, or deposition in, the viscera (Hicks et al. 2014). As such, dAd5GNE vaccination may prevent some of the systemic toxicities associated with cocaine overdose, including arrhythmia and cardiovascular collapse (Derlet and Albertson 1989; Lange and Hillis 2001; Lipton et al. 2000).

13.10 dAd5GNE-Induced Suppression of Cocaine-Induced Behavior

When a weight-adjusted typical human dose of cocaine (1 mg/kg) was delivered intravenously to naive mice, there was a marked increase in the locomotor activity. In dAd5GNC- and dAd5GNE-vaccinated mice, this increase was abrogated (Hicks et al. 2011) (see Fig. 13.2 for an example). The relative distribution of movement behaviors, including ambulation, stereotypy, vertical, and resting time, in vaccinated animals challenged with cocaine showed no significant difference relative to PBS-challenged controls. Behavior studies of dAd5GNE-vaccinated rats challenged intraperitoneally with 15 mg/kg cocaine demonstrated significant vaccine-mediated reduction of cocaine-induced locomotor activity (Wee et al. 2012). Cocaine-challenged naive rats traveled farther and spent more time exhibiting a vertical rearing behavior than vaccinated rats, which were similar to naive PBS-treated controls.

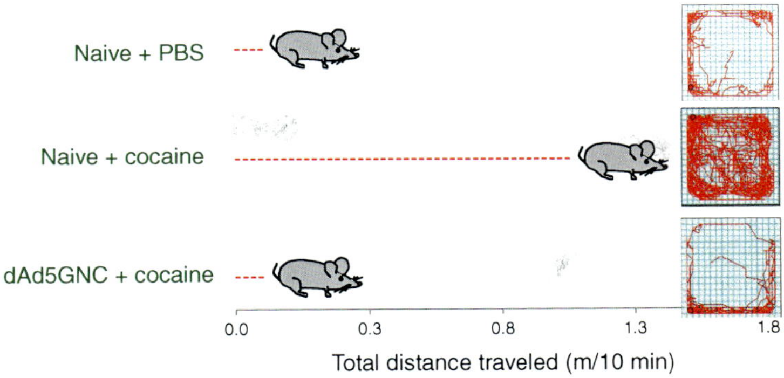

Fig. 13.2 dAd5GNE-mediated abrogation of cocaine-mediated hyper-locomotor activity. Naive or vaccinated mice were administered with cocaine, and the distance traveled over 10 min was measured in a rodent ambulatory behavior box. As a control, naive mice were treated with PBS (no cocaine). The cocaine-treated vaccinated mice were indistinguishable from the PBS controls and significantly different from the cocaine-treated naive mice. Shown at *left* is the total distance traveled for each group and at *right* the tracing of the mouse movement in the behavior box

13.11 dAd5GNE Protection in Binge Drug Use

An issue for the use of therapeutic vaccines to treat addictive drugs is the concern that the use of multiple administrations of the addictive drug or an increase in the dose will be used to overwhelm the antibody-mediated protection and leave vaccinated individuals vulnerable to binge drug use and its associated adverse effects (Orson et al. 2009; Kosten et al. 2002; Martell et al. 2009). In studies that address these concerns, dAd5GNE-vaccinated mice and NHPs retained high anti-cocaine titers 15 min following cocaine administration. Similarly, dAd5GNE-vaccinated non-human primates that received cocaine on a daily basis were compared with cocaine-naive NHPs, and the two groups exhibited no significant differences in anti-cocaine antibody titer half-life, suggesting that continuous cocaine use will not lead to antibody exhaustion and that vaccination likely remains protective soon after cocaine use. Notably, dAd5GNE protected the brain of vaccinated mice equally well whether cocaine was administered on a weekly or daily basis, and while naive mice exhibited marked hyperactivity following a daily and bihourly cocaine "binge," vaccinated mice did not (Havlicek et al. 2014). Cocaine dose escalation produced increasing levels of hyperactivity in naive mice, but did not significantly affect the activity of vaccinated mice. Finally, vaccinated mice receiving high intravenous doses of cocaine had fewer cocaine-induced seizures, suggesting that vaccination not only prevents the behavior associated with high-dose cocaine use but also reduces the toxicity of high-dose use.

13.12 dAd5GNE-Induced Reductions in Cocaine Self-Administration

The ultimate goal of an anti-cocaine vaccine is to decrease motivation to self-administer cocaine; if vaccination removes the reward of drug use, it is expected that the reinforcing effects of addiction will fall off as well. While successful achievement of these end points will require evaluation in clinical trials, preclinical experiments with dAd5GNE suggest that vaccination can reduce cocaine self-administration in rodents and non-human primates. In rats trained to self-administer cocaine, vaccination did not reduce the frequency of 0.5 mg/kg intravenous cocaine self-administration, but when the effort to access cocaine was elevated, vaccinated animals self-administered less frequently than naive animals (Wee et al. 2012). Importantly, when access to cocaine was suspended, naive rats primed with cocaine resumed self-administration whereas the vaccinated rats did not, suggesting that dAd5GNE vaccination significantly reduced the reinforcing effects of cocaine use and may be effective at preventing recidivism.

Studies with dAd5GNE-vaccinated and non-vaccinated control non-human primates that were trained to self-administer cocaine and candy and become "addicted" were deprived of access to the cocaine with the candy alternative remaining (Evans et al. 2012). Subsequent reinstatement of cocaine was followed by a relatively fast return to self-administration in the control monkeys but not in those that were dAd5GNE vaccinated. Most of the vaccinated monkeys resisted the option of cocaine, even in the contexts of removal of the candy alternative, reduced work required for cocaine access, or administration of a cocaine prime. These three manipulations were required for reinstatement, and the time until reinstatement correlated with anti-cocaine antibody titer. Taken together, this evidence suggests that dAd5GNE vaccination may be effective for recovering cocaine addicts.

13.13 Safety of dAd5GNE

Prior to translation to the clinic, formal safety and toxicology studies are required for any drug product. During the preclinical efficacy studies, it was established that the vaccine-mediated redistribution of cocaine served to protect peripheral organs from the drug. Additionally, concerns that the vaccine may drive "binge" use were addressed by the protection of mice from seizures induced by very high doses of cocaine. These important findings complement our formal IND-enabling toxicology studies in mice and non-human primates.

A dose-ranging, placebo-controlled, murine study evaluated potential vaccine-mediated changes in serum chemistry, hematology, organ weight, gross pathology, histopathology, and general health over the course of six months. Aside from minor localized inflammation in mice, which was associated with repeated administrations of the adjuvant at the local site of injection, no adverse effects related to the intramuscular administration of dAd5GNE were observed. This local inflammation was due to the required large dose of adjuvant, which did not scale with body weight as did the active ingredient dAd5GNE. In contrast to the mice, a dose-ranging, placebo-controlled, toxicology study in non-human primates evaluating similar parameters over the course of six months showed no toxicity, including no local toxicity at the site of vaccine administration. Finally, these animals were challenged with cocaine on each of the 3 days leading up to sacrifice as a model to evaluate vaccine safety in the context of cocaine use.

13.14 Adenovirus-Based Anti-nicotine Vaccine HexonAM1

In light of efficacy demonstrated with the adenovirus-based anti-cocaine vaccine dAd5GNE, we have developed adenovirus-based vaccines against other highly addictive molecules. With the goal of improved efficacy with an easily characterized product, a single component of the adenovirus capsid, hexon, was chosen as the immunogen for its established high immunopotency. Thus, the nicotine vaccine HexonAM1 was developed as a potential immunotherapy for smoking cessation. Similar in design to the cocaine vaccine dAd5GNE, HexonAM1 uses conjugation of a non-immunogenic nicotine analog (AM1) to hexon to evoke an anti-nicotine immune response, sufficient to abrogate systemically administered nicotine. As with the anti-cocaine vaccine, the strategy is to block the transfer of nicotine across the blood–brain barrier to the CNS nicotinic acetylcholine receptors (nAChR). This immunotherapy, with many parallel concepts to the dAd5GNE cocaine vaccine, targets the nicotine molecule in order to block reward to drug cravings.

Similar to cocaine, nicotine is a small addictive molecule that evades immune surveillance and must be coupled to larger immunogenic proteins to evoke an immune response (Cerny and Cerny 2009; Moreno et al. 2010). Since conjugating the nicotine molecule to proteins requires the addition of reactive free carboxyl groups, nicotine analogs have been developed to mimic the chemical characteristics of nicotine while providing a handle for chemical conjugation (Moreno et al. 2010; Carrera et al. 2004; Isomura et al. 2001; Meijler et al. 2003). In studies comparing a series of these analogs (Nic, CNI, and AM1), we found that only AM1 produced a high-titer relevant response in mice, and thus, this hapten was used for all further studies.

Our first-generation adenovirus-based nicotine vaccine dAd5AM1 utilized the same immunogenic disrupted adenovirus (dAd5) platform as dAd5GNE (De et al. 2013). Studies with dAd5AM1 demonstrated that the vaccine produced high anti-nicotine titers in mice within 4 weeks (De et al. 2013). Further, anti-nicotine titers remained high throughout the course of the study and were not hindered by preexisting adenovirus immunity (De et al. 2013). However, the potency was not sufficient to protect rodents from high levels of nicotine, leading our laboratory to explore the individual adenoviral capsid proteins hexon, penton, and fiber as potential immunogenic carriers (Rosenberg et al. 2013). Prior studies have evaluated these adenoviral capsid components and have found that the hexon proteins elicit the highest anti-Ad antibody titers in mice and humans (Molinier-Frenkel et al. 2002). To apply this potency to the nicotine analog, purified hexon protein was conjugated to AM1 with the same reagents used for dAd5GNE production.

Studies in mice showed that HexonAM1 triggered persistently higher anti-nicotine titers than dAd5AM1 (~1.0×10^6). As an initial measure of efficacy, the capacity of HexonAM1-evoked anti-nicotine antibodies to rapidly bind nicotine and block access to the CNS was evaluated (Rosenberg et al. 2013). Vaccinated and non-vaccinated mice were challenged with radioactive ^{3}H-nicotine and sacrificed 1 min later to evaluate the partition of nicotine in the blood (IgG bound and free) and CNS. Nicotine levels in the brain of HexonAM1-vaccinated mice were 53 % lower than naive control mice, generating a 3.4-fold reduction in the brain to blood nicotine ratio. In the serum 83 % of the nicotine was IgG bound, indicating that this was an immune-mediated effect.

The mice required preconditioning (sensitization) with nicotine before typical weight-adjusted human doses of nicotine produced changes in locomotor activity (Rosenberg et al. 2013). HexonAM1-vaccinated and control, non-vaccinated, sensitized mice were challenged daily with subcutaneously administered nicotine (0.5 mg/kg) and assessed for ambulatory activity. While control mice displayed typical nicotine-induced hypo-locomotion during each nicotine challenge, the behavior of HexonAM1-vaccinated mice was indistinguishable from control mice challenged with PBS. Repeat assessment over 5 weeks demonstrated that HexonAM1-mediated immunity abrogated nearly all nicotine-induced hypo-locomotor activity, i.e., the HexonAM1-mediated blockade of nicotine was sufficient to prevent nicotine-induced behavior in mice.

13.15 The Potential of Adenovirus-Based Vaccines

The adenovirus capsid protein-based vaccines to cocaine and nicotine hold promise as therapeutics for the treatment of these substance use disorders. Designed to leverage the potent immunity of the adenovirus capsid and redirect it to the conjugated small drug analogs, these vaccines blocked administered drugs from reaching their CNS receptors and abrogated drug-induced physiological responses. For the disrupted capsid platform applied to the cocaine target, formal safety and toxicology studies led to the conclusion of an excellent safety profile, and therefore, the vaccine platform is ready to be evaluated in clinical trials. Careful consideration of clinical trial design includes specifying the target population, the dosing regimen, safety and efficacy phenotypes, and a reasonable prospective definition of successful end points.

Targeting cocaine offers the risk/benefit advantage of having no competing, currently approved pharmacological therapy, and therefore, there is motivation to meet a clear-cut societal need. Clinical success of an adenovirus-based vaccine against cocaine will justify rapid application to other addictive substances such as nicotine, opiates, and methamphetamine.

References

Aguilar LK, Guzik BW, Aguilar-Cordova E. Cytotoxic immunotherapy strategies for cancer: mechanisms and clinical development. J Cell Biochem. 2011;112:1969–77.

Anton B, Leff P. A novel bivalent morphine/heroin vaccine that prevents relapse to heroin addiction in rodents. Vaccine. 2006;24:3232–40.

Aurisicchio L, Ciliberto G. Genetic cancer vaccines: current status and perspectives. Expert Opin Biol Ther. 2012;12:1043–58.

Barouch DH, Picker LJ. Novel vaccine vectors for HIV-1. Nat Rev Microbiol. 2014;12:765–71.

Benowitz NL. Clinical pharmacology and toxicology of cocaine. Pharmacol Toxicol. 1993;72:3–12.

Berkowitz B, Spector S. Evidence for active immunity to morphine in mice. Science. 1972;178:1290–2.

Bonese KF, Wainer BH, Fitch FW, Rothberg RM, Schuster CR. Changes in heroin self-administration by a rhesus monkey after morphine immunisation. Nature. 1974;252:708–10.

Boyer JL, Kobinger G, Wilson JM, Crystal RG. Adenovirus-based genetic vaccines for biodefense. Hum Gene Ther. 2005;16:157–68.

Brimijoin S, Shen X, Orson F, Kosten T. Prospects, promise and problems on the road to effective vaccines and related therapies for substance abuse. Expert Rev Vaccines. 2013;12:323–32.

Brody SL, Slovis CM, Wrenn KD. Cocaine-related medical problems: consecutive series of 233 patients. Am J Med. 1990;88:325–31.

Byrnes-Blake KA, Carroll FI, Abraham P, Owens SM. Generation of anti-(+)methamphetamine antibodies is not impeded by (+)methamphetamine administration during active immunization of rats. Int Immunopharmacol. 2001;1:329–38.

Carrera MR, Ashley JA, Parsons LH, Wirsching P, Koob GF, Janda KD. Suppression of psychoactive effects of cocaine by active immunization. Nature. 1995;378:727–30.

Carrera MR, Ashley JA, Hoffman TZ, Isomura S, Wirsching P, Koob GF, et al. Investigations using immunization to attenuate the psychoactive effects of nicotine. Bioorg Med Chem. 2004;12:563–70.

Cerny EH, Cerny T. Vaccines against nicotine. Hum Vaccin. 2009;5:200–5.

Chirmule N, Propert K, Magosin S, Qian Y, Qian R, Wilson J. Immune responses to adenovirus and adeno-associated virus in humans. Gene Ther. 1999;6:1574–83.

Chiuchiolo MJ, Boyer JL, Krause A, Senina S, Hackett NR, Crystal RG. Protective immunity against respiratory tract challenge with Yersinia pestis in mice immunized with an adenovirus-based vaccine vector expressing V antigen. J Infect Dis. 2006;194:1249–57.

Choi JW, Lee JS, Kim SW, Yun CO. Evolution of oncolytic adenovirus for cancer treatment. Adv Drug Deliv Rev. 2012;64:720–9.

Cornuz J, Zwahlen S, Jungi WF, Osterwalder J, Klingler K, Van Melle G, et al. A vaccine against nicotine for smoking cessation: a randomized controlled trial. PLoS One. 2008;3:e2547.

Crystal RG. Adenovirus: the first effective in vivo gene delivery vector. Hum Gene Ther. 2014;25:3–11.

Crystal RG, McElvaney NG, Rosenfeld MA, Chu CS, Mastrangeli A, Hay JG, et al. Administration of an adenovirus containing the human CFTR cDNA to the respiratory tract of individuals with cystic fibrosis. Nat Genet. 1994;8:42–51.

Crystal RG, Harvey BG, Wisnivesky JP, O'Donoghue KA, Chu KW, Maroni J, et al. Analysis of risk factors for local delivery of low- and intermediate-dose adenovirus gene transfer vectors to individuals with a spectrum of comorbid conditions. Hum Gene Ther. 2002;13:65–100.

Crystal RG, Kaminsky SM, Hackett NR, Rosengart TK. Double-blinded, placebo-controlled, randomized gene therapy using surgery for vector delivery. Hum Gene Ther. 2012;23:438–41.

Cytos Biotechnology ZS. CYT002 Nic Qb: a novel vaccine for nicotine addiction. 2006. www.cytos.com/doc/NicQb_June06_E_fv.pdf.

D'Ambrosio E, Del GN, Chicca A, Midulla M. Neutralizing antibodies against 33 human adenoviruses in normal children in Rome. J Hyg (Lond). 1982;89:155–61.

de Villiers SH, Lindblom N, Kalayanov G, Gordon S, Malmerfelt A, Johansson AM, et al. Active immunization against nicotine suppresses nicotine-induced dopamine release in the rat nucleus accumbens shell. Respiration. 2002;69:247–53.

de Villiers SH, Lindblom N, Kalayanov G, Gordon S, Baraznenok I, Malmerfelt A, et al. Nicotine hapten structure, antibody selectivity and effect relationships: results from a nicotine vaccine screening procedure. Vaccine. 2010;28:2161–8.

De BP, Pagovich OE, Hicks MJ, Rosenberg JB, Moreno AY, Janda KD, et al. Disrupted adenovirus-based vaccines against small addictive molecules circumvent anti-adenovirus immunity. Hum Gene Ther. 2013;24:58–66.

Degenhardt L, Chiu WT, Sampson N, Kessler RC, Anthony JC, Angermeyer M, et al. Toward a global view of alcohol, tobacco, cannabis, and cocaine use: findings from the WHO World Mental Health Surveys. PLoS Med. 2008;5:e141.

Deisseroth A, Tang Y, Zhang L, Akbulut H, Habib N. TAA/ecdCD40L adenoviral prime-protein boost vaccine for cancer and infectious diseases. Cancer Gene Ther. 2013;20:65–9.

Derlet RW, Albertson TE. Emergency department presentation of cocaine intoxication. Ann Emerg Med. 1989;18:182–6.

Duarte S, Carle G, Faneca H, de Lima MC, Pierrefite-Carle V. Suicide gene therapy in cancer: where do we stand now? Cancer Lett. 2012;324:160–70.

Evans SM, Foltin RW, Hicks MJ, Rosenberg JB, De BP, Janda KD, et al. The efficacy of an adenovirus-based anti-cocaine vaccine to reduce preference for cocaine self-administration in rhesus monkeys. Am Coll Neuropsychopharm. 2012;38 Suppl T196.

Fahim RE, Kessler PD, Kalnik MW. Therapeutic vaccines against tobacco addiction. Expert Rev Vaccines. 2013;12:333–42.

Fox BS. Development of a therapeutic vaccine for the treatment of cocaine addiction. Drug Alcohol Depend. 1997;48:153–8.

Fox BS, Kantak KM, Edwards MA, Black KM, Bollinger BK, Botka AJ, et al. Efficacy of a therapeutic cocaine vaccine in rodent models. Nat Med. 1996;2:1129–32.

Fukazawa T, Matsuoka J, Yamatsuji T, Maeda Y, Durbin ML, Naomoto Y. Adenovirus-mediated cancer gene therapy and virotherapy (review). Int J Mol Med. 2010;25:3–10.

Ginsberg HS. The adenoviruses. New York: Plenum Press; 1984.

Hackett NR, Crystal RG. Adenovirus vectors for gene therapy. In: Lasic D, Templeton NS, editors. Gene therapy: therapeutic mechanisms and strategies. 3rd ed. New York: CRC Press; 2008. p. 39–68.

Hackett NR, Kaminsky SM, Sondhi D, Crystal RG. Antivector and antitransgene host responses in gene therapy. Curr Opin Mol Ther. 2000;2:376–82.

Haney M, Gunderson EW, Jiang H, Collins ED, Foltin RW. Cocaine-specific antibodies blunt the subjective effects of smoked cocaine in humans. Biol Psychiatry. 2010;67:59–65.

Hartman ZC, Appledorn DM, Amalfitano A. Adenovirus vector induced innate immune responses: impact upon efficacy and toxicity in gene therapy and vaccine applications. Virus Res. 2008;132:1–14.

Harvey BG, Hackett NR, El-Sawy T, Rosengart TK, Hirschowitz EA, Lieberman MD, et al. Variability of human systemic humoral immune responses to adenovirus gene transfer vectors administered to different organs. J Virol. 1999;73:6729–42.

Harvey BG, Maroni J, O'Donoghue KA, Chu KW, Muscat JC, Pippo AL, et al. Safety of local delivery of low- and intermediate-dose adenovirus gene transfer vectors to individuals with a spectrum of morbid conditions. Hum Gene Ther. 2002;13:15–63.

Hashimoto M, Boyer JL, Hackett NR, Wilson JM, Crystal RG. Induction of protective immunity to anthrax lethal toxin with a nonhuman primate adenovirus-based vaccine in the presence of preexisting anti-human adenovirus immunity. Infect Immun. 2005;73:6885–91.

Hatsukami DK, Rennard S, Jorenby D, Fiore M, Koopmeiners J, de Vos A, et al. Safety and immunogenicity of a nicotine conjugate vaccine in current smokers. Clin Pharmacol Ther. 2005;78:456–67.

Hatsukami DK, Jorenby DE, Gonzales D, Rigotti NA, Glover ED, Oncken CA, et al. Immunogenicity and smoking-cessation outcomes for a novel nicotine immunotherapeutic. Clin Pharmacol Ther. 2011;89:392–9.

Havlicek DF, Hicks MJ, De BP, Rosenberg JB, Kaminsky SM, Janda KD, et al. Efficacy of the dAd5GNE anti-cocaine vaccine in models of "binge" cocaine use. Mol Ther. 2014;22:S302.

Hicks MJ, De BP, Rosenberg JB, Davidson JT, Moreno AY, Janda KD, et al. Cocaine analog coupled to disrupted adenovirus: a vaccine strategy to evoke high-titer immunity against addictive drugs. Mol Ther. 2011;19:612–9.

Hicks MJ, Kaminsky SM, De BP, Rosenberg JB, Evans SM, Foltin RW, et al. Fate of systemically administered cocaine in nonhuman primates treated with the dAd5GNE anticocaine vaccine. Hum Gene Ther Clin Dev. 2014;25:40–9.

Hoke Jr CH, Snyder Jr CE. History of the restoration of adenovirus type 4 and type 7 vaccine, live oral (adenovirus vaccine) in the context of the Department of Defense acquisition system. Vaccine. 2013;31:1623–32.

Hollander JE, Hoffman RS, Burstein JL, Shih RD, Thode Jr HC. Cocaine-associated myocardial infarction. Mortality and complications. Cocaine-Associated Myocardial Infarction Study Group. Arch Intern Med. 1995;155:1081–6.

Isomura S, Wirsching P, Janda KD. An immunotherapeutic program for the treatment of nicotine addiction: hapten design and synthesis. J Org Chem. 2001;66:4115–21.

Jooss K, Chirmule N. Immunity to adenovirus and adeno-associated viral vectors: implications for gene therapy. Gene Ther. 2003;10:955–63.

Jupp B, Lawrence AJ. New horizons for therapeutics in drug and alcohol abuse. Pharmacol Ther. 2010;125:138–68.

Kantak KM, Collins SL, Lipman EG, Bond J, Giovanoni K, Fox BS. Evaluation of anti-cocaine antibodies and a cocaine vaccine in a rat self-administration model. Psychopharmacology (Berl). 2000;148:251–62.

Kantak KM, Collins SL, Bond J, Fox BS. Time course of changes in cocaine self-administration behavior in rats during immunization with the cocaine vaccine IPC-1010. Psychopharmacology (Berl). 2001;153:334–40.

Kinsey B. Vaccines against drugs of abuse: where are we now? Ther Adv Vaccines. 2014;2:106–17.

Kinsey BM, Jackson DC, Orson FM. Anti-drug vaccines to treat substance abuse. Immunol Cell Biol. 2009;87:309–14.

Kloss MW, Rosen GM, Rauckman EJ. Cocaine-mediated hepatotoxicity. A critical review. Biochem Pharmacol. 1984;33:169–73.

Kosten TR, Rosen M, Bond J, Settles M, Roberts JS, Shields J, et al. Human therapeutic cocaine vaccine: safety and immunogenicity. Vaccine. 2002;20:1196–204.

Kosten TR, Domingo CB, Shorter D, Orson F, Green C, Somoza E, et al. Vaccine for cocaine dependence: a randomized double-blind placebo-controlled efficacy trial. Drug Alcohol Depend. 2014;140:42–7.

Krause A, Worgall S. Delivery of antigens by viral vectors for vaccination. Ther Deliv. 2011;2:51–70.

Lange RA, Hillis LD. Cardiovascular complications of cocaine use. N Engl J Med. 2001;345:351–8.

Leshner AI. Molecular mechanisms of cocaine addiction. N Engl J Med. 1996;335:128–9.

Lindblom N, de Villiers SH, Kalayanov G, Gordon S, Johansson AM, Svensson TH. Active immunization against nicotine prevents reinstatement of nicotine-seeking behavior in rats. Respiration. 2002;69:254–60.

Lipton JW, Mangan KP, Silvestri JM. Acute cocaine toxicity: pharmacology and clinical presentations in adult and pediatric populations. J Pharm Pract. 2000;13:159–69.

Mack CA, Magovern CJ, Budenbender KT, Patel SR, Schwarz EA, Zanzonico P, et al. Salvage angiogenesis induced by adenovirus-mediated gene transfer of vascular endothelial growth factor protects against ischemic vascular occlusion. J Vasc Surg. 1998;27:699–709.

Maoz A, Hicks MJ, Vallabhjosula S, Synan M, Kothari PJ, Dyke JP, et al. Adenovirus capsid-based anti-cocaine vaccine prevents cocaine from binding to the nonhuman primate CNS dopamine transporter. Neuropsychopharmacology. 2013;38:2170–8.

Martell BA, Mitchell E, Poling J, Gonsai K, Kosten TR. Vaccine pharmacotherapy for the treatment of cocaine dependence. Biol Psychiatry. 2005;58:158–64.

Martell BA, Orson FM, Poling J, Mitchell E, Rossen RD, Gardner T, et al. Cocaine vaccine for the treatment of cocaine dependence in methadone-maintained patients: a randomized, double-blind, placebo-controlled efficacy trial. Arch Gen Psychiatry. 2009;66:1116–23.

Mast TC, Kierstead L, Gupta SB, Nikas AA, Kallas EG, Novitsky V, et al. International epidemiology of human pre-existing adenovirus (Ad) type-5, type-6, type-26 and type-36 neutralizing antibodies: correlates of high Ad5 titers and implications for potential HIV vaccine trials. Vaccine. 2010;28:950–7.

Matthews KS, Alvarez RD, Curiel DT. Advancements in adenoviral based virotherapy for ovarian cancer. Adv Drug Deliv Rev. 2009;61:836–41.

Maurer P, Jennings GT, Willers J, Rohner F, Lindman Y, Roubicek K, et al. A therapeutic vaccine for nicotine dependence: preclinical efficacy, and Phase I safety and immunogenicity. Eur J Immunol. 2005;35:2031–40.

Meijler MM, Matsushita M, Altobell III LJ, Wirsching P, Janda KD. A new strategy for improved nicotine vaccines using conformationally constrained haptens. J Am Chem Soc. 2003;125:7164–5.

Molinier-Frenkel V, Lengagne R, Gaden F, Hong SS, Choppin J, Gahery-Segard H, et al. Adenovirus hexon protein is a potent adjuvant for activation of a cellular immune response. J Virol. 2002;76:127–35.

Moreno AY, Azar MR, Warren NA, Dickerson TJ, Koob GF, Janda KD. A critical evaluation of a nicotine vaccine within a self-administration behavioral model. Mol Pharm. 2010;7:431–41.

Muscholl E. Effect of cocaine and related drugs on the uptake of noradrenaline by heart and spleen. Br J Pharmacol Chemother. 1961;16:352–9.

Nabi.com. Nabi Biopharmaceuticals Announces Results of First NicVAX(R) Phase III Clinical Trial. Smoking cessation immunotherapy failed to meet primary endpoint. 2011. http://globenewswire.com/news-release/2011/07/18/451456/226731/en/Nabi-Biopharmaceuticals-Announces-Results-of-First-NicVAX-R-Phase-III-Clinical-Trial.html.

Nemerow GR. A new link between virus cell entry and inflammation: adenovirus interaction with integrins induces specific proinflammatory responses. Mol Ther. 2009;17:1490–1.

Nicotine Conjugate Vaccine. Clinical Trials NicVAX. 2015. http://www.nabi.com/pipeline/clinicaltrials.php.

Nwanegbo E, Vardas E, Gao W, Whittle H, Sun H, Rowe D, et al. Prevalence of neutralizing antibodies to adenoviral serotypes 5 and 35 in the adult populations of The Gambia, South Africa, and the United States. Clin Diagn Lab Immunol. 2004;11:351–7.

Orson FM, Kinsey BM, Singh RA, Wu Y, Kosten TR. Vaccines for cocaine abuse. Hum Vaccin. 2009;5:194–9.

Orson FM, Rossen RD, Shen X, Lopez AY, Wu Y, Kosten TR. Spontaneous development of IgM anti-cocaine antibodies in habitual cocaine users: effect on IgG antibody responses to a cocaine cholera toxin B conjugate vaccine. Am J Addict. 2013;22:169–74.

Patel SR, Lee LY, Mack CA, Polce DR, El-Sawy T, Hackett NR, et al. Safety of direct myocardial administration of an adenovirus vector encoding vascular endothelial growth factor 121. Hum Gene Ther. 1999;10:1331–48.

Piedra PA, Poveda GA, Ramsey B, McCoy K, Hiatt PW. Incidence and prevalence of neutralizing antibodies to the common adenoviruses in children with cystic fibrosis: implication for gene therapy with adenovirus vectors. Pediatrics. 1998;101:1013–9.

Pittet L, Altreuter D, Ilyinskii P, Praser C, Gao Y, Baldwin S, et al. Development and preclinical evaluation of SEL-068, a novel targeted Synthetic Vaccine Particle (tSVP™) for smoking cessation and relapse prevention that generates high titers of antibodies against nicotine. J Immunol. 2012;188 (Meeting Abstracts):75.11.

Rein DT, Breidenbach M, Curiel DT. Current developments in adenovirus-based cancer gene therapy. Future Oncol. 2006;2:137–43.

Restrepo CS, Carrillo JA, Martinez S, Ojeda P, Rivera AL, Hatta A. Pulmonary complications from cocaine and cocaine-based substances: imaging manifestations. Radiographics. 2007;27:941–56.

Rosenberg JB, De BP, Hicks MJ, Janda KD, Kaminsky SM, Worgall S, et al. Suppression of nicotine-induced pathophysiology by an adenovirus hexon-based antinicotine vaccine. Hum Gene Ther. 2013;24:595–603.

Rosenfeld MA, Yoshimura K, Trapnell BC, Yoneyama K, Rosenthal ER, Dalemans W, et al. In vivo transfer of the human cystic fibrosis transmembrane conductance regulator gene to the airway epithelium. Cell. 1992;68:143–55.

Rosengart TK, Lee LY, Patel SR, Kligfield PD, Okin PM, Hackett NR, et al. Six-month assessment of a phase I trial of angiogenic gene therapy for the treatment of coronary artery disease using direct intramyocardial administration of an adenovirus vector expressing the VEGF121 cDNA. Ann Surg. 1999a;230:466–70.

Rosengart TK, Lee LY, Patel SR, Sanborn TA, Parikh M, Bergman GW, et al. Angiogenesis gene therapy: phase I assessment of direct intramyocardial administration of an adenovirus vector expressing VEGF121 cDNA to individuals with clinically significant severe coronary artery disease. Circulation. 1999b;100:468–74.

Ross S, Peselow E. Pharmacotherapy of addictive disorders. Clin Neuropharmacol. 2009;32:277–89.

Rump AF, Theisohn M, Klaus W. The pathophysiology of cocaine cardiotoxicity. Forensic Sci Int. 1995;71:103–15.

Russell WC. Adenoviruses: update on structure and function. J Gen Virol. 2009;90:1–20.

Schroeder Jr HW, Cavacini L. Structure and function of immunoglobulins. J Allergy Clin Immunol. 2010;125:S41–52.

Shayakhmetov DM. Virus infection recognition and early innate responses to non-enveloped viral vectors. Viruses. 2010;2:244–61.

Shen XY, Orson FM, Kosten TR. Vaccines against drug abuse. Clin Pharmacol Ther. 2012;91:60–70.

Shen XY, Kosten TA, Lopez AY, Kinsey BM, Kosten TR, Orson FM. A vaccine against methamphetamine attenuates its behavioral effects in mice. Drug Alcohol Depend. 2013;129:41–8.

Short JJ, Curiel DT. Oncolytic adenoviruses targeted to cancer stem cells. Mol Cancer Ther. 2009;8:2096–102.

Silva MO, Roth D, Reddy KR, Fernandez JA, Albores-Saavedra J, Schiff ER. Hepatic dysfunction accompanying acute cocaine intoxication. J Hepatol. 1991;12:312–5.

Song W, Kong HL, Carpenter H, Torii H, Granstein R, Rafii S, et al. Dendritic cells genetically modified with an adenovirus vector encoding the cDNA for a model antigen induce protective and therapeutic antitumor immunity. J Exp Med. 1997;186:1247–56.

Spector S, Berkowitz B, Flynn EJ, Peskar B. Antibodies to morphine, barbiturates, and serotonin. Pharmacol Rev. 1973;25:281–91.

St.Clair Roberts J, Akers C, Vanhinsbergh L, McKenna K, Wood D. Longitudinal safety and immunogenicity data of TA-NIC, a novel nicotine vaccine. Presented at: Ninth annual meeting of the society for research on nicotine and tobacco, New Orleans, 2003.

Stowe GN, Vendruscolo LF, Edwards S, Schlosburg JE, Misra KK, Schulteis G, et al. A vaccine strategy that induces protective immunity against heroin. J Med Chem. 2011;54:5195–204.

Tagawa M, Kawamura K, Ueyama T, Nakamura M, Tada Y, Ma G, et al. Cancer therapy with local oncolysis and topical cytokine secretion. Front Biosci. 2008;13:2578–87.

Tan Y, Hackett NR, Boyer JL, Crystal RG. Protective immunity evoked against anthrax lethal toxin after a single intramuscular administration of an adenovirus-based vaccine encoding humanized protective antigen. Hum Gene Ther. 2003;14:1673–82.

Thaci B, Ulasov IV, Wainwright DA, Lesniak MS. The challenge for gene therapy: innate immune response to adenoviruses. Oncotarget. 2011;2:113–21.

Volkow ND, Wang GJ, Fischman MW, Foltin RW, Fowler JS, Abumrad NN, et al. Relationship between subjective effects of cocaine and dopamine transporter occupancy. Nature. 1997;386:827–30.

Wagena EJ, de Vos A, Horwith G, van Schayck CP. The immunogenicity and safety of a nicotine vaccine in smokers and nonsmokers: results of a randomized, placebo-controlled phase 1/2 trial. Nicotine Tob Res. 2008;10:213–8.

Wee S, Hicks MJ, De BP, Rosenberg JB, Moreno AY, Kaminsky SM, et al. Novel cocaine vaccine linked to a disrupted adenovirus gene transfer vector blocks cocaine psychostimulant and reinforcing effects. Neuropsychopharmacology. 2012;37:1083–91.

Wilson JM. Adenoviruses as gene-delivery vehicles. N Engl J Med. 1996;334:1185–7.

Wold WS, Doronin K, Toth K, Kuppuswamy M, Lichtenstein DL, Tollefson AE. Immune responses to adenoviruses: viral evasion mechanisms and their implications for the clinic. Curr Opin Immunol. 1999;11:380–6.

Worgall S, Leopold PL, Wolff G, Ferris B, Van RN, Crystal RG. Role of alveolar macrophages in rapid elimination of adenovirus vectors administered to the epithelial surface of the respiratory tract. Hum Gene Ther. 1997;8:1675–84.

Wu Q, Xia D, Carlsen S, Xiang J. Adenovirus-mediated transgene-engineered dendritic cell vaccine of cancer. Curr Gene Ther. 2005;5:237–47.

Yahyavi-Firouz-Abadi N, See RE. Anti-relapse medications: preclinical models for drug addiction treatment. Pharmacol Ther. 2009;124:235–47.

Yang Y, Nunes FA, Berencsi K, Furth EE, Gonczol E, Wilson JM. Cellular immunity to viral antigens limits E1-deleted adenoviruses for gene therapy. Proc Natl Acad Sci U S A. 1994; 91:4407–11.

Yang Y, Jooss KU, Su Q, Ertl HC, Wilson JM. Immune responses to viral antigens versus transgene product in the elimination of recombinant adenovirus-infected hepatocytes in vivo. Gene Ther. 1996;3:137–44.

Zabner J, Couture LA, Gregory RJ, Graham SM, Smith AE, Welsh MJ. Adenovirus-mediated gene transfer transiently corrects the chloride transport defect in nasal epithelia of patients with cystic fibrosis. Cell. 1993;75:207–16.

Zaiss AK, Machado HB, Herschman HR. The influence of innate and pre-existing immunity on adenovirus therapy. J Cell Biochem. 2009;108:778–90.

Zeyaullah M, Patro M, Ahmad I, Ibraheem K, Sultan P, Nehal M, et al. Oncolytic viruses in the treatment of cancer: a review of current strategies. Pathol Oncol Res. 2012;18:771–81.

Zuckerman JB, Robinson CB, McCoy KS, Shell R, Sferra TJ, Chirmule N, et al. A phase I study of adenovirus-mediated transfer of the human cystic fibrosis transmembrane conductance regulator gene to a lung segment of individuals with cystic fibrosis. Hum Gene Ther. 1999;10: 2973–85.

Chapter 14
Nanoparticle-Based Nicotine Vaccine

Petr O. Ilyinskii and Lloyd P.M. Johnston

14.1 Introduction

Nicotine addiction due to cigarette smoking is a global public health problem with few and relatively inefficient treatment options. The Centers for Disease Control and Prevention estimates that in the United States, smoking is responsible for $96 billion a year in direct health care costs and an additional $97 billion a year in lost productivity (Centers for Disease Control and Prevention 2008). Current approved therapies result, at most, in only 1 in 5 patients abstaining from smoking for 1 year (Oncken et al. 2006). Nicotine vaccines could provide a powerful new tool to facilitate smoking cessation as stand-alone therapy or in combination with other treatment modalities.

Nicotine vaccines cause the body to raise nicotine antibodies that are able to bind to the nicotine as it enters the bloodstream and prevent nicotine from crossing the blood–brain barrier and exerting its addictive affect. All nicotine vaccines described to date are conjugates of nicotine attached to a carrier protein that is intended to make nicotine "visible" to the immune system and an adjuvant, which enhances immune responses leading to increased antibody production (Hatsukami et al. 2011; Escobar-Chávez et al. 2011). Phase 2 clinical data with nicotine vaccines have demonstrated a correlation between nicotine antibody titer and smoking cessation. However, the majority of the patients treated with two different developmental vaccines (Cytos Biotechnology, NicQb; NABI Biopharmaceuticals, NicVAX™) failed to achieve adequate titers to affect smoking cessation. In a Phase IIb trial conducted by Cytos, it was demonstrated that continuous abstinence rates can be increased by vaccination. The subjects with nicotine antibody titers in the top 1/3 of all responders

P.O. Ilyinskii (✉) • L.P.M. Johnston
Selecta Biosciences, Inc., Watertown, MA, USA
e-mail: PIlyinskii@selectabio.com

I.D. Montoya (ed.), *Biologics to Treat Substance Use Disorders: Vaccines, Monoclonal Antibodies, and Enzymes*, DOI 10.1007/978-3-319-23150-1_14

achieved one-year smoking cessation rates of 42 %. The bottom 2/3 of responders had smoking cessation rates that were no different than placebo (~21 %) (Cornuz et al. 2008). Similarly, post hoc analysis of clinical trials of NicVax by Nabi demonstrated a correlation between nicotine antibody levels and smoking cessation (Fahim et al. 2011). Two Phase 3 trials of NicVax both failed to meet the primary endpoint of a statistically significant higher 1-year smoking cessation rate over placebo (Fahim et al. 2013). Despite the positive correlation with smoking cessation observed in the minority of subjects that achieved high antibody levels, the majority of subjects failed to differentiate from placebo in pivotal trials likely due to insufficient immunogenicity (Fahim et al. 2011).

The available preclinical and clinical literature on nicotine vaccines allows the following conclusions:

1. Nicotine vaccines are generally well tolerated; adverse events while best avoided are mostly short-lived and likely due to proinflammatory adjuvant effects.
2. Inducible antibodies are highly specific for nicotine and do not appear to cross-react with the major nicotine metabolites or acetylcholine (Hatsukami et al. 2011; Escobar-Chávez et al. 2011; Castro et al. 1980; Bjercke et al. 1986).
3. In preclinical animal models, sequestration of nicotine in the blood compartment and thus inhibition of movement to the brain were highly correlated with anti-nicotine titers.
4. Clinical efficacy requires high antibody levels, which existing vaccines achieve only in a minority of vaccinees.

Hartman-Boyce et al. published a review of nicotine vaccines for smoking cessation in 2012 in which they conclude that there is no current evidence that nicotine vaccines enhance long-term smoking cessation but that further trials of nicotine vaccines are needed, to look not only at smoking cessation but also at relapse prevention (Hartmann-Boyce et al. 2012). At the same time, while analyzing clinical data from human trials conducted to date, subgroup analyses showed enhanced long-term abstinence rate compared to placebo in smokers with the highest antibody levels (Hatsukami et al. 2011; Cornuz et al. 2008). Thus, it is generally accepted in the field that an improved nicotine vaccine, that can increase the immune response compared to the failed first-generation clinical candidates while exhibiting good safety in a majority of subjects, should have a significant clinical impact on smoking cessation rates (Lockner et al. 2015; Pryde et al. 2013).

It is difficult to raise antibodies to small molecules, such as nicotine and many other drugs of addiction. As noted above, the general strategy (as with many other haptens, which are not immunogenic per se) is to attach nicotine to a highly immunogenic carrier protein (Hatsukami et al. 2011; Escobar-Chávez et al. 2011; Cornuz et al. 2008). The immune system responds to the protein carrier, and at the same time antibodies are raised against the attached nicotine. This can lead to a significant so-called vector effect where the immune response to the carrier dominates over the immune response to the desired antigen. The result can be a weaker immune response to the desired antigen, requiring numerous booster shots to get a sustained effect. The efficacy of such booster shots can be further compromised by the strong immune response against the carrier, which can lead to rapid clearance of the vaccine.

Encapsulation of antigens and adjuvants into micro- and nanocarriers, such as viruslike particles (VLP), liposomes, and biodegradable polymeric particles, such as those comprised of PLGA, is a powerful means to augment an immune response. Of these, synthetic polymer-based vaccines have potential advantages with respect to antigen (or epitope) specificity, safety, and ease of manufacturing. In this chapter we will describe a novel platform of synthetic, self-assembling nanoparticle-based vaccines or synthetic vaccine particles (SVP) that precisely deliver antigens and adjuvant to antigen-presenting cells (APC) and induce potent immune responses. Moreover, this SVP technology enables surface display of B-cell antigens, including haptens, and additional encapsulation of T-cell helper antigens as well as TLR agonists. This provides several immunological advantages, since encapsulation of adjuvants reduces systemic exposure of the adjuvant (and hence its undesired reactogenicity) and enhances its uptake by APCs in the local draining lymph node resulting in focused and prolonged cytokine induction. Furthermore, co-encapsulation of both antigen and adjuvant in SVP nanoparticulate carriers enables synergistic effects by targeting both antigen and adjuvant to the endosomal compartment of APCs.

One potential application field for this technology is a development of vaccines for smoking cessation as well as against other addictions. Nicotine, being non-immunogenic, previously had to be attached to a high molecular weight carrier to induce a humoral response in vivo. Traditionally, such carrier was a protein or proteinaceous particle. Such an approach that has been undertaken by several groups using naturally derived virus particles, Qβ phage, or various protein carriers, but all of the above, has not been proven to induce high level of antibody response in humans.

In contrast, synthetic nanoparticle approach has a potential to overcome many of the problems exhibited by first-generation nicotine vaccines. The following are advantages of nanoparticulate vaccines that make them highly attractive as a basis for the next generation of vaccines:

1. Particulate antigens are more efficiently captured and presented by APCs than soluble antigens.
2. Co-encapsulation and surface co-localization of multiple antigens, targeting moieties and adjuvants, are feasible, thus allowing for much more efficient targeting of immunological information and minimizing off-target activity.
3. Nanocarriers themselves can be non-immunogenic and don't elicit the undesired misdirected responses (vector effect).
4. Polymeric nanoparticles enable protracted antigen and adjuvant release profiles and may act as an intracellular depot of antigen and adjuvant to provide sustained immunological responses.
5. Polymeric-based nanoparticles are likely to be stable at ambient temperature, which simplifies vaccine storage, shipping, handling, and use.
6. Synthetic nanoparticles can be made in a scalable and reproducible process under Good Manufacturing Practices (GMP).

In this chapter we describe the SVP technology (including covalent attachment of nicotine and adjuvant to polymers and development of a broadly active T helper peptide) to induce antibodies to nicotine.

14.2 Nicotine Vaccines: General Background

Development of vaccines against infectious diseases constituted one of the greatest public health advancements of the last century (Plotkin et al. 2012). There are several major types of vaccines, which mostly prevent disease via generation of neutralizing antibodies: attenuated or killed infectious agents, inactivated toxins (toxoids), polysaccharide–protein conjugates, and viruslike particles (VLP) (Plotkin et al. 2012; Barrett and Stanberry 2009) with the latter being, in essence, proteinaceous self-assembling nanoparticles which preserve virion structure, but are incapable of replicating in vivo due to absence of genetic material (Barrett and Stanberry 2009).

It has been realized long ago that protein-based carriers, in particular toxoids, bacterial membrane components (e.g., exoprotein of *P. aeruginosa*), and VLP, have a significant potential to augment an immunogenicity of low- or non-immunogenic entity such as hapten, peptide, or polysaccharide. Several polysaccharide–protein conjugate vaccines have entered clinical practice, and a number of peptide–VLP vaccine constructs are in development or clinical testing. Notably, all of these approaches, namely, conjugation to a protein carrier, membrane complex, or VLP, have been utilized to generate an immune response to nicotine with the aim of creating a therapeutic drug for smoking cessation and relapse prevention (Fahim et al. 2013).

14.3 Non-particulate Nicotine Vaccines in Clinical Development

Among protein-based vaccines, the best studied are those developed by Nabi Biopharmaceuticals (Rockville, MD, USA) and by Pfizer (NY, USA). The first one, 3'-amino-methyl-nicotine conjugate to detoxified exoprotein A of *P. aeruginosa* (3'-AmNic-rEPA), also known as NicVAX, failed to demonstrate efficacy over placebo in two and Phase III trials whether alone or in combination with approved nicotine cessation drug, partial nicotine receptor agonist varenicline (Hatsukami et al. 2011; Fahim et al. 2011, 2013; Hoogsteder et al. 2012). The second one, NIC7-DT, comprises trans-3'-aminomethylnicotine (3'-AmNic) conjugated to diphtheria toxoid (DT, its mutant nontoxic form, known as CRM_{197}), which originally showed high antibody-inducing activity in mice and non-human primates when used in combination with two adjuvants, aluminum hydroxide (alum) and CpG oligodeoxynucleotide (CpG ODN), but showed only modest effects in preventing brain entry by nicotine, similar to those observed in unsuccessful clinical studies with NicVAX (Esterlis et al. 2013; McCluskie et al. 2013). Later, NIC7-DT developers tested a series of nicotine-like haptens, with varying attachment sites on nicotine, type of protein-hapten linker, and the handle used to attach the nicotine to DT. Based on Ab titers, affinity, and function (using the radiolabeled nicotine challenge model in mouse), 5-amino-ethoxy-nicotine was selected and further used with the DT carrier to evaluate the influence of linker polarity, rigidity, and length on immunogenicity (Pryde et al. 2013). High Ab concentrations and nicotine binding efficiencies were reported in mice and non-human primates (Pryde et al. 2013; McCluskie et al. 2013, 2015). In the latest study 27 variants of a candidate vaccine, now designated NIC7–CRM, were evaluated (McCluskie et al. 2015). These lots differed in hapten load (number of haptens conjugated to each molecule of CRM_{197}), degree of conjugate aggregation, and presence of adducts (small molecules attached to CRM_{197} during conjugation). Authors focused on functional responses (reduced nicotine brain entry) induced by said conjugates adjuvanted with aluminum hydroxide and CpG. Trends for better functional responses in mice were obtained with conjugates having a hapten load of 11 to 18, being non-aggregated and containing a low level of adducts. Similar trends were observed in cynomolgus monkeys in which three conjugates were tested with two of them showing the suppression of nicotine brain entry within 50–60 % range (McCluskie et al. 2015). Currently, two formulations of DT-based conjugate nicotine vaccine, NIC7-001 and NIC7-003, are in clinical trials [ClinicalTrials.gov identifier: NCT01672645; accessed July 17, 2015]. Clinical test of yet another nicotine conjugate vaccine based on tetanus toxoid was completely unsuccessful (Tonstad et al. 2013).

14.4 Nanoparticle-Based Vaccines Against Nicotine: Utilization of VLP

VLPs are composed of viral proteins expressed in vitro upon which the self-assembly forms regularly structured particles in the 20–100 nm size range (Ghasparian et al. 2011). Several VLP-based products have successfully entered medical practice (Plotkin et al. 2012), and a several dozen of VLP-based vaccine candidates are either in clinical trials or undergoing preclinical evaluation (Clinicaltrials.gov 2015). Moreover, VLPs have been shown to be a suitable carrier for other antigenic determinants, and there are several vaccines in development that are aiming to exploit this feature (De Filette et al. 2008; Cruz et al. 2009; Woo et al. 2006). Generally, VLP showed a strong induction of humoral immunity, especially in rodent models (Tan et al. 2011; Parez et al. 2006; Quan et al. 2007; Slupetzky et al. 2007; Akahata et al. 2010). One of the main reasons for this strong immunogenicity stems from VLPs presenting epitopes in a repetitive, high-density display (Vicente et al. 2011). However, many VLPs require the coadministration of adjuvants (Qian et al. 2006; Storni et al. 2002; Young et al. 2006), and antibodies induced by them do not always possess a strong neutralizing activity (Schneemann et al. 2012). VLP-based vaccines also have significant bioprocess challenges associated with large-scale production and purification (Vicente et al. 2011).

One candidate vaccine against nicotine, CYT002-NicQb or Nic002, has been based on a VLP-nicotine conjugate (Maurer et al. 2005) and reached several Phase I/II trials (Cornuz et al. 2008; Fahim et al. 2013). In this case nicotine was chemically coupled to VLP formed by the coat protein of the RNA bacteriophage Qb, a relatively small (25 nm) capsid virus (Kozlovska et al. 1993). Like NicVAX, Nic002 utilized nicotine conjugation via the 3'-position on the pyrrolidine ring using a succinimate linker and induced strong and specific IgG responses in preclinical animal studies including high antibody affinity and reduced nicotine brain entry after intravenous challenge (Maurer et al. 2005). However, the Phase II trials of Nic002 showed efficacy only in the minority of subjects who achieved the highest antibody levels, not dissimilar to later results with NicVAX (Hatsukami et al. 2011; Cornuz et al. 2008; Pentel and LeSage 2014) despite the 100 % antibody responder rate. There were several explanations given for Nic002 ultimate failure such as sequestration of nicotine by antibodies simply being not sufficient to increase abstinence or that average antibody levels which Nic002 induces (not unlike protein-based vaccines) may be insufficient for smoking cessation (Cornuz et al. 2008). It has been noted that in Phase II clinical trials of the NicVAX, a peak geometric mean serum IgG concentration of 45 μg/ml was associated with higher smoking cessation rates (Hatsukami et al. 2011), which aligns reasonably well with data showing that subjects with serum antibody levels of 40–160 μg/mL have some reduction in occupancy of brain nicotinic cholinergic receptors (Esterlis et al. 2013).

This may indicate that the level of serum antibody against nicotine needs to be at least at 50–100 μg/mL range to provide a minimum effective concentration (Pentel and LeSage 2014). Furthermore, it has been calculated that a serum antibody concentration of 100 μg/ml would provide ~6 μM of binding sites for nicotine while smoking one cigarette provides an absorbed nicotine dose of about 5–7 μM, meaning that proposed minimum effective nicotine antibody concentration in human serum would provide the binding capacity for at most one cigarette (Pentel and LeSage 2014).

Collectively, clinical data on nicotine vaccine development are at the same time promising and disappointing: it has been generally accepted that high levels of antibodies to nicotine will aid smoking cessation, but there is no product which seems to hold enough potential to pass a very high bar of systemic IgG induction necessary to see a clear clinical benefit. This propels the search for new alternatives in nicotine vaccine development, such as utilization of synthetic polymer-based nanoparticles. Such particles, mostly manufactured using biodegradable materials, have been long viewed as an extremely promising avenue of vaccine development and have performed well in many experimental and preclinical settings.

14.5 Development of Polymer Nanoparticle-Based Nicotine Vaccine, Synthetic Vaccine Particle (SVP)

14.5.1 Rationale for Nanoparticle-Based Vaccine Development: General Considerations

Clinical data from the first generation of nicotine vaccines demonstrated a statistically significant correlation between anti-nicotine antibody concentration and sustained smoking cessation (Cornuz et al. 2008; Fahim et al. 2011). These results suggest the therapeutic potential for a vaccine that can induce high anti-nicotine antibody levels in a majority of treated subjects. Several lines of research indicate that modular polymer-based biodegradable nanoparticles have an ability to overcome immunogenicity hurdles delineated above.

It is well known that many antigens are more immunogenic in particulate form (Manolova et al. 2008). This is most likely due to the higher antigen uptake after particularization and antigen processing and presentation (Bachmann and Jennings 2010). However, a simple hapten attachment to a nanoparticle is unlikely to provide a sufficient immunogenicity. Moreover, even a coadministration of a known adjuvant may not suffice in this case since hapten-exhibiting nanoparticles will have a high potential of inducing a transient (IgM-based) humoral response without affinity maturation and class switching (not unlike antibodies to bacterial polysaccharides, LPS or PEG). Similarly to conjugated vaccines, T helper cell activation is essential for robust and long-term antibody responses. This activity is initiated when a protein- or peptide-based vaccine is taken up by APCs, its contents are proteolytically processed, and resulting peptides presented to naive CD4 T cells in MHC class II context. After that, a committed T helper will be able to recognize nicotine-specific B cells (which also act as APC) displaying this same peptide. This interaction, especially if occurring in the presence of an adjuvant, will further activate nicotine-specific B cells and enable their affinity maturation.

Collectively, strong immunogenicity against a hapten presented in a particulate form may be reached only if all the essential vaccine components, hapten antigen, adjuvant, and T helper activator, are effectively co-delivered to professional APC. This task can be effectively met via encapsulation of the abovementioned components within biodegradable polymer nanoparticles (Heit et al. 2008). Such immunogens will provide for continuous hapten presentation, improve adjuvant pharmacokinetics, and, if effectively constructed, are likely to be capable of inducing $CD4^+$ cell expansion comparable to that of live vectors (Bachmann and Jennings 2010; Jennings and Bachmann 2009).

14.5.2 Nanoparticle Design

14.5.2.1 General Parameters (Multiple Target Elements)

The following design criteria have been used to develop a platform of synthetic vaccine particles (SVP):

(a) Use of polymers that are biocompatible and biodegradable and used in products previously approved by the FDA (i.e., PLA-/PLGA-based polymers)
(b) Development of "stealth" vehicles capable of delivering an immunogenic payload to APCs while being non-immunogenic themselves
(c) Incorporation of adjuvants that may be integrated, delivered, and released in a tunable manner, to elicit an optimal immune response while minimizing systemic reactions

(d) Presenting a dense array of hapten-based B-cell antigen on the surface of the particles to engage and cross-link B-cell receptors
(e) Development and incorporation of a universal CD4+ helper T-cell antigen to drive antibody affinity maturation and B-cell memory

Finally, all of these components need to be efficiently co-delivered to APC.

14.5.2.2 Integrated Immunologic Design (Efficient Immunologic Communication)

Lymph nodes (LNs) are strategically positioned to filter the afferent lymph for nano-sized particles, such as viruses, where they can be captured by APCs which process and present microbial antigens to the adaptive immune system. Selecta's SVPs were designed to mimic key recognition features of highly immunogenic microbial pathogens (Figs. 14.1 and 14.2):

(a) A particulate form
(b) Nano-scale size for unimpeded access to lymph vessels and travel to LNs
(c) Pathogen-associated molecular patterns that serve as adjuvant by stimulating APC-expressed receptors, such as TLRs
(d) Densely arrayed surface molecules that are capable of cross-linking B-cell receptors (BCRs) on antigen-specific B cells
(e) Incorporation of protein sequences that can be processed and presented in diverse major histocompatibility (MHC) class II complexes for recognition by CD4+ T cells

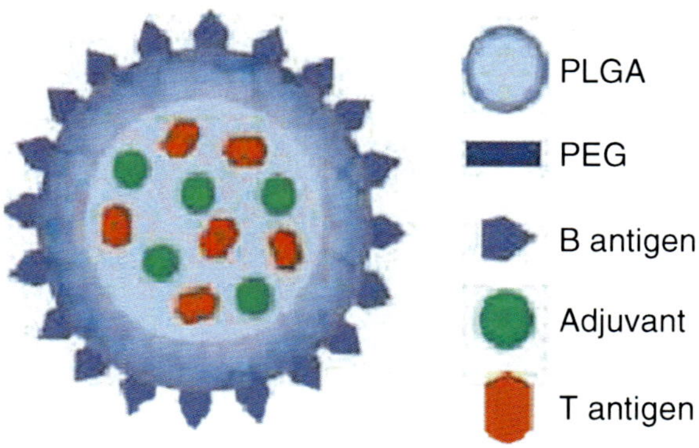

Fig. 14.1 Schematic of Selecta's SVP nanoparticle platform SVP nanoparticles are created from polymers [poly(lactic-co-glycolic acid) (*PLGA*) and polyethylene glycol (*PEG*) (as *PLGA-PEG*)] that are present in multiple FDA-approved products. Targeted nanoparticles carry a dense array of surface B-cell antigen (e.g., nicotine) for high avidity B-cell receptor triggering. A TLR agonist adjuvant and a universal T-cell help peptide (TCHP) are encapsulated in the particle core and designed to be released in the endosomal compartment of antigen-presenting cells (APC) where they can trigger TLR receptors and be loaded onto MHC class II complexes, respectively. The physicochemical properties (e.g., size and surface properties) of the nanoparticles target them to desired cell types (APCs) and anatomic locations (lymph nodes)

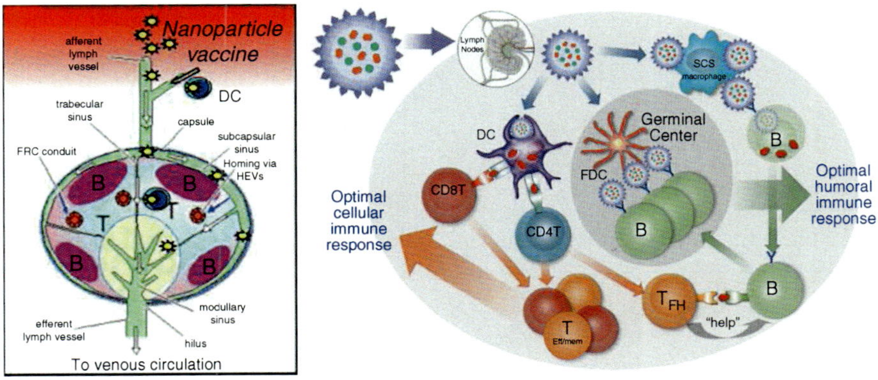

Fig. 14.2 Stylized schematic of local draining lymph node and the interaction among immune cells. (**a**) Pathogens or particles move via the afferent lymphatics to local draining LNs where they enter through the subcapsular sinus. (**b**) Once particles have moved into the lymph node, they are captured by dendritic cells (*DCs*) and subcapsular sinus (SCS) macrophages. DCs internalize and digest the nanoparticles and present payload-derived antigenic peptides in MHC classes I and II to CD8⁺ and CD4⁺ T cells, respectively. Activated T cells differentiate into effector/memory ($T_{Eff/Mem}$) cells that mediate cellular immune responses. Activated CD4⁺ T cells also give rise to follicular T helper cells (T_{FH}). They provide help to B cells that were initially stimulated by surface antigen on nanoparticles captured by SCS macrophages. Following the initial antigen encounter, B cells acquire and process T-cell antigen for restimulation of T_{FH} cells. The action of T_{FH} cells allows the development of a germinal center reaction during which B cells interact with nanoparticles on follicular dendritic cells (*FDCs*). This induces them to proliferate, generate high-affinity IgG antibodies, and differentiate into memory and plasma cells. All the key players must be provided with the proper information and instruction to generate the highest possible antibody titer and durability

14.5.2.3 Hapten Selection

Low molecular weight haptens, such as nicotine (Mw = 162), are not immunogenic and must be attached to high molecular weight carriers or displayed on a nanoparticulate in order to induce an immune response. Earlier studies have shown that nicotine coupled to protein carriers is immunogenic (Pentel et al. 2000; Cerny 2005). In our initial developmental studies, we demonstrated that presentation of nicotine as an antigen covalently attached to SVP results in a potent anti-nicotine antibody response. The self-assembly nature of the SVP platform effectively and efficiently displays the nicotine on the surface of the SVP in a controllable and tunable manner. Nicotine is conjugated to the hydrophilic PEG end of the amphiphilic polymer PLGA–PEG, creating PLGA–PEG–Nic. The SVP nanoparticles are produced by an oil-in-water emulsion process, in which nano-sized oil droplets containing the PLGA–PEG–Nic and other agents are formed. The PLGA–PEG–Nic molecules move by Brownian motion in the oil droplet, and when it nears the oil water interface, the hydrophilic PEG–Nic end of the polymer orients into the water phase where it now stays. In this way the PLGA–PEG–Nic is oriented to display the PEG–Nic end on the surface of the particle, allowing for presentation to B cells. In addition, by varying the amount of the PLGA–PEG–Nic in the formulation, the density of nicotine on the surface of the particle can be varied and optimized to achieve a maximal immune response to nicotine.

14.5.2.4 Adjuvant Selection and Development

Nanoparticles targeted to dendritic cells (DC) may result in more efficient B- and T-cell priming, especially if containing TLR agonists which act via pattern recognition receptors (PRRs), thus serving as signals for DC maturation (Andersen and Ohlfest 2012). Upon being activated through various PRRs, professional APC starts to actively migrate into secondary lymphoid organs, capture antigens, process, and present them, thus driving T- and B-cell activation. In particular, $CD4^+$ cells ensure optimal responses by many other lymphocyte classes, including antibody-producing B cells (Swain et al. 2012).

Several lines of evidence point that effective antigen exposure on the surface of VLP or NP leads to an augmented immunogenicity of a poorly immunogenic epitope (De Filette et al. 2008; Denis et al. 2008; Hashemi et al. 2012). Additionally, utilization of a modular nanoparticle platform makes it possible to accommodate a variety of antigenic iterations for their rapid testing and development. Nanoparticles are typically prepared from organic building blocks and polymers, such as polylactide-co-glycolide (PLGA), or inorganic and metallic elements. Biodegradable NP made from PLGA or polylactic acid (PLA) has especially attracted much attention as vehicle for delivery of drugs and vaccines in vivo (Mahapatro and Singh 2011). It has been demonstrated that nanoparticles may target distinct APC with smaller (20–200 nm) particles being able to drain freely to LN-resident DC and macrophages (Manolova et al. 2008; Reddy et al. 2007).

Over the last decades, many strong novel adjuvants have been described, but only one TLR agonist-based composition, AS04, has become in an approved product in the United States (Alving et al. 2012). The main reason for this is the inability to formulate these adjuvants in such a way that their systemic effects are minimized. Since APCs preferentially take up micro- and nanoparticles, using particle-encapsulated adjuvants may solve this safety versus efficacy issue. In fact, many TLR agonists are known to have potent adjuvant properties, but their clinical use has been limited by systemic adverse reactions or insufficient breadth of immune response (e.g., TLR4 agonists are more biased toward Th2 response). It is apparent that efficient encapsulation of adjuvants within the SVPs may enable the safe use of potent TLR agonists.

TLRs are widely expressed on dendritic cells (DC) and other professional APCs such as macrophages and B cells. While some TLRs are expressed on the cell surface and act as sensors for extracellular PAMPs (e.g., lipopolysaccharides), a subset of TLR molecules (TLR3, TLR7, TLR8, and TLR9) are expressed on endosomal membranes and bind nucleic acid-derived molecules, such as single-stranded RNA of viral origin for TLR7 and TLR8 (Hemmi et al. 2002; Jurk et al. 2002; Edwards 2003; Diebold 2004, 2008; Heil et al. 2004) and bacterial unmethylated DNA oligonucleotides (ODNs) containing CpG motifs (CpG ODNs) for TLR9 (Krieg et al.

1995; Sato 1996; Roman et al. 1997; Sparwasser et al. 1997; Hemmi et al. 2000). TLR ligands of natural and synthetic origin are potent inducers of innate immune responses and have been shown to effectively stimulate the transition from an innate immune response to an adaptive immune response. As such, TLR agonists have been evaluated as potential adjuvants in a variety of applications (Wang and Singh 2011).

To date, only one PRR ligand, *3*-O-desacyl-4'-monophosphoryl lipid A (MPL), a TLR4 agonist, has been included as an adjuvant in an FDA- or EMA-licensed vaccine. MPL adsorbed onto alum is utilized in the HPV vaccine Cervarix, licensed in the United States and Europe (Harper 2009), and the hepatitis B vaccine Fendrix, licensed in Europe (Johnson 2008). Imiquimod, a topically administered TLR7 agonist, has been approved for treatment of genital warts, actinic keratosis, and basal cell carcinoma (Basith et al. 2011). Other TLR agonists, such as poly (I:C) (TLR3), imidazoquinolines other than imiquimod (TLR7, TLR8, or TLR7/TLR8), and CpG ODNs (TLR9), have failed thus far to enter clinical practice as parenteral adjuvants despite a multitude of promising data obtained in preclinical and clinical studies (Wang et al. 2005; Krieg 2006; Wille-Reece et al. 2006; Karan et al. 2007; Krieg 2007). One of the main reasons for this failure is the delicate balance between the induction of augmented immunogenicity by TLR agonists and safety concerns, which are often related to the generation of systemic inflammatory responses (Hemmi et al. 2002; Vasilakos et al. 2000; Doxsee et al. 2003; Pockros 2007).

Several groups have utilized micro- and nanocarriers, such as viruslike particles, liposomes, and PLGA particles, to encapsulate adjuvants (Bachmann and Jennings 2010; Malyala et al. 2009; Kasturi et al. 2011). Encapsulation of adjuvants reduces systemic exposure of adjuvant and enhances uptake by APCs. Nano-sized viruses and particles distribute rapidly to the local draining lymph node where they are taken up by subcapsular macrophages and dendritic cells (Manolova et al. 2008; Bachmann and Jennings 2010; Junt 2007). Antigens can also be delivered in particles to target efficient uptake by APCs (Bachmann and Jennings 2010; Krieg 2007; Singh et al. 2006; Wagner 2009). Recent studies show that co-encapsulation of both antigen and adjuvant in nanoparticulate carriers has synergistic effects in augmenting immunity by targeting antigen and adjuvant to the endosomal compartment of APCs (Krieg 2007; Kasturi et al. 2011; Wagner 2009).

We evaluated the immune responses induced by synthetic vaccine particles (SVP) carrying covalently bound or entrapped TLR agonist co-delivered with encapsulated antigen (either in the same or in separate nanoparticle preparations). We hypothesized that such an approach may provide a two-pronged benefit by enabling a focused delivery of antigen and adjuvant and hence enhancing immunogenicity while preventing systemic exposure of the TLR agonist, which can result in excessive systemic cytokine release. We were able to demonstrate that the SVPs deliver their payloads directly to APCs in lymph nodes, as evidenced by the local production of cytokines in draining lymph nodes and the lack of systemic inflammatory cytokines that are typically associated with adverse reactions.

Nanoparticle Encapsulation of TLR Agonists Changes the Pattern of Inflammatory Cytokine Induction In Vitro

TLR7/TLR8 (resiquimod also known as R848) and TLR9 (CpG ODN 1826; mouse-specific B-type CpG ODN) agonists were encapsulated in synthetic polymer nanoparticles and tested for their ability to induce cytokines in vitro. R848 was chemically conjugated to PLGA and used for SVP formulation as PLGA-R848, and CpG ODN was passively entrapped into SVP as described by Ilyinskii et al. (Ilyinskii et al. 2014). Natural oligonucleotide sequences contain a phosphodiester (PO) backbone, which is susceptible to rapid hydrolytic cleavage by nucleases in vivo. Nuclease-resistant CpG sequences with a phosphorothioate (PS) backbone have been shown to have superior activity to PO-CpG in vivo. Both PS and PO forms of the immunostimulatory CpG ODN 1826 sequence (PS-CpG 1826 and PO-CpG 1826) were evaluated. SVP-encapsulated R848 induced lower levels of TNF-α from splenocytes and especially from murine macrophages than identical amounts of free R848 (Fig. 14.3a, b). Similar profiles were seen when PS-CpG 1826 and PO-CpG 1826 sequences were tested in free or SVP-encapsulated form. Not surprisingly, PO-CpG 1826 was a less potent inducer of TNF-α production than PS-CpG 1826, with its SVP-encapsulated form being nearly inactive, even in the

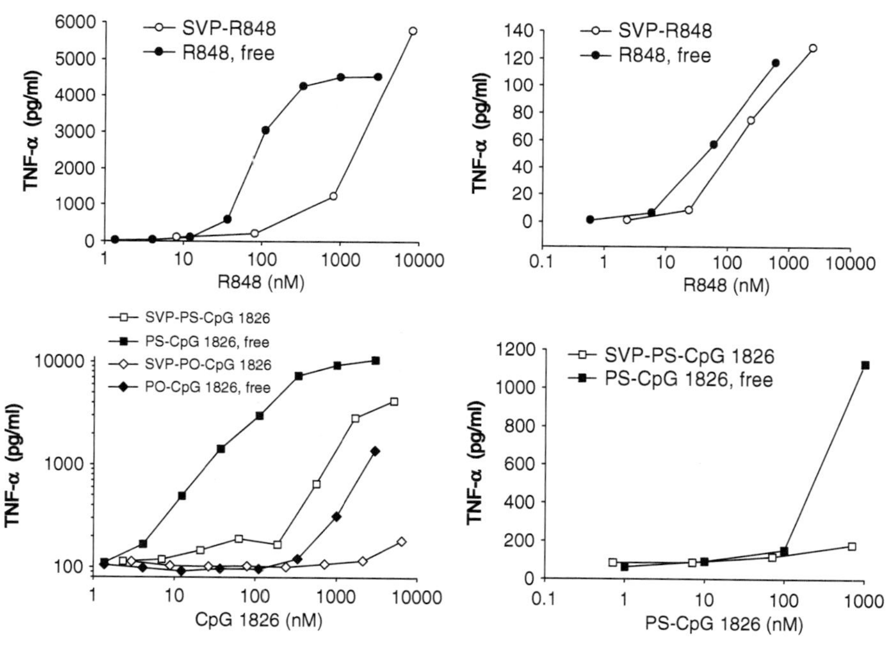

Fig. 14.3 Adjuvant encapsulation in nanoparticles (*SVP*) results in suppressed TNF-α induction in murine cells in vitro. SVP containing TLR7/TLR8 agonist R848 (**a**, **b**) or TLR9 agonists PO-CpG 1826 (**c**) or PS-CpG1826 (**d**) were added to J774 cells (**a**, **c**) or fresh mouse splenocyte cultures (**b**, **d**) in parallel with free adjuvants in triplicates. The amount of TNF-α in culture supernatants was measured 6 h (splenocytes) or 16 h (J774) after incubation. Representative results out of two separate experiments with groups of three mice are shown

more sensitive J774 cells (Fig. 14.3c, d). IL-6 production in vitro followed the same pattern as TNF-α (data not shown). However, a static in vitro system does not capture potential differences in biodistribution and pharmacokinetics of free adjuvant versus nanoparticle-encapsulated adjuvant that is expected in vivo.

Rapid Infiltration of Draining Lymph Nodes by Innate and Adaptive Immune Cells Upon Injection of Nanoparticle-Encapsulated R848

As reported by Ilyinskii et al. (Ilyinskii et al. 2014), R848-bearing nanoparticles induced a profound increase in cellularity within the draining lymph nodes at 4 days after a single inoculation (Fig. 14.4). Further analysis of cellularity within the draining lymph nodes after s.c. injection showed that LN infiltration starts as early as 1 day after inoculation, reaches a peak at 7–8 days, and is maintained for at least 3 weeks (Tables 14.1 and 14.2). The increase in lymph node cellularity was even more rapid and pronounced in mice that were previously immunized

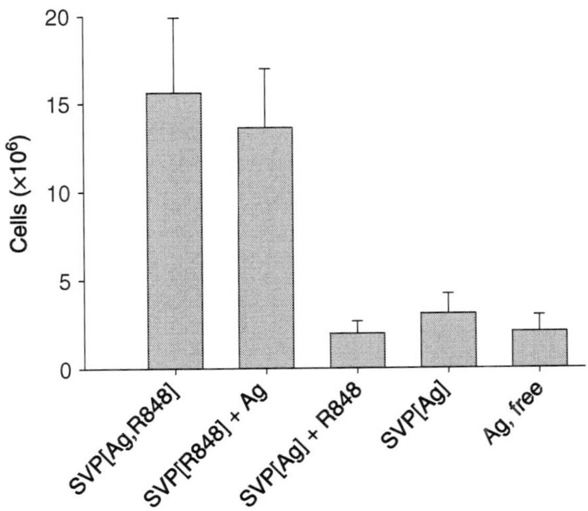

Fig. 14.4 Nanoparticle encapsulation of TLR7/TLR8 agonist (adjuvant) results in higher local immune infiltration than utilization of free adjuvant. Total draining lymph node (*LN*) cell count is presented at 4 days after s.c. injection. The total dose of antigen (*Ag*) was the same across all treatment groups, and the total dose of R848 was the same for all groups receiving R848

Table 14.1 Local lymphadenopathy induction by administration of SVP-encapsulated but not free TLR7/TLR8 agonist

Day	SVP-R848	SVP (no adjuvant)	SVP (no adjuvant) + R848
0	1.00	1.00	1.00
1	1.50	1.36	1.08
4	3.19	1.53	1.03
7	8.06	1.53	0.84

Mice were injected subcutaneously (hind limb) with SVP-R848, SVP (no adjuvant), or SVP (no adjuvant) admixed with free R848. Popliteal LNs were taken at various times as indicated. Total lymph node cells (normalized to day 0 values) in all groups (average of 3 mice per time point) are shown

Table 14.2 Local lymphadenopathy after administration of SVP-encapsulated TLR7/TLR8 agonist and nicotine antigen in naive vs. pre-immunized mice

	SVP-R848, total cells in LN	
Day	Naive mice	Immune mice
0	1.00	1.00
3	4.33	10.14
8	8.04	9.86
14	5.36	6.93
21	4.14	6.60

Naive or previously immunized mice were injected with SVP-R848 with co-encapsulated nicotine antigen (hind limb, s.c.). Popliteal LNs were taken at various times as indicated. Total lymph node cell counts (normalized to day 0 values) in all groups (average of 3 mice per time point) are shown

with SVP (tenfold increase in the popliteal LN cell count at 3 days after inoculation, Table 14.2). No significant cell infiltration of the draining lymph node was seen if SVP lacking R848 were used either alone or admixed with free R848 (Table 14.1).

A detailed analysis of intranodal cell populations after injection of SVP containing both encapsulated R848 and nicotine antigen (Nic) showed a rapid increase in the number of innate immune cells, such as granulocytes and myeloid DC, in the draining LN, with their numbers increasing threefold within 24 h after a single injection (Table 14.3). There was also an early elevation in macrophage cell numbers in the draining lymph node, while increases in other APC subtypes (plasmacytoid DC and B cells) were observed at a slightly later time point. Interestingly, among the populations analyzed, only effector cells of the adaptive immune response (T and B cells) showed a continued expansion from day 4 to day 7 (Table 14.3). Presence of nicotine antigen within the SVP had no influence on LN cellularity.

Nanoparticle Encapsulation of TLR7/TLR8 Agonist Induces Strong Local Cytokine Production

Strong local immune activation by nanoparticle-encapsulated R848 was further manifested by cytokine production in the draining LN milieu (Figs. 14.5 and 14.6). At 4 h after subcutaneous injection, high levels of IFN-γ, RANTES, IL-12(p40), and IL-1β were secreted by LNs from animals injected with SVP[Ag,R848] (encapsulated R848 and antigen), while the production of these cytokines by LNs from mice injected with free R848 was close to the background level (Fig. 14.5). In particular, the amount of IFN-γ secreted by LNs from mice injected with SVP[Ag,R848] at 4 h was more than 100-fold higher than that from the LNs of mice injected with SVP[Ag] and an equal amount of free R848 (Fig. 14.5a), while RANTES was elevated more than 27-fold (Fig. 14.5b). Production of all of these cytokines in the LN was maintained for at least 72 h after injection of SVP[Ag,R848], with levels of IL-12(p40) and IL-1β remaining nearly stable (Fig. 14.5c, d) and levels of IFN-γ and RANTES, while decreasing, remaining 4- to 20-fold higher than the

Table 14.3 Local lymphadenopathy and immune cell population expansion after administration of SVP-encapsulated TLR7/TLR8 agonist irrespective of nicotine presence

Day	Total cells	CD11c$^+$ B220$^-$ (mDC)	CD11c$^+$B220$^+$ (pDC)	B220$^+$ CD11c$^-$ (B cells)	F4/80$^+$ GR1$^-$ (Mø)	F4/80$^-$ GR1$^+$ (Gran)	CD3$^+$ (T cells)	CD3$^-$CD49b$^+$ (NK)	CD3$^+$ CD49b$^+$ (NKT)
0	1.00	1.00	1.00	1.00	1.000	1.00	1.00	1.00	1.00
1	1.50	3.15	1.36	0.98	1.97	3.52	1.52	1.03	0.62
4	3.19	6.50	8.14	3.56	1.16	14.20	2.54	9.64	6.72
7	8.06	7.00	7.77	11.09	2.51	18.43	4.39	8.57	8.25

Mice were injected s.c. (hind limb) with SVP[Nic,R848], SVP (Nic, no adjuvant), or SVP (Nic, no adjuvant) admixed with free R848. Popliteal LNs were taken at times indicated. Total lymph node cells were counted; stained for various surface markers, as indicated; and analyzed by flow cytometry. Cell numbers were normalized to day 0 values. Data shown in table are from SVP[Nic,R848]-injected mice. No marked variation in LN cell populations was seen in mice injected with "no adjuvant"-SVP[Nic] or "no adjuvant"-SVP[Nic] admixed with free R848 (not shown)

Mø macrophages, *mDC and pDC* myeloid and plasmacytoid DC, *Gran* granulocytes, *NKT* NK T cells

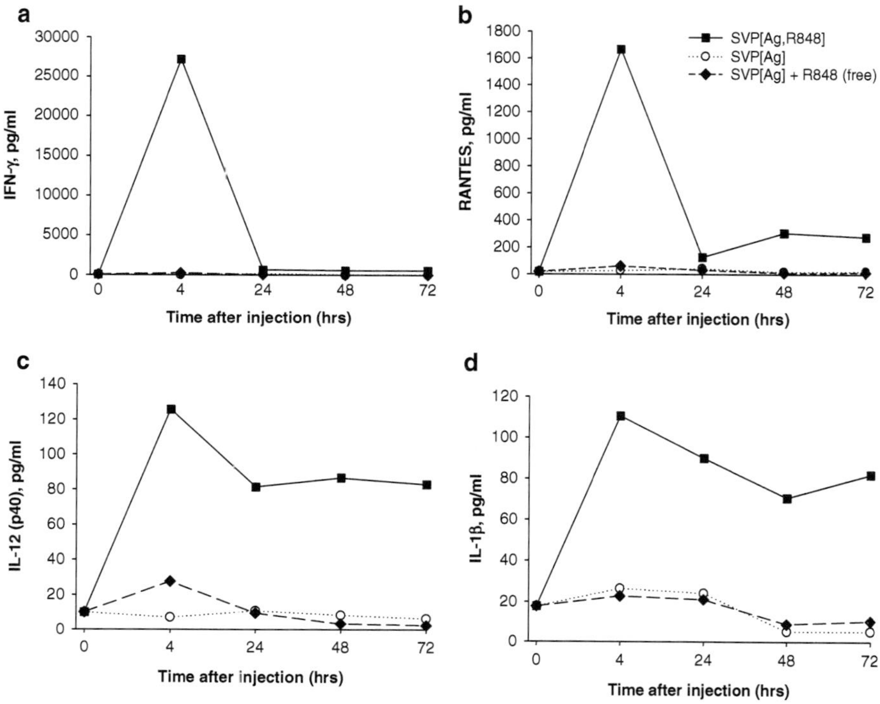

Fig. 14.5 Local cytokines are induced by SVP-encapsulated, but not free, TLR7/TLR8 agonist R848. Mice were injected s.c. in both hind limbs with either SVP-OVA-R848, SVP-OVA, or SVP-OVA admixed with free R848. At the times indicated, popliteal LNs were taken and incubated in vitro overnight. Culture supernatants were collected and analyzed for the presence of specific cytokines by ELISA. (**a**) IFN-γ, (**b**) RANTES, (**c**) IL-12(p40), (**d**) IL-1β. Average of four LNs per time point is shown

background. In contrast, inoculation of free R848 led to only a modest increase of local cytokine production at 4 h, which returned to background levels by 24 h after administration (Ilyinskii et al. 2014). Levels of IP-10 and MCP-1 in LNs from SVP[Ag,R848]-injected animals were also elevated in a similar fashion (data not shown).

The striking difference in local cytokine production after administration of nanoparticle-encapsulated versus free R848 (Fig. 14.5) was also evident by comparing cytokine production in the ipsilateral draining lymph node versus the contralateral lymph node after injection in a single hind limb (Figs. 14.6a, b). The sustained expression of IFN-γ, IL-12(p40), and IL-1β was seen in the ipsilateral LN at 4–48 h after injection of SVP-R848, but not in the contralateral lymph node. In contrast, free R848 induced a modest elevation of IL-12(p40) and IFN-γ in both the ipsilateral and contralateral lymph nodes (Fig. 14.6b). The level of IFN-γ observed in the ipsilateral lymph node following injection of free R848 was 50-fold lower than that induced by SVP-R848 (Fig. 14.6a). No induction of IL-1β by free R848 was seen (Fig. 14.6c) (Ilyinskii et al. 2014).

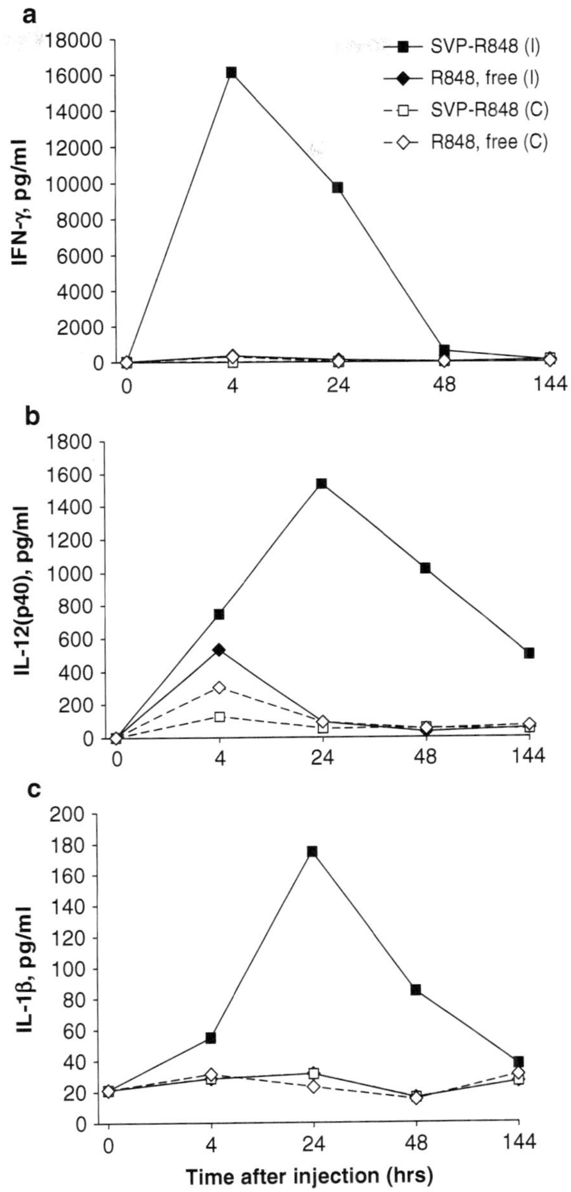

Fig. 14.6 Focused local cytokine induction after a single-site injection with SVP encapsulated, but not free, TLR7/TLR8 agonist R848. Mice were injected s.c. in a single hind limb with either SVP-R848 or free R848. At the times indicated, popliteal LNs from the injection side (ipsilateral, *I*) and from the opposite side (contralateral, *C*) were collected and incubated in vitro overnight. Culture supernatants were analyzed for the presence of specific cytokines by ELISA. (**a**) IFN-γ, (**b**) IL-12(p40), (**c**) IL-1β. Average of two mice per time point is shown

Nanoparticle Encapsulation of TLR7/TLR8 Agonist R848 Attenuates the Production of Systemic Inflammatory Cytokines

While nanoparticle encapsulation of R848 enhanced immunogenicity and local induction of immune cytokines, the production of systemic inflammatory cytokines by SVP-R848 was markedly suppressed compared to that observed with

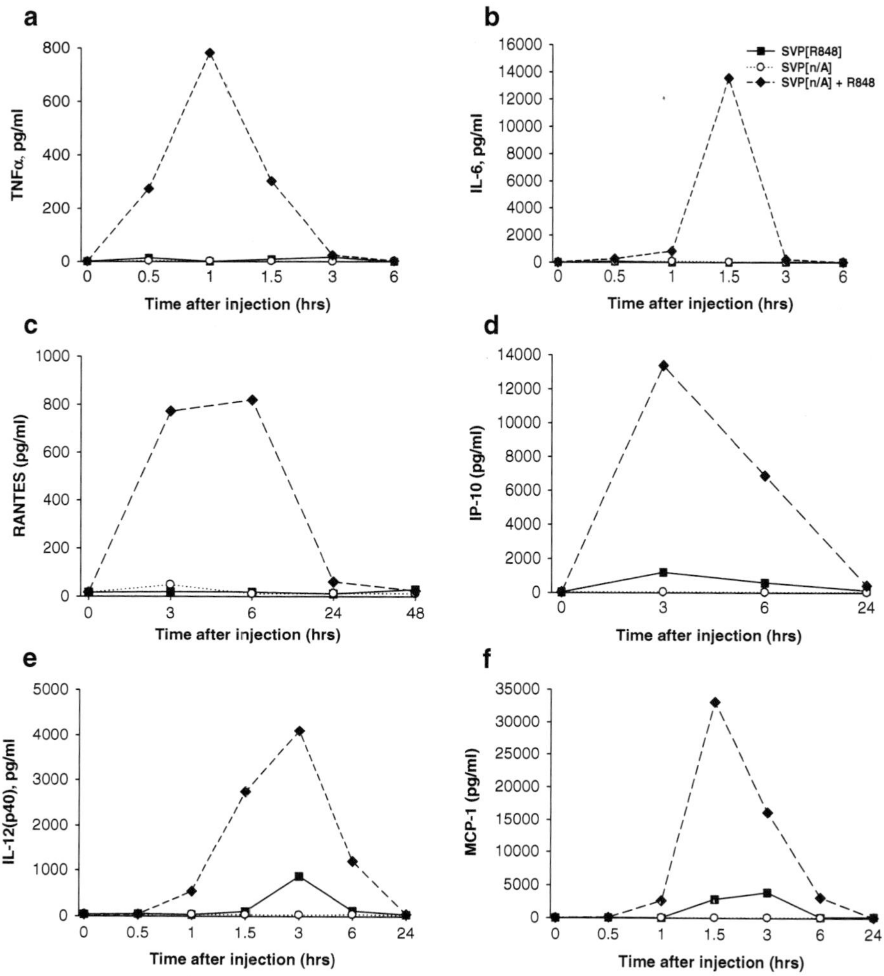

Fig. 14.7 Strong systemic cytokine induction after injection of free, but not SVP-encapsulated TLR7/TLR8 agonist R848. Mice were injected s.c. with either SVP[R848], SVP without adjuvant (SVP[n/A]), or SVP[n/A] admixed with free R848 and bled at times indicated. The same amount of free or SVP-encapsulated R848 was used for each group (6.8 μg). Serum samples were collected at the times indicated and analyzed for individual cytokines by ELISA. Average cytokine concentration is shown (three samples per group per each time point). (**a**) TNF-α, (**b**) IL-6, (**c**) RANTES, (**d**) IP-10, (**e**) IL-12(p40), (**f**) MCP-1

free R848 after either subcutaneous or intranasal inoculation (Figs. 14.7 and 14.8, respectively). In particular, 4 h after subcutaneous inoculation, serum concentrations of early inflammatory cytokines TNF-α and IL-6 were 50–200 times higher if free R848 was used (Fig. 14.7a, b). Serum cytokine levels were similar in animals inoculated with SVP[Ag] (antigen-containing SVP) with or without encapsulated R848. Similar differences were observed with systemic production of

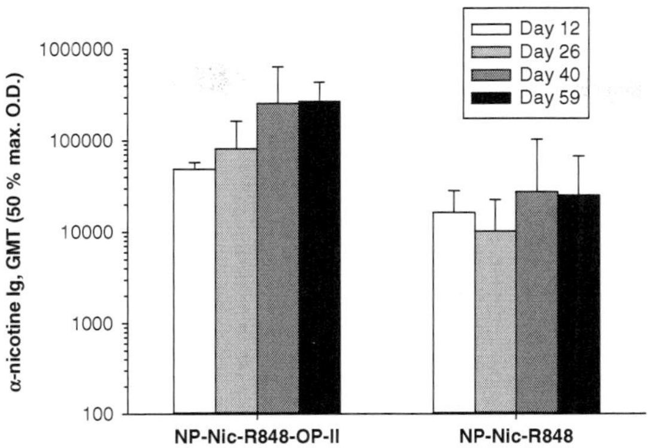

Fig. 14.8 T helper peptide OP-II provides for stronger immunogenicity upon prime and boost with SVP. Mice were immunized subcutaneously with either NP[Nic,R848] or NP[Nic,R848,OP-II] on days 0, 14, and 28. Serum was collected at days 12, 26, 40, and 59, and antibody titers to nicotine were measured by ELISA. NP[Nic,R848,OP-II] induced a significantly higher anti-nicotine antibody response than NP[Nic,R848] without OP-II (Mann–Whitney rank sum test, $p<0.005$). Bars on graph represent anti-nicotine antibody geometric mean titers (*GMT*) with standard deviations ($n=5$ mice/group)

RANTES (Fig. 14.7c). SVP[Ag,R848] induced modest levels of IP-10, IL-12(p40), and MCP-1, which were approximately five to ten times lower than that observed after injection of SVP[Ag] admixed with free R848 (Figs. 14.7d–f) (Ilyinskii et al. 2014).

14.5.2.5 T Helper Peptide Development

A T-cell helper antigen is required for effective generation of anti-nicotine antibodies by SVP since in the absence of so-called T-cell help, IgG affinity maturation and Ig class switching do not occur. Briefly, T lymphocytes can be separated into two subpopulations based on their expression of the cell surface markers CD4 and CD8. The $CD4^+$ subset is primarily responsible for providing "help" to stimulate and activate other immune cells through direct cell–cell interactions and/or the secretion of cytokines. Collaboration with B cells leads to an antibody isotype switch and enhanced antibody production. The T-cell receptors of $CD4^+$ T cells recognize peptide antigens presented by MHC class II molecules on APCs, such as DCs. MHC class II molecules generally present peptides derived from exogenous antigens. Exogenous antigens are captured by DCs and trafficked into the endo-/lysosomal compartment for processing. The resulting peptides are loaded onto MHC class II molecules and presented to MHC class II-restricted $CD4^+$ helper T cells in the draining lymph nodes.

Initially, it was demonstrated in principle that SVP can provide antigen to the MHC class II pathway for T-cell activation. For this, a well-known MHC class II-restricted peptide from ovalbumin (OVA 323–339, designated as OP-II) was used. OP-II was encapsulated into the SVP as a mouse CD4⁺ T-cell helper peptide together with nicotine antigen and R848 adjuvant and tested for nicotine antibody induction against a similar SVP without OP-II. Postvaccination, the OP-II-specific response can be detected in two ways: (1) OP-II-specific $CD4^+$ T cells can be recalled to produce interferon (IFN)-γ by co-culture in vitro with peptide-pulsed DCs and (2) indirectly by providing T-cell help to antigen-specific B cells for improved anti-nicotine antibody production. To assess the latter, two groups of mice were either immunized with SVP containing nicotine antigen and R848 or, in addition, formulated with OP-II (Fig. 14.8). Both initial immunogenicity (post-prime, d12) and, especially, further development of antibody response (post-boost) were affected by OP-II presence with animals immunized with SVP containing OP-II demonstrating approximately tenfold higher antibody titer after three injections compared to those injected with SVP without OP-II (Fig. 14.8).

OP-II is a peptide containing a dominant mouse T-cell epitope and is effectively presented by the MHC class II pathway in two mouse strains, C57BL/6 and BALB/c (the latter strain was used for T helper peptide development for SVP-based nicotine vaccine to enable comparison between OP-II and newly developed peptides). MHC class II presentation in the human population is highly varied due to allelic diversity. Thus, the most broadly recognized single pathogen-derived peptide epitopes are only recalled by approximately 70 % of individuals (Diethelm-Okita et al. 2000; James et al. 2007). Therefore, we designed and successfully tested an MHC class II-presented memory peptide with promiscuous coverage of MHC class II alleles to which the vast majority of patients are expected to respond, based on our testing of random human blood samples.

As described by Fraser et al. (Fraser et al. 2014), we screened over 30 known peptides from tetanus, adenovirus, diphtheria, respiratory syncytial virus, measles, and others, all of which are expected to be broadly recognized as memory epitopes in the human population. We used computational algorithms to determine the predicted frequency of MHC class II alleles and their affinities for peptides and selected candidates based on their affinity and cross-reactivity between alleles. Because no single epitope has been documented to generate a recall response in more than 70 % of individuals, several chimeras of two or more epitopes linked into one peptide sequence optimized for MHC class II coverage were screened (Table 14.4). We additionally engineered proteolytic cleavage sites between the epitopes of the best performing chimeras (Table 14.4). This development effort resulted in the discovery of several candidate human $CD4^+$ memory T-cell helper peptides that appear to be universal as they have elicited strong recall responses in human blood samples from random donors at near 100 % frequency. The best performing T-cell helper peptide (TCHP) was TT830DTt, designated as S-320, which was capable of efficiently inducing a helper T-cell memory recall response in 20 of 20 human donors tested (Fig. 14.9). In non-human primates vaccinated with SVP containing S-320, PBMC demonstrated efficient T-cell memory recall to the S-320 peptide (Fig. 14.10), while in BALB/c mice, nanoparticle (NP)-encapsulated S-320

Table 14.4 Single and chimeric epitopes tested for memory recall in human donors

1. ILMQYIKANSKFIGI (15, TT830)
2. IDKISDVSTIVPYIGPALNI (20, TT632)
3. NNFTVSFWLRVPKVSASHLET (21, TT950)
4. QSIALSSLMVAQAIPLVGEL (20, DT); QSIALSSLMVAQ (12, DTt)
5. TLLYVLFEV (9, AdV)
6. TLLYVLFEVNNFTVSFWLRVPKVSASHLET (30, AdVTT950)
7. ILMQYIKANSKFIGIQSIALSSLMVAQAIPLVGEL (35, TT830DT)
8. ILMQYIKANSKFIGIQSIALSSLMVAQ (27, TT830DTtrunc)
9. TLLYVLFEVILMQYIKANSKFIGI (24, AdVTT830)
10. TLLYVLFEV**PMGLP**ILMQYIKANSKFIGI (29, AdVpTT830)
11. TLLYVLFEV**KVSVR**ILMQYIKANSKFIGI (29, AdVkTT830)
12. ILMQYIKANSKFIGI**PMGLP**QSIALSSLMVAQ (32, TT830pDTt)
13. ILMQYIKANSKFIGI**KVSVR**QSIALSSLMVAQ (32, TT830kDTt)

Cathepsin cleavage sites are shown in bold
TT tetanus toxoid, *DT* diphtheria toxoid, *AdV* adenovirus

demonstrated T-cell help for anti-nicotine antibody induction to an extent comparable with OP-II (Fig. 14.11). Based on these results, S-320 was chosen as the T-cell helper peptide.

14.5.3 Production of Synthetic Vaccine Particles (SVPs)

All of the SVPs were prepared for mouse studies at a 100 mg particle scale using a double emulsion water/oil/water system (Astete and Sabliov 2006). Briefly, the polymers were dissolved in CH_2Cl_2, and S-320 was prepared in PBS. Emulsification via sonication was performed using a Branson Digital Sonifier model 250 equipped with a model 102C converter and a 1/8" tapered microtip from Branson Ultrasonics (Danbury, CT, USA). Centrifugation was carried out using a Beckman Coulter J-30I centrifuge with a JA-30.50 rotor (Beckman Coulter, Brea, CA, USA). The primary emulsion was carried out in a thick-walled glass pressure tube with an aqueous to organic phase ratio of 1:5. Following a brief sonication step, Emprove PVA aqueous solution was added to the polymer organic solution, vortex mixed, and emulsified by sonication. The resultant double emulsion was then transferred into a beaker under stirring containing 70 mM phosphate buffer pH 8.0 at a volume

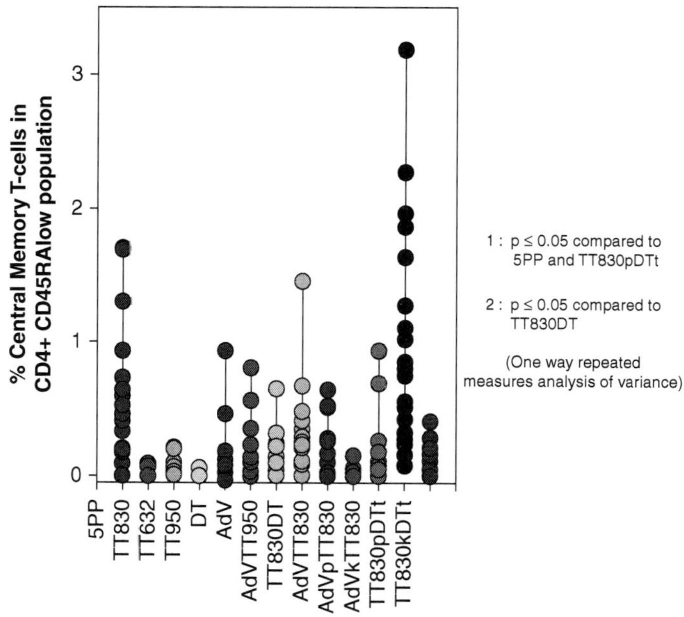

Fig. 14.9 Robust CD4 central memory T cell recall response in human donors by class II peptide chimeras derived from adenovirus, tetanus, or diphtheria toxoids. PBMCs were isolated by Ficoll density gradient centrifugation, cryopreserved, thawed, and plated at 5×10^6/mL, and peptides were added at a final concentration of 4 mM. PBMC controls were non-stimulated or stimulated with a pool of 5 peptides (5PP), respectively, and returned to 5 % CO_2 at 37 °C for 2 h, and 1 mg/mL brefeldin A was added. 6 h later the cells are transferred to a 5 % CO_2 at 25 °C and left overnight. Prior to cytometric analysis, the cells were stained with CD4-FITC, CD45RA-PE, and CD62LPE/Cy7. The cells were then permeabilized, fixed, and stained with IFN-γ. Central memory T cells were designated as CD4+/CD45RA$_{low}$/CD62L+/IFN-γ+. The values shown are the percent of CD62L+/IFN-γ+cells found in a CD4+/CD62L gate and normalized by subtracting the values for a non-stimulated control for each donor

ratio of 1 part double emulsion to 7.5 parts buffer. The organic solvent (CH_2Cl_2) was allowed to evaporate for two hours under stirring, and the nanoparticles were recovered via centrifugation at 75,600 rcf with two wash steps. PBS was used for the wash solutions and the final resuspension media. The washed SVP suspension was stored at -20 °C.

R848 and CpG loading were each determined by SVP hydrolysis followed by reversed-phase HPLC analysis. Briefly, nanoparticle solutions were centrifuged, and the pellets were subjected to base hydrolysis to release the adjuvant. R848 hydrolysis was carried out at room temperature using concentrated ammonium hydroxide. Results were quantified from the absorption of R848 at 254 nm using mobile phases comprised of water/acetonitrile/TFA. For CpG analysis, NaOH was used at elevated temperature, with results quantified from the absorption of CpG at 260 nm. The HPLC mobile phases for CpG analysis used acetonitrile/water/TEA.

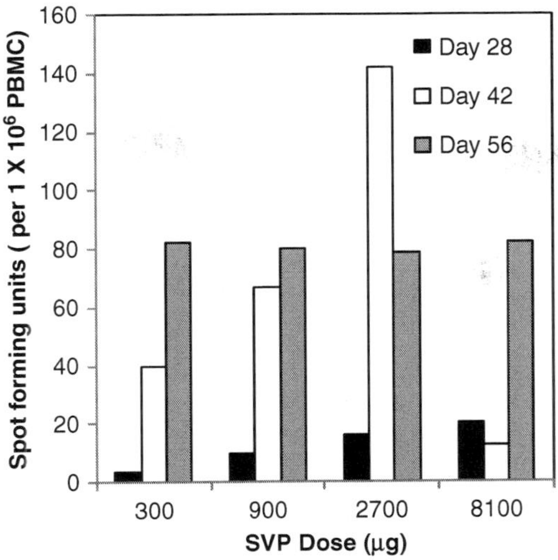

Fig. 14.10 MHC class II peptide S-320 produces a robust CD4 memory T-cell recall response in SVP-immunized non-human primates. Rhesus macaques were immunized with SVP dose levels of 300, 900, 2700, or 8100 μg of PLA–PEG–Nic per injection (shown in *X*-axis) at days 0, 28, and 56 (groups 1–4, respectively). Macaque PBMCs were isolated at days 28, 42, and 56 and stimulated with S-320 peptide, and expression of IFN-γ was measured by ELISpot. The values shown are the number of spots observed (spot-forming units) per 1×10^6 cells. PBMC analyzed from blood taken prior to the first immunization showed less than 1 SFU per 1×10^6 cells

14.5.4 Overview of Test Results in Mouse and Non-human Primate Models

Initially, 30–300 μg doses of nicotine-containing nanoparticles were evaluated for mouse studies. It was determined that the dose of 100 μg nanoparticles per injection consistently results in strong immunogenicity with no observed side effects. Therefore, mouse studies were conducted using 100 μg dose of nanoparticles at each injection. As a final test in a mouse model, animals were immunized with SVP containing all three components: nicotine antigen in the form of PLA-PEG-nicotine, TCHP S-320, and R848 adjuvant, in SVP-encapsulated form, or with several SVP/component combinations containing at least one of these component in the free form (Fig. 14.11). None of the tested combinations was equal to the SVP with all three components in the capacity to induce antibodies to nicotine.

The first non-human primate pharmacology study involved ten animals at each of 0.5 mg, 2 mg, 8 mg, and 16 mg of SVP for a prime and four boosts at 28-day intervals. A strong and specific anti-nicotine response was induced (Fig. 14.12),

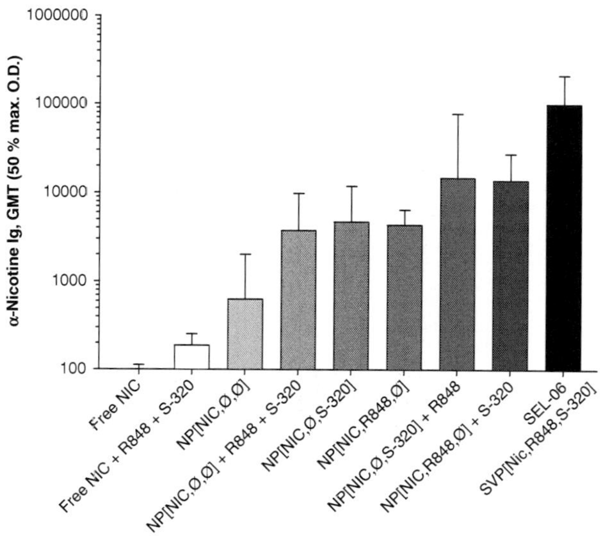

Fig. 14.11 All components are essential for induction of optimal immune response to nicotine. Mice were immunized subcutaneously with free nicotine; a mixture of free nicotine, resiquimod, and S-320 or the following SVP: NP[NIC,Ø,Ø] (SVP[Nic]), NP[NIC,Ø,S-320] (SVP[Nic, S-320]); NP[NIC,R848,Ø] (SVP[Nic,R848]) or the complete SVP vaccine SVP[Nic, R848,S-320] combined with free components as described in the legend on days 0, 14, and 28. Serum was collected at day 40, and antibody titers to nicotine measured by ELISA. The SVP with all components (nicotine nanoparticles with entrapped resiquimod and S-320) induced a significantly higher anti-nicotine antibody response than any of the other formulations (Mann–Whitney rank sum test, $p<0.005$). Bars on graph represent anti-nicotine antibody GMT with standard deviations ($n=10$ mice/group)

and the vaccine was well tolerated by the animals at all doses. Equilibrium dialysis measurement of nicotine antibodies affinity and concentration in NHP group immunized with 8 mg of SVP yielded values for B_{max} of 310.04 nM (46.51 μg/mL) and of 13.78 nM for K_d.

Collectively, in the preclinical studies of the SVP nicotine vaccine, we observed the following:

- A strong and specific anti-nicotine response is induced by immunization of non-human primates.
- A strong and specific anti-nicotine response is induced by immunization of mice with nicotine SVP carrying an adjuvant and a T-cell helper peptide, both of which are essential for generation of potent anti-nicotine antibody responses.
- Immunization with SVP-encapsulated resiquimod does not induce systemic inflammatory cytokines in mice.
- Antibodies induced by immunization with nicotine SVP possess high affinity for nicotine.
- S-320, a peptide capable of stimulating helper T-cell recall responses in humans, has been developed, and it contributes to a potent anti-nicotine antibody response in vivo in mouse and non-human primate immunization models.

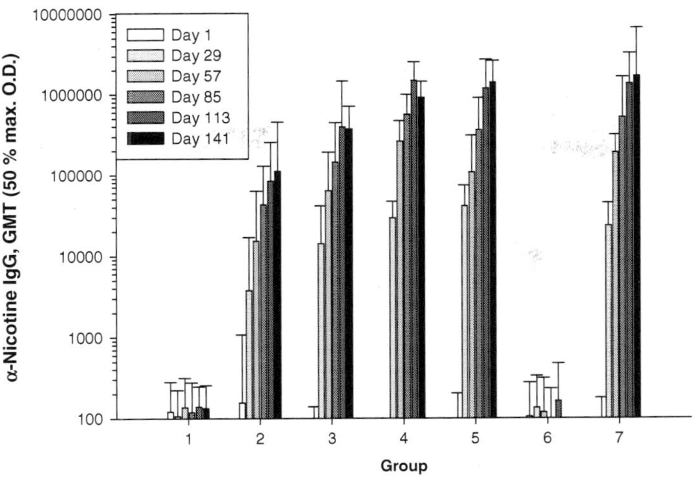

Fig. 14.12 SVP generates anti-nicotine antibodies in a dose-dependent manner, and additional injections of SVP boost this response. Cynomolgus monkeys were injected with saline (group 1), or SVP doses of 0.5, 2, 8, or 16 mg (groups 2–5, respectively), at each of days 1, 29, 57, 85, and 113. Two groups of cynomolgus monkeys were preexposed to nicotine by oral gavage prior to injection, one group received saline injection post-gavage (group 6), and the other an SVP dose of 8 mg PLA–PEG–nicotine per injection (group 7) at days 1, 29, 57, 85, and 113. Blood was collected and sera isolated prior to each injection and prior to recovery necropsy. Anti-nicotine antibody titers were measured by ELISA. Bars on graph represent anti-nicotine antibody GMT with standard deviations

14.6 Conclusion

Since so few promising novel vaccines against drug addiction are now close to clinical application, it has been convincingly argued that utilization of completely novel paradigms may be necessary, including the use of synthetic nanoparticle (NP) platforms as opposed to modified VLP and protein-based carriers. Among the most exciting aspects of nanoparticles is their potential to mimic features of pathogens such as viruses. Since NPs can encapsulate or be decorated with protein, peptide, and haptens along with other immune-potentiating components, they may be viewed by the immune system as real pathogens (Mamo and Poland 2012). Over the course of recent wide-ranging studies by many research groups, no significant safety or toxicity concerns have been detected (Mahapatro and Singh 2011; Galloway et al. 2013; Su et al. 2011; Taha et al. 2012; Voltan et al. 2007). It is apparent that synthetic polymer-based platforms may provide augmented immunogenicity by efficient adjuvant delivery, surface exposure of conserved antigens, and T-cell response induction (Bachmann and Jennings 2010; Jennings and Bachmann 2009). Additionally, modular production may permit manufacturing of ready-to-use polymeric NPs with various active groups exposed on their surface, in effect using them as "platforms" for the presentation of foreign epitopes. These particles will potentially have a long shelf life, and there is even a possibility of immunogenic nanoparticles being successfully stored for months or potentially, even years at ambient temperatures, without refrigeration (Sloat et al. 2010).

Therefore, synthetic polymeric NPs have a potential to provide a solution for several pressing issues in developing vaccines for drug addiction: induce T-cell memory response, augment immunogenicity of non-immunogenic hapten antigens, and alleviate safety concerns regarding novel adjuvants, thus permitting their clinical utilization. Collectively, polymer NP-based vaccines may eventually pave the new avenues for discovery, testing, manufacturing, and clinical application of vaccines against drug addiction.

References

Akahata W, Yang ZY, Andersen H, Sun S, Holdaway HA, et al. A virus-like particle vaccine for epidemic Chikungunya virus protects nonhuman primates against infection. Nat Med. 2010;16(3):334–8.

Alving CR, Peachman KK, Rao M, Reed SG. Adjuvants for human vaccines. Curr Opin Immunol. 2012;24(3):310–5.

Andersen BM, Ohlfest JR. Increasing the efficacy of tumor cell vaccines by enhancing cross priming. Cancer Lett. 2012;325(2):155–64.

Astete C, Sabliov C. Synthesis and characterization of PLGA nanoparticles. J Biomater Sci Polymer Ed. 2006;17:247–89.

Bachmann MF, Jennings GT. Vaccine delivery: a matter of size, geometry, kinetics and molecular patterns. Nat Rev Immunol. 2010;10:787–96.

Barrett ADT, Stanberry LR. Vaccines for biodefense and emerging and neglected diseases. San Diego: Academic; 2009.

Basith S, Manavalan B, Lee G, Kim SG, Choi S. Toll-like receptor modulators: a patent review (2006-2010). Expert Opin Ther Pat. 2011;21:927–44.

Bjercke RJ, Cook G, Rychlik N, Gjika HB, Van Vunakis H, Langone JJ. Stereospecific monoclonal antibodies to nicotine and cotinine and their use in enzyme-linked immunosorbent assays. J Immunol Methods. 1986;90(2):203–13.

Castro A, Monji N, Ali H, Yi JM, Bowman ER, McKennis Jr H. Nicotine antibodies: comparison of ligand specificities of antibodies produced against two nicotine conjugates. Eur J Biochem. 1980;104(2):331–40.

Centers for Disease Control and Prevention. Smoking-attributable mortality, years of potential life lost, and productivity losses—United States, 2000–2004. Morb Mortal Wkly Rep. 2008;57(45): 1226–8.

Cerny T. Anti-nicotine vaccination: where are we? Recent Results Cancer Res. 2005;166:167–75.

Clinicaltrials.gov. 2015. Accessed 18 July 2015.

Cornuz J, Zwahlen S, Jungi WF, Osterwalder J, Klingler K, van Melle G, et al. A vaccine against nicotine for smoking cessation: a randomized controlled trial. PLoS One. 2008;3(6), e2547.

Cruz LJ, Cabrales A, Iglesias E, Aguilar JC, González LJ, Reyes O. Enhanced immunogenicity and cross-reactivity of HIV-1 V3-peptide and multiple antigen peptides conjugated to distinct carrier proteins. Int Immunopharmacol. 2009;9(12):1452–9.

De Filette M, Martens W, Smet A, Schotsaert M, Birkett A, et al. Universal influenza A M2e-HBc vaccine protects against disease even in the presence of pre-existing anti-HBc antibodies. Vaccine. 2008;26(51):6503–7.

Denis J, Acosta-Ramirez E, Zhao Y, Hamelin ME, Koukavica I, et al. Development of a universal influenza A vaccine based on the M2e peptide fused to the papaya mosaic virus (PapMV) vaccine platform. Vaccine. 2008;26(27-28):3395–403.

Diebold SS, Kaisho T, Hemmi H, Akira S, Reis e Sousa C. Innate antiviral responses by means of TLR7-mediated recognition of single-stranded RNA. Science. 2004;303:1529–31.

Diebold SS. Recognition of viral single-stranded RNA by Toll-like receptors. Adv Drug Deliv Rev. 2008;60:813–23.

Diethelm-Okita BM, Okita DK, Banaszak L, Conti-Fine BM. Universal epitopes for human CD4+ cells on tetanus and diphtheria toxins. J Infect Dis. 2000;181(3):1001–9.

Doxsee CL, Riter TR, Reiter MJ, Gibson SJ, Vasilakos JP, Kedl RM. The immune response modifier and Toll-like receptor 7 agonist S-27609 selectively induces IL-12 and TNF-alpha production in CD11c+CD11b+CD8- dendritic cells. J Immunol. 2003;71:1156–63.

Edwards AD, Diebold SS, Slack EM, Tomizawa H, Hemmi H, Kaisho T, Akira S, Reis e Sousa C. Toll-like receptor expression in murine DC subsets: lack of TLR7 expression by CD8 alpha+DC correlates with unresponsiveness to imidazoquinolines. Eur J Immunol. 2003;33:827–33.

Escobar-Chávez JJ, Domínguez-Delgado CL, Rodríguez-Cruz IM. Targeting nicotine addiction: the possibility of a therapeutic vaccine. Drug Des Devel Ther. 2011;5:211–24.

Esterlis I, Hannestad JO, Perkins E, Bois F, D'Souza DC, et al. Effect of a nicotine vaccine on nicotine binding to b2*-Nicotinic acetylcholine receptors in vivo in human tobacco smokers. Am J Psychiatry. 2013;170(4):399–407.

Fahim RE, Kessler PD, Fuller SA, Kalnik MW. Nicotine vaccines. CNS Neurol Disord Drug Targets. 2011;10(8):905–15.

Fahim RE, Kessler PD, Kalnik MW. Therapeutic vaccines against tobacco addiction. Expert Rev Vaccines. 2013;12(3):333–42.

Fraser CC, Altreuter DH, Ilyinskii P, Pittet L, LaMothe RA, et al. Generation of a universal CD4 memory T cell recall peptide effective in humans, mice and non-human primates. Vaccine. 2014;32(24):2896–903.

Galloway AL, Murphy A, DeSimone JM, Di J, Herrmann JP, Hunter ME, et al. Development of a nanoparticle-based influenza vaccine using the PRINT technology. Nanomedicine. 2013;9(4): 523–31.

Ghasparian A, Riedel T, Koomullil J, Moehle K, Gorba C, et al. Engineered synthetic virus-like particles and their use in vaccine delivery. Chembiochem. 2011;12:100–9.

Harper DM. Currently approved prophylactic HPV vaccines. Expert Rev Vaccines. 2009;8:1663–79.

Hartmann-Boyce J, Cahill K, Hatsukami D, Cornuz J. Nicotine vaccines for smoking cessation. Cochrane Database Syst Rev. 2012;(8):CD007072. doi:10.1002/14651858.

Hashemi H, Pouyanfard S, Bandehpour M, Noroozbabaei Z, Kazemi B, et al. Immunization with M2e-displaying T7 bacteriophage nanoparticles protects against influenza A virus challenge. PLoS One. 2012;7(9), e45765.

Hatsukami DK, Jorenby DE, Gonzales D, Rigotti NA, Glover ED, et al. Immunogenicity and smoking-cessation outcomes for a novel nicotine immunotherapeutic. Clin Pharmacol Ther. 2011;89:392–9.

Heil F, Hemmi H, Hochrein H, Ampenberger F, Kirschning C, Akira S, Lipford G, Wagner H, Bauer S. Species-specific recognition of single-stranded RNA via toll-like receptor 7 and 8. Science. 2004;303:1526–9.

Heit A, Busch DH, Wagner H, Schmitz F. Vaccine protocols for enhanced immunogenicity of exogenous antigens. Int J Med Microbiol. 2008;298(1-2):27–32.

Hemmi H, Takeuchi O, Kawai T, Kaisho T, Sato S, Sanjo H, Matsumoto M, Hoshino K, Wagner H, Takeda K, Akira S. A toll-like receptor recognizes bacterial DNA. Nature. 2000;408:740–5.

Hemmi H, Kaisho T, Takeuchi O, Sato S, Sanjo H, Hoshino K, Horiuchi T, Tomizawa H, Takeda K, Akira S. Small anti-viral compounds activate immune cells via the TLR7 MyD88-dependent signaling pathway. Nat Immunol. 2002;3:196–200.

Hoogsteder PH, Kotz D, van Spiegel PI, Viechtbauer W, Brauer R, et al. The efficacy and safety of a nicotine conjugate vaccine (NicVAX®) or placebo co-administered with varenicline (Champix®) for smoking cessation: study protocol of a phase IIb, double blind, randomized, placebo controlled trial. BMC Public Health. 2012;12:1052. doi:10.1186/1471-2458-12-1052.

Ilyinskii PO, Roy CJ, O'Neil CP, Browning EA, Pittet LA, et al. Adjuvant-carrying synthetic vaccine particles augment the immune response to encapsulated antigen and exhibit strong local immune activation without inducing systemic cytokine release. Vaccine. 2014;32(24): 2882–95.

James EA, Bui J, Berger D, Huston L, Roti M, Kwok WW. Tetramer-guided epitope mapping reveals broad, individualized repertoires of tetanus toxin-specificCD4+ T cells and suggests HLA-based differences in epitope recognition. Int Immunol. 2007;19(11):1291–301.

Jennings GT, Bachmann MF. Immunodrugs: therapeutic VLP-based vaccines for chronic diseases. Annu Rev Pharmacol Toxicol. 2009;49:303–26.

Johnson DA. Synthetic TLR4-active glycolipids as vaccine adjuvants and stand-alone immunotherapeutics. Curr Top Med Chem. 2008;8:64–79.

Junt T, Moseman EA, Iannacone M, Massberg S, Lang PA, et al. Subcapsular sinus macrophages in lymph nodes clear lymph-borne viruses and present them to antiviral B cells. Nature. 2007;450:110–4.

Jurk M, Heil F, Vollmer J, Schetter C, Krieg AM, Wagner H, Lipford G, Bauer S. Human TLR7 or TLR8 independently confer responsiveness to the antiviral compound R-848. Nat Immunol. 2002;3:499.

Karan D, Krieg AM, Lubaroff DM. Paradoxical enhancement of CD8 T cell-dependent anti-tumor protection despite reduced CD8 T cell responses with addition of a TLR9 agonist to a tumor vaccine. Int J Cancer. 2007;121:1520–8.

Kasturi SP, Skountzou I, Albrecht RA, Koutsonanos D, Hua T, et al. Programming the magnitude and persistence of antibody responses with innate immunity. Nature. 2011;470:543–7.

Kozlovska TM, Cielens I, Dreilinņa D, Dislers A, Baumanis V, et al. Recombinant RNA phage Q beta capsid particles synthesized and self-assembled in Escherichia coli. Gene. 1993;137(1):133–7.

Krieg AM. Therapeutic potential of Toll-like receptor 9 activation. Nat Rev Drug Discov. 2006;5:471–84.

Krieg AM. Antiinfective applications of Toll-like receptor 9 agonists. Proc Am Thorac Soc. 2007;4:289–94.

Krieg AM, Yi AK, Matson S, Waldschmidt TJ, Bishop GA, Teasdale R, Koretzky GA, Klinman DM. CpG motifs in bacterial DNA trigger direct B-cell activation. Nature. 1995;374:546–9.

Lockner JW, Lively JM, Collins KC, Vendruscolo JC, Azar MR, Janda KD. A conjugate vaccine using enantiopure hapten imparts superior nicotine-binding capacity. J Med Chem. 2015;58:1005–11.

Mahapatro A, Singh DK. Biodegradable nanoparticles are excellent vehicle for site directed in-vivo delivery of drugs and vaccines. J Nanobiotechnol. 2011;9:55.

Malyala P, O'Hagan DT, Singh M. Enhancing the therapeutic efficacy of CpG oligonucleotides using biodegradable microparticles. Adv Drug Deliv Rev. 2009;61:218–25.

Mamo T, Poland GA. Nanovaccinology: the next generation of vaccines meets 21st century materials science and engineering. Vaccine. 2012;30(47):6609–11.

Manolova V, Flace A, Bauer M, Schwarz K, Saudan P, Bachmann MF. Nanoparticles target distinct dendritic cell populations according to their size. Eur J Immunol. 2008;38(5):1404–13.

Maurer P, Jennings GT, Willers J, Rohner F, Lindman Y, et al. A therapeutic vaccine for nicotine dependence: preclinical efficacy, and Phase I safety and immunogenicity. Eur J Immunol. 2005;35(7):2031–40.

McCluskie MJ, Pryde DC, Gervais DP, Stead DR, Zhang N, et al. Enhancing immunogenicity of a 3′aminomethylnicotine-DT-conjugate anti-nicotine vaccine with CpG adjuvant in mice and non-human primates. Int Immunopharmacol. 2013;16(1):50–6.

McCluskie MJ, Thorn J, Mehelic PR, Kolhe P, Bhattacharya K, et al. Molecular attributes of conjugate antigen influence function of antibodies induced by anti-nicotine vaccine in mice and non-human primates. Int Immunopharmacol. 2015;25(2):518–27.

Oncken C, Gonzales D, Nides M, Rennard S, Watsky E, Billing CB, et al. Efficacy and safety of the novel selective nicotinic acetylcholine receptor partial agonist, varenicline, for smoking cessation. Arch Intern Med. 2006;166:1571–7.

Parez N, Fourgeux C, Mohamed A, Dubuquoy C, Pillot M, et al. Rectal immunization with rotavirus virus-like particles induces systemic and mucosal humoral immune responses and protects mice against rotavirus infection. J Virol. 2006;80(4):1752–61.

Pentel PR, LeSage MG. New directions in nicotine vaccine design and use. Adv Pharmacol. 2014;69:553–80.

Pentel PR, Malin DH, Ennifar S, Hieda Y, Keyler DE, et al. A nicotine conjugate vaccine reduces nicotine distribution to brain and attenuates its behavioral and cardiovascular effects in rats. Pharmacol Biochem Behav. 2000;65(1):191–8.

Plotkin S, Orenstein W, Offit P. Vaccines. 6th ed. Philadelphia: Elsevier Saunders; 2012.

Pockros PJ, Guyader D, Patton H, Tong MJ, Wright T, McHutchison JG, Meng TC. Oral resiquimod in chronic HCV infection: safety and efficacy in 2 placebo-controlled, double-blind phase IIa studies. J Hepatol. 2007;47:174–82.

Pryde DC, Jones LH, Gervais DP, Stead DR, Blakemore DC. Selection of a novel anti-nicotine vaccine: influence of antigen design on antibody function in mice. PLoS One. 2013;8(100), e76557.

Qian J, Dong Y, Pang YY, Ibrahim R, Berzofsky JA, et al. Combined prophylactic and therapeutic cancer vaccine: enhancing CTL responses to HPV16 E2 using a chimeric VLP in HLA-A2 mice. Int J Cancer. 2006;118(12):3022–9.

Quan FS, Huang C, Compans RW, Kang SM. Virus-like particle vaccine induces protective immunity against homologous and heterologous strains of influenza virus. J Virol. 2007;81(7):3514–24.

Reddy ST, van der Vlies AJ, Simeoni E, Angeli V, Randolph GJ, et al. Exploiting lymphatic transport and complement activation in nanoparticle vaccines. Nat Biotechnol. 2007;25(10):1159–64.

Roman M, Martin-Orozco E, Goodman JS, Nguyen MD, Sato Y, Ronaghy A, Kornbluth RS, Richman DD, Carson DA, Raz E. Immunostimulatory DNA sequences function as T helper-1-promoting adjuvants. Nat Med. 1997;3:849–54.

Sato Y, Roman M, Tighe H, Lee D, Corr M, et al. Immunostimulatory DNA sequences necessary for effective intradermal gene immunization. Science. 1996;273:352–4.

Schneemann A, Speir JA, Tan GS, Khayat R, Ekiert DC, et al. A virus-like particle that elicits cross-reactive antibodies to the conserved stem of influenza virus hemagglutinin. J Virol. 2012;86(21):11686–97.

Singh M, Kazzaz J, Ugozzoli M, Malyala P, Chesko J, O'Hagan DT. Polylactide-co-glycolide microparticles with surface adsorbed antigens as vaccine delivery systems. Curr Drug Deliv. 2006;3:115–20.

Sloat BR, Sandoval MA, Cui Z. Towards preserving the immunogenicity of protein antigens carried by nanoparticles while avoiding the cold chain. Int J Pharm. 2010;393(1-2):197–202.

Slupetzky K, Gambhira R, Culp TD, Shafti-Keramat S, Schellenbacher C, et al. A papillomavirus-like particle (VLP) vaccine displaying HPV16 L2 epitopes induces cross-neutralizing antibodies to HPV11. Vaccine. 2007;25(11):2001–10.

Sparwasser T, Miethke T, Lipford G, Borschert K, Häcker H, Heeg K, Wagner H. Bacterial DNA causes septic shock. Nature. 1997;386:336–7.

Storni T, Lechner F, Erdmann I, Bächi T, Jegerlehner A, et al. Critical role for activation of antigen-presenting cells in priming of cytotoxic T cell responses after vaccination with virus-like particles. J Immunol. 2002;168(6):2880–6.

Su X, Fricke J, Kavanagh DG, Irvine DJ. In vitro and in vivo mRNA delivery using lipid-enveloped pH-responsive polymer nanoparticles. Mol Pharm. 2011;8(3):774–87.

Swain SL, McKinstry KK, Strutt TM. Expanding roles for $CD4^+$ T cells in immunity to viruses. Nat Rev Immunol. 2012;12(2):136–48.

Taha MA, Singh SR, Dennis VA. Biodegradable PLGA85/15 nanoparticles as a delivery vehicle for Chlamydia trachomatis recombinant MOMP-187 peptide. Nanotechnology. 2012;23(32):325101.

Tan M, Huang P, Xia M, Fang PA, Zhong W, et al. Norovirus P particle, a novel platform for vaccine development and antibody production. J Virol. 2011;85(2):753–64.

Tonstad S, Heggen E, Giljam H, Lagerbäck PÅ, Tønnesen P, et al. Niccine®, a nicotine vaccine, for relapse prevention: a phase II, randomized, placebo-controlled, multicenter clinical trial. Nicotine Tob Res. 2013;15(9):1492–501.

Vasilakos JP, Smith RMA, Gibson SJ, Lindh JM, Pederson LK, et al. Adjuvant activities of immune response modifier R-848: comparison with CpG ODN. Cell Immunol. 2000;204:64–74.

Vicente T, Roldão A, Peixoto C, Carrondo MJ, Alves PM. Large-scale production and purification of VLP-based vaccines. J Invertebr Pathol. 2011;107(Suppl):S42–8.

Voltan R, Castaldello A, Brocca-Cofano E, Altavilla G, Caputo A, et al. Preparation and characterization of innovative protein-coated poly(methylmethacrylate) core-shell nanoparticles for vaccine purposes. Pharm Res. 2007;24(10):1870–82.

Wagner H. The immunogenicity of CpG-antigen conjugates. Adv Drug Deliv Rev. 2009; 61:243–7.

Wang W, Singh M. Selection of adjuvants for enhanced vaccine potency. World J Vaccines. 2011;1:33–78.

Wang Y, Abel K, Lantz K, Krieg AM, McChesney MB, Miller CJ. The toll-like receptor 7 (TLR7) agonist, imiquimod, and the TLR9 agonist, CpG ODN, induce antiviral cytokines and chemokines but do not prevent vaginal transmission of simian immunodeficiency virus when applied intravaginally to rhesus macaques. J Virol. 2005;79:14355–70.

Wille-Reece U, Flynn BJ, Loré K, Koup RA, Miles AP, Saul A, Kedl RM, Mattapallil JJ, Weiss WR, Roederer M, Seder RA. Toll-like receptor agonists influence the magnitude and quality of memory T cell responses after prime-boost immunization in nonhuman primates. J Exp Med. 2006;203:1249–58.

Woo WP, Doan T, Herd KA, Netter HJ, Tindle RW. Hepatitis B surface antigen vector delivers protective cytotoxic T-lymphocyte responses to disease-relevant foreign epitopes. J Virol. 2006;80(8):3975–84.

Young SL, Wilson M, Wilson S, Beagley KW, Ward V, Baird MA. Transcutaneous vaccination with virus-like particles. Vaccine. 2006;24(26):5406–12.

Chapter 15
Exploration of DNA Nanostructures for Rational Design of Vaccines

Xiaowei Liu, Sidney M. Hecht, Hao Yan, Paul R. Pentel, and Yung Chang

Abbreviations

APCs	Antigen-presenting cells
BCRs	B-cell receptors
cGAMP	Cyclic GMP-AMP

X. Liu
Center for Infectious Diseases and Vaccinology, The Biodesign Institute, Arizona State University, Tempe, AZ 85287, USA

S.M. Hecht
Center for BioEnergetics, The Biodesign Institute, Arizona State University, Tempe, AZ 85287, USA

Department of Chemistry and Biochemistry, Arizona State University, Tempe, AZ 85287, USA

H. Yan
Center for Molecular Design and Biomimetics, The Biodesign Institute, Arizona State University, Tempe, AZ 85287, USA

Department of Chemistry and Biochemistry, Arizona State University, Tempe, AZ 85287, USA

P.R. Pentel
Minneapolis Medical Research Foundation, Minneapolis, MN 55404, USA

Department of Medicine, University of Minnesota Medical School, Minneapolis, MN 55415, USA

Y. Chang (✉)
Center for Infectious Diseases and Vaccinology, The Biodesign Institute, Arizona State University, Tempe, AZ 85287, USA

School of Life Sciences, Arizona State University, Tempe, AZ 85287, USA
e-mail: yung.chang@asu.edu

I.D. Montoya (ed.), *Biologics to Treat Substance Use Disorders: Vaccines, Monoclonal Antibodies, and Enzymes*, DOI 10.1007/978-3-319-23150-1_15

cGAS	Cyclic GMP-AMP synthase
CpG ODN	Cytosine-phosphodiester-guanine oligonucleotide
DC	Dendritic cells
DNase	Deoxyribonuclease
FDC	Follicular dendritic cells
GC	Germinal center
IDO	Indoleamine-2, 3-dioxygenase
IFN	Interferon
LLPCs	Long-lived plasma cells
MYD88	Myeloid differentiation primary response 88
Nic	Nicotine
Nic-KLH	Nicotine-keyhole limpet hemocyanin conjugates
Nic-SA-CpG	Nicotine-streptavidin-biotin-CpG conjugates
Nic-SA-TH-CpG	Tetrahedron DNA assembled with Nic-SA conjugates and CpG
OVA	Ovalbumin
PAMP	Pathogen-associated molecular patterns
SA	Streptavidin
STING	Stimulator of interferon genes
T_{FH}	T follicular helper cells
TH	Tetrahedron DNA
TH-CpG	Tetrahedron DNA assembled with CpG
TLR	Toll-like receptor
VLPs	Virus-like particles

15.1 Introduction

Vaccines specific to drugs of abuse have been explored as one type of biologics for treating drug addiction. Vaccine efficacy is dependent on durable production of high-titered and high-affinity antibodies that can bind to these small chemical compounds and block their entrance into the brain. Many studies on B-cell biology have shown that high-quality antibody responses result from the persistence of memory B cells and long-lived plasma cells (LLPCs) that produce high-affinity antibodies (Tarlinton and Good-Jacobson 2013). Recently, several memory B-cell subsets, generated either from germinal centers (GCs) or independently of GCs, were identified and the mechanisms underlying their production, maintenance, and selection for high antibody affinity have been extensively studied (Pape et al. 2011; Taylor et al. 2012; Elgueta et al. 2010; McHeyzer-Williams et al. 2012; Zuccarino-Catania et al. 2014). Essentially, two signals are required for effective B-cell responses. One is an antigen-dependent activation signal induced upon antigen interaction with the membrane immunoglobulin, an important component of B-cell receptors (BCRs) expressed by antigen-specific B cells, while the other is an accessory signal integrated from the concerted actions of various cell types in response to the antigen and adjuvants, including dendritic cells (DCs), cognate follicular T helper (T_{FH}) cells, follicular dendritic cells (FDCs), non-cognate B cells, and many others (Heesters et al. 2014; Rawlings et al. 2012). Thus, ideal antigens should activate both of these signaling pathways for the generation of high-quality B-cell responses.

It has long been recognized that particulate antigens, such as virus or virus-like particles (VLPs), can induce a long-term production of antibodies specific to many proteins displayed on the surface of these viral particles, yet immunization with the same proteins often results in a low-level and short-lived production of antibodies (Bachmann and Jennings 2010; Slifka and Amanna 2014). The high immunogenicity of particulate antigens has been ascribed to (1) increased antigen transport to and retention within secondary lymphoid tissues, (2) repetitive display of multivalent antigenic epitopes for cross-linking BCRs, and (3) adjuvant activity either intrinsic to particulate structures or attributed to the presence of pathogen-associated molecular pattern (PAMP) molecules (Bachmann and Jennings 2010). Nanotechnology and nanomaterials harness the engineering potential of particulate antigens for rational design and construction of effective nanoparticle-based vaccines by mimicking biophysical and biochemical cues from viruses and VLPs (Irvine et al. 2013; Zhao et al. 2014; Mora-Solano and Collier 2014; Swartz et al. 2012; Smith et al. 2013a).

Many synthetic micro/nanoparticles have been explored as vaccine carriers to induce B-cell responses (Swartz et al. 2012). For example, as reported by Moon et al, the malaria antigen displayed by nanoparticles that are composed of interbilayer-cross-linked multilamellar lipid vesicles (ICMVs) was found to elicit strong humoral responses, presumably by promoting germinal center formation and expansion of T_{FH} cells (Moon et al. 2012). Biodegradable polymer micro- or nanoparticles, such as poly(L-lactic-co-glycolic acid (PLGA), have been investigated for their action in antigen delivery (Swartz et al. 2012; Gregory et al. 2013; Pavot et al. 2014). The PLGA polymer encapsulated with various purified proteins or peptides in combination with Toll-like receptor (TLR) ligands has been shown by many groups to induce strong and persistent antibody responses (Kasturi et al. 2011; Jewell et al. 2011). Research involving particles such as PLGA, liposome, and VLPs has also been extended to the construction of vaccines against nicotine although the efficacy of these vaccines has been mixed, especially in comparison to the conventional hapten-protein conjugate vaccines (Lockner et al. 2013; Hu et al. 2014; Fraser et al. 2014).

DNA nanostructures have emerged as a new nanomaterial, which has been explored for biomedical application (Nishikawa et al. 2010; Smith et al. 2013b; Charoenphol and Bermudez 2014). Here, we highlight the feasibility and potential of using DNA nanostructures for rational design and construction of synthetic vaccines. We demonstrate that a potent and long-lasting anti-nicotine antibody response could be elicited by an appropriate priming/boost combination of DNA-directed nicotine vaccines with nicotine-protein conjugates and is effective in blocking nicotine entry into the brain. Due to the robust assembly and programmability of DNA nanostructures, DNA-assembled nicotine vaccines can be readily optimized in a modular fashion to further enhance nicotine immunogenicity.

15.2 Self-Assembly DNA Nanostructures and Their Biomedical Applications

In addition to encoding genetic information, DNA is also an excellent structural material (Seeman 2003, 2010; Lin et al. 2009). Various DNA nanostructures have been built, ranging from two-dimensional DNA bricks and nanoarrays to highly ordered three-dimensional DNA devices with defined shapes and sizes (Fig. 15.1) (Pinheiro et al. 2011; Seeman 1982; Yan et al. 2003; Bath and Turberfield 2007; Rothemund 2006; Dietz et al. 2009; Douglas et al. 2010; Han et al. 2010, 2011, 2013). All of these DNA nanostructures are self-assembled autonomously

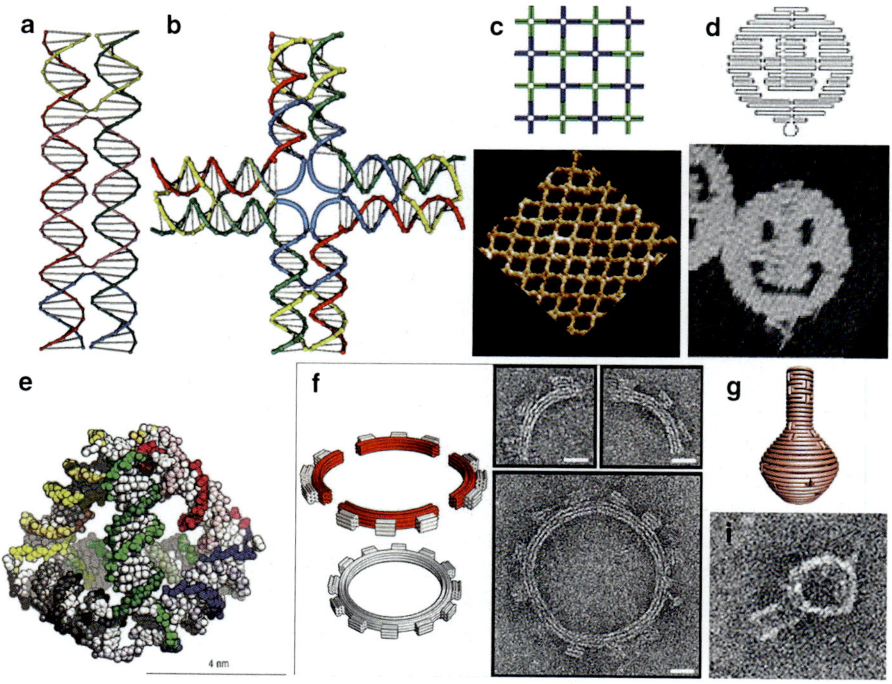

Fig. 15.1 Representative DNA nanostructures. (**a**) Representative DNA double crossover, known as DAE (double crossover in antiparallel with even number of helical half turns between crossovers) (Lin et al. 2009; Seeman 1982) (Adapted with permission from (Lin et al. 2009), copyright (2009) American Chemical Society). (**b**) Four-way DNA tile built of Holliday junction-like DNA junctions, which may assemble into two-dimensional DNA arrays as shown in (**c**) (Adapted from (Yan et al. 2003). Reprinted with permission from AAAS). (**d**) DNA origami assembled from about 7 kilobase circular M13 genomic DNA that is folded by about 200 short DNA "staple" strands (From (Rothemund 2006). Reprinted with permission from AAAS). (**e**) Tetrahedral-shaped DNA (Reproduced with permission from (Bath and Turberfield 2007)). (**f**) Curved DNA bundle with non-bent teeth, four of which assembles into a twelve-tooth gear (From (Dietz et al. 2009). Reprinted with permission from AAAS). (**g**) Vase-shaped DNA origami with curvature (From (Han et al. 2011). Reprinted with permission from AAAS)

following the simple rule of Watson-Crick base pairing, and the basis for such assembly lies in the sequence design of individual synthetic oligonucleotides, and manufacture is facilitated by computational design programs (Williams et al. 2010; Douglas et al. 2009). The design of DNA nanostructures is therefore rational and assembly is robust and programmable. Any functional group that is prelabeled on certain component oligonucleotides can be placed at predefined positions on the assembled nanostructure (Ke et al. 2008; Rinker et al. 2008; Zhao et al. 2011; Liu et al. 2011). Moreover, the existence of various DNA crossovers within the nanostructures provides control over desired structural rigidity, which contributes to the controlled configuration of these functional groups. All these features allow easy incorporation, organization, and subsequent release of various cargos. Due to the recent development of DNA conjugation techniques, a diverse set of functional groups can be attached to DNA oligonucleotides covalently or non-covalently, expediting construction of customized DNA platforms for multiple purposes including but not limited to fluorescence-based multiplexed imaging and/or DNA detection devices (Ke et al. 2008; Lin et al. 2006; Liang et al. 2014; Campolongo et al. 2010).

Aside from regular double-strand DNA in plasmid or other transfectant vectors, DNA nanostructures are more compact, which may facilitate their cellular uptake and may help enhance nuclease resistance due to steric hindrance (Keum and Bermudez 2009; Mei et al. 2011). There are many reports demonstrating the feasibility of DNA nanostructures as nano-vehicles for therapeutic cargo transportation ranging from imaging agents and chemical compounds (Jiang et al. 2012; Kim et al. 2013; Li et al. 2013a; Zhang et al. 2014; Yan et al. 2015) to functional nucleic acid motifs (e.g., aptamer, antisense oligonucleotides, siRNA, miRNA, and CpG ODN) (Keum et al. 2011; Li et al. 2011; Schüller et al. 2011; Mohri et al. 2012; Lee et al. 2012). Furthermore, changes in pH or cation concentration within the cellular environment may trigger conformational changes of DNA motifs, forming such structures as i-motifs and G-quadruplexes, which, when used in combination with various DNA nanostructures, has proven to be effective for controlled release of drugs in anticancer therapy (Yang et al. 2012; Dong et al. 2014; Li and Famulok 2013).

Composed of mostly natural biological components, DNA nanostructures are considered to be biocompatible. Despite the enhanced nuclease resistance of DNA nanostructures compared to conventional double-stranded DNA (Keum and Bermudez 2009; Mei et al. 2011), they are still susceptible to degradation in biological systems, due both to nuclease digestion and component strand dissociation caused by changes in cation concentrations (Hahn et al. 2014). While such biodegradable features reduce the risk of DNA-associated toxicity during prolonged circulation, sufficient stability within the nanostructure is required to carry out the designed biological function. Thus, new efforts are needed to design and program DNA nanostructures with the expressed purpose of exhibiting optimal stability, a feature critical to the proper function of DNA-based nanomaterials in vivo.

15.3 Immune Stimulatory Activity of DNA Molecules and Their Feedback Regulation

In a live eukaryotic cell, DNA molecules outside their natural nuclear or mitochondrial compartments are considered PAMPs, which alert the host cell to an invasion by microbial pathogens or the presence of damaged cells (Barber 2011; Desmet and Ishii 2012). PAMPs function as potent activators of the innate immune system, resulting in production of a battery of proinflammatory cytokines, leading to the removal of infectious microbes or the clearance of damaged cells (Kumar et al. 2011). Two major signaling pathways have been identified to sense DNA "danger" signals and transduce them into sterile inflammation (Wu and Chen 2014). Unmethylated CpG motifs, which are common to bacterial and viral DNA but rarely found in the mammalian genome, are major ligands of TLR9 localized in the endoplasmic reticulum (Vollmer and Krieg 2009). Upon interaction with the internalized CpG DNA, TLR9 is translocated to the endolysosomal compartment, activating the myeloid differentiation primary response 88 (MYD88)-mediated signaling pathway and resulting production of type I interferon (IFN) and other proinflammatory cytokines (Latz et al. 2004). This pathway operates primarily in phagocytic and antigen-presenting cells (APCs) and serves as the critical host defense system against virus and bacteria. However, the DNA-mediated signaling pathway that controls IFN production was also found in cells lacking TLR9, such as many non-immune cell types, in which intracellular DNA devoid of the CpG motif still bears immune stimulatory activity (Ishii and Akira 2006; Vilaysane and Muruve 2009). Several DNA receptors have been identified in various cell types. Recently, it has been discovered that the signaling cascade of these DNA sensors is mediated by an adaptor protein, known as stimulator of interferon genes (STINGs), which leads to the production of type I IFN (IFN-alpha) (Abe et al. 2013; Konno and Barber 2014). Furthermore, cyclic GMP-AMP synthase (cGAS) was identified as a non-redundant and universal cytosolic DNA sensor (Wu et al. 2013; Li et al. 2013b). Upon binding to DNA, cGAS catalyzes the conversion of ATP and GTP into cyclic GMP-AMPs (cGAMP), which function as a second message to activate STING (Wu et al. 2013). The cGAS-cGAMP-STING signaling pathway is functional in many different cell types.

In addition to rendering immediate innate immunity against microbial DNA and damaged endogenous genome, the inflammation induced by both TLR9 and STING signaling pathways helps activate the body's adaptive immunity against those targets. For the past two decades, CpG DNA has been extensively developed as a vaccine adjuvant to increase immunity against cancer and infectious agents (Vollmer and Krieg 2009; Murad and Clay 2009). Recently, it has been demonstrated that dendritic cells activate the STING signaling pathway to induce antitumor immunity by sensing DNA derived from apoptotic tumor cells upon irradiation or chemical therapy (Deng et al. 2012; Woo et al. 2014). Thus, similar to TLR9 ligands, extracellular DNA molecules, possibly including synthetic DNA nanostructures, could also be explored as adjuvants to induce both innate and adaptive immunities.

Although type I IFN is critical to host defense against invading pathogens, its excessive production can cause inflammation and provoke autoimmune diseases (Choubey 2012), such as systemic lupus erythematosus (SLE). To avoid this dire consequence, mammalian cells are equipped with several regulatory mechanisms to ensure that the inflammatory pathway is activated only transiently. First, both foreign DNA and self-DNA released from nuclear or mitochondrial compartments are usually degraded rapidly by several DNA-degrading nucleases, including DNAse I, DNAse II (lysosomal endonuclease), and DNAse III (3' repair exonuclease, also known as Trex1). Defects in DNAse I and III have been associated with autoimmune diseases (Ablasser et al. 2014; Tsukumo and Yasutomo 2004), while DNAse II-deficient mice die late in embryogenesis, due to overproduction of type I IFN (Ahn et al. 2012; Yoshida et al. 2005). Second, both TLR9-MYD88 and cGAS-cGAMP-STING signaling pathways are stringently regulated to prevent overt activation. For example, type I/II IFN has been shown to induce indoleamine-2, 3-dioxygenase (IDO), an enzyme that catalyzes oxidative catabolism of tryptophan into kynurenine (Puccetti 2007). By depleting tryptophan, an essential amino acid, and producing kynurenine, IDO exerts metabolic immune regulation, promoting tolerance and immunosuppression (Grohmann et al. 2003). Thus, the IDO-mediated negative regulation may be intrinsically coupled to the DNA-sensing pathways to enforce homeostasis of immune stimulation and tolerance (Munn and Mellor 2013; Lemos et al. 2014). This regulation ensures a transient activation of innate immunity in response to extracellular DNA. Therefore, although multiple DNA-sensing pathways promote an immediate containment of invasion as well as long-term protection against pathogens, they are tightly regulated from overreaction, therefore minimizing the risk of DNA-mediated autoimmunity. Conceivably, exogenous DNA, such as those widely tested in gene therapy and vaccination, may bind to various DNA sensors for TLR9-dependent and cGAS-cGAMP-STING-mediated signaling pathways and trigger a transient activation of the innate system, imposing minimal toxicity in a host with functional nucleases and a DNA regulatory mechanism. This argument is in line with the general safety record of DNA vaccines tested in vivo, including both animal and clinical studies (Stenler et al. 2014; Hayton et al. 2014).

DNA nanostructures are readily taken up by macrophages and dendritic cells (Li et al. 2013a; Liu et al. 2012). The internalized DNA molecules were often found within endolysomal compartments (Mohri et al. 2012; Liu et al. 2012), which are likely sensed by the TLR9 signaling pathway for the activation of APCs. We and many other groups have shown that DNA nanostructures assembled with multiple copies of CpG demonstrated potent stimulation of macrophages and dendritic cells (Liang et al. 2014; Li et al. 2011; Mohri et al. 2012). Thus, DNA nanostructures can be customized by incorporation of CpG for enhanced adjuvant activity, which has been harnessed for anticancer therapy (Nishikawa et al. 2010, 2011; Kim et al. 2013; Zhang et al. 2014; Lee et al. 2012) and vaccine development (Liu et al. 2012; Rattanakiat et al. 2012; Nishikawa et al. 2014). Meanwhile, DNA-mediated activation should be controlled at an appropriate level and duration to avoid persistent inflammation and autoimmune reaction.

15.4 DNA-Nanoscaffolded Vaccines

Owing to robust engineering capability and intrinsic adjuvant activity, DNA represents an ideal platform for assembling both antigen and adjuvants on the same complex. With their particulate structures, the assembled DNA vaccine particles, like many nanomaterial-based vaccines, have the potential to facilitate the antigen delivery and antigen retention in the secondary lymphoid tissues and mediate co-delivery of both antigen and adjuvants to antigen-presenting cells. This functionality is critical to the initiation of adaptive immunity. For example, as reported recently by Nishikawa et al., a model antigen, ovalbumin (OVA), upon incorporation *via* physical trapping into self-assembled CpG nanoparticles or DNA nanogels, was found to induce antigen-specific antibodies (Rattanakiat et al. 2012; Nishikawa et al. 2014). Thus, these DNA nanoparticles or nanogels composed of 50–100 μg OVA and 100–2,200 μg CpG-containing DNA potently induced T-cell-dependent antibody responses (Rattanakiat et al. 2012; Nishikawa et al. 2014).

Given the current understanding of DNA sensing, attention should be focused toward minimizing autoreactivity of self-DNA molecules. Due to the programmability of DNA nanostructures, improved design of more stable complexes of DNA-based vaccines may afford good immunogenicity with a small amount of antigens. To test this hypothesis, we took advantage of the three-dimensional DNA-tetrahedron structure as our vaccine platform, a design initially developed by Mao's group (Zhang et al. 2012). This structure has several unique features that enable rational assembly of the vaccine: (1) simple assembly from four DNA strands, (2) well-defined particulate structures with 15–20 nm in size, (3) sufficient lattice for antigen/adjuvant attachment, and (4) presence of streptavidin (SA) that not only stabilizes three-dimensional DNA nanostructures but also serves as a model antigen for eliciting T-cell-dependent humoral responses.

We tested the immunogenicity of SA-specific antibody responses since SA antigens were assembled within DNA nanostructures, as illustrated in Fig. 15.2a. Immunogenicity of these vaccines was examined under a low dosage of antigens and CpG (5.5 μg and 2 μg CpG administered per mouse) (Liu et al. 2012). As a control, the mice were immunized with a mixture comprised of the same amount of antigen and adjuvant. As shown in Fig. 15.2b, the SA linked to DNA tetrahedrons engineered with CpG molecules is highly immunogenic, generating strong and long-lasting anti-SA antibody responses, much more potent than the one induced by SA mixed with CpG. Meanwhile, none of the immunized mice showed any anti-DNA reactivity (Liu et al. 2012). Thus, DNA tetrahedron presents a good platform to induce effective antibody responses. Furthermore, compared to other nanomaterials, the tunable DNA nanostructure offers more structural complexity and flexibility for modifications in order to further improve immunogenicity of the antigen.

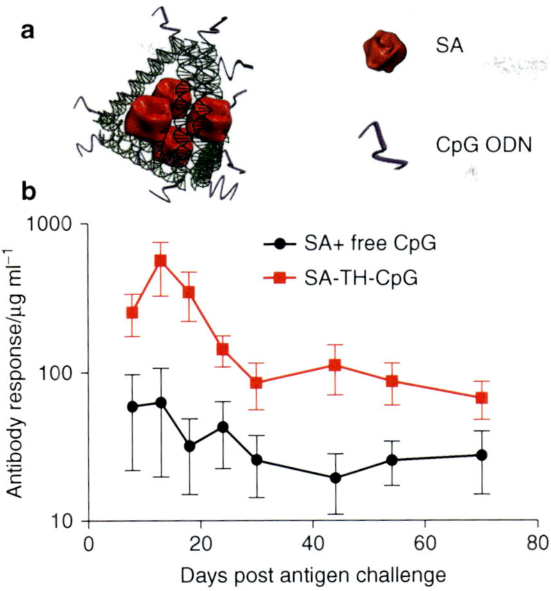

Fig. 15.2 DNA-scaffolded streptavidin (*SA*) vaccine and its antibody response in BALB/C mice. (**a**) Cartoon of the tetrahedron DNA-scaffolded vaccine complex. The antigen, SA, and adjuvant, CpG ODN, are assembled onto the same DNA-tetrahedron nanostructure to form the vaccine complex. (**b**) Anti-SA IgG antibody level in mice after challenge with free SA protein. Mice were immunized twice with different vaccines and challenged with the same free SA. The averages are calculated from at least eight mice, and the error bar represents standard deviation (Reprinted with permission from (Liu et al. 2012). Copyright (2012) American Chemical Society)

15.5 DNA-Tetrahedron-SA Platform for Self-Assembly of Nicotine Vaccine Particles

Given the promising response elicited by DNA-tetrahedron-SA, we decided to extend this vaccine platform to the design and construction of nicotine vaccines. The well-characterized structural information in both SA and DNA tetrahedron makes it possible to engineer vaccine complexes with predefined valences and configuration of nicotine epitopes and CpG molecules.

To create vaccines that allow co-delivery of antigen and adjuvants, two forms of CpG-containing nicotine vaccines were constructed, a soluble antigen, nicotine-SA conjugate linked to biotinylated CpG (Nic-SA-CpG), and a DNA-scaffolded nanoparticle 15–20 nm in diameter. The same nicotine-SA conjugate was attached to a DNA tetrahedron that was self-assembled from biotinylated DNA strands, CpG-containing oligonucleotides, and other strands, leading to the same antigen to adjuvant ratio as that of nicotine-SA-CpG conjugate, as depicted in Fig. 15.3a. Thus, these two types of nicotine vaccines have identical hapten-

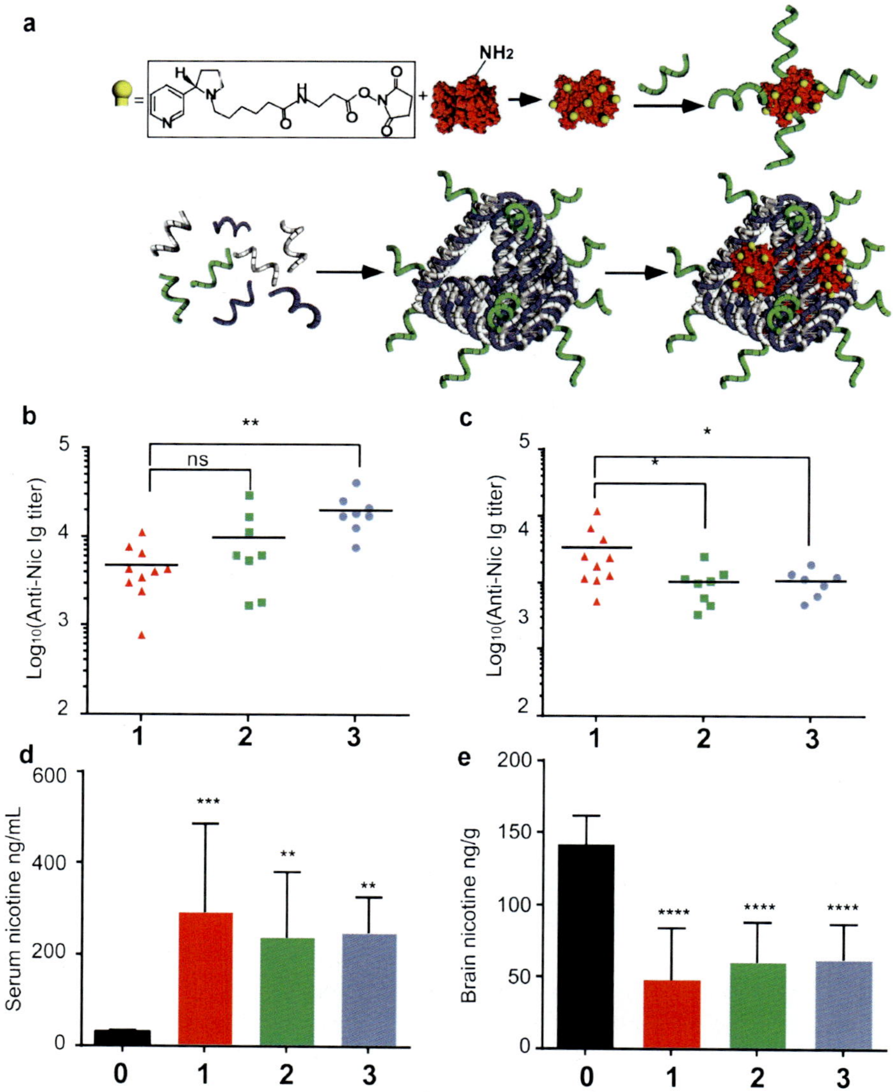

Fig. 15.3 DNA-scaffolded nicotine vaccines, structural features, immunogenicity, and pharmacokinetics. (**a**) Nicotine hapten (sphere-cylinder symbol) is conjugated to streptavidin (SA) through reaction between NHS ester and primary amine. The conjugated form, Nic-SA, was linked to biotinylated CpG ODN (helical symbol) to form Nic-SA-CpG conjugates. Tetrahedron DNA (TH) is assembled from its component strands, including that containing CpG, through base pairing, and Nic-SA was loaded to the assembled DNA product, TH-CpG, via biotin binding, thereby forming a Nic-SA-TH-CpG vaccine complex. (**b**, **c**) Anti-Nic antibody level after the third immunization. (**b**) 9-day post-third immunization; (**c**) 78-day post-third immunization. Group 1, prime-boost group; group 2, direct linkage group; group 3, KLH/Nic mixed with CpG group. * represents $p<0.05$ compared to prime-boost group, and ** represents $p<0.01$, as measured by t-test with Welch's correction. (**d**, **e**) pharmacokinetic analysis of s.c. injected nicotine distribution in mouse serum and brain. (**d**) shows serum nicotine concentration and (**e**) shows brain nicotine concentration. Group 0 represents naïve mice without immunization. ** represents $p<0.01$, and **** represents $p<0.0001$ compared to naïve mice, all as measured by one-way ANOVA with Dunnett's correction

protein conjugates and the same stoichiometry of antigen and CpG. Their immunogenicity can be directly compared. In addition, given the recently reported finding of an innate stimulatory effect of particulate antigens during the priming, but not boosting process (Link et al. 2012), we inquired whether priming with our particulate nicotine vaccines followed by boosting with soluble Nic-SA-CpG conjugates would elicit stronger nicotine-specific antibody responses. Although soluble Nic-SA-CpG conjugates gave rise to a potent anti-nicotine response (Fig. 15.3b), the priming with DNA-based vaccines followed by challenging with Nic-SA-CpG conjugates rendered a much more durable response as the antibody titer remains elevated 10-week post-third immunization and even surpasses the level of our positive control, nicotine-KLH (Nic-KLH) conjugates mixed with CpG (Fig. 15.3c). The high antibody titers resulted in significant sequestration of nicotine within the serum and blocked the nicotine from entering into the brain. Upon further analysis of the quality of antibody responses, the quantity and affinity of nicotine-specific antibodies were found to be higher in the prime-boost group than in the group immunized with Nic-SA-CpG conjugates and the positive control (although there is no statistically significant difference among these groups). Nevertheless, the promising trend of this immunization regime validates the feasibility of our DNA-based vaccines as a priming agent to induce a high-quality nicotine-specific antibody response. More importantly, the well-defined composition and structural information of soluble and particulate vaccine formulations and the flexibility of combining the two for priming and boosting open opportunities for further optimization of nicotine vaccines and immunization regimes. Finally, the application of DNA-based vaccines as priming agents reduces the chances of adverse autoimmune effects resulting from overt activation in response to synthetic DNA scaffolds.

DNA nanostructures are feasible as a platform for construction of vaccines against nicotine, a small molecule hapten. Certainly, further experimentation is needed to improve nicotine immunogenicity. According to recent understanding of B-cell responses to particulate antigens, various parameters, including particle size, display and density of antigenic epitopes, and attachment of adjuvant molecules, should be considered in future design of effective B-cell vaccines. Given their robust assembly, precision control, and facile introduction of functional groups, tunable DNA nanostructures offer a versatile platform for modular optimizations on all these parameters. In particular, we are focusing on the following tasks: (1) modifying the size and stability of DNA nanoparticles to enhance particle delivery to FDC to promote direct interaction with nicotine-specific B cells; (2) increasing epitope density by incorporating nicotine to DNA molecules at predefined positions and valences for better BCR cross-linking; and (3) optimizing the number and presentation of CpG moiety to enhance adjuvant activity. Furthermore, our finding of DNA-based vaccines as a promising agent in priming simplifies the screening of various DNA nanostructures on the basis of their immunogenicity. Informed application of programmable DNA nanostructures empowers the development of optimized nicotine vaccines.

References

Abe T et al. STING recognition of cytoplasmic DNA instigates cellular defense. Mol Cell. 2013;50(1):5–15.

Ablasser A et al. TREX1 deficiency triggers cell-autonomous immunity in a cGAS-dependent manner. J Immunol. 2014;192(12):5993–7.

Ahn J et al. STING manifests self DNA-dependent inflammatory disease. Proc Natl Acad Sci U S A. 2012;109(47):19386–91.

Bachmann MF, Jennings GT. Vaccine delivery: a matter of size, geometry, kinetics and molecular patterns. Nat Rev Immunol. 2010;10(11):787–96.

Barber GN. Cytoplasmic DNA innate immune pathways. Immunol Rev. 2011;243(1):99–108.

Bath J, Turberfield AJ. DNA nanomachines. Nat Nanotechnol. 2007;2(5):275–84.

Campolongo MJ et al. DNA nanomedicine: engineering DNA as a polymer for therapeutic and diagnostic applications. Adv Drug Deliv Rev. 2010;62(6):606–16.

Charoenphol P, Bermudez H. Design and application of multifunctional DNA nanocarriers for therapeutic delivery. Acta Biomater. 2014;10(4):1683–91.

Choubey D. DNA-responsive inflammasomes and their regulators in autoimmunity. Clin Immunol. 2012;142(3):223–31.

Deng Z et al. Robust DNA-functionalized core/shell quantum dots with fluorescent emission spanning from UV-vis to near-IR and compatible with DNA-directed self-assembly. J Am Chem Soc. 2012;134(42):17424–7.

Desmet CJ, Ishii KJ. Nucleic acid sensing at the interface between innate and adaptive immunity in vaccination. Nat Rev Immunol. 2012;12(7):479–91.

Dietz H, Douglas SM, Shih WM. Folding DNA into twisted and curved nanoscale shapes. Science. 2009;325(5941):725–30.

Dong Y, Yang Z, Liu D. DNA nanotechnology based on i-motif structures. Acc Chem Res. 2014;47(6):1853–60.

Douglas SM et al. Rapid prototyping of 3D DNA-origami shapes with caDNAno. Nucleic Acids Res. 2009;37(15):5001–6.

Douglas SM et al. Self-assembly of DNA into nanoscale three-dimensional shapes. Nature. 2010;459:414–8.

Elgueta R, de Vries VC, Noelle RJ. The immortality of humoral immunity. Immunol Rev. 2010;236:139–50.

Fraser CC et al. Generation of a universal CD4 memory T cell recall peptide effective in humans, mice and non-human primates. Vaccine. 2014;32(24):2896–903.

Gregory AE, Titball R, Williamson D. Vaccine delivery using nanoparticles. Front Cell Infect Microbiol. 2013;3.

Grohmann U, Fallarino F, Puccetti P. Tolerance, DCs and tryptophan: much ado about IDO. Trends Immunol. 2003;24(5):242–8.

Hahn J et al. Addressing the instability of DNA nanostructures in tissue culture. ACS Nano. 2014;8(9):8765–75.

Han D et al. Folding and cutting DNA into reconfigurable topological nanostructures. Nat Nanotechnol. 2010;5(10):712–7.

Han D et al. DNA origami with complex curvatures in three-dimensional space. Science. 2011;332(6027):342–6.

Han D et al. DNA gridiron nanostructures based on four-arm junctions. Science. 2013;339(6126):1412–5.

Hayton EJ et al. Safety and tolerability of conserved region vaccines vectored by plasmid DNA, simian adenovirus and modified vaccinia virus ankara administered to human immunodeficiency virus type 1-uninfected adults in a randomized, single-blind phase I trial. PLoS One. 2014;9(7), e101591.

Heesters BA, Myers RC, Carroll MC. Follicular dendritic cells: dynamic antigen libraries. Nat Rev Immunol. 2014;14(7):495–504.

Hu Y et al. A novel and efficient nicotine vaccine using nano-lipoplex as a delivery vehicle. Hum Vaccin Immunother. 2014;10(1):64–72.

Irvine DJ, Swartz MA, Szeto GL. Engineering synthetic vaccines using cues from natural immunity. Nat Mater. 2013;12(11):978–90.

Ishii KJ, Akira S. Innate immune recognition of, and regulation by. DNA Trends Immunol. 2006;27(11):525–32.

Jewell CM, Lopez SC, Irvine DJ. In situ engineering of the lymph node microenvironment via intranodal injection of adjuvant-releasing polymer particles. Proc Natl Acad Sci U S A. 2011;108(38):15745–50.

Jiang Q et al. DNA origami as a carrier for circumvention of drug resistance. J Am Chem Soc. 2012;134(32):13396–403.

Kasturi SP et al. Programming the magnitude and persistence of antibody responses with innate immunity. Nature. 2011;470(7335):543–7.

Ke Y et al. Self-assembled water-soluble nucleic acid probe tiles for label-free RNA hybridization assays. Science. 2008;319(5860):180–3.

Keum JW, Bermudez H. Enhanced resistance of DNA nanostructures to enzymatic digestion. Chem Commun (Camb). 2009;45:7036–8.

Keum JW, Ahn JH, Bermudez H. Design, assembly, and activity of antisense DNA nanostructures. Small. 2011;7(24):3529–35.

Kim KR et al. Drug delivery by a self-assembled DNA tetrahedron for overcoming drug resistance in breast cancer cells. Chem Commun (Camb). 2013;49(20):2010–2.

Konno H, Barber GN. The STING controlled cytosolic-DNA activated innate immune pathway and microbial disease. Microbes Infect. 2014;16(12):998–1001.

Kumar H, Kawai T, Akira S. Pathogen recognition by the innate immune system. Int Rev Immunol. 2011;30(1):16–34.

Latz E et al. TLR9 signals after translocating from the ER to CpG DNA in the lysosome. Nat Immunol. 2004;5(2):190–8.

Lee H et al. Molecularly self-assembled nucleic acid nanoparticles for targeted in vivo siRNA delivery. Nat Nanotechnol. 2012;7(6):389–93.

Lemos H et al. Cytosolic DNA sensing via the stimulator of interferon genes adaptor: Yin and Yang of immune responses to DNA. Eur J Immunol. 2014;44(10):2847–53.

Li T, Famulok M. I-motif-programmed functionalization of DNA nanocircles. J Am Chem Soc. 2013;135(4):1593–9.

Li J et al. Self-assembled multivalent DNA nanostructures for noninvasive intracellular delivery of immunostimulatory CpG oligonucleotides. ACS Nano. 2011;5(11):8783–9.

Li J et al. Smart drug delivery nanocarriers with self-assembled DNA nanostructures. Adv Mater. 2013a;25(32):4386–96.

Li XD et al. Pivotal roles of cGAS-cGAMP signaling in antiviral defense and immune adjuvant effects. Science. 2013b;341(6152):1390–4.

Liang L et al. Single-particle tracking and modulation of cell entry pathways of a tetrahedral DNA nanostructure in live cells. Angew Chem Int Ed Engl. 2014;53(30):7745–50.

Lin C et al. Self-assembled signaling aptamer DNA arrays for protein detection. Angew Chem Int Ed Engl. 2006;45(32):5296–301.

Lin C, Liu Y, Yan H. Designer DNA Nanoarchitectures†. Biochemistry. 2009;48(8):1663–74.

Link A et al. Innate immunity mediates follicular transport of particulate but not soluble protein antigen. J Immunol. 2012;188(8):3724–33.

Liu X et al. Targeted cell-cell interactions by DNA nanoscaffold-templated multivalent bispecific aptamers. Small. 2011;7(12):1673–82.

Liu X et al. A DNA nanostructure platform for directed assembly of synthetic vaccines. Nano Lett. 2012;12(8):4254–9.

Lockner JW et al. Enhancing nicotine vaccine immunogenicity with liposomes. Bioorg Med Chem Lett. 2013;23(4):975–8.

McHeyzer-Williams M et al. Molecular programming of B cell memory. Nat Rev Immunol. 2012;12(1):24–34.

Mei Q et al. Stability of DNA origami nanoarrays in cell lysate. Nano Lett. 2011;11(4):1477–82.
Mohri K et al. Design and development of nanosized DNA assemblies in polypod-like structures as efficient vehicles for immunostimulatory CpG motifs to immune cells. ACS Nano. 2012;6(7):5931–40.
Moon JJ et al. Enhancing humoral responses to a malaria antigen with nanoparticle vaccines that expand Tfh cells and promote germinal center induction. Proc Natl Acad Sci U S A. 2012;109(4):1080–5.
Mora-Solano C, Collier JH. Engaging adaptive immunity with biomaterials. J Mater Chem B Mater Biol Med. 2014;2(17):2409–21.
Munn DH, Mellor AL. Indoleamine 2,3 dioxygenase and metabolic control of immune responses. Trends Immunol. 2013;34(3):137–43.
Murad YM, Clay TM. CpG oligodeoxynucleotides as TLR9 agonists: therapeutic applications in cancer. BioDrugs. 2009;23(6):361–75.
Nishikawa M, Rattanakiat S, Takakura Y. DNA-based nano-sized systems for pharmaceutical and biomedical applications. Adv Drug Deliv Rev. 2010;62(6):626–32.
Nishikawa M et al. Biodegradable CpG DNA hydrogels for sustained delivery of doxorubicin and immunostimulatory signals in tumor-bearing mice. Biomaterials. 2011;32(2):488–94.
Nishikawa M et al. Injectable, self-gelling, biodegradable, and immunomodulatory DNA hydrogel for antigen delivery. J Control Release. 2014;180:25–32.
Pape KA et al. Different B cell populations mediate early and late memory during an endogenous immune response. Science. 2011;331(6021):1203–7.
Pavot V et al. Poly(lactic acid) and poly(lactic-co-glycolic acid) particles as versatile carrier platforms for vaccine delivery. Nanomedicine (Lond). 2014;9(17):2703–18.
Pinheiro AV et al. Challenges and opportunities for structural DNA nanotechnology. Nat Nanotechnol. 2011;6(12):763–72.
Puccetti P. On watching the watchers: IDO and type I/II IFN. Eur J Immunol. 2007;37(4):876–9.
Rattanakiat S, Nishikawa M, Takakura Y. Self-assembling CpG DNA nanoparticles for efficient antigen delivery and immunostimulation. Eur J Pharm Sci. 2012;47(2):352–8.
Rawlings DJ et al. Integration of B cell responses through Toll-like receptors and antigen receptors. Nat Rev Immunol. 2012;12(4):282–94.
Rinker S et al. Self-assembled DNA nanostructures for distance-dependent multivalent ligand-protein binding. Nat Nanotechnol. 2008;3(7):418–22.
Rothemund PWK. Folding DNA to create nanoscale shapes and patterns. Nature. 2006;440(7082):297–302.
Schüller VJ et al. Cellular immunostimulation by CpG-sequence-coated DNA origami structures. ACS Nano. 2011;5(12):9696–702.
Seeman NC. Nucleic-acid junctions and lattices. J Theor Biol. 1982;99(2):237–47.
Seeman NC. DNA in a material world. Nature. 2003;421(6921):427–31.
Seeman NC. Nanomaterials based on DNA. Annu Rev Biochem. 2010;79:65–87.
Slifka MK, Amanna I. How advances in immunology provide insight into improving vaccine efficacy. Vaccine. 2014;32(25):2948–57.
Smith DM, Simon JK, Baker JR. Applications of nanotechnology for immunology. Nat Rev Immunol. 2013a;13(8):592–605.
Smith D et al. Nucleic acid nanostructures for biomedical applications. Nanomedicine (Lond). 2013b;8(1):105–21.
Stenler S, Blomberg P, Smith CI. Safety and efficacy of DNA vaccines: plasmids vs. minicircles. Hum Vaccin Immunother. 2014;10(5):1306–8.
Swartz MA, Hirosue S, Hubbell JA. Engineering approaches to immunotherapy. Sci Transl Med. 2012;4(148):148rv9.
Tarlinton D, Good-Jacobson K. Diversity among memory B cells: origin, consequences, and utility. Science. 2013;341(6151):1205–11.
Taylor JJ, Jenkins MK, Pape KA. Heterogeneity in the differentiation and function of memory B cells. Trends Immunol. 2012;33(12):590–7.

Tsukumo S, Yasutomo K. DNaseI in pathogenesis of systemic lupus erythematosus. Clin Immunol. 2004;113(1):14–8.

Vilaysane A, Muruve DA. The innate immune response to DNA. Semin Immunol. 2009;21(4):208–14.

Vollmer J, Krieg AM. Immunotherapeutic applications of CpG oligodeoxynucleotide TLR9 agonists. Adv Drug Deliv Rev. 2009;61(3):195–204.

Williams S et al. Tiamat: a three dimensional editing tool for complex DNA structures. DNA Comput Lect Notes Comp Sci. 2010;5347:90–101.

Woo SR et al. STING-dependent cytosolic DNA sensing mediates innate immune recognition of immunogenic tumors. Immunity. 2014;41(5):830–42.

Wu J, Chen ZJ. Innate immune sensing and signaling of cytosolic nucleic acids. Annu Rev Immunol. 2014;32:461–88.

Wu J et al. Cyclic GMP-AMP is an endogenous second messenger in innate immune signaling by cytosolic DNA. Science. 2013;339(6121):826–30.

Yan H et al. DNA-templated self-assembly of protein arrays and highly conductive nanowires. Science. 2003;301(5641):1882–4.

Yan J et al. Growth and origami folding of DNA on nanoparticles for high-efficiency molecular transport in cellular imaging and drug delivery. Angew Chem Int Ed Engl. 2015;54(8):2431–5.

Yang Y et al. DNA pillars constructed from an i-motif stem and duplex branches. Small. 2012;8(4):552–6.

Yoshida H et al. Lethal anemia caused by interferon-beta produced in mouse embryos carrying undigested DNA. Nat Immunol. 2005;6(1):49–56.

Zhang C et al. DNA-directed three-dimensional protein organization. Angew Chem Int Ed Engl. 2012;51(14):3382–5.

Zhang Q et al. DNA origami as an in vivo drug delivery vehicle for cancer therapy. ACS Nano. 2014;8(7):6633–43.

Zhao Z et al. Encapsulation of gold nanoparticles in a DNA origami cage. Angew Chem Int Ed Engl. 2011;50(9):2041–4.

Zhao L et al. Nanoparticle vaccines. Vaccine. 2014;32(3):327–37.

Zuccarino-Catania GV et al. CD80 and PD-L2 define functionally distinct memory B cell subsets that are independent of antibody isotype. Nat Immunol. 2014;15(7):631–7.

Chapter 16
Adjuvants for Substance Abuse Vaccines

Frank M. Orson, Berma M. Kinsey, Reetakshi Arora, Muthu Ramakrishnan, and Thomas R. Kosten

16.1 Introduction

While all vaccines require the immune system to respond with effector molecules and cells in order to protect the body against a threat, most typically a toxin or microorganism, substance abuse vaccines have a special requirement that the effector molecules (antibodies in this case) be especially abundant (Orson et al. 2008). Although antibodies against tetanus toxin, for example, can be completely protective in the 1–2 μg/mL range (Stevens and Saxon 1979), antibodies against cocaine, methamphetamine, or morphine must be substantially higher. To bind a sufficient fraction of cocaine molecules to block or slow entry into the brain and thus inhibit the basic pharmacological

F.M. Orson, MD (✉)
Departments of Medicine, Pathology and Immunology, and Molecular Virology and Microbiology, Center for Translational Research in Inflammatory Diseases, Baylor College of Medicine, Houston, TX, USA

Allergy, Immunology, and Rheumatology Service, Veterans Affairs Medical Center, Bldg. 109, Rm. 234, 2002 Holcombe Blvd., Houston, TX 77030, USA
forson@bcm.edu

B.M. Kinsey, PhD • M. Ramakrishnan, PhD
Department of Medicine, Baylor College of Medicine, 2002 Holcombe, Houston, TX, USA
Research Service, Veterans Administration Medical Center, 2002 Holcombe, Houston, TX, USA

R. Arora, PhD
Research Service, Veterans Administration Medical Center, 2002 Holcombe, Houston, TX, USA

Department of Psychiatry, Baylor College of Medicine, 2002 Holcombe, Houston, TX, USA

T.R. Kosten, MD
Psychiatry Service, Veterans Administration Medical Center, 2002 Holcombe, Houston, TX, USA

Departments of Medicine, Psychiatry & Neuroscience, Baylor College of Medicine, 2002 Holcombe, Houston, TX, USA

I.D. Montoya (ed.), *Biologics to Treat Substance Use Disorders: Vaccines, Monoclonal Antibodies, and Enzymes*, DOI 10.1007/978-3-319-23150-1_16

effects of typical recreational doses of the drug, at least 40 μg/mL of anti-cocaine antibodies must be in circulation (Orson et al. 2009). Furthermore, the antibodies need to be of sufficient binding affinity with a rapid on-rate in order to sequester the drug in the bloodstream and reduce its entry rate into the brain (Ramakrishnan et al. 2012). As a result, it is essential to optimize substance abuse vaccine responses, and adjuvants will be a necessary component of any drug vaccine formulation.

16.2 Protein Vaccines Are Generally Combinations of Antigen and Adjuvant

Most individual proteins are perceived by the immune system as relatively bland molecules from the perspective of the immune system (Hawiger et al. 2001), though virtually any foreign or modified native protein may eventually be recognized as such with at least low-level reactions if administered in purified form and in sufficient quantity, e.g., insulins (Witters et al. 1977). It is only with costimulation of additional immune system signaling pathways that the immune system produces robust reactions to these molecules. However, some conjugate molecules already in clinical use have costimulatory properties. In some cases, these properties are very well explored, e.g., the outer membrane protein complex (OMPC) of *Neisseria meningitidis*. For OMPC, a major part of the costimulation comes from a retained partially hidden lipopolysaccharide (LPS) (Donnelly et al. 1990). Although humans are too sensitive to LPS for it to be used directly, the exposed portions of LPS in OMPC are stimulatory without being toxic and, as a result, have been very useful for pneumococcal polysaccharide and *Haemophilus influenzae* B polysaccharide vaccines (Heath 1998; Zangwill et al. 2003). More commonly, this costimulation can come through added chemicals, specific inflammatory proteins (e.g., cytokines), or in some cases from components associated with the antigens, e.g., lipids (Bublin et al. 2014) or in a few cases from structures of the protein itself (e.g., flagellin, which will be discussed in more detail later). Furthermore the direction and strength of these immune responses are guided by the types and quantities of the signaling molecules elicited by these co-stimuli. In recent years the multiplicity of signals and the complex interactions of these signals have become more appreciated and then continue to be intensely investigated, as reflected in numerous detailed reviews (Brito and O'Hagan 2014; Buonaguro et al. 2011; Harandi et al. 2009; Wilson-Welder et al. 2009).

16.3 Costimulatory Pathways: TLRs, RIHs, NLPs, Inflammasome, Cytokines, and Chemokines

As the innate immune system has become more thoroughly investigate, the numerous interactions of the signaling pathways in the component cells of this system as well as within the adaptive immune system cells have gradually been uncovered.

Toll-like receptors (TLRs) comprise one of the most prominent costimulatory systems for immunity, and these signaling molecules have been under intensive investigation in the past few decades (Iwasaki and Medzhitov 2004; Kawasaki and Kawai 2014; Qian and Cao 2013). Other pathways, including retinoic acid-inducible gene-like helicases (RIHs) (Hall et al. 2011), nucleotide-binding oligomerization domain (NOD)-like receptors (NLRs) (Motta et al. 2015), and inflammasomes (Lamkanfi and Dixit 2014), have also become more clearly elucidated, in addition to the better know cytokine and chemokine immunoregulatory pathways. In every immune response, it is the balance of all these signals that finally determines the resulting immune activities, and thus the fundamental properties of each receptor, its intracellular pathway components, and the cellular and genetic responses to the signaling are all highly variable with genetic differences on both a population and individual basis (Chen et al. 2011; Dhiman et al. 2008; Ovsyannikova et al. 2012; Ovsyannikova et al. 2011).

16.4 Individual Adjuvants in or Near Clinical Use

16.4.1 Alum

The adjuvant that was first established as clinically usable was alum, and it continues to be the adjuvant used for most clinical protein-based vaccines and a few polysaccharide conjugate vaccines (Kumru et al. 2014). Although its actual functions were not understood and misattributed to a simple "depot" function for many years, recent work has illuminated the complex effects of the variable amorphous suspension of crystalline material that is alum (aluminum hydroxide, aluminum phosphate, a mixture of the two, or in one case an aluminum hydroxyphosphate sulfate) (Hem and Hogenesch 2007). Protein-based antigens are generally adsorbed to the aluminum hydroxide crystals (Johnston et al. 2002) or aluminum phosphate amorphous precipitate structures (Ramesh et al. 2007) before administration. However, under physiological conditions, proteins generally are fairly rapidly desorbed from the alum particles (Hansen et al. 2007), taken up by antigen-presenting cells and transported to appropriate immune tissue locations. In fact, ablation of the injection site on the same day as the injection (eliminating any depot effect contribution) had no negative effect on the magnitude or quality of the immune response in certain mouse experiments (Hutchison et al. 2012).

If there is not a significant depot effect from alum, then what are the mechanisms of adjuvant action for alum? There have been numerous recent investigations into this question in recent years, and it has become clear that there are many contributing factors, rather than a single mechanism. This has been thoroughly reviewed recently (Brito and O'Hagan 2014), but in brief, these effects include inflammatory responses at the injection site with cell infiltration (Calabro et al. 2011; Kool et al. 2008; McKee et al. 2008), cytokine production (McKee et al. 2009; Mosca et al. 2008), and increased antigen uptake by antigen-presenting cells (Gupta 1998) and transport from the injection site to lymph nodes (Calabro et al. 2011). One of the more interesting aspects of these recent studies is the demonstration of the production of IL-1b, via activation of the inflammasome due to the crystalline structure of alum. Since a similar process occurs in the inflammation that occurs from uric acid crystals in clinical gout and calcium pyrophosphate crystals in pseudogout (Martinon et al. 2006), the inflammatory and febrile reactions that can occur with vaccines, especially in children, are now more clearly understood. In any case, it is quite obvious now that there is no single mechanism by which alum potentiates immune responses, but rather a complex series of events that, as a result, can vary considerably between individuals.

16.4.2 MF59

This adjuvant was the first non-alum adjuvant to be approved for human use (1997, in Europe), though only with influenza vaccines. It is a squalene emulsion in water adjuvant that has an extensive safety record thus far (O'Hagan et al. 2013), although as with even long-established vaccines, there have been claims of injury from squalene in vaccines (Asa et al. 2000), later shown to be unsubstantiated (Phillips et al. 2009). The mechanism of action of MF59 has some similarities to alum, in that cell infiltration, cell activation, enhanced antigen uptake, and cytokine and chemokine production are induced, and there is no substantive "depot" function (O'Hagan et al. 2012). Furthermore, there is no association of the antigen with the emulsion droplets, at least in influenza vaccines (O'Hagan et al. 2012).

16.4.3 ASO3 and ASO4

ASO3 is an adjuvant composed of squalene and alpha tocopherol that was approved for use with the flu vaccine for the pandemic H1N1 influenza A virus in 2009 (Morel et al. 2011). Unfortunately, this was found to be associated with a rare incidence of narcolepsy among recipients (Nohynek et al. 2012), unlike any other vaccines of related composition (e.g., MF59). The difference appears to be the alpha tocopherol, which can elicit nonspecific immune activation (Morel et al. 2011), unlike squalene alone. AS04 has a different composition and immunostimulants, using alum-adsorbed monophosphoryl lipid A, a TLR4 agonist (Mata-Haro et al. 2007; Vandepapeliere et al. 2008). This adjuvant was approved for inclusion in a human papillomavirus vaccine formulation that has been shown to be very effective (Garcon et al. 2011).

16.4.4 Adjuvants in Current Development

There are numerous agents in evaluation as potential vaccine adjuvants at early stages of evaluation and development (Brito and O'Hagan 2014). Some of the adjuvants are potentially attractive for substance abuse vaccine conjugates, but others have more promise in other applications. For example, CpG oligonucleotides are especially useful in directing immunity toward a Th1-biased response (Krieg 2000), that will be valuable for eliciting T-cell-mediated responses to cancers (He et al. 2014) and certain parasites (Mullen et al. 2008; Wu et al. 2010), or redirecting responses away from allergy (Beeh et al. 2013). Although this redirection can be very valuable for certain vaccine targets, Th1 responses in general have lower total antibody responses than do Th2 responses and the main problem for anti-substance abuse vaccines at this juncture is the total level of specific IgG antibodies that have sufficient affinity for binding drugs in the proper concentration range (Orson et al. 2014; Ramakrishnan et al. 2012).

One of the new adjuvants that has shown considerable promise for substance abuse vaccines is the TLR5 agonist derived from bacterial flagellin. The intact protein itself is an effective TLR5 stimulant, but antibodies against the intact specific protein can inhibit its function as an adjuvant (Terron-Exposito et al. 2012). In addition, injection of high doses of flagellin administered systemically were reported by some groups to have some toxic effects (Xiao et al. 2014). Recent studies from numerous labs, however, have shown that modifying the protein by truncation of the hypervariable domain, fusion to antigens, or conjugation to drugs can enhance activity and in some cases minimize the induction of neutralizing antibodies and toxicity.

Flagellin was recognized as a potential tool for enhancing responses against antigens other than itself in the previous decade (Honko and Mizel 2005; Mizel and Bates 2010), and numerous experimental vaccines have been developed against various targets, e.g., influenza (Treanor et al. 2010), but also including cocaine (Lockner et al. 2015). The latter studies showed a number of important findings. First, haptenization of the recombinant flagellin (FliC) did not reduce TLR5 activation until hapten densities exceeded ~10 haptens per molecule. Second, doses of conjugated FliC were not toxic (as measured by failure of weight gain in the mice) until the dosage was 50 μg or higher. Third, antibody production was limited in low dosing (10 μg/dose, but at higher doses (50 μg/dose and 100 μg/dose); robust antibody production was observed, with modest enhancement of responses (~40 %) at the highest dose with added alum, compared with alum alone and a KLH conjugate. However, a reduction in antibody production was observed with addition of monophosphoryl A to the 50 μg FliC conjugate dose.

Attachment of antigens and immunogenic epitopes has been thought to be required for adjuvant activity of flagellin (Huleatt et al. 2007); however our lab has shown that when combined with alum, enhancement of antibody production against a conjugate drug vaccine beyond optimized alum alone clearly occurs (Table 16.1). It is likely that delivery to the same or nearby antigen-presenting cells occurs due to co-adsorption of both the conjugate vaccine and the flagellin molecule.

A more recent advance utilizes entolimod (previously termed CBLB502, developed by Cleveland Biolabs Inc, CBLI (Burdelya et al. 2008), a truncated and pharmacologically optimized derivative form of salmonella flagellin. As an adjuvant for a drug conjugate vaccine, coadministration of Entolimod with alum results in higher responses than alum alone or alum plus intact flagellin (even at tenfold lower dosing, Table 16.1). Entolimod was developed as a treatment for radiation poisoning due to its immunostimulatory function and in fact is the only TLR5 agonist that has

Table 16.1 Alum plus flagellin or Entolimod increases anti-cocaine IgG

Formulation	μg flagellin or Entolimod	%[a]
Alum	0	100
Alum + flagellin	10	149
Alum + Entolimod	1	254

[a]Antibody response of pooled sera from 5 mice in each group 6 weeks after immunization, expressed as a ratio percentage of the response to IM injection of succinylnorcocaine conjugated to tetanus toxoid and adsorbed to alum. The optimal dose for each condition was selected for presentation. Other adjuvants (flagellin, kindly provided by Rongfu Wang, The Methodist Hospital Research Institute, Houston, TX) and Entolimod, kindly provided by Cleveland BioLabs, Inc., Buffalo, NY) were added to the alum and conjugate vaccine mix before injection.

been tested in humans, as it is currently in early-stage clinical development as a prospective immunotherapy drug (http://clinicaltrials.gov/show/NCT01527136). Adjuvant properties have also been demonstrated in animal models against tumors (Burdelya et al. 2013) and viruses (Hossain et al. 2014).

Due to internal truncation of D2-D3 hypervariable flagellin domains, entolimod (combined with Alum) showed maximal adjuvant activity at low doses (≤1 mg / injection), while inducing undesirable anti-flagellin antibodies only at higher doses (> 3 mg / injection) (Vadim Mett, Cleveland Biolabs, personal communication). As a result, such formulations should be able to be readministered in booster doses to maintain antidrug antibody levels for more prolonged periods of time.

16.4.5 Adjuvant Combinations

Recent experiments from many laboratories have shown that combinations of adjuvants are often much more effective than single adjuvants in stimulating robust immune responses. However, achieving this result is not merely a simple process of adding optimal concentrations of each adjuvant. As the understanding of immunoregulatory signaling has developed, the reasons underlying the challenges of multiple costimulation have become more apparent. The TLR signaling pathways were studied singly and in pairs in an extensive study (Makela et al. 2009), demonstrating that while additive or synergistic stimulation of cytokine production was achievable in some combinations, others resulted in a reduction in cytokine production. Given the number of combinations studied, it is understandable that dose-response curves for each agonist for each combination could not be examined, but this is precisely the problem facing optimization of costimulation. The number of combinations with different dosings is very prohibitive to study in a simple systematic fashion. Even stimulation of TLR4 alone is complex, due to the MyD88 and TRIF pathways being both activated (Shen et al. 2008) for maximal cytokine production, although this may not necessarily elicit maximal antibody, and there are additional recently described inhibitory components in TLR4 function involved as well (Daringer et al. 2015). However, individual TLR4 agonists do not activate both pathways equivalently. For example, MPL dominantly activates the TRIF pathway (Mata-Haro et al. 2007), while E6020 strongly activates both pathways. In any case, it is clear that there are differential effects of these pathways on B-cell differentiation and function (Yanagibashi et al. 2015).

In our laboratory, we have found that combinations of co-stimuli can have significantly different effects depending on the doses and specific combinations that are used. For example, the addition of alum to the TLR4 agonist monophosphoryl lipid A (MPL) markedly reduced antibody production compared to stimulation by either adjuvant alone (Orson, unpublished), as also observed with other conjugate vaccines (Pravetoni et al. 2014), although in other formulations of alum and MPL (ASO4) have shown no inhibition (and no enhancement) of antibody responses with alum (Didierlaurent et al. 2009). On the other hand, addition of alum to other selected agents markedly enhances production of antibody, e.g., the TLR9 agonist CPG (Mullen et al. 2008) and small molecule agonists of TLR7 (Wu et al. 2014). Similarly, a TLR5 agonist (flagellin) markedly increases antibody production at intermediate doses, but combining E6020 and flagellin with alum results in a substantial decrease in antibody production (Table 16.2).

16.5 Humanized Mice as a Tool for Adjuvant Evaluation

It remains unclear whether humanized mice (HM, immunodeficient mice stably engrafted with human hematopoietic stem cells) will provide an avenue to break through the problems with evaluating these complex systems in the mouse or other animal models which often do not accurately reflect the subsequent clinical responses and problems that may develop in human testing or widespread use. As noted above, even with human screening of adjuvants, promising data in animals has all too frequently resulted in disappointing results or unacceptable side effects. Certainly, the HM is not the answer to all such problems, but may provide some guidance by permitting relative comparisons on immune responses from replicates in individual donor HM and measurements of cytokine and other mediator production in the in vivo context.

Table 16.2 Combination of alum and flagellin derivative (Entolimod)

Formulation	μg E6020	μg Entolimod	%[a]
Alum	0	0	100
Alum + E6020	3	0	259
Alum + Entolimod	0	1	254
Aum + both	3	1	209

[a]Antibody response of pooled sera from 5 mice in each group 6 weeks after immunization, expressed as a ratio percentage of the alum only response to 32 μg of succinylnorcocaine conjugated to tetanus toxoid (injected IM). E6020 was kindly provided by Eisai Co., Ltd

With any model system for developing vaccines, but in particular with HM (Akkina 2013), it is important that responses be sufficiently robust and consistent in individual animals. With the NOD-Rag1^{null}IL2rγ^{null} mouse, a strain of relatively long-lived immunodeficient radioresistant nonobese diabetic mice (NOD), efficient engraftment with human hematopoietic stem cells occurs since these mice lack the common IL2rγ chain cytokine receptor component blocking natural killer cell development. There are no murine T cells or B cells due to the Rag1 gene deletion, and since human antigen-presenting cells are required for effective antigen presentation to human lymphocytes, the full function of immune activation for vaccines is present. Our laboratory has shown that features essential for vaccine evaluation are present in the NOD-Rag1^{null}IL2rγ^{null} mouse (Orson et al. 2014). These include consistent responses to single vaccine formulations for replicate mice of individual donors, distinct differences between groups of mice engrafted with different donor stem cells to the same formulations, and critically significant differences between different formulations in groups of mice all engrafted with stem cells from a single donor.

16.6 Formulation Complexities

Unfortunately, this complexity is often underappreciated in that experimental observations are sometimes thought to be more generalizable than they really are. This can be due to inappropriate controls for evaluating the relative strength of costimulatory signals on immune responses. As an example of this, certain adjuvants may be described as stimulating orders of magnitude, better antibody responses than controls. However, if those control formulations include only the antigen without any adjuvant (e.g., not using alum for a protein antigen under standard conditions), then the value of the studied material may or may not have a significant impact in practical terms. Immune responses to specific conditions are highly dependent on the exact concentrations of co-stimuli, concurrent antigen exposures, and balance of cytokines and other immune signaling molecules that result (Pulendran 2015; Schenten and Medzhitov 2011). Furthermore, certain antigenic molecules and/or carrier molecules may have intrinsic properties of co-stimuli (e.g., bacterial proteins that directly activate TLR5 or lipid molecules that are incorporated into carrier proteins derived from natural sources activating TLR4) that may not recognized as part of the adjuvant effects with these vaccines. Even though differences for clinically approved carriers like TT and CTB are rather modest when used with alum adjuvant alone (Ramakrishnan et al. 2014), addition of another costimulant can alter this limited difference. For example, we have observed that the anti-hapten response to a conjugate vaccine and costimulation of alum and e6020 is substantially stronger for the norcocaine hapten when conjugated to CTB than when conjugated to TT (Orson, unpublished).

16.7 Conclusions

The improved understanding of immunoregulation and costimulatory pathways' current status of adjuvant development has opened new opportunities for novel and improved vaccine development. To be most effective, substance abuse vaccines will require much higher antibody levels than most clinical vaccines currently in use, as well as a larger proportion of high-response recipients. New adjuvants, but particularly combinations of adjuvants, will not only permit the high antibody production required but will also prolong the persistence of the antibody responses to enhance their clinical effectiveness. Determining the formulations that can achieve these results will require an understanding of both positive and negative signaling immunoregulatory pathways. In fact, it is likely that future studies will demonstrate the need to use different formulations at initial and booster doses. Demonstration of these issues will require careful and thorough testing of adjuvant dosing and booster timing, as well as the formulation issues.

Acknowledgments This work was supported by the National Institute on Drug Abuse (NIDA) grants R01 DA030338, R01 DA023979, DA025223, and DA035591 and the Michael E. DeBakey Veterans Affairs Medical Center Research Program and the Department of Veterans Affairs Merit Review Program.

References

Akkina R. Human immune responses and potential for vaccine assessment in humanized mice. Curr Opin Immunol. 2013;25(3):403–9.

Asa PB, Cao Y, Garry RF. Antibodies to squalene in Gulf War syndrome. Exp Mol Pathol. 2000;68(1):55–64. doi:10.1006/exmp.1999.2295.

Beeh KM, Kanniess F, Wagner F, Schilder C, Naudts I, Hammann-Haenni A, Willers J, Stocker H, Mueller P, Bachmann MF, Renner WA. The novel TLR-9 agonist QbG10 shows clinical efficacy in persistent allergic asthma. J Allergy Clin Immunol. 2013;131(3):866–74. doi:10.1016/j.jaci.2012.12.1561.

Brito LA, O'Hagan DT. Designing and building the next generation of improved vaccine adjuvants. J Control Release: Off J Control Release Soc. 2014;190:563–79. doi:10.1016/j.jconrel.2014.06.027.

Bublin M, Eiwegger T, Breiteneder H. Do lipids influence the allergic sensitization process? J Allergy Clin Immunol. 2014;134(3):521–9. doi:10.1016/j.jaci.2014.04.015.

Buonaguro FM, Tornesello ML, Buonaguro L. New adjuvants in evolving vaccine strategies. Expert Opin Biol Ther. 2011;11(7):827–32.

Burdelya LG, et al. An agonist of toll-like receptor 5 has radioprotective activity in mouse and primate models. Science. 2008;320(5873):226–30.

Burdelya LG, Brackett CM, Kojouharov B, Gitlin II, Leonova KI, Gleiberman AS, Aygun-Sunar S, Veith J, Johnson C, Haderski GJ, Stanhope-Baker P, Allamaneni S, Skitzki J, Zeng M, Martsen E, Medvedev A, Scheblyakov D, Artemicheva NM, Logunov DY, Gintsburg AL, Naroditsky BS, Makarov SS, Gudkov AV. Central role of liver in anticancer and radioprotective activities of toll-like receptor 5 agonist. Proc Natl Acad Sci U S A. 2013;110(20):E1857–66. doi:10.1073/pnas.1222805110.

Calabro S, Tortoli M, Baudner BC, Pacitto A, Cortese M, O'Hagan DT, De Gregorio E, Seubert A, Wack A. Vaccine adjuvants alum and MF59 induce rapid recruitment of neutrophils and monocytes that participate in antigen transport to draining lymph nodes. Vaccine. 2011;29(9):1812–23. doi:10.1016/j.vaccine.2010.12.090.

Chen J, Liang Z, Lu F, Fang X, Liu S, Zeng Y, Zhu F, Chen X, Shen T, Li J, Zhuang H. Toll-like receptors and cytokines/cytokine receptors polymorphisms associate with non-response to hepatitis B vaccine. Vaccine. 2011;29(4):706–11.

Daringer NM, Schwarz KA, Leonard JN. Contributions of unique intracellular domains to switch-like biosensing by toll-like receptor 4. J Biol Chem. 2015. doi:10.1074/jbc.M114.610063.

Dhiman N, Ovsyannikova IG, Vierkant RA, Pankratz VS, Jacobson RM, Poland GA. Associations between cytokine/cytokine receptor single nucleotide polymorphisms and humoral immunity to measles, mumps and rubella in a Somali population. Tissue Antigens. 2008;72(3):211–20.

Didierlaurent AM, Morel S, Lockman L, Giannini SL, Bisteau M, Carlsen H, Kielland A, Vosters O, Vanderheyde N, Schiavetti F, Larocque D, Van Mechelen M, Garcon N. AS04, an aluminum salt- and TLR4 agonist-based adjuvant system, induces a transient localized innate immune response leading to enhanced adaptive immunity. J Immunol. 2009;183(10):6186–97.

Donnelly JJ, Deck RR, Liu MA. Immunogenicity of a Haemophilus influenzae polysaccharide-Neisseria meningitidis outer membrane protein complex conjugate vaccine. J Immunol. 1990;145(9):3071–9.

Garcon N, Morel S, Didierlaurent A, Descamps D, Wettendorff M, Van Mechelen M. Development of an AS04-adjuvanted HPV vaccine with the adjuvant system approach. BioDrugs: Clinical Immunother Biopharmaceuticals Gene Ther. 2011;25(4):217–26. doi:10.2165/11591760-000000000-00000.

Gupta RK. Aluminum compounds as vaccine adjuvants. Adv Drug Deliv Rev. 1998;32(3):155–72.

Hall JA, Grainger JR, Spencer SP, Belkaid Y. The role of retinoic acid in tolerance and immunity. Immunity. 2011;35(1):13–22. doi:10.1016/j.immuni.2011.07.002.

Hansen B, Sokolovska A, HogenEsch H, Hem SL. Relationship between the strength of antigen adsorption to an aluminum-containing adjuvant and the immune response. Vaccine. 2007;25(36):6618–24. doi:10.1016/j.vaccine.2007.06.049.

Harandi AM, Davies G, Olesen OF. Vaccine adjuvants: scientific challenges and strategic initiatives. Expert Rev Vaccines. 2009;8(3):293–8.

Hawiger D, Inaba K, Dorsett Y, Guo M, Mahnke K, Rivera M, Ravetch JV, Steinman RM, Nussenzweig MC. Dendritic cells induce peripheral T cell unresponsiveness under steady state conditions in vivo. J Exp Med. 2001;194(6):769–79.

He LZ, Weidlick J, Sisson C, Marsh HC, Keler T. Toll-like receptor agonists shape the immune responses to a mannose receptor-targeted cancer vaccine. Cell Mol Immunol. 2014. doi:10.1038/cmi.2014.100.

Heath PT. Haemophilus influenzae type b conjugate vaccines: a review of efficacy data. Pediatr Infect Dis J. 1998;17(9 Suppl):S117–22.

Hem SL, Hogenesch H. Relationship between physical and chemical properties of aluminum-containing adjuvants and immunopotentiation. Expert Rev Vaccines. 2007;6(5):685–98. doi:10.1586/14760584.6.5.685.

Honko AN, Mizel SB. Effects of flagellin on innate and adaptive immunity. Immunol Res. 2005;33(1):83–101. doi:10.1385/IR:33:1:083.

Hossain MS, Ramachandiran S, Gewirtz AT, Waller EK. Recombinant TLR5 agonist CBLB502 promotes NK cell-mediated anti-CMV immunity in mice. PLoS One. 2014;9(5), e96165. doi:10.1371/journal.pone.0096165.

Huleatt JW, Jacobs AR, Tang J, Desai P, Kopp EB, Huang Y, Song L, Nakaar V, Powell TJ. Vaccination with recombinant fusion proteins incorporating Toll-like receptor ligands induces rapid cellular and humoral immunity. Vaccine. 2007;25(4):763–75. doi:10.1016/j.vaccine.2006.08.013.

Hutchison S, Benson RA, Gibson VB, Pollock AH, Garside P, Brewer JM. Antigen depot is not required for alum adjuvanticity. FASEB J: Off Publ Fed Am Soc Exp Biol. 2012;26(3):1272–9. doi:10.1096/fj.11-184556.

Iwasaki A, Medzhitov R. Toll-like receptor control of the adaptive immune responses. Nat Immunol. 2004;5(10):987–95.

Johnston CT, Wang SL, Hem SL. Measuring the surface area of aluminum hydroxide adjuvant. J Pharm Sci. 2002;91(7):1702–6. doi:10.1002/jps.10166.

Kawasaki T, Kawai T. Toll-like receptor signaling pathways. Front Immunol. 2014;5:461. doi:10.3389/fimmu.2014.00461.

Kool M, Soullie T, van Nimwegen M, Willart MA, Muskens F, Jung S, Hoogsteden HC, Hammad H, Lambrecht BN. Alum adjuvant boosts adaptive immunity by inducing uric acid and activating inflammatory dendritic cells. J Exp Med. 2008;205(4):869–82. doi:10.1084/jem.20071087.

Krieg AM. Immune effects and mechanisms of action of CpG motifs. Vaccine. 2000;19(6):618–22.

Kumru OS, Joshi SB, Smith DE, Middaugh CR, Prusik T, Volkin DB. Vaccine instability in the cold chain: mechanisms, analysis and formulation strategies. Biologicals: J Int Assoc Biol Stand. 2014;42(5):237–59. doi:10.1016/j.biologicals.2014.05.007.

Lamkanfi M, Dixit VM. Mechanisms and functions of inflammasomes. Cell. 2014;157(5):1013–22. doi:10.1016/j.cell.2014.04.007.

Lockner JW, Eubanks LM, Choi JL, Lively JM, Schlosburg JE, Collins KC, Globisch D, Rosenfeld-Gunn RJ, Wilson IA, Janda KD. Flagellin as carrier and adjuvant in cocaine vaccine development. Mol Pharm. 2015;12(2):653–62. doi:10.1021/mp500520r.

Makela SM, Strengell M, Pietila TE, Osterlund P, Julkunen I. Multiple signaling pathways contribute to synergistic TLR ligand-dependent cytokine gene expression in human monocyte-derived macrophages and dendritic cells. J Leukoc Biol. 2009;85(4):664–72. doi:10.1189/jlb.0808503.

Martinon F, Petrilli V, Mayor A, Tardivel A, Tschopp J. Gout-associated uric acid crystals activate the NALP3 inflammasome. Nature. 2006;440(7081):237–41. doi:10.1038/nature04516.

Mata-Haro V, Cekic C, Martin M, Chilton PM, Casella CR, Mitchell TC. The vaccine adjuvant monophosphoryl lipid A as a TRIF-biased agonist of TLR4. Science. 2007;316(5831):1628–32.

McKee AS, MacLeod M, White J, Crawford F, Kappler JW, Marrack P. Gr1+IL-4-producing innate cells are induced in response to Th2 stimuli and suppress Th1-dependent antibody responses. Int Immunol. 2008;20(5):659–69. doi:10.1093/intimm/dxn025.

McKee AS, Munks MW, MacLeod MK, Fleenor CJ, Van Rooijen N, Kappler JW, Marrack P. Alum induces innate immune responses through macrophage and mast cell sensors, but these sensors are not required for alum to act as an adjuvant for specific immunity. J Immunol. 2009;183(7):4403–14.

Mizel SB, Bates JT. Flagellin as an adjuvant: cellular mechanisms and potential. J Immunol. 2010;185(10):5677–82. doi:10.4049/jimmunol.1002156.

Morel S, Didierlaurent A, Bourguignon P, Delhaye S, Baras B, Jacob V, Planty C, Elouahabi A, Harvengt P, Carlsen H, Kielland A, Chomez P, Garcon N, Van Mechelen M. Adjuvant System AS03 containing alpha-tocopherol modulates innate immune response and leads to improved adaptive immunity. Vaccine. 2011;29(13):2461–73. doi:10.1016/j.vaccine.2011.01.011.

Mosca F, Tritto E, Muzzi A, Monaci E, Bagnoli F, Iavarone C, O'Hagan D, Rappuoli R, De Gregorio E. Molecular and cellular signatures of human vaccine adjuvants. Proc Natl Acad Sci U S A. 2008;105(30):10501–6.

Motta V, Soares F, Sun T, Philpott DJ. NOD-like receptors: versatile cytosolic sentinels. Physiol Rev. 2015;95(1):149–78. doi:10.1152/physrev.00009.2014.

Mullen GE, Ellis RD, Miura K, Malkin E, Nolan C, Hay M, Fay MP, Saul A, Zhu D, Rausch K, Moretz S, Zhou H, Long CA, Miller LH, Treanor J. Phase 1 trial of AMA1-C1/Alhydrogel plus CPG 7909: an asexual blood-stage vaccine for Plasmodium falciparum malaria. PLoS One. 2008;3(8), e2940. doi:10.1371/journal.pone.0002940.

Nohynek H, Jokinen J, Partinen M, Vaarala O, Kirjavainen T, Sundman J, Himanen SL, Hublin C, Julkunen I, Olsen P, Saarenpaa-Heikkila O, Kilpi T. AS03 adjuvanted AH1N1 vaccine associated with an abrupt increase in the incidence of childhood narcolepsy in Finland. PLoS One. 2012;7(3), e33536. doi:10.1371/journal.pone.0033536.

O'Hagan DT, Ott GS, De Gregorio E, Seubert A. The mechanism of action of MF59 – an innately attractive adjuvant formulation. Vaccine. 2012;30(29):4341–8. doi:10.1016/j.vaccine.2011.09.061.

O'Hagan DT, Ott GS, Nest GV, Rappuoli R, Giudice GD. The history of MF59((R)) adjuvant: a phoenix that arose from the ashes. Expert Rev Vaccines. 2013;12(1):13–30. doi:10.1586/erv.12.140.

Orson FM, Kinsey BM, Singh RA, Wu Y, Gardner T, Kosten TR. Substance abuse vaccines. Ann N Y Acad Sci. 2008;1141:257–69. doi:10.1196/annals.1441.027.

Orson FM, Kinsey BM, Singh RA, Wu Y, Kosten TR. Vaccines for cocaine abuse. Hum Vaccin. 2009;5(4):194–9.

Orson FM, Wang R, Brimijoin S, Kinsey BM, Singh RA, Ramakrishnan M, Wang HY, Kosten TR. The future potential for cocaine vaccines. Expert Opin Biol Ther. 2014;14(9):1271–83. doi:10.1517/14712598.2014.920319.

Ovsyannikova IG, Haralambieva IH, Vierkant RA, Pankratz VS, Jacobson RM, Poland GA. The role of polymorphisms in toll-like receptors and their associated intracellular signaling genes in measles vaccine immunity. Hum Genet. 2011;130(4):547–61.

Ovsyannikova IG, Haralambieva IH, Kennedy RB, Pankratz VS, Vierkant RA, Jacobson RM, Poland GA. Impact of cytokine and cytokine receptor gene polymorphisms on cellular immunity after smallpox vaccination. Gene. 2012;510(1):59–65.

Phillips CJ, Matyas GR, Hansen CJ, Alving CR, Smith TC, Ryan MA. Antibodies to squalene in US Navy Persian Gulf War veterans with chronic multisymptom illness. Vaccine. 2009;27(29):3921–6. doi:10.1016/j.vaccine.2009.03.091.

Pravetoni M, Pentel PR, Potter DN, Chartoff EH, Tally L, LeSage MG. Effects of an oxycodone conjugate vaccine on oxycodone self-administration and oxycodone-induced brain gene expression in rats. PLoS One. 2014;9(7), e101807. doi:10.1371/journal.pone.0101807.

Pulendran B. The varieties of immunological experience: of pathogens, stress, and dendritic cells. Annu Rev Immunol. 2015. doi:10.1146/annurev-immunol-020711-075049.

Qian C, Cao X. Regulation of toll-like receptor signaling pathways in innate immune responses. Ann N Y Acad Sci. 2013;1283:67–74. doi:10.1111/j.1749-6632.2012.06786.x.

Ramakrishnan M, Alves De Melo F, Kinsey BM, Ladbury JE, Kosten TR, Orson FM. Probing cocaine-antibody interactions in buffer and human serum. PLoS One. 2012;7(7), e40518.

Ramakrishnan M, Kinsey BM, Singh RA, Kosten TR, Orson FM. Hapten optimization for cocaine vaccine with improved cocaine recognition. Chem Biol Drug Des. 2014;84(3):354–63. doi:10.1111/cbdd.12326.

Ramesh M, Turner LF, Yadav R, Rajan TV, Vella AT, Kuhn LT. Effects of the physico-chemical nature of two biomimetic crystals on the innate immune response. Int Immunopharmacol. 2007;7(13):1617–29. doi:10.1016/j.intimp.2007.08.011.

Schenten D, Medzhitov R. The control of adaptive immune responses by the innate immune system. Adv Immunol. 2011;109:87–124. doi:10.1016/B978-0-12-387664-5.00003-0.

Shen H, Tesar BM, Walker WE, Goldstein DR. Dual signaling of MyD88 and TRIF is critical for maximal TLR4-induced dendritic cell maturation. J Immunol. 2008;181(3):1849–58.

Stevens RH, Saxon A. Reduced in vitro production of anti-tetanus toxoid antibody after repeated in vivo immunization with tetanus toxoid. J Immunol. 1979;122(2):592–8.

Terron-Exposito R, Dudognon B, Galindo I, Quetglas JI, Coll JM, Escribano JM, Gomez-Casado E. Antibodies against Marinobacter algicola and Salmonella typhimurium flagellins do not cross-neutralize TLR5 activation. PLoS One. 2012;7(11), e48466. doi:10.1371/journal.pone.0048466.

Treanor JJ, Taylor DN, Tussey L, Hay C, Nolan C, Fitzgerald T, Liu G, Kavita U, Song L, Dark I, Shaw A. Safety and immunogenicity of a recombinant hemagglutinin influenza-flagellin fusion vaccine (VAX125) in healthy young adults. Vaccine. 2010;28(52):8268–74. doi:10.1016/j.vaccine.2010.10.009.

Vandepapeliere P, Horsmans Y, Moris P, Van Mechelen M, Janssens M, Koutsoukos M, Van Belle P, Clement F, Hanon E, Wettendorff M, Garcon N, Leroux-Roels G. Vaccine adjuvant systems containing monophosphoryl lipid A and QS21 induce strong and persistent humoral and T cell responses against hepatitis B surface antigen in healthy adult volunteers. Vaccine. 2008;26(10):1375–86.

Wilson-Welder JH, Torres MP, Kipper MJ, Mallapragada SK, Wannemuehler MJ, Narasimhan B. Vaccine adjuvants: current challenges and future approaches. J Pharm Sci. 2009;98(4):1278–316.

Witters LA, Ohman JL, Weir GC, Raymond LW, Lowell FC. Insulin antibodies in the pathogenesis of insulin allergy and resistance. Am J Med. 1977;63(5):703–9.

Wu W, Huang L, Mendez S. A live Leishmania major vaccine containing CpG motifs induces the de novo generation of Th17 cells in C57BL/6 mice. Eur J Immunol. 2010;40(9):2517–27. doi:10.1002/eji.201040484.

Wu TY, Singh M, Miller AT, De Gregorio E, Doro F, D'Oro U, Skibinski DA, Mbow ML, Bufali S, Herman AE, Cortez A, Li Y, Nayak BP, Tritto E, Filippi CM, Otten GR, Brito LA, Monaci E, Li C, Aprea S, Valentini S, Calabromicron S, Laera D, Brunelli B, Caproni E, Malyala P, Panchal RG, Warren TK, Bavari S, O'Hagan DT, Cooke MP, Valiante NM. Rational design of small molecules as vaccine adjuvants. Sci Transl. 2014;6(263):263ra160. doi:10.1126/scitranslmed.3009980.

Xiao Y, Liu F, Yang J, Zhong M, Zhang E, Li Y, Zhou D, Cao Y, Li W, Yu J, Yang Y, Yan H. Over-activation of TLR5 signaling by high-dose flagellin induces liver injury in mice. Cell Mol Immunol. 2014. doi:10.1038/cmi.2014.110.

Yanagibashi T, Nagai Y, Watanabe Y, Ikutani M, Hirai Y, Takatsu K. Differential requirements of MyD88 and TRIF pathways in TLR4-mediated immune responses in murine B cells. Immunol Lett. 2015;163(1):22–31. doi:10.1016/j.imlet.2014.11.012.

Zangwill KM, Greenberg DP, Chiu CY, Mendelman P, Wong VK, Chang SJ, Partridge S, Ward JI. Safety and immunogenicity of a heptavalent pneumococcal conjugate vaccine in infants. Vaccine. 2003;21(17-18):1894–900.

Chapter 17
Skin Vaccination Against Nicotine Addiction

Xinyuan Chen, Ji Wang, Jeffrey H. Wu, and Mei X. Wu

17.1 Introduction

In 2014, the Surgeon General of the United States released a report revealing that an estimated 480,000 premature deaths occurred annually between 2005 and 2009 due to cigarette smoking and the associated secondhand smoke, a measure that did not account for cigar, pipe, or e-cigarette uses (Hallquist 2014). Meanwhile, 8.6 million people in the United States live with serious smoking attributable-medical conditions such as cancers and cardiovascular, metabolic, and pulmonary diseases (Hallquist 2014). The combined economic costs of direct medical care and loss of productivity are estimated to be $289–332.5 billion a year (Hallquist 2014). Thus, while attitudes toward smoking have changed over the last 50 years, smoking remains an enormous health problem in the United States. Furthermore it is a global pandemic, each year resulting in 6 million deaths worldwide (Cerny and Cerny 2009).

Cessation can save former smokers 10, 9, or 6 years of life if they quit from ages 25–34, 35–44, or 45–59, respectively (Jha and Peto 2014). Yet of the 68.9 % of daily smokers who want to quit, only 4–7 % successfully do so without aids, and another 2–3.5 % with some combination of behavioral counseling, medication, and replacement therapy (Moreno and Janda 2009). Hence, there is an urgent demand for

X. Chen (✉) • J. Wang • J.H. Wu
Department of Dermatology, Wellman Center for Photomedicine,
Massachusetts General Hospital, Harvard Medical School, Boston, MA, USA
e-mail: xchen14@partners.org

M.X. Wu (✉)
Department of Dermatology, Wellman Center for Photomedicine,
Massachusetts General Hospital, Harvard Medical School, Boston, MA, USA

Harvard-MIT Division of Health Sciences and Technology,
Cambridge, MA, USA
e-mail: mwu2@partners.org

I.D. Montoya (ed.), *Biologics to Treat Substance Use Disorders: Vaccines, Monoclonal Antibodies, and Enzymes*, DOI 10.1007/978-3-319-23150-1_17

innovative treatment strategies such as nicotine vaccines. Nicotine vaccines are often produced by conjugation of nicotine hapten to carrier proteins and nicotine vaccines act by stimulation of anti-nicotine antibodies (NicAb) to bind with and prevent nicotine from crossing the blood-brain barrier (Fahim et al. 2011). In this way, smoking will not cause reinforcing effects. In order to generate an effective antibody response, nicotine vaccines must include a B-cell epitope, T-cell epitope, and an optimal adjuvant (Pentel and LeSage 2014a). Nicotine hapten serves as the B-cell epitope to stimulate nicotine-specific B cells to secret NicAb, while the carrier protein provides T-cell epitopes, which activate carrier-specific T cells to assist nicotine-specific B cells to differentiate into plasma cells and secret NicAb. Adjuvants boost carrier-specific T-cell and nicotine-specific B-cell responses in generation of high-level and high-affinity NicAb.

Various nicotine vaccines have been generated and explored in preclinical animal models and several of them, like NicVAX, NicQb, and Niccine, have entered clinical trials due to the good tolerability and safety in smokers (Cornuz et al. 2008; Hatsukami et al. 2011; Maurer et al. 2005; Tonstad et al. 2013). Yet, all these vaccines failed to induce significantly higher abstinence rate as compared to placebo (Cornuz et al. 2008; Hatsukami et al. 2011; Maurer et al. 2005; Tonstad et al. 2013). As an example, NicVAX generated by conjugation of nicotine hapten to recombinant exoprotein A (rEPA) represents the most advanced nicotine vaccine ever developed (Fahim et al. 2013). Despite promising data in phase II clinical trial, NicVAX failed in the first phase III trial, which explored NicVAX alone as a therapy for nicotine addiction, and then in the second phase III trial, which explored combination of NicVAX with varenicline, a prescription medication that competes with nicotine to bind to nicotine acetylcholine receptor in the brain (Hatsukami et al. 2011; Hoogsteder et al. 2012a, 2014).

Nicotine vaccines differ considerably from conventional vaccines used to prevent infectious diseases in the following aspects. Firstly, cigarettes contain large amounts of nicotine, often in the range of milligrams, to be targeted by the immune system, which is only NicAb. In comparison, pathogens at the early phase of infection are in relatively low amounts and thus can be readily targeted by the immune system, which includes pathogen-specific antibodies and T cells. Secondly, vaccine-induced memory T and B cells can be quickly expanded after pathogen invasion, while the immune system totally depends on the existing NicAb at the time of smoking to sequester and block an entrance of nicotine into the brain. Such a blockade must be in high efficiency. Even a low-nicotine Quest cigarette with 5 % the nicotine content of standard cigarettes can result in 26 % occupation of the brain's nicotinic acetylcholine receptors (Pentel and LeSage 2014a), and low-affinity antibodies have been found to increase nicotine acetylcholine receptor occupancy rather than decrease it (Alexey et al. 2013).

Despite these failures and challenges, 30 % vaccines in the early-phase trials were able to develop relatively high NicAb titers and show significantly increased abstinence rates as compared to placebo, providing important validation for the nicotine vaccine concept (Cornuz et al. 2008; Hoogsteder et al. 2012b). From these studies, a successful nicotine vaccine should be high immunogenic and capable of generating high NicAb titers for a prolonged time in a majority of smokers. The nicotine vaccine would also require easy-to-use delivery technologies to enhance patient compliance and clinical acceptance due to the multidose immunization regimen to induce and periodical boosts to maintain a high level of NicAb. Various strategies, like optimization of linker and hapten designs, incorporation of more potent adjuvants, and so on, have been or are being pursued toward a successful nicotine vaccine, discussion of which can be found elsewhere in this book. This chapter focuses on skin vaccination and novel skin delivery technologies aimed at improving not only nicotine vaccine immunogenicity but also patient compliance and vaccine acceptance in the clinics.

17.2 High Immunogenic Skin Vaccination

Skin covers external body surface, prevents environmental pathogen invasion, and is considered a crucial part of our defense system. The defense barrier is attributed first to the outermost layer of the skin, called stratum corneum (SC) (Prausnitz and Langer 2008). Human SC is about 10–20 μm in thickness and packed with highly specialized lipid structures, impermeable to most of the hydrophilic molecules (Prausnitz and Langer 2008). Aside from the physical barrier, skin is a highly immunogenic organ with large amounts of antigen-presenting cells (APCs) residing, including epidermal Langerhans cells (LCs) and various types of dermal dendritic cells (DCs) (Romani et al. 2012a). These innate immune cells occupy ~30 % surface area and function as immune sentinels for invading pathogens (Chen and Wu 2011). LCs and dermal DCs are capable of efficiently taking up invading pathogens, migrating to the draining lymph nodes, and eliciting adaptive immune responses. Skin is also enriched with blood and lymphatic vessel networks, which facilitate immune cell migration into and out of the skin.

Delivery of vaccines into the skin simulates natural infection of many pathogens and often elicits potent immune responses. For instance, the fist human vaccine, called smallpox vaccine, was delivered into the skin by scarification, in which a bifurcated needle was used to scratch and deposit vaccine solutions into the superficial skin (Lofquist et al. 2003). Scarification contributes to the early control and later eradication of this once deadliest disease in human history (Lofquist et al. 2003). Recent studies corroborated that scarification was superior to different routes of vaccination, like intramuscular (IM), subcutaneous, and intradermal (ID) injections, in induction of poxvirus-specific immune responses (Liu et al. 2010). Yet, scarification is rarely used in the modern world due to the development of skin lesions and an increased risk of local infections. For convenience, the majority of modern vaccines are delivered into the muscular tissue by hypodermic needles, which drastically reduces incidence of various infectious diseases, like measles, diphtheria, and influenza (Barnighausen et al. 2014; Chen et al. 2013). Yet, IM vaccination elicits relatively weak immune responses partly due to few APCs in the muscular tissue and may not be suitable for vaccines with weak immunogenicity, like nicotine vaccines, or immunization at extreme ages, like newborns and the elderly, when these populations need vaccines the most (Chen et al. 2013; Siegrist and Aspinall 2009). The inferior immune responses elicited by IM vaccination lead to millions of vaccine-preventable deaths in newborns and more than 90 % influenza-associated morbidity and mortality in the elderly (PrabhuDas et al. 2011; Nichol 2005). In pursuit of more potent immune responses, vaccines have been delivered into the dermal tissue by hypodermic needles, exhibiting significantly improved vaccine immunogenicity (Romani et al. 2012b; Glenn et al. 2003). However, ID vaccination requires special training due to the thin skin tissue, which limits its widespread use especially in resource-poor countries. With the advent of a novel ID microinjection system, the same dose of seasonal influenza vaccine was approved for ID delivery in the elderly in Europe (Intanza®, 15 μg) and a reduced dose (9 μg) was approved for ID delivery in young adults in Europe (Intanza®, 9 μg) and the United States (Fluzone Intradermal®) (Foy et al. 2013; Duggan and Plosker 2010; Nougarede et al. 2014). To reduce the cost or address the shortage of human diploid cell rabies vaccine, the World Health Organization (WHO) recommends ID rabies vaccination for postexposure prophylaxis, in which 1/10th vaccine dose is intradermally injected to generate seroconversion rates and antibody levels comparable to those of full-dose IM vaccination (Verma et al. 2011). Besides influenza and rabies vaccine, hepatitis B vaccine (NCT02186977) and a novel tuberculosis vaccine (MVA85A, NCT01954563) are under clinical trials for ID vaccination to improve immunogenicity and efficacy.

Similar to the majority of other vaccines, nicotine vaccines were delivered into the muscular tissue in clinical trials (Cornuz et al. 2008; Hatsukami et al. 2011; Maurer et al. 2005; Tonstad et al. 2013; Hoogsteder et al. 2012a, 2014). To explore whether ID vaccination induced more potent immune responses, a preclinical nicotine vaccine Nic-KLH generated by conjugation of nicotine hapten (6-carboxymethylureido nicotine, abbreviated as 6-CMUNic) to keyhole limpet hemocyanin (KLH) was either intradermally or intramuscularly injected into BALB/c mice (Chen et al. 2012). We found that ID vaccination induced at least 5 times higher NicAb titer than IM vaccination after a single dose (Chen et al. 2012). Three ID vaccinations were able to generate comparable NicAb titer to 7 IM vaccinations (Chen et al. 2012). Brain nicotine levels were comparable between 3 ID and 7 IM vaccinations after nicotine challenge (Chen et al. 2012). These results indicate that nicotine vaccine immunogenicity can be greatly improved by a mere change of the route of vaccination.

17.3 Adjuvants for Skin Vaccination

17.3.1 Conventional Adjuvants

Although skin is a more immunogenic site for vaccination as compared to the muscle, ID nicotine vaccination needs adjuvant to induce the most potent immune responses (Pentel and LeSage 2014b). Unfortunately, most of conventional adjuvants are too toxic to use in skin vaccination (Chen and Wu 2011). As shown in

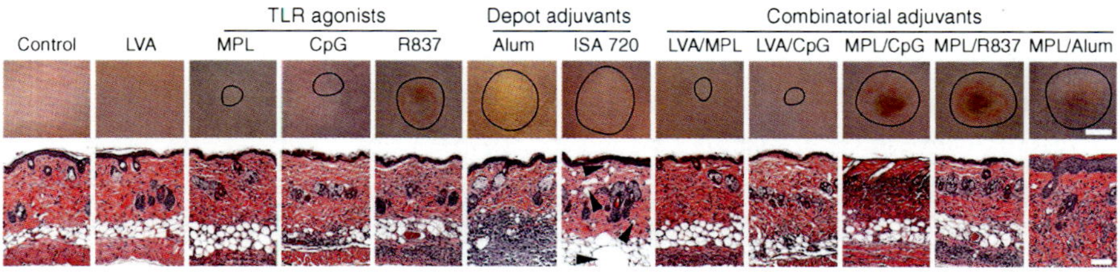

Fig. 17.1 Reactogenicity of adjuvant-treated skin. The low back skin of BALB/c mice was treated with a laser defined in 17.3.2.1, TLR agonist-based adjuvants (MPL, R837, CpG), depot adjuvants (alum, Montanide ISA 720), and combinatorial adjuvants (LVA/MPL, LVA/CpG, MPL/CpG, MPL/R837, MPL/alum). Five days later, photos of adjuvant-treated sites were taken (*upper panel*; scale bar, 2 mm), followed by histological examination (*lower panel*; scale bar, 100 μm). The lesion in the skin is outlined by a circle in the upper panel. Arrows in the lower panel in Montanide ISA 720-injected skin point to void bulbs preoccupied by the water-in-oil adjuvant

Fig. 17.1, Toll-like receptor 7 (TLR7) agonist R837, combinatorial TLR4 agonist monophosphoryl lipid A (MPL) and TLR9 agonist CpG (MPL/CpG), MPL/R837, and MPL/alum induced the most severe local reactions with a lesion size of 4–6 mm in diameter, concurrent with skin ulceration (upper panels), which was persistent for weeks. Histological examination revealed a heavy infiltration of inflammatory cells into adjuvant-injected site (lower panel). The strong and persistent local reactions can potentially breach the integrity of the skin and cause local and systemic infections. Alum and Montanide ISA 720 induced a similar lesion size as above with infiltration of inflammatory cells evoked by alum stronger than Montanide ISA 720 (Fig. 17.1). Deposition of alum, Montanide ISA 720, and MPL/alum was readily visible at the injection site, appearing as an abscess owing to white/silver color of the adjuvant, and did not go away for months. Although only two emulsion adjuvants are tested, it is likely that other emulsion adjuvants (e.g., AS02, MF59, and AS03) may have similar depositions in the skin in light of their similar physiochemical properties. The unpleasant "abscess" and persistent inflammation in the skin question the use of any antigen-depot adjuvants for skin vaccination. In comparison, MPL and CpG alone induced mild local reactions with a lesion size of about 2 mm in diameter that were completely resolved within 2 weeks (Fig. 17.1). MPL and CpG may potentially be safe adjuvants for skin vaccination.

17.3.2 Laser Vaccine Adjuvants

Apart from conventional adjuvants, we, alongside others, took a totally different approach in developing physical type laser adjuvants to specifically boost skin vaccination (Kashiwagi et al. 2013, 2014; Wang et al. 2014; Chen et al. 2010). Two kinds of laser adjuvants have been developed to boost ID vaccination with the first causing no skin damage or inflammation and the second generating microscopic skin damage (Kashiwagi et al. 2013; Wang et al. 2014; Chen et al. 2010). The unique feature of the laser adjuvants is the superb local safety and no potential systemic or long-term side effects since no foreign materials are injected into the body with laser adjuvantation (Chen and Wu 2011; Chen et al. 2013; Kashiwagi et al. 2013, 2014; Wang et al. 2014; Chen et al. 2010).

17.3.2.1 Laser Vaccine Adjuvant (LVA)

A Q-switched 532 nm Nd: YAG laser was first demonstrated to possess adjuvant effects (Chen et al. 2010). Laser illumination (0.3 W, 2 min) of a small area of the skin (<1 cm^2) followed by ID injection of model antigen ovalbumin (OVA) into laser-illuminated site significantly enhanced OVA-specific humoral immunity without skin damage or inflammation (Chen et al. 2010). LVA is also able to augment immune responses induced by seasonal influenza vaccine, recombinant malarial liver-stage antigen 1, hepatitis B surface antigen (HBsAg), and nicotine vaccine (Chen and Wu 2011; Chen et al. 2010). Since laser at 532 nm can be strongly absorbed by melanin, laser adjuvant effect might vary with skin colors. To overcome this, near-infrared (NIR) laser was also tested for its adjuvant effect (Kashiwagi et al. 2013). Similar to 532 nm laser, NIR laser significantly enhanced OVA and influenza vaccine-induced immune responses (Kashiwagi et al. 2013). Laser adjuvants can be used alone or combined with other conventional adjuvants to synergistically or additively augment vaccine-induced immune responses (Chen and Wu 2011; Chen et al. 2012). We showed that a combination of LVA and MPL augmented NicAb titer by 33-fold, while LVA or MPL only increased NicAb titers by 4-fold or 13-fold, respectively (Chen et al. 2012). Importantly, the combination did not induce overt skin reactions (Fig. 17.1), holding great promise for clinical use (Chen and Wu 2011; Chen et al. 2012).

The mechanism underlying laser-induced adjuvanicity is not completely understood, but it is clear that tissue damage or inflammation is not responsible for the adjuvant effect, in contrast to the majority of conventional adjuvants (Chen and Wu 2011; Kashiwagi et al. 2013, 2014; Chen et al. 2010). It is reported that laser treatment at 2–20-fold higher power can induce production of extracellular heat-shock protein (HSP) 70 and inflammatory response (Mackanos and Contag 2011). But, neither HSP70 nor proinflammatory cytokines were detected at the site of laser illumination (Chen and Wu 2011; Chen et al. 2010). Rather, we found that laser treatment accelerated the motility of APC, presumably due to alteration of the dense connective tissue of the skin (Chen and Wu 2011; Chen et al. 2010). The loosely connected micro-architecture of the skin after laser illumination permits free movement of APCs in the dermal tissue and allows them to survey a greater area and better sample antigens (Chen and Wu 2011; Chen et al. 2010). The impact on APCs was also found with the NIR laser, although the enhanced recruitment and migration of APCs may be ascribed to local cytokine and chemokine production (Kashiwagi et al. 2013, 2014). Further investigation of the underlying mechanism will help to improve and apply the laser adjuvant in the clinics.

17.3.2.2 Non-ablative Fractional Laser (NAFL)

NAFL represents a second type of laser adjuvant (Wang et al. 2014). Sterile inflammation is well known to be induced by "danger" signals released from dying cells as a natural response to pathogen invasion or tissue damage (Chen and Nunez 2010). This inflammatory response also plays a crucial role in the adjuvant effect of alum and MF59 because the adjuvants induce cell death at the site of inoculation (Vono et al. 2013; Lambrecht et al. 2009; Kool et al. 2008). But the sterile inflammation provoked by the adjuvants often causes significant local reactions due to too much unwanted cell death that stimulates bulk, persistent skin inflammation as indicated in Fig. 17.1. Utilization of NAFL is not to detour sterile inflammation, but to reduce the side effects of this process by segregation of the sterile inflammation into hundreds of micro-zones (Wang et al. 2014). Each of these micro-inflammation zones can be quickly resolved before it can spread into the nearby tissue, provided that distances between nearby zones are large enough (Wang et al. 2014). Our investigations clearly demonstrated that quick resolution of the inflammation in each micro-zone effectively averted skin lesion while evoking transient, yet sufficient innate immunity to augment immune responses against the vaccine (Wang et al. 2014). Moreover, the laser treatment does not damage the SC layer, so that the barrier function of skin was well preserved, minimizing the risk of skin infections (Wang et al. 2014). The superb safety of NAFL is further warranted as the technology has been broadly employed in the clinics or at home for cosmetic wrinkle removal and skin resurfacing in the past decade (Preissig et al. 2012). The 1,410 nm laser works in a stamp/scanning fashion and is equally effective regardless of skin colors (Wang et al. 2014). It emits high-energy laser beams onto skin surface and generates an array of self-healing microthermal zones (MTZ) beneath skin surface (Wang et al. 2014). The dying cells within MTZs release "danger" signals also called damage associated molecule patterns (DAMPs) to alert the immune system (Wang et al. 2014). Thus, each MTZ can be regarded as a mini adjuvant zone and hundreds of such mini adjuvant zones could be very effective in augmenting vaccine-induced immune responses (Wang et al. 2014). Indeed, illumination of the inoculation site with NAFL prior to ID vaccination significantly enhanced immune responses against OVA, HBsAg, and seasonal influenza vaccine (Wang et al. 2014). The adjuvant effect has been also confirmed in swine, in which the immune responses are augmented by eight-, five-, and twofolds for HBsAg, influenza vaccine, and nicotine vaccine, respectively (Wang et al. 2014).

Intravital confocal microscopy revealed an increase in the motility of APCs around each MTZ soon after laser illumination (Wang et al. 2014). These APCs were actively recruited into the vicinity of MTZs, forming a micro-sterile inflammation array (Wang et al. 2014). The recruitment is likely directed by various chemokines including CCL2, CCL3, CCL7, CCL20, CXCL9, CXCL10, and CXCL2 that are expressed at high levels at the inoculation site following NAFL treatment (Wang et al. 2014). Over a 48 h period, these APCs were activated around individual MTZs, and upon activation, the cells migrated into the draining lymph nodes (Wang et al. 2014). Accelerated emigration of activated APCs into the draining lymph nodes was crucial for augmentation of vaccine-induced immunity as well as for reduction of local inflammation (Wang et al. 2014). In this regard, a smaller number of activated APCs at the inoculation site can speed up resolution of inflammation, whereas a higher number of mature APCs in draining lymph nodes are pivotal for heightened immune responses. One of the crucial “danger” signals was recently identified to be double-strand DNA (dsDNA) released from laser-damaged cells (Wang et al. 2014). Thus, mice deficient in STING, a key protein in DNA sensing pathway, could not respond to NAFL treatment and failed to augment immune responses against influenza vaccines (Wang et al. 2014). In comparison, mice deficient in other immune pathways, including TLRs and inflammasome, responded to NAFL treatment similarly to wild-type mice (Wang et al. 2014).

17.4 Adjuvant-Incorporated ID Nicotine Vaccination

Several adjuvants, like LVA and MPL adjuvants that cause little skin irritation and a highly potent MPL/CpG adjuvant, were tested in ID nicotine vaccination. As can be seen in Fig. 17.2a, incorporation of LVA only in the primary immunization in a 3-dose regimen significantly increased NicAb titer by 2.5 and 18.5 times as compared to the same doses of ID and IM immunization, respectively. Two ID immunizations in the presence of MPL induced 5.0 times higher NicAb titer than 3 ID immunizations or 6.8 times higher NicAb titer than 7 IM immunizations (Fig. 17.2a). Two ID immunizations in the presence of MPL/CpG further increased NicAb titer that was 9.3 times higher than 3 ID immunizations and 12.6 times higher than 7 IM immunizations (Fig. 17.2a). NicAb titer after 3 ID immunizations in the presence of LVA or 2 immunizations in the presence of MPL or MPL/CpG was 1.9, 3.5, or 6.9 times higher than that induced by 4 IM immunizations in the presence of alum adjuvant, respectively (Fig. 17.2a). The latter is a vaccination regimen similar to the clinical trial. Incorporation of adjuvants into ID immunization also significantly prolonged a high NicAb titer for more than 3 months as compared to ID group (Fig. 17.2a). Increased NicAb titers after incorporation of adjuvants into ID immunization more significantly inhibited nicotine entry into the brain after nicotine challenge (Fig. 17.2b). Decreases in brain nicotine levels by 34 %, 48 %, or 62 % were attained after incorporation of LVA, MPL, and MPL/CpG into ID immunization, respectively (Fig. 17.2b). Among the 3 adjuvants tested, MPL/CpG adjuvant is the most potent and brain nicotine levels after 2 ID immunizations in the presence of MPL/CpG were only half of those after 4 IM immunizations in the presence of alum adjuvant (Fig. 17.2b). As compared to ID vaccination alone, serum nicotine level was increased by 167 %, 130 %, and 294 % after incorporation of LVA, MPL, and MPL/CpG adjuvant, respectively (Fig. 17.2c). Serum nicotine level was comparable between LVA + ID and alum + IM group (Fig. 17.2c). The more significant inhibition of nicotine entry into the brain with a fewer doses of MPL/CpG-incorporated ID immunization strongly indicates the advantages of MPL/CpG adjuvant in adjuvantation of nicotine vaccines.

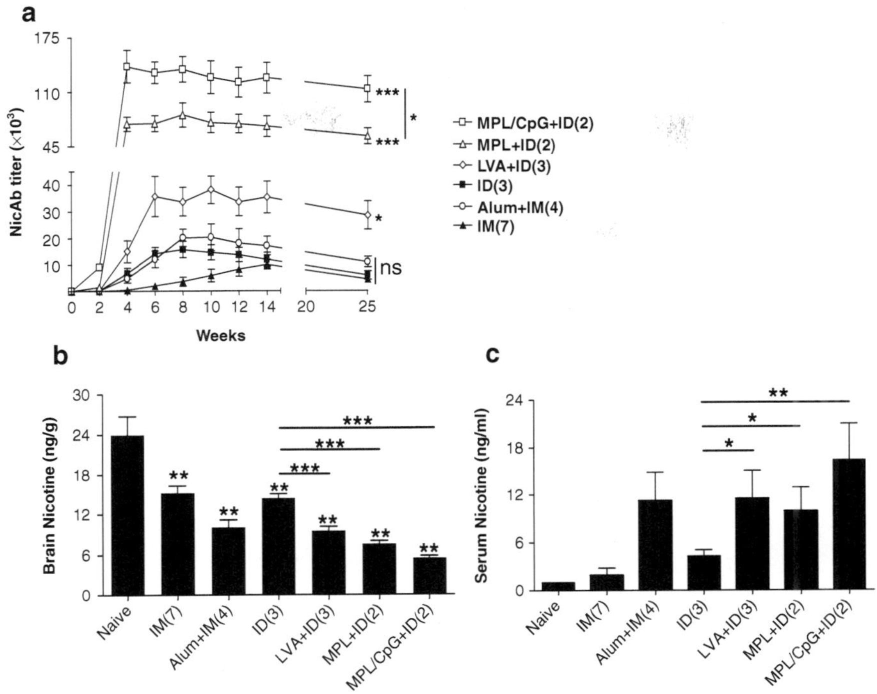

Fig. 17.2 Superior ID nicotine vaccine immunization with various adjuvants. (**a**) BALB/c mice were IM immunized with Nic-KLH alone (*filled triangle*) or in combination with alum (*circle*) or ID immunized with Nic-KLH alone (*filled rectangle*) or in combination with LVA (*diamond*), MPL (*triangle*), and MPL/CpG (*rectangle*). The number of immunizations is shown in the parentheses behind the group name. Serum NicAb titer was measured one day before each immunization and 2 and 13 weeks after the last immunization. NicAb titer in the alum + IM group was compared with the IM group, while NicAb titers in LVA + ID, MPL + ID, and MPL/CpG + ID group were compared with the ID group. (**b**, **c**) Brain and blood nicotine levels following nicotine challenge. Nonimmunized or nicotine vaccine-immunized mice were intravenously challenged with 0.01 mg/kg nicotine, and 5 min later, brain and blood were harvested and brain (**b**) and serum nicotine levels (**c**) were quantified by gas chromatography. Two-tailed student t-test was used to compare difference between various immunization groups and nonimmunized control group or between LVA-, MPL-, and MPL/CpG-incorporated ID immunization group and ID immunization alone in (**b**). One-tailed Mann-Whitney test was used to compare difference between LVA-, MPL-, and MPL/CpG-incorporated ID immunization and ID immunization alone in (**c**). $n = 4–6$. *, **, ***, $p < 0.05$, 0.01, and 0.001, respectively

17.5 Novel Skin Delivery Technologies

Apart from safe adjuvants for skin vaccination, how to deliver vaccines and adjuvants into the skin without overt skin reactions remains a significant challenge. This is particularly true for nicotine vaccines considering nicotine vaccines require potent adjuvants to be effective. For instance, the aforementioned MPL/CpG adjuvant profoundly improved immunogenicity of ID nicotine vaccine, yet caused severe local reactions (Fig. 17.1). Aside from adjuvant-induced local reactions, it is well documented in the clinics that ID vaccination alone often causes more frequent and severer local reactions than IM vaccination (Leroux-Roels et al. 2008; Sticchi et al. 2010). For instance, the live-attenuated *Mycobacterium bovis* Bacillus Calmette-Guerin (BCG) vaccine induced severe local reactions that ended with permanent scars in more than 90 % vaccinees (Jeena et al. 2001). ID rabies vaccine induced much higher rates of erythema, pruritus, and other local reactions than IM vaccination (Lang et al. 1999). ID influenza vaccine induced an overall 30–75 % erythema, induration, edema, and pruritus at local injection site, while IM injection induced only <10 % of these local reactions (Leroux-Roels et al. 2008). Because of more unwanted skin irritation associated with ID vaccination, BCG vaccine, rabies vaccine, and seasonal influenza vaccine are the only vaccines approved for ID delivery, among which BCG vaccine has to be administered into the dermal tissue to avoid abscesses and the other two vaccines are delivered into the dermal tissue for dose sparing and cost saving (Leroux-Roels et al. 2008; Jeena et al. 2001; Lang et al. 1999). Thus, development of novel ID or skin delivery technologies with minimized local reactions are urgently needed. Next we introduce recent advances in developing reliable ID delivery technologies and novel skin delivery technologies that are needle-free, painless, and potentially lesion-free.

17.5.1 ID Immunization

Due to the thin skin tissue, special techniques are required to accurately deliver vaccines into the skin. Currently, Mantoux technique, developed by Charles Mantoux in the early twentieth century, has been used for ID delivery of BCG vaccine and tuberculin for tuberculosis (TB) prevention and diagnosis, respectively (Roth et al. 2005). For accurate ID delivery, needle bevel in Mantoux method is inserted at a 5–15° angle into the skin, and after advancing ~3 mm until the entire bevel is covered by the skin, vaccine or tuberculin is slowly injected and a tense, pale wheal will appear around the needle bevel (Kim et al. 2012a). Mantoux technique has been also used for ID delivery of rabies vaccine. Although Mantoux technique can accurately deliver vaccines into the skin, this method requires specially trained personnel and faces significant challenges for use in resource-poor areas (Kim et al. 2012a). Mantoux technique also generates pain because relatively big needles (26th–27th gauge) are used to avoid the curving of the needle during insertion and to ensure the right positioning of the needle bevel within the dermal tissue. Mantoux-based ID injection hasn't been broadly practiced for mass immunization in the clinics despite the advantage of improved vaccine immunogenicity so far.

To facilitate reliable ID injection, an ID adapter is designed to fit traditional 1 cc syringe and ½ inch needle (Norman et al. 2014). By sitting around the ½ inch needle, the ID adapter guides the injection depth and angles in avoid of needle penetration across the dermal layer. The ID adapter was approved by FDA in 2013 for readily ID injection with minimal training. A microneedle (MN)-based device, called MicronJet 600 (NanoPass), equipped with three hollow pyramid-shaped MNs, each with 250 μm tall, is also developed to replace hypodermic needles to fit with traditional syringes for readily ID injection (Donnelly et al. 2010).

In 2009, a microinjection technique, called ID microinjection system (Soluvia™, BD), was approved for delivering a reduced dose of seasonal influenza vaccine in adults (Leroux-Roels et al. 2008; Laurent et al. 2007). The microinjection system is a prefilled syringe equipped with an ultrashort (1.5 mm) and ultrafine (30th gauge) needle (Laurent et al. 2007). Different from Mantoux technique, the needle in the microinjection system is perpendicularly inserted into the skin. The human skin is about 2–3 mm in thickness and the microinjection system can accurately deliver vaccine into the dermal tissue with minimal training. In addition, an ~40 % thinner needle in the microinjection system causes less pain during insertion as compared to traditional needles. More than 80 % adults reported no or hardly any pain at the time of microinjection, as compared to ~75 % reported obvious pain in Mantoux-based ID injection (Leroux-Roels et al. 2008; Laurent et al. 2007; Kenney et al. 2004; Belshe et al. 2004). It also causes less pain when compared with IM injection (Leroux-Roels et al. 2008; Laurent et al. 2007; Kenney et al. 2004; Belshe et al. 2004). The microinjection system has been approved for a reduced dose of seasonal influenza vaccine in Europe and the United States today. The clinical test of using the microinjection system in place of a traditional needle to deliver tuberculin has been completed (trial #NCT01611844). Due to the minimal training and pain, the microinjection system holds great promise for ID delivery of vaccines, like hepatitis B vaccine, inactivated polio vaccine, yellow fever vaccine, hepatitis A vaccine, and the like.

Besides the microinjection system, an ID Needle-free Injection System (PharmaJet) has been developed as an alternative to Mantoux-based ID injection (Kwilas et al. 2014). The PharmaJet ID System uses high pressure to generate a narrow, high-velocity fluid to penetrate and deposit liquid vaccines into the dermal tissue (Kim et al. 2012a; Kwilas et al. 2014). To eliminate contamination risks, the contact part with patients in the PharmaJet ID system is a sterile, single-use, disposable needle-free syringe. This system represents the first FDA-approved needle-free injection system that greatly reduces biohazardous sharp waste in association with vaccination. Besides ID injection, PharmaJet needle-free injection system has been also approved as an alternative to traditional syringes and needles for subcutaneous or IM injection.

17.5.2 Novel Technologies for Lesion-Free Skin Vaccination

The aforementioned ID delivery technologies largely ease the technical hurdles of ID injection. Yet, these technologies deliver liquid vaccines into the dermal tissue, causing skin wheals, and are not absolutely painless due to the existence of nerve ends in the dermis. Although only 0.1 ml vaccine liquids are delivered into the dermal tissue (vs. 0.5 ml in IM vaccination), significant skin morphology change occurs to accommodate the vaccine liquids (Laurent et al. 2007). Moreover, these technologies don't necessarily limit local reactogenicity of vaccines and adjuvants. We next introduce a micro-fractional epidermal powder delivery (EPD) for needle-free, painless vaccination, concurrent with little local reactogenicity (Chen et al. 2014).

It is well known that skin injury is healed by expansion of surrounding healthy epithelial cells into injured area (Shaw and Martin 2009). The larger the skin injury is, the longer the healing takes. On the contrary, if separated micro-injuries are generated in the skin surface with an equivalent area to a bulk injury, these micro-injuries would be healed much quicker than the bulk injury (e.g., days vs. weeks). This fully repairing capacity forms the basis of ablative fractional laser- and MN-based cosmetic skin resurfacing (Manstein et al. 2004). We extend the quick recovery of micro-injuries to transdermal vaccine delivery aimed at minimizing vaccine-induced local reactions. One of these technologies is called micro-fractional epidermal powder delivery, abbreviated as EPD, based on pretreatment of the skin with ablative fractional laser or MN to generate an array of microchannels (MC) in the epidermis followed by topical application of powder vaccine-coated array patches to deliver vaccines into skin via MCs (Chen et al. 2014). Our investigation shows that EPD generates more than 80 % delivery efficiency within 1 h (Chen et al. 2014). Efflux of interstitial fluid into the MCs probably plays a crucial role in laser- or MN-based EPD (Chen et al. 2014). It can be envisioned that topically applied vaccine powder would be dissolved by the efflux fluid, and after dissolution, the vaccine diffuses from patches into MCs and then the surrounding tissue along the concentration gradient (Chen et al. 2014). Laser- and MN-generated MCs can be quickly healed by the surrounding normal tissue, thus warranting lesion-free (Chen et al. 2014). While profoundly reducing skin reactions, fractional delivery did not compromise vaccine immunogenicity and adjuvant potency (Chen et al. 2014). As mentioned early, combined MPL and CpG vigorously augmented ID nicotine vaccination, but it caused unacceptable skin lesion (Chen et al. 2012). If the adjuvant is delivered via the EPD technology, the skin lesion is expected to be largely averted. As can be seen in Fig. 17.3, ID delivery of lipopolysaccharide (LPS), similar in structure but more potent than MPL, and CpG adjuvants (LPS/CpG) induced significant local reactions, like erythema, swelling, and ulceration, which peaked on day 4 in mice (Fig. 17.3a) or day 2 in pigs (Fig. 17.3b) (Chen et al. 2014). Although the skin was gradually healed, it was unable to fully recover during the experimental period, as evidenced by the obvious skin morphology change observed 21 days later in mice and 35 days later in pigs (Fig. 17.3). In contrast, EPD of LPS/CpG induced minimal local reactions with little erythema, swelling, or ulceration, and the skin completely recovered within 2–3 weeks (Fig. 17.3). Similarly, ID delivery of the highly reactive BCG vaccine induced severe local reactions, while EPD of BCG vaccine induced minimal local reactions and the skin obtained a full recovery within 10 days (Chen et al. 2014). In addition to the micro-fractional delivery, reduced local reactions and a full skin recovery following EPD may also be ascribed to a slow release of vaccines and adjuvants from laser-generated MCs (Chen et al. 2014). In accordance to this, we found a significant amount of AF647-OVA remained inside MCs and slowly released for >7 days (Chen et al. 2014). In contrast, ID injection acutely releases all vaccine/adjuvant content into the skin and induces robust inflammation at the inoculation

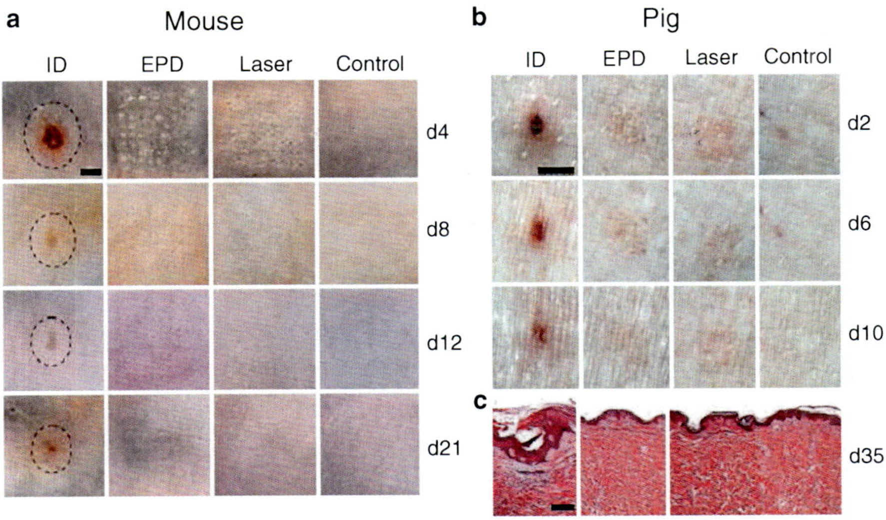

Fig. 17.3 EPD reduces local reactogenicity of LPS/CpG adjuvant. (**a**) Mice were treated with laser followed by topical application of powder LPS/CpG (20 μg each)-coated array patches (*EPD*), or intradermally injected with patch extracts (ID), or treated with laser alone, or left untreated. Skin pictures were taken on days 4, 8, 12, and 21 and representative local reactions were shown. The edges of the local reactions in ID group were outlined by dashed lines. Scale: 1.5 mm. (**b–c**) Pigs were treated with laser followed by topical application of powder LPS/CpG (20 μg each)-coated array patches, or intradermally injected with LPS/CpG from patch extracts, or treated with laser alone, or intradermally injected with PBS. Representative local reactions on days 2, 6, and 10 were shown (**b**, scale: 3 mm). Pigs were sacrificed on day 35 and skin samples were collected and subjected to histological analysis. Representative skin H&E sections were shown (**c**, scale: 200 μm)

site. The local reactions following ID injection occur in the entire skin surface with a few millimeters in diameter, which takes much longer time and is more difficult for new tissue to grow and replace the damaged skin (Chen et al. 2014).

Conceivably, the novel EPD would allow the safe delivery of many potent adjuvants, like MPL/CpG, to robustly improve nicotine vaccine immunogenicity and success rate in the clinics. Besides traditional adjuvants, EPD can be conveniently combined with laser adjuvants, like the previously described LVA and NAFL, to boost nicotine vaccine immunogenicity with minimal local reactions. The novel EPD potentially offers the following advantages for nicotine vaccine delivery. Firstly, powder nicotine vaccines are more stable than liquid vaccines and might eliminate cold-chain storage, enabling cost-effective anti-nicotine immunotherapy in developing countries, where 84 % smokers reside (McAdams et al. 2012). Secondly, EPD is expected to significantly improve patient compliance and vaccine acceptance due to its needle-free, painless delivery. Thirdly, adjuvant-incorporated EPD is able to maintain a high NicAb titer and induce a long abstinence rate with fewer boosters, as indicated in our previous report (Chen et al. 2012). Fourthly, with a handheld laser- or MN-based EPD device, smokers may be able to do self-administration of nicotine vaccines at home. The handheld device can be engineered to integrate laser ablation and patch application for clinical or home use. Alternatively, powder array patch delivery may be accomplished with skin-piercing MNs, which might provide a more simple and cost-effective EPD. Besides nicotine vaccines, EPD can be used to deliver many other vaccines considering the fact that many current vaccines are already manufactured, shipped, and stored in a lyophilized powder form and various technologies are available to transform liquid vaccines into a dry form, like freeze-drying, spray-drying, and spray-freeze-drying (McAdams et al. 2012; Alcock et al. 2010; Sou et al. 2011; Chen and Kristensen 2009). Clearly, EPD opens a new avenue for safer and more effective skin vaccination.

Besides EPD, MNs represent another micro-fractional delivery technology under active development for various drug and vaccine deliveries (Donnelly et al. 2010; Kim et al. 2012b). With sufficient distances between nearby MNs, MN technology is promising to also reduce local side effects of vaccines and adjuvants. The potential use of MN technology for nicotine vaccine delivery and adjuvantation warrants further investigation.

17.6 Summary

Despite recent setbacks in the field, much can be improved, like nicotine vaccine design, immunization protocol, delivery, and adjuvants, toward a successful anti-nicotine immunotherapy. This chapter introduces highly immunogenic ID route in combination with safe cutaneous adjuvants to improve nicotine vaccine immunogenicity and novel ID delivery technologies to facilitate clinical translation of this approach. In address of local reactogenicity associated with ID vaccination and patient compliance, this chapter also introduces a needle-free, painless EPD with minimized local reactions for nicotine vaccine delivery and effective adjuvantation, because EPD allows incorporation of potent adjuvants. Besides nicotine vaccine, EPD also holds great promise to significantly improve efficacy of other addiction vaccines.

Acknowledgments This work is supported in part by the National Institutes of Health grants RC1 DA028378 and AI089779 (to M.X.W.) and DA033371 and AI107678 (to X.Y.C.).

Conflict of Interest The authors have no conflict of interest to declare.

References

Alcock R, Cottingham MG, Rollier CS, Furze J, De Costa SD, Hanlon M, Spencer AJ, Honeycutt JD, Wyllie DH, Gilbert SC, Bregu M, Hill AV. Long-term thermostabilization of live poxviral and adenoviral vaccine vectors at supraphysiological temperatures in carbohydrate glass. Sci Transl Med. 2010;2:19ra12.

Alexey M, Sudha G, Yantao Z, Rachid N, Frederique B, Ivan B, Jed R, Pradeep G. Effect of anti-nicotine immunization with NIC-002 vaccine on brain nicotine accumulation during cigarette smoking. J Nucl Med. 2013;54:30.

Barnighausen T, Bloom DE, Cafiero-Fonseca ET, O'Brien JC. Valuing vaccination. Proc Natl Acad Sci U S A. 2014;111:12313–9.

Belshe RB, Newman FK, Cannon J, Duane C, Treanor J, Van Hoecke C, Howe BJ, Dubin G. Serum antibody responses after intradermal vaccination against influenza. N Engl J Med. 2004;351:2286–94.

Cerny EH, Cerny T. Vaccines against nicotine. Hum Vaccin. 2009;5:200–5.

Chen D, Kristensen D. Opportunities and challenges of developing thermostable vaccines. Expert Rev Vaccines. 2009;8:547–57.

Chen GY, Nunez G. Sterile inflammation: sensing and reacting to damage. Nat Rev Immunol. 2010;10:826–37.

Chen X, Wu MX. Laser vaccine adjuvant for cutaneous immunization. Expert Rev Vaccines. 2011;10:1397–403.

Chen X, Kim P, Farinelli B, Doukas A, Yun SH, Gelfand JA, Anderson RR, Wu MX. A novel laser vaccine adjuvant increases the motility of antigen presenting cells. PLoS One. 2010;5, e13776.

Chen X, Pravetoni M, Bhayana B, Pentel PR, Wu MX. High immunogenicity of nicotine vaccines obtained by intradermal delivery with safe adjuvants. Vaccine. 2012;31:159–64.

Chen X, Wang J, Shah D, Wu MX. An update on the use of laser technology in skin vaccination. Expert Rev Vaccines. 2013;12:1313–23.

Chen X, Kositratna G, Zhou C, Manstein D, Wu MX. Micro-fractional epidermal powder delivery for improved skin vaccination. J Control Release. 2014;192:310–6.

Cornuz J, Zwahlen S, Jungi WF, Osterwalder J, Klingler K, van Melle G, Bangala Y, Guessous I, Muller P, Willers J, Maurer P, Bachmann MF, Cerny T. A vaccine against nicotine for smoking cessation: a randomized controlled trial. PLoS One. 2008;3, e2547.

Donnelly RF, Raj Singh TR, Woolfson AD. Microneedle-based drug delivery systems: microfabrication, drug delivery, and safety. Drug Deliv. 2010;17:187–207.

Duggan ST, Plosker GL. Intanza 15 microg intradermal seasonal influenza vaccine: in older adults (aged>or=60 years). Drugs Aging. 2010;27:597–605.

Fahim RE, Kessler PD, Fuller SA, Kalnik MW. Nicotine vaccines. CNS Neurol Disord Drug Targets. 2011;10:905–15.

Fahim RE, Kessler PD, Kalnik MW. Therapeutic vaccines against tobacco addiction. Expert Rev Vaccines. 2013;12:333–42.

Foy JE, Hendriksz T, Malouf P, Tobin A. Acceptability of fluzone intradermal vaccine to patients and vaccine administrators. J Am Osteopath Assoc. 2013;113:134–43.

Glenn GM, Kenney RT, Ellingsworth LR, Frech SA, Hammond SA, Zoeteweij JP. Transcutaneous immunization and immunostimulant strategies: capitalizing on the immunocompetence of the skin. Expert Rev Vaccines. 2003;2:253–67.

Hallquist VP. Thank you for NOT smoking. J Adv Pract Oncol. 2014;5:161–2.

Hatsukami DK, Jorenby DE, Gonzales D, Rigotti NA, Glover ED, Oncken CA, Tashkin DP, Reus VI, Akhavain RC, Fahim RE, Kessler PD, Niknian M, Kalnik MW, Rennard SI. Immunogenicity and smoking-cessation outcomes for a novel nicotine immunotherapeutic. Clin Pharmacol Ther. 2011;89:392–9.

Hoogsteder PH, Kotz D, van Spiegel PI, Viechtbauer W, Brauer R, Kessler PD, Kalnik MW, Fahim RE, van Schayck OC. The efficacy and safety of a nicotine conjugate vaccine (NicVAX(R)) or placebo co-administered with varenicline (Champix(R)) for smoking cessation: study protocol of a phase IIb, double blind, randomized, placebo controlled trial. BMC Public Health. 2012a;12:1052.

Hoogsteder PH, Kotz D, van Spiegel PI, Viechtbauer W, Brauer R, Kessler PD, Kalnik MW, Fahim RE, van Schayck OC. The efficacy and safety of a nicotine conjugate vaccine (NicVAX(R)) or placebo co-administered with varenicline (Champix(R)) for smoking cessation: study protocol of a phase IIb, double blind, randomized, placebo controlled trial. BMC Public Health. 2012b;12:1052.

Hoogsteder PH, Kotz D, van Spiegel PI, Viechtbauer W, van Schayck OC. Efficacy of the nicotine vaccine 3'-AmNic-rEPA (NicVAX) co-administered with varenicline and counselling for smoking cessation: a randomized placebo-controlled trial. Addiction. 2014;109:1252–9.

Jeena PM, Chhagan MK, Topley J, Coovadia HM. Safety of the intradermal Copenhagen 1331 BCG vaccine in neonates in Durban. South Africa Bull World Health Organ. 2001;79:337–43.

Jha P, Peto R. Global effects of smoking, of quitting, and of taxing tobacco. N Engl J Med. 2014;370:60–8.

Kashiwagi S, Yuan J, Forbes B, Hibert ML, Lee EL, Whicher L, Goudie C, Yang Y, Chen T, Edelblute B, Collette B, Edington L, Trussler J, Nezivar J, Leblanc P, Bronson R, Tsukada K, Suematsu M, Dover J, Brauns T, Gelfand J, Poznansky MC. Near-infrared laser adjuvant for influenza vaccine. PLoS One. 2013;8, e82899.

Kashiwagi S, Brauns T, Gelfand J, Poznansky MC. Laser vaccine adjuvants. History, progress, and potential. Hum Vaccin Immunother. 2014;10:1892–907.

Kenney RT, Frech SA, Muenz LR, Villar CP, Glenn GM. Dose sparing with intradermal injection of influenza vaccine. N Engl J Med. 2004;351:2295–301.

Kim YC, Jarrahian C, Zehrung D, Mitragotri S, Prausnitz MR. Delivery systems for intradermal vaccination. Curr Top Microbiol Immunol. 2012a;351:77–112.

Kim YC, Park JH, Prausnitz MR. Microneedles for drug and vaccine delivery. Adv Drug Deliv Rev. 2012b;64:1547–68.

Kool M, Soullie T, van Nimwegen M, Willart MA, Muskens F, Jung S, Hoogsteden HC, Hammad H, Lambrecht BN. Alum adjuvant boosts adaptive immunity by inducing uric acid and activating inflammatory dendritic cells. J Exp Med. 2008;205:869–82.

Kwilas S, Kishimori JM, Josleyn M, Jerke K, Ballantyne J, Royals M, Hooper JW. A hantavirus pulmonary syndrome (HPS) DNA vaccine delivered using a spring-powered jet injector elicits a potent neutralizing antibody response in rabbits and nonhuman primates. Curr Gene Ther. 2014;14:200–10.

Lambrecht BN, Kool M, Willart MA, Hammad H. Mechanism of action of clinically approved adjuvants. Curr Opin Immunol. 2009;21:23–9.

Lang J, Hoa DQ, Gioi NV, Vien NC, Nguyen CV, Rouyrre N, Forrat R. Immunogenicity and safety of low-dose intradermal rabies vaccination given during an expanded programme on immunization session in Viet Nam: results of a comparative randomized trial. Trans R Soc Trop Med Hyg. 1999;93:208–13.

Laurent PE, Bonnet S, Alchas P, Regolini P, Mikszta JA, Pettis R, Harvey NG. Evaluation of the clinical performance of a new intradermal vaccine administration technique and associated delivery system. Vaccine. 2007;25:8833–42.

Leroux-Roels I, Vets E, Freese R, Seiberling M, Weber F, Salamand C, Leroux-Roels G. Seasonal influenza vaccine delivered by intradermal microinjection: a randomised controlled safety and immunogenicity trial in adults. Vaccine. 2008;26:6614–9.

Liu L, Zhong Q, Tian T, Dubin K, Athale SK, Kupper TS. Epidermal injury and infection during poxvirus immunization is crucial for the generation of highly protective T cell-mediated immunity. Nat Med. 2010;16:224–7.

Lofquist JM, Weimert NA, Hayney MS. Smallpox: a review of clinical disease and vaccination. Am J Health Syst Pharm. 2003;60:749–56.

Mackanos MA, Contag CH. Pulse duration determines levels of Hsp70 induction in tissues following laser irradiation. J Biomed Opt. 2011;16:078002.

Manstein D, Herron GS, Sink RK, Tanner H, Anderson RR. Fractional photothermolysis: a new concept for cutaneous remodeling using microscopic patterns of thermal injury. Lasers Surg Med. 2004;34:426–38.

Maurer P, Jennings GT, Willers J, Rohner F, Lindman Y, Roubicek K, Renner WA, Muller P, Bachmann MF. A therapeutic vaccine for nicotine dependence: preclinical efficacy, and Phase I safety and immunogenicity. Eur J Immunol. 2005;35:2031–40.

McAdams D, Chen D, Kristensen D. Spray drying and vaccine stabilization. Expert Rev Vaccines. 2012;11:1211–9.

Moreno AY, Janda KD. Immunopharmacotherapy: vaccination strategies as a treatment for drug abuse and dependence. Pharmacol Biochem Behav. 2009;92:199–205.

Nichol KL. Influenza vaccination in the elderly: impact on hospitalisation and mortality. Drugs Aging. 2005;22:495–515.

Norman JJ, Jyoti G, Patel SR, Sara P, Courtney J, Darin Z, Prausnitz MR. Reliability and accuracy of intradermal injection by Mantoux technique, hypodermic needle adapter, and hollow microneedle in pigs. Drug Deliv Transl Res. 2014;4:126–30.

Nougarede N, Bisceglia H, Rozieres A, Goujon C, Boudet F, Laurent P, Vanbervliet B, Rodet K, Hennino A, Nicolas JF. Nine mug intradermal influenza vaccine and 15 mug intramuscular influenza vaccine induce similar cellular and humoral immune responses in adults. Hum Vaccin Immunother. 2014;10:2713–20.

Pentel PR, LeSage MG. New directions in nicotine vaccine design and use. Adv Pharmacol. 2014a;69:553–80.

Pentel PR, LeSage MG. New directions in nicotine vaccine design and use. Adv Pharmacol. 2014b;69:553–80.

PrabhuDas M, Adkins B, Gans H, King C, Levy O, Ramilo O, Siegrist CA. Challenges in infant immunity: implications for responses to infection and vaccines. Nat Immunol. 2011;12: 189–94.

Prausnitz MR, Langer R. Transdermal drug delivery. Nat Biotechnol. 2008;26:1261–8.

Preissig J, Hamilton K, Markus R. Current laser resurfacing technologies: a review that delves beneath the surface. Semin Plast Surg. 2012;26:109–16.

Romani N, Flacher V, Tripp CH, Sparber F, Ebner S, Stoitzner P. Targeting skin dendritic cells to improve intradermal vaccination. Curr Top Microbiol Immunol. 2012a;351:113–38.

Romani N, Flacher V, Tripp CH, Sparber F, Ebner S, Stoitzner P. Targeting skin dendritic cells to improve intradermal vaccination. Curr Top Microbiol Immunol. 2012b;351:113–38.

Roth A, Sodemann M, Jensen H, Poulsen A, Gustafson P, Gomes J, Djana Q, Jakobsen M, Garly ML, Rodrigues A, Aaby P. Vaccination technique, PPD reaction and BCG scarring in a cohort of children born in Guinea-Bissau 2000-2002. Vaccine. 2005;23:3991–8.

Shaw TJ, Martin P. Wound repair at a glance. J Cell Sci. 2009;122:3209–13.

Siegrist CA, Aspinall R. B-cell responses to vaccination at the extremes of age. Nat Rev Immunol. 2009;9:185–94.

Sou T, Meeusen EN, de Veer M, Morton DA, Kaminskas LM, McIntosh MP. New developments in dry powder pulmonary vaccine delivery. Trends Biotechnol. 2011;29:191–8.

Sticchi L, Alberti M, Alicino C, Crovari P. The intradermal vaccination: past experiences and current perspectives. J Prev Med Hyg. 2010;51:7–14.

Tonstad S, Heggen E, Giljam H, Lagerback PA, Tonnesen P, Wikingsson LD, Lindblom N, de Villiers S, Svensson TH, Fagerstrom KO. Niccine(R), a nicotine vaccine, for relapse prevention: a phase II, randomized, placebo-controlled, multicenter clinical trial. Nicotine Tob Res. 2013;15:1492–501.

Verma R, Khanna P, Prinja S, Rajput M. Intra-dermal administration of rabies vaccines in developing countries: at an affordable cost. Hum Vaccin. 2011;7:792–4.

Vono M, Taccone M, Caccin P, Gallotta M, Donvito G, Falzoni S, Palmieri E, Pallaoro M, Rappuoli R, Di Virgilio F, De Gregorio E, Montecucco C, Seubert A. The adjuvant MF59 induces ATP release from muscle that potentiates response to vaccination. Proc Natl Acad Sci U S A. 2013;110:21095–100.

Wang J, Shah D, Chen X, Anderson RR, Wu MX. A micro-sterile inflammation array as an adjuvant for influenza vaccines. Nat Commun. 2014;5:4447.

Chapter 18
Hapten Design for Anti-addiction Vaccine Development

Karen C. Collins and Kim D. Janda

The success of a drug of abuse vaccine is contingent on obtaining significant concentrations of high-affinity antibodies that are specific to the targeted drug(s), and the structural identity of the hapten used to elicit the immune response is a crucial determinant of these key vaccine properties (LeSage and Pentel 2010; Berzofsky and Schechter 1981; Nowak 1996; Langman 2000). Although the exact structure of the targeted drug is the theoretically ideal template for antibody production, drugs of abuse are low-molecular-weight molecules that cannot themselves elicit an immune response, instead requiring conjugation to a protein or peptide carrier to allow them to be recognized. Furthermore, not all drugs are stable; for example, both cocaine and heroin are metabolized/hydrolyzed rapidly in vivo to give multiple metabolites, which themselves can be bioactive or bioinactive. This instability and resulting multidrug mixture is a key strategic consideration in hapten design. Most drugs of abuse are also taken in enantiopure form, introducing hapten enantiopurity as another potentially important variable. Finally, the hapten must of course be tractable to synthesis and suitably functionalized to allow chemoselective conjugation to the carrier.

This review will predominantly focus on vaccines against the four main targets in this area, namely, those against opioids (including heroin and oxycodone), cocaine, nicotine, and methamphetamine (Fig. 18.1). Ideally, cross comparison between vaccination studies would allow definitive critical analysis of the key hapten design elements listed above, using quantitative data on antibody affinities, concentrations, and specificities. However, the nascent field of drugs of abuse vaccines has yet to reach a generally accepted methodology for experimental design to allow comparison between studies, and at this point, attempted analysis of that type is greatly flawed. Differences abound in vaccination schedule, choice of animals, analytical methods, and other practical aspects. Furthermore, in addition to the hapten

K.C. Collins • K.D. Janda (✉)
Department of Chemistry, The Scripps Research Institute, 10550 North Torrey Pines Road, La Jolla, CA 92037, USA
e-mail: kdjanda@scripps.edu

I.D. Montoya (ed.), *Biologics to Treat Substance Use Disorders: Vaccines, Monoclonal Antibodies, and Enzymes*, DOI 10.1007/978-3-319-23150-1_18

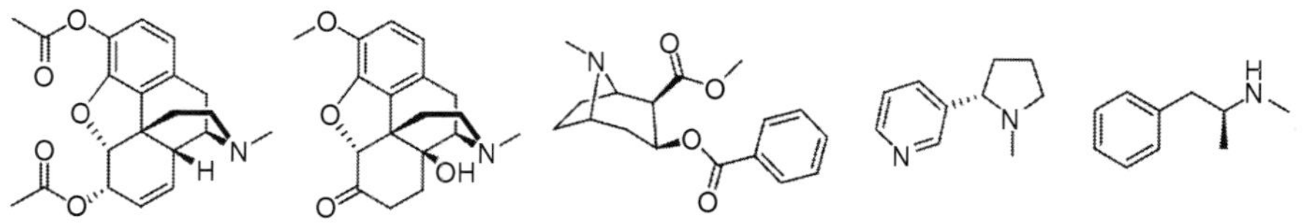

Fig. 18.1 Major drugs of abuse targets for immunopharmacotherapy

design, the carrier protein, adjuvant, and formulation are all critical variables in the overall success of the vaccine and are rarely consistent across different studies. Finally, high variability is observed and accepted in the field even between repeated experiments. The examples selected and discussed in this analysis are therefore primarily considered in relation to direct analogs studied in the same experiment. This review provides a general overview of hapten design considerations, by no means exhaustive, to illustrate the current strategies employed in the field.

18.1 Drug Target Consideration for Hapten Design

Many of the principles of hapten design are generally applicable to any target drug vaccine: adhere as close to the structure of the natural drug molecule as possible, attach the linker (used to conjugate to the carrier protein) such that appropriate epitopes are displayed for recognition by the immune system, and attempt to minimize any inherent linker-derived immunogenicity. However, other design factors require consideration of the structure and pharmacology of the target drug, including metabolic or hydrolytic instability, the requirement for target selectivity, and the ease of hapten synthesis. In this section, the choice of hapten for each of the five main targets for drugs of abuse vaccines is discussed in the context of the specific challenges faced in obtaining the desired immunological response (Fig. 18.2).

18.1.1 Heroin

Heroin provides a complex example that highlights the wide range of challenges involved in hapten design. The acetyl groups of heroin are rapidly hydrolyzed in vivo to give 6-acetylmorphine (6-AM) and subsequently morphine, before glucuronidation to give morphine-6-glucuronide or its 3-isomer (Fig. 18.2a). The parent drug itself is pharmacologically inactive (Inturrisi et al. 1983), but all the major metabolites (bar morphine-3-glucuronide) are active to various extents and have different pharmacokinetic profiles. There are therefore multiple factors to consider when selecting a hapten or haptens for a heroin vaccine. A strategy targeting heroin would attempt to sequester the parent before it could be hydrolyzed, but should sequestration by the antibody not be fast enough, this would result in an ineffective vaccine. A hapten targeting 6-AM, the more stable first metabolic intermediate exhibiting the

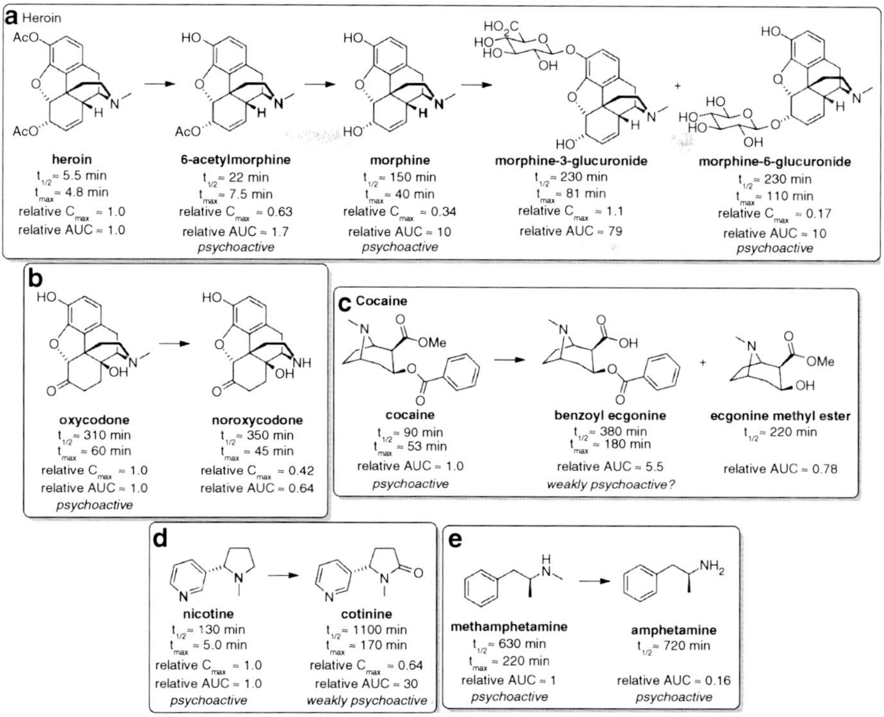

Fig. 18.2 Major metabolites of heroin (Skopp et al. 1997; Osborne et al. 1992; Rook et al. 2006a, b), oxycodone (Pöyhiä et al. 1992), cocaine (Jeffcoat et al. 1989; Jufer et al. 2000; Kolbrich et al. 2006), nicotine (Hukkanen et al. 2005; Yuki et al. 2013) and methamphetamine (Schep et al. 2010; Barceloux 2012) in humans

initial psychoactive pharmacology, may therefore be a more realistic and effective strategy. An important consideration is that heroin can rapidly pass through the blood–brain barrier (BBB), more so than its metabolites, potentially escaping the clutches of protective antibodies circulating in the plasma prior to its hydrolysis to the active species (Janda and Treweek 2012). In fact, however, antibody binding is believed to occur on a much more rapid timescale than brain localization (Orson et al. 2014). Morphine could also be considered an important target since it is the first stable, long-lived intermediate, with a much higher plasma exposure than both heroin and 6-AM (Cook et al. 1993). However, due to its higher polarity and reduced brain penetration, the concentrations of morphine observed in the brain are more likely a result of hydrolysis of heroin and/or 6-AM within the brain rather than BBB passage of morphine itself; in this event, sequestering morphine in the bloodstream may not substantially alter the brain concentration of morphine, and no significant modulation of behavioral effects would be achieved (Seleman et al. 2014).

Janda and Koob attempted to delineate the most favorable drug target for an anti-heroin vaccine through direct comparison of heroin and morphine haptens (Schlosburg et al. 2013) (Fig. 18.3). Vaccination with **Her** resulted in a substantial increase in binding of both heroin and 6-AM in the blood, thus reducing the amount

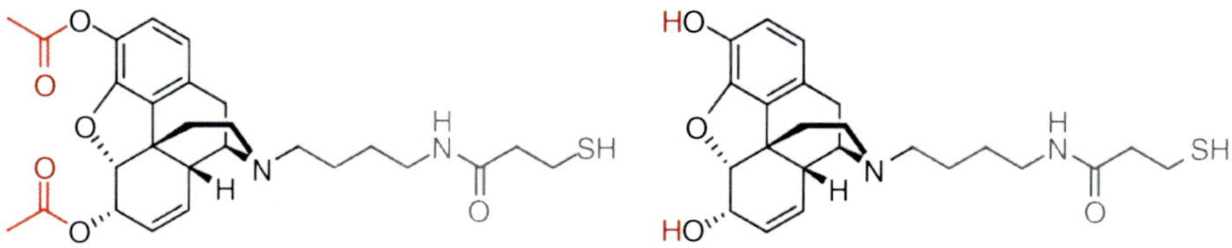

Fig. 18.3 Janda's comparison of heroin and morphine haptens (Schlosburg et al. 2013)

of unbound drug able to enter the brain, but essentially no binding of morphine was seen, whereas **Mor** vaccination resulted in selective morphine sequestration. Supporting this data, **Her** has been shown to elicit antibodies against both heroin and 6-AM, but not towards morphine, suggesting that **Her** presents only heroin- and 6-AM-like epitopes to the immune system (Bremer and Janda 2012). In key behavioral studies, **Her** elicited protection against heroin-induced antinociception, but no significant effect was observed for **Mor**-vaccinated rats. These data taken together strongly suggest that although protection against heroin is important, protection against 6-AM appears to be a key driver in obtaining overall protection against the effects of heroin, and morphine-selective vaccines are relatively ineffective.

18.1.2 Oxycodone

The choice of hapten for oxycodone is much more straightforward than heroin. There is only one major metabolite, noroxycodone, which is not believed to contribute to the pharmacological effects in humans (Kim Pei and Smith 1994; Lalovic et al. 2006) (Fig. 18.2b). A key study used pharmacokinetic–pharmacodynamic modeling to show that pupil constriction in humans, a centrally mediated effect, is fully attributable to levels of the parent oxycodone. However, noroxycodone still has significant plasma exposure, and therefore, selectivity of the antibodies for the parent drug may be important to achieve maximal efficacy.

18.1.3 Cocaine

Although cocaine has similarly unstable ester functionalities as heroin, its hydrolysis is slower (Schramm et al. 1993) (Fig. 18.2c). The major metabolites, benzoyl ecgonine and ecgonine methyl ester, are believed to have limited psychoactivity, although there is some debate over whether benzoyl ecgonine is responsible for some of the effects of cocaine administration (Morishima et al. 1999; Brust 2004). However, since benzoyl ecgonine has much greater plasma exposure than cocaine, accumulating over time due to its long half-life (Ambre et al. 1988), this species has the potential to limit binding of nonselective antibodies to the parent drug, especially after repeated cocaine administration. It therefore may be important to develop an anti-cocaine immune response that is selective for cocaine (Schramm et al. 1993).

One other complicating factor is that abuse of cocaine with alcohol has been shown to result in an additional metabolite, cocaethylene, resulting from transesterification of the methyl ester with ethanol (McCance et al. 1995). This metabolite is also psychoactive and results in longer-lasting effects than when cocaine is taken alone. This may therefore be an important practical consideration when predicting the selectivity of antibodies generated by an anti-cocaine vaccine that will be required for efficacy beyond the clinic.

18.1.4 Nicotine

Nicotine is much more stable than heroin or cocaine, with only one major metabolite, cotinine (Hukkanen et al. 2005; Yuki et al. 2013). Although it possesses some psychoactive properties, cotinine is a much weaker agonist of acetylcholine receptors (Dwoskin et al. 1999) and appears to have no pharmacological effect at feasibly attainable levels in the blood after smoking (Hatsukami et al. 1997) (Fig. 18.2d). However, cotinine can antagonize the effects of nicotine (Keenan et al. 1994) and has comparatively higher serum concentrations due to a substantially longer half-life (Yuki et al. 2013). A nonselective vaccine would therefore likely be less efficacious than a vaccine that was selective for nicotine.

Conversely, it has been suggested that this antagonistic activity of cotinine may actually make it a viable target for an anti-smoking vaccine as the presence of cotinine increases withdrawal during nicotine replacement therapy (NRT) (Oliver et al. 2007). However, given that maintained abstinence from nicotine is required for complete smoking cessation, increasing its pharmacological efficacy would appear to be a risky approach, and nicotine itself is the more popular target of anti-smoking vaccination. In any case, it appears crucial to obtain antibody selectivity for one of these two molecules.

18.1.5 Methamphetamine

Methamphetamine, like nicotine, is relatively stable, with amphetamine being the only appreciable metabolite (Schep et al. 2010; Barceloux 2012) (Fig. 18.2e). Although amphetamine is also psychoactive, it only reaches relatively low plasma concentrations and therefore has a negligible effect following methamphetamine administration (Perez-Reyes et al. 1991; Cook et al. 1993). Methamphetamine therefore represents the simplest scenario for hapten choice, as neither targeting multiple species nor obtaining selectivity for the parent drug is likely necessary to achieve high efficacy.

18.2 Structure Modification for Linker Introduction

The structure of the target drug must inevitably be modified by the attachment of the linker that covalently connects it to the requisite carrier protein or peptide. As discussed above, modification of the structure should ideally be achieved without significantly impacting the antibody recognition of the drug, thus avoiding generation of antibodies that may have high affinity for the hapten but poor affinity to the soluble drug. This is theoretically achieved by the strategic position of the linker at a distal location on the drug to the optimal epitope, although in practice, the latter is difficult to predict and define. Given that antibody binding is a result of multiple molecular interactions with polar and hydrophobic surfaces, multiple attachment points may need to be tested in order to identify the optimal linker location. Furthermore, the synthetic complexity must also be considered; if the resulting hapten is fairly intractable to synthesis, it may preclude its therapeutic use even if it demonstrates high efficacy.

The previous section illustrated that the stability and/or metabolic lability of the drug is another key factor. In the case of heroin, there are multiple, rapidly formed metabolites that the immune response may need to be directed against in order to block the effects of the drug. However in the case of nicotine, the primary metabolite cotinine is essentially inactive yet is present at much higher concentrations in the blood after smoking (Hukkanen et al. 2005), and thus, a linker position ideally should be selected to provide an immune response targeted specifically towards the parent drug.

There are several positions on each drug structure that have been commonly used for linker attachment (Fig. 18.4). The majority of these were chosen due to ease of synthetic derivatization, although stability and epitope presentation are also key considerations.

18.2.1 Heroin

Heroin and cocaine are rigid molecules, with arguably three key chemical motifs that may comprise the critical pharmacophore for antibody recognition: the bridgehead nitrogen and the two esters. Derivatization of these functional groups is far less synthetically challenging than alternative strategies given that syntheses of haptens for these drugs start from the corresponding naturally derived precursors, and thus, the majority of heroin and cocaine haptens link off of these positions.

As discussed previously, heroin hydrolyzes to give psychoactive metabolites 6-AM and morphine, and obtaining effective protection following heroin administra-

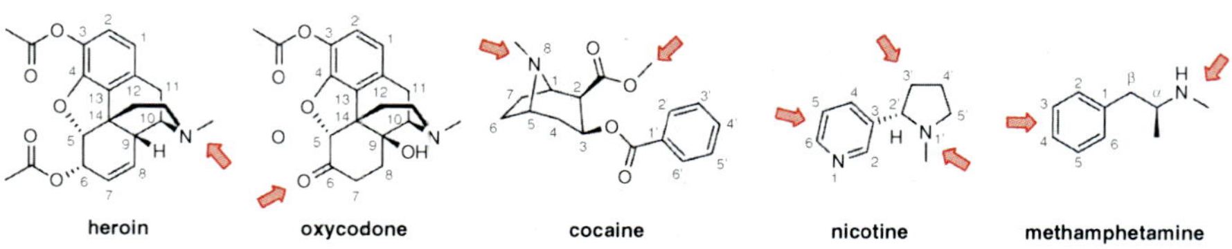

Fig. 18.4 Commonly used sites for linker attachment

tion appears to require antibodies that are directed towards both 6-AM and heroin. Given the comparatively larger size and rigid three-dimensional shape of heroin compared to other drugs of abuse, it can be argued that heroin can display multiple chemical epitopes to the immune system (Matyas et al. 2014). It therefore follows that haptens linked through different locations should provide alternative faces of the molecule as the binding epitope and thus generate antibodies with differing selectivity. However, exploration of alternative linker positions on heroin has been limited, with all examples utilizing stable linkage through the bridgehead nitrogen (Schlosburg et al. 2013; Bremer and Janda 2012; Matyas et al. 2014; Li et al. 2014). A wider variety of linking positions have been explored for morphine haptens; derivatization of the bridgehead nitrogen appears to elicit the most selective anti-morphine antibodies, with antibodies with equivalent affinities towards heroin, 6-AM, and morphine being raised against haptens linked through the 6' alcohol (Stowe et al. 2011).

18.2.2 Oxycodone

Oxycodone mostly shares the structural considerations discussed for heroin, but its pharmacokinetic profile is much simpler, with only the parent drug showing appreciable activity. Again, only one linkage position has been explored for haptens targeting oxycodone, namely, by derivatization of the C6 ketone (Pravetoni et al. 2012b, 2013). One could envisage that linking through the bridgehead nitrogen, thereby presenting the ketone as part of the epitope, may provide greater selectivity over heroin and morphine, although as will be discussed in Sect. 18.6.2 that is not necessarily desired.

18.2.3 Cocaine

As with heroin, there are three functional motifs that can potentially provide strong interactions with an antibody. Linking through the bridgehead amine has been most extensively investigated for cocaine (Cai et al. 2013a, b, c; Fox et al. 1996; Ramakrishnan et al. 2014), but derivatization of the C2 ester has also been explored (Carrera et al. 1995, 2001; Cai et al. 2013b).

Janda carried out a comparative study of two positions for cocaine hapten linkage (Cai et al. 2013c): attachment to the protein *via* the C2 ester in **GNC** (Carrera et al. 1995), a hapten known to elicit antibodies that result in a protective effect, or through the bridgehead nitrogen in **GNNS**, a linkage position previously shown to be effective in a parallel catalytic antibody approach (see Sect. 5.11) (Matsushita et al. 2001) (Fig. 18.5). Both haptens elicited a comparable immune response, with **GNC** generating slightly higher-affinity antibodies, albeit at a slightly lower concentration. **GNE** and **GNNA**, two alternative haptens which utilize the same linker positions as **GNC** and **GNNS**, respectively, but are stabilized through bioisosteric replacement of the C2 ester, gave similar results, albeit with the nitrogen-linked

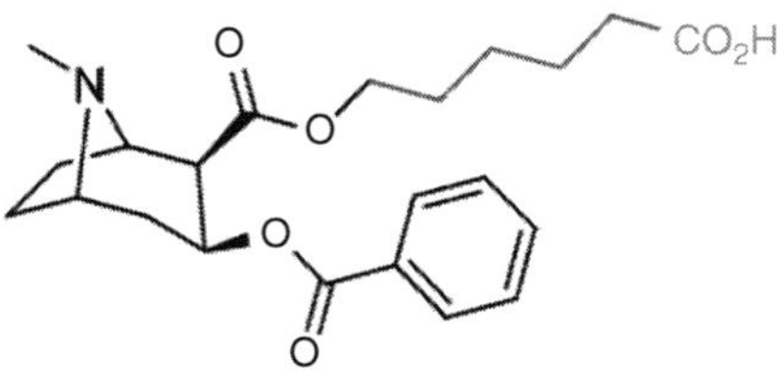

GNC

K_d = 0.79 nM
[Ab] = 48 μg/mL

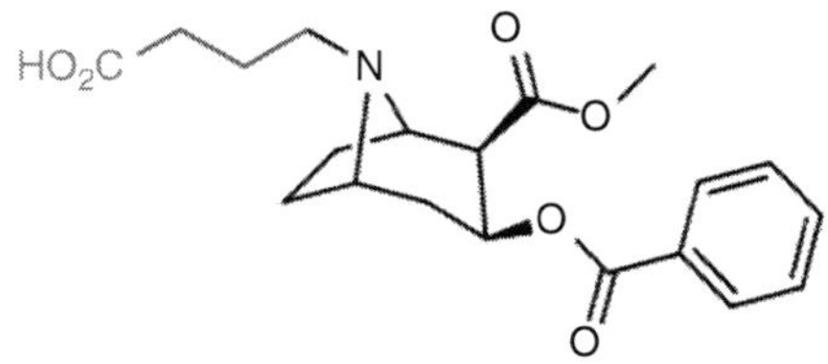

GNNS

K_d = 2.1 nM
[Ab] = 65 μg/mL

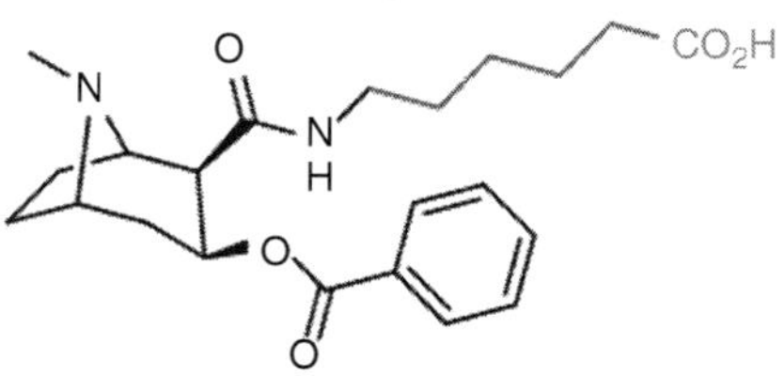

GNE

K_d = 5.7 nM
[Ab] = 120 μg/mL

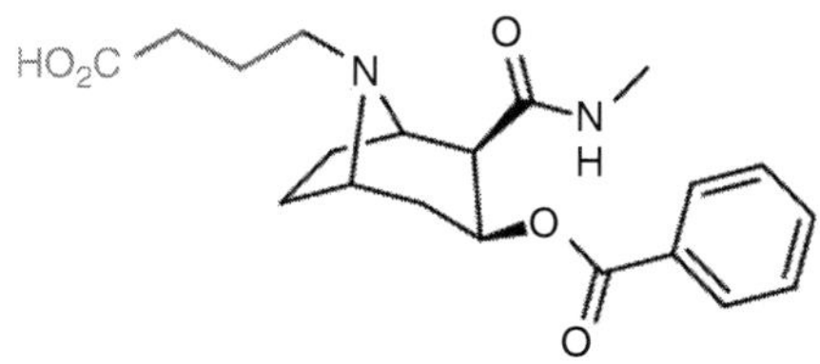

GNNA

K_d = 3.6 nM
[Ab] = 73 μg/mL

Fig. 18.5 Janda's investigation of C2-linked and bridgehead nitrogen-linked cocaine haptens (Cai et al. 2013c)

hapten giving slightly higher-affinity antibodies at a lower concentration. These results suggest that there is no real preference for linker location between these two positions in conferring greater immunogenicity. However, **GNE** was shown to grant greater protection than **GNNA** (and **GNC**) upon cocaine-induced psychomotor stimulation, which could suggest that antibody concentration may be the crucial factor is eliciting an effective anti-cocaine immune response and thus linker location may not have a significant impact. Alternatively, there was no data obtained for the selectivity of the antibodies raised for cocaine over benzoyl ecgonine, which may be the key to understanding the superior protective effect displayed for **GNE**.

18.2.4 Nicotine

The simple molecular structure of nicotine affords few potential binding interactions for the generation of high-affinity antibodies (relative to cocaine and the opioids), and this is a primary concern when attempting to determine an innocuous linker attachment position. Multiple locations have therefore been investigated, including the pyrrolidine amine (Meijler et al. 2003; Pravetoni et al. 2012a), the 3'-position on the pyrrolidine ring (Langone et al. 1973; Pentel et al. 2000), and various positions on the aromatic ring (Hieda et al. 1997; Pryde et al. 2013; de Villiers et al. 2010, 2002).

Conjugation through the 3' position has been investigated with Langone's **(±)-3'-EstNic** (Langone et al. 1973) hapten and Pentel's **(±)-3'-AmNic** hapten (Pentel et al. 2000) (Fig. 18.6). Both demonstrated the ability to elicit a robust immune response with moderate affinity antibodies at high concentrations that were able to promote a reduction of nicotine concentrations in the brain (Cerny et al. 2002; Maurer et al. 2005; Pentel et al. 2000; Hieda et al. 2000; Pravetoni et al. 2011). These haptens result in antibodies with high selectivity over cotinine, as would be expected due to the distal location of the linker from the site of oxidation. However, it is possible that the proximity of the linker to the ring junction may perturb the structure from the natural conformation, which would render this position suboptimal for the generation of high-affinity antibodies.

Janda has investigated linking from the pyrrolidine nitrogen using **NIC**, which in one study in mice was found to elicit poor affinity anti-nicotine antibodies (Meijler et al. 2003) (Fig. 18.7). However, in a repeat study in rats using a different adjuvant and different schedule, **(±)-NIC** elicited very high antibody affinities for nicotine (Moreno et al. 2012). Unfortunately, only limited behavioral effects were observed, possibly a result of the low antibody concentration elicited. It would be anticipated

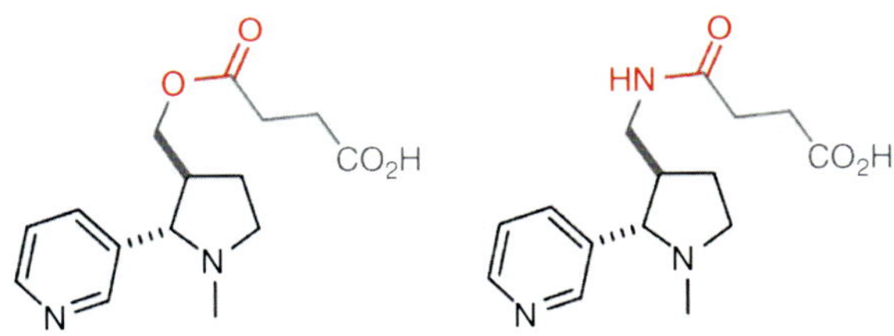

(±)-**3'-EstNic**
(bacteriophage Qβ conjugate with Freund's adjuvant)
K_d = 10-40 nM
[Ab] = 280 μg/mL
brain reduction = 66%

(±)-**3'-AmNic**
(rEPA conjugate with alum)
K_d = 46 nM
[Ab] = 160 μg/mL
brain reduction = 57%

Fig. 18.6 3'-Substituted nicotine haptens (Cerny et al. 2002; Maurer et al. 2005; Pentel et al. 2000; Hieda et al. 2000; Pravetoni et al. 2011)

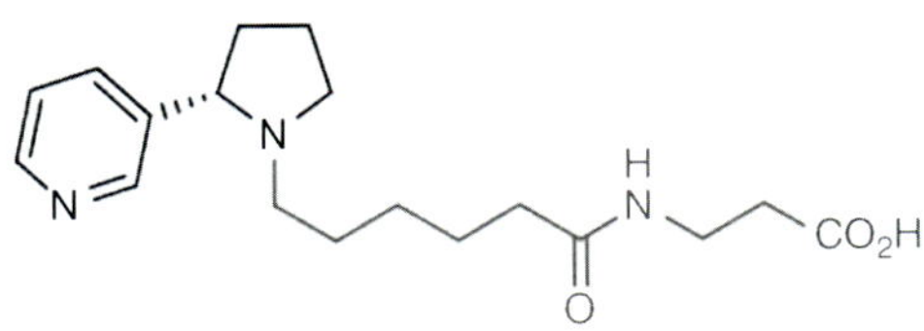

NIC

Merjler et al. 2003 K_d = 1,700 nM

Moreno et al. 2012 K_d = 3.1 nM, [Ab] = 56 μg/mL

Fig. 18.7 Janda's pyrrolidine nitrogen-linked nicotine vaccine (Meijler et al. 2003; Moreno et al. 2012)

that the close proximity of the linker to the position of the additional carbonyl group that differentiates cotinine resulted in antibodies that were unselective for nicotine over its metabolite. However, in a different study, mAbs raised against **NIC** showed no cross-reactivity with a cotinine hapten also linked at the pyrrolidine nitrogen (Isomura et al. 2001), suggesting that selectivity is possible using this linkage position.

McKluskie investigated a range of nicotine haptens linked at different positions on the pyridine ring (Pryde et al. 2013) (Fig. 18.8a). Haptens 2, 3, and 7 from that study allowed direct comparison as they obtained similar hapten densities and all utilized the same linker strategy. Competitive ELISA data suggested that the C6-linked **Hapten 2** was slightly superior, with C5-linked **Hapten 7** showing the lowest affinity to nicotine of the three. However, **Hapten 7** was able to reduce brain concentrations of nicotine to a greater extent than **Hapten 2**, which was in turn superior to **Hapten 3**. This is the first example discussed that demonstrates a common hazard in small molecule vaccine research. The antibody affinities measured by competitive ELISA are dependent on the serum binding to the hapten, not the soluble drug, and thus do not necessarily give a true indication of the vaccine efficacy. The direct measurement of nicotine brain concentrations is a simple yet powerful method to assess how much is actually being sequestered in the bloodstream, and this study therefore suggests that linking off the C5 position can give more effective anti-nicotine protection than either the C2 or C6 positions, due to either spatial or electronic effects. The poor results for **Hapten 3** could potentially be due to the close proximity of the linker to both the pyrrolidine and pyridine nitrogens, shielding the only two functionalities in the nicotine molecule able to form strong and specific interactions with antibodies.

In the work of de Villiers, a similar trend was observed for affinities to nicotine, again using competitive ELISA, but the situation was less clear when analyzing vaccine impact (Fig. 18.8b) (de Villiers et al. 2010). C6-linked GK60 showed a reduc-

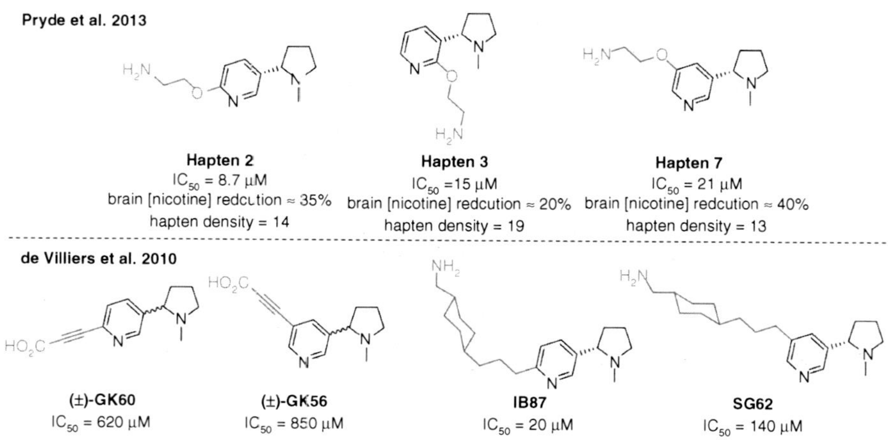

Fig. 18.8 McKluskie and de Villiers comparison of linker attachment on the pyridine ring of nicotine (de Villiers et al. 2010; Pryde et al. 2013)

tion in nicotine-induced dopamine overflow, whereas vaccination using GK56 actually showed an increased response. However, the reverse was seen when comparing SG62 and IB87, where the C5-linked hapten appeared superior.

The disparity in results between the groups of nicotine haptens linked through the pyridine ring may be a result of the effect of the linker on immunogenicity. However, the difficulty in rationalizing this disparity demonstrates a consistent issue with hapten design; experimental testing against metabolites is ultimately required to understand relative efficacy.

18.2.5 Methamphetamine

Methamphetamine is the simplest of all the major drugs of abuse, with a flexible structure and only one major chemical motif: the secondary amine. This could therefore be considered the toughest drug against which to develop high-affinity antibodies. Many positions on methamphetamine have been derivatized for conjugation to carrier proteins, albeit mostly for the generation of mAbs in passive immunization approaches.

Attachment sites that have been examined for active vaccines include the *N*-methyl group, simply performed through direct derivatization of amphetamine (Moreno et al. 2011; Miller et al. 2013) and the amine itself, to form a 3° amine (Collins et al. 2014) or amide (Shen et al. 2013), and functionalization of the aromatic ring at both the *meta*- (Carroll et al. 2011) and *para*-positions (Byrnes-Blake et al. 2001; Moreno et al. 2011; Duryee et al. 2009) (Fig. 18.4). All the haptens tested have shown some efficacy; however, there are currently few comparative studies between haptens directed towards methamphetamine.

Janda directly compared **MH6** and **MH7**, haptens conjugated through the *N*-methyl group and the *para*-position of the aromatic ring, respectively (Fig. 18.9). An initial study in mice showed that both haptens elicited similar concentrations of antibodies with similar affinities. In rats using a different vaccination schedule, comparable affinities were again observed, but **MH6** was found to elicit higher antibody concentrations, resulting in a reduction in locomotor activity that was not observed for **MH7**.

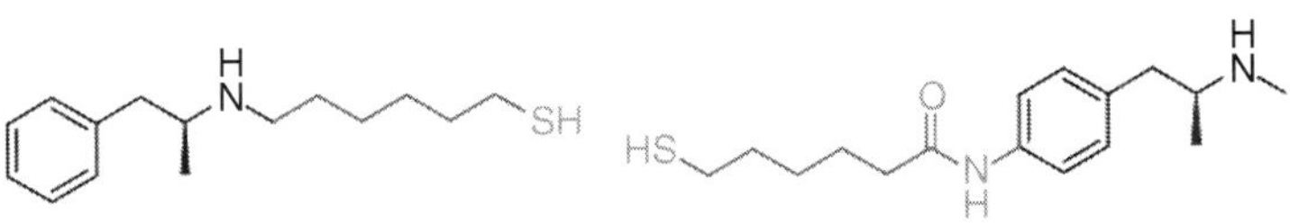

	MH6	**MH7**
Moreno et al. 2011	K_d = 130 nM [Ab] = 110 μg/mL	K_d = 170 nM [Ab] = 90 μg/mL
Miller et al. 2013	K_d = 30 nM [Ab] = 270 μg/mL	K_d = 26 nM [Ab] = 95 μg/mL

Fig. 18.9 Janda's comparison of linker attachment on methamphetamine (Moreno et al. 2011; Miller et al. 2013)

18.3 Linker Composition

Once the optimal position for the linker attachment to the hapten has been identified that minimizes any negative effect on antigen presentation, the composition of the linker must also be considered as an important factor that can affect the immune response. Firstly, a stable linkage is a necessity to avoid loss of the hapten from the carrier protein during both preparation and vaccination. Secondly, in order to achieve effective presentation in the MHCII complex and recognition by B cell receptors (BCRs), it is vital that the hapten be spatially displayed in an effective manner, and the nature, length, and rigidity of the linker are likely crucial components in achieving this. The choice of linker will likely also impact the preparation of the carrier–hapten vaccine by determining the conjugation efficiency and potentially even the tertiary structure of the modified protein. Finally, it is of course vital that the linker not be part of the epitope and contribute to the binding of the resultant antibodies; this additional unwanted immunogenicity will likely produce greater affinity to the hapten at the expense of the target soluble drug.

18.3.1 Nicotine

In the case of Pentel's nicotine vaccine CMUNic, the antibodies elicited bound the hapten with substantially higher affinity than nicotine, likely due in part to the choice of a urea-containing linker (Hieda et al. 1997) (Fig. 18.10). Ureas are conformationally rigid and display a powerful hydrogen-bonding pattern for potential recognition as an epitope. Even so, the vaccine was still able to demonstrate efficacy, altering the blood–brain distribution of nicotine by partial sequestration in the blood (Hieda et al. 1999).

Originally developed by Langone for the development of antibody-based diagnostic assays for nicotine (Langone et al. 1973), **(±)-3'-EstNic** has become one of the most widely used haptens for nicotine vaccines (Fig. 18.11). It had been found to effectively reduce nicotine concentrations in the brain (Cerny et al. 2002; Maurer et al. 2005) and was progressed into human clinical trials. However, ultimately

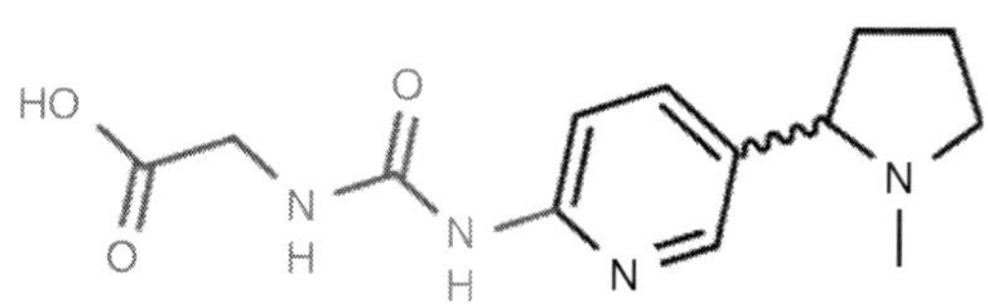

(±)-6-CMUNic

IC_{50}((±)-6-CMUNic) = 1.5 μM

IC_{50} (nicotine) = 580 μM

Fig. 18.10 Pentel's (±)-6-CMUNic hapten elicited preferential binding of the hapten over nicotine (Hieda et al. 1997)

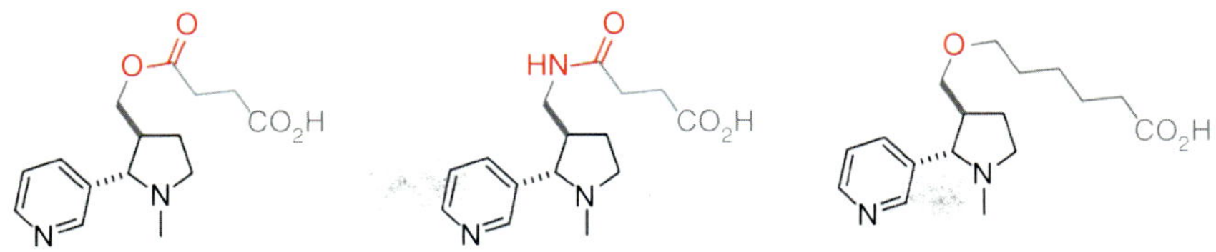

(±)-3'-EstNic
(bacteriophage Qβ conjugate with Freund's adjunt)
K_d = 10-40 nM
[Ab] = 280 μg/mL
brain [nicotine] reduction = 66%

(±)-3'-AmNic
(rEPA conjugate with alum)
K_d = 46 nM
[Ab] = 160 μg/mL
brain [nicotine] reduction = 57%

(±)-Am1
(TT conjugate with AS-03)
K_d = 5.7 nM
[Ab] = 40 μg/mL

Fig. 18.11 Evolution of 3′-substituted nicotine haptens (Cerny et al. 2002; Maurer et al. 2005; Pentel et al. 2000; Hieda et al. 2000; Pravetoni et al. 2011; Moreno et al. 2010)

(±)-3'-EstNic was found to elicit a highly variable response, only delivering long-term abstinence in the limited number of individuals that obtained high antibody titers (Maurer et al. 2005; Cornuz et al. 2008). **(±)-3'-EstNic** contains a potentially labile ester linkage, and one hypothesis was that this could result in uncontrolled and unpredictable hydrolysis, reducing hapten density and vaccine efficacy. Pentel sought to stabilize the hapten using a bioisosteric amide, giving **(±)-3'-AmNic**, which was again able to effectively reduce nicotine concentrations in the brain (Pentel et al. 2000; Hieda et al. 2000; Pravetoni et al. 2011). However, the undesirably high variability between individuals was still observed in clinical trials (Hatsukami et al. 2005, 2011; Wagena et al. 2008).

The proximity of functionality within the linker to the intended drug epitope may also be a source of additional, unwanted immunogenicity. Janda therefore developed **(±)-AM1**, a version of the hapten with an ether linkage that is both stable and should exhibit minimal unwanted immunogenicity. **(±)-AM1** was shown to elicit antibodies with high affinity for nicotine, but at a much lower concentration, and an increase in self-administration relative to unvaccinated mice suggests that the protective effects were surmountable (Moreno et al. 2010).

Although it can be rationalized that **AM1** should result in antibodies with reduced linker-derived immunogenicity and thus elicit antibodies with greater affinity to the target nicotine, the three 3'-linked nicotine haptens have not been directly compared. Given the huge disparity between the methods employed in the studies performed, there is no experimental data to determine which is superior. As alluded to previously, this is an ongoing issue within the drugs of abuse field, and unless direct comparison is performed, it is not possible to actually test the hypotheses that inspire the design of the next generation of haptens.

As before, it is possible to extract interesting comparative data from the rigorous study conducted by McKluskie, this time analyzing the properties of linkers attached to C5-modified nicotine haptens (Pryde et al. 2013) (Fig. 18.12a). All three haptens with similar hapten densities elicited antibodies that showed similar affinities for nicotine using competitive ELISA, but **Hapten 7**, appended *via* an electron-donating

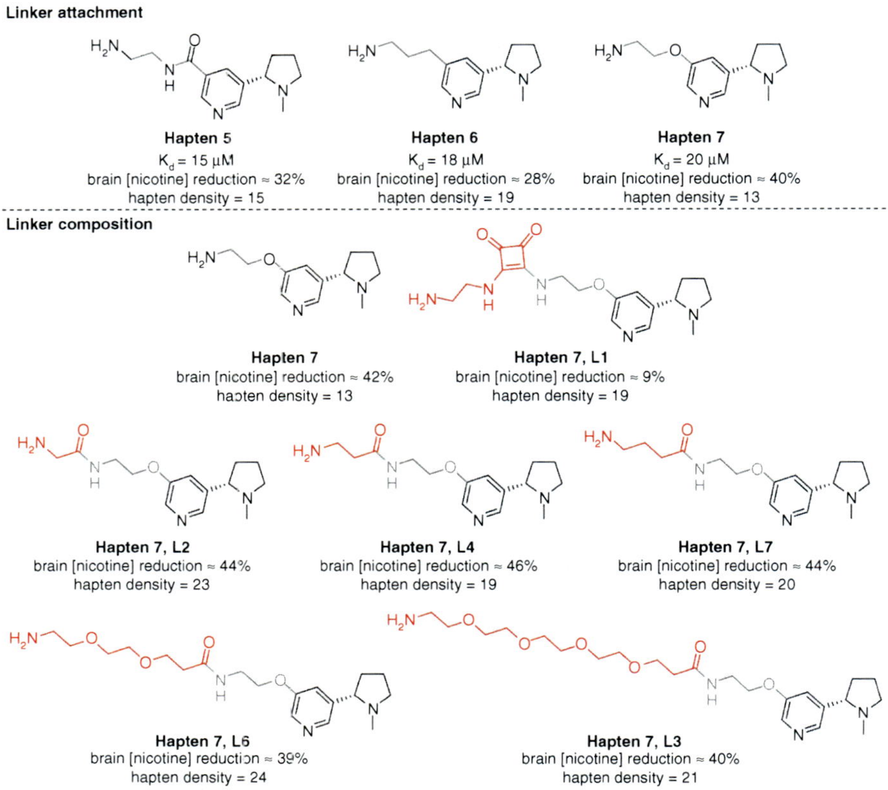

Fig. 18.12 McKluskie's C5-linked nicotine hapten comparison (Pryde et al. 2013)

ether linker, showed greater efficacy in reducing brain concentrations of nicotine than both electron-withdrawing amide **Hapten 5** and alkyl-linked **Hapten 6**. The effect of the linker composition was then further investigated through modification of **Hapten 7** (Fig. 18.12b). This revealed that the amide-containing linkers **L2**, **L4**, and **L7** gave comparable reduction in brain concentrations of nicotine to the original linker in **Hapten 7** and PEG linkers in **L6** and **L3** only conferred a marginal decrease in efficacy. The conformationally rigid squaramide linker in **L1** proved to substantially decrease the ability to reduce nicotine concentrations in the brain, suggesting that flexibility may be required for effective epitope recognition.

18.3.2 Cocaine

Orson's use of bridgehead amine-linked cocaine haptens **HNC**, **BNC**, and **SBNC** serves to demonstrate that the linker composition can have a distinct and unexpected impact on the chemical stability (Ramakrishnan et al. 2014) (Fig. 18.13). **HNC** and

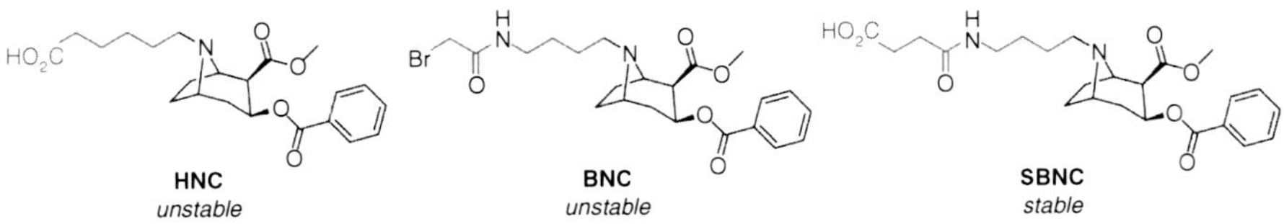

Fig. 18.13 Orson's stabilized cocaine haptens (Ramakrishnan et al. 2014)

BNC showed substantial C2-ester hydrolysis during synthesis and thus elicited an immune response skewed towards benzoyl ecgonine, whereas **SBNC** apparently remained intact during synthesis and was able to elicit antibodies that showed no appreciable binding to benzoyl ecgonine (discussed in more detail in Sect. 18.7.2, Fig. 18.26). It is difficult to rationalize this improved stability given the minor structural differences between **BNC** and **SBNC**, and as such, this does not appear to be a general solution even within the cocaine vaccine field, but this study does demonstrate that the linker composition may have a greater impact on the hapten than anticipated.

18.3.3 Peptidic Linkers

The biological processing that results in MHCII presentation of an immunogen requires a peptidic substrate. As discussed previously, since drugs of abuse antigens are not peptidic, they require conjugation to a carrier protein or peptide. It would therefore follow that a more peptidic conjugate vaccine might facilitate efficient binding within the MHCII complex and recognition by the immune system. Despite this, linkers used for protein conjugation are predominantly composed of hydrophobic aliphatic chains, presumably to allow minimal immunogenicity, good flexibility, and ease of synthesis, which by the logic above may negatively impact on binding to the MHCII protein. Increasing the peptidic nature of the linker may therefore be expected to increase the immune response to the attached hapten, and this hypothesis has begun to be explored. The use of polyglycine linkers, first investigated in vaccinations against *Bacillus anthracis* (Schneerson et al. 2003; Kubler-Kielb et al. 2006), has been employed in both opioid and nicotine vaccines (Pravetoni et al. 2012b, 2013; Collins and Janda 2014).

Pentel found that the introduction of a tetraglycine unit in an oxycodone vaccine, **OXY(Gly)$_4$**, elicited substantially higher anti-oxycodone antibody titers than the corresponding hapten **OXY(HS)** (Pravetoni et al. 2012b) (Fig. 18.14a). However, the use of different linker attachment chemistry in the two haptens may have been partially responsible for this effect. Later work by Pentel used both hapten linkers with the same linking chemistry in both oxycodone and hydrocodone vaccines, demonstrating for the tetraglycine analogs both higher titers and reduced brain concentrations of oxycodone in vaccinated animals (Pravetoni et al. 2013) (Fig. 18.14b). However again a direct comparison cannot be made since, in this case, the tetraglycine haptens were conjugated through amide bond formation, whereas the comparators were linked to the carrier protein through maleimide conjugation,

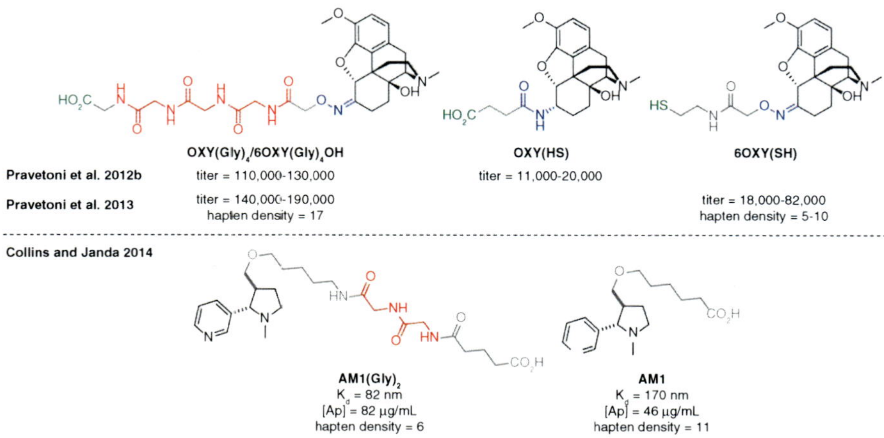

Fig. 18.14 Pentel and Janda's application of polyglycine linkers within oxycodone and nicotine vaccines (Pravetoni et al. 2012b; Pravetoni et al. 2013; Collins and Janda 2014)

resulting in substantially lower hapten densities. The tetraglycine linker was reported by Pentel to be more effective than the corresponding diglycine or non-peptidic linker for a morphine vaccine, although no comparative data to support this conclusion was shown (Pravetoni et al. 2013).

In a more closely controlled example, the application of a diglycine linker to a nicotine vaccine was carried out by Janda (Fig. 18.14c) (Collins and Janda 2014). An increase in both antibody concentration and affinity was observed for the diglycine-containing hapten **AM1(Gly)$_2$** than corresponding hapten **AM1**. Although the structures and conjugation chemistry were the same in this case, there was still a disparity in hapten densities; however on this occasion, there were fewer copies of hapten in the superior vaccine. Given that it is generally considered that higher hapten densities correlate with increased immune response (Marco et al. 1995), this data strongly suggests that the **AM1(Gly)$_2$** hapten elicits a superior response due to the inclusion of the diglycine motif.

Further work will determine the optimal length and composition of peptidic linkers based on these promising initial findings using di- and tetraglycine, providing a modular and generally applicable solution to increase the efficacy of vaccines against any drug of abuse. However, the inconsistent hapten densities obtained within these studies attempting to directly compare linkers again highlight the difficulties in performing a controlled comparison of hapten or linker structure.

18.4 Choice of Conjugation Method

Another important design element for the linker is the functionality through which the hapten will be attached to the carrier. It is crucial that the linkage be stable and use orthogonal conjugation chemistry to avoid side reactions with either the carrier or the hapten itself. The two most frequently utilized conjugation methods append the hapten to surface-exposed lysine residues, which are abundant in carrier proteins and peptides. Direct amide bond formation requires the activation of a carboxylic acid hapten, usually using EDC/NHS chemistry (Fig. 18.15a). This requires that there are no other carboxylic acids in the hapten or reactive amines with which the resulting activated ester can couple. The stability of the activated intermediate ("OAct" in Fig. 18.15a) can potentially be tuned to give the desired reactivity.

Alternatively, the protein lysine residues can be functionalized for reaction with a thiol-containing hapten by initial coupling with a maleimide-containing activated carboxylic acid (Fig. 18.15b). The thiol–maleimide conjugate addition is rapid and highly orthogonal to other functionality. However, it has been observed that maleimide conjugation tends to give lower hapten densities than the corresponding amide bond formation (Collins et al. 2014). The requirement for a linker between the carrier and the maleimide introduces additional chemical matter between the hapten and the carrier, potentially affecting the resulting immune response. Furthermore, since conjugation of thiols to maleimides is usually not quantitative, a surfeit of unreacted linker–maleimide appendages will be decorating the protein surface, possibly proving detrimental to stability and immunological efficacy. The precursor thiols are also unstable, forming disulfides upon storage. Although this can be reversed by performing the conjugation reaction under reductive conditions, this is potentially incompatible with carrier proteins containing disulfide bridges. Finally, it has been shown that thiol addition to maleimide can be reversible, leading to unexpected loss of the hapten from the carrier (Fontaine et al. 2014).

Less frequently, the reverse amide bond formation is performed for hapten conjugation (Fig. 18.15c). It is possible to conjugate to the intrinsic surface aspartate and glutamate residues, but the lysines can also be modified to incorporate additional carboxylic acids for conjugation to an amine-containing hapten, usually using succinic anhydride. However, analysis post-conjugation can be complicated by a

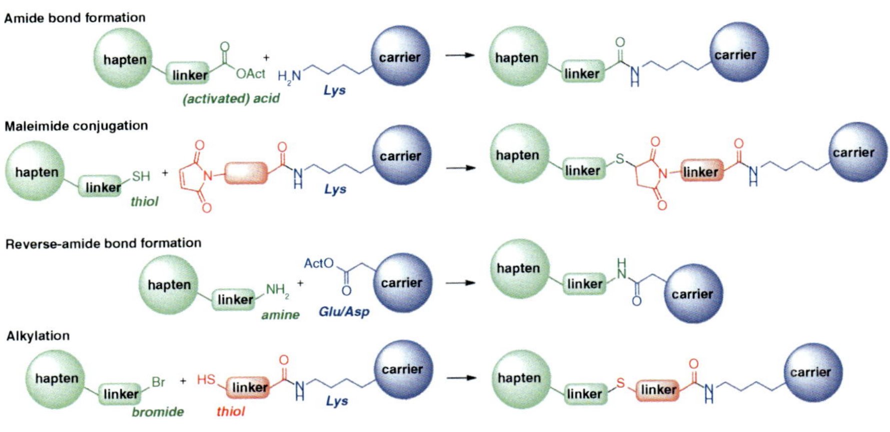

Fig. 18.15 Standard methods of hapten–protein conjugation. "OAct" refers to the activated ester intermediate, usually an *N*-hydroxysuccinimide ester or equivalent

side reaction resulting from the activation of the acids, namely, irreversible *O*-acylisourea to *N*-acylurea rearrangement (DeTar and Silverstein 1966), which results in an increase in protein mass without concomitant hapten conjugation.

Rarely, bromide-derivatized haptens can be used in combination with carrier proteins that have been decorated with thiols through addition to the protein lysine residues (Duncan et al. 1983) (Fig. 18.15d). Although this alkylation should be orthogonal to other functionalities that may be in the hapten, there is potential to introduce disulfide bridges both intra- and intermolecularly, which can complicate the resulting conjugates.

Other types of conjugation method have been explored, including the production of squaric acid diamides from the corresponding hapten amines and lysines (Tietze et al. 1991), Huisgen [3+2] cycloadditions from azides and terminal alkynes (Rostovtsev et al. 2002; Tornøe et al. 2002; Agard et al. 2004), traceless Staudinger reactions from azides and esters (Grandjean et al. 2005), and oxime ligations from hydroxylamines and aldehydes (Ulrich et al. 2014); these may be required where standard conjugation chemistry is incompatible with the functionalities in the haptens. These alternative approaches are rarely utilized in drugs of abuse vaccines; the chemistry involved is often more complicated, the linkages can be less stable, and some require the use of relatively bulky or functionalized linkers which would be considered too intrusive for conjugation of small molecules with low inherent size and immunogenicity.

18.5 Multivalent Haptens

Combination vaccines are well established in the arena of infectious diseases, either using multiple immunogens for the same target (e.g., pneumococcal disease vaccines) or multiple unrelated immunogens, for example, against measles, mumps, and rubella (MMR) or diphtheria, pertussis, and tetanus (DPT). In these cases, no compromising effects on the response to the individual immunogens have been observed (Skibinski et al. 2011; Andrews et al. 2012). Combination vaccines for drugs of abuse have therefore been explored as a potential solution to problems of poor selectivity and efficacy.

18.5.1 Multivalent Haptens Targeting Multiple Species

As discussed, designing an efficacious hapten to target the complex family of heroin metabolites has significant challenges, and targeting multiple species may prove to be the most effective strategy. Co-vaccination using haptens that mimic multiple species is an alternative strategy that may give superior results.

Janda investigated co-vaccination of the two haptens, **Her** and **Mor**, that had shown effective stimulation of heroin and anti-6-AM and anti-morphine antibodies, respectively (Stowe et al. 2011) (Fig. 18.3). Given the rapid hydrolysis of heroin to morphine and its greater AUC than heroin and 6-AM, it was proposed that the addition of anti-morphine antibodies to those generated by **Her** may elicit enhanced protection following heroin administration (Cook et al. 1993) (Fig. 18.16). However, the co-vaccination of both **Her** and **Mor** haptens appeared to drastically affect the overall immune response, resulting in a far lower antibody titer and reduced protection against the antinociceptive effects of heroin when compared to **Her** alone, with no prevention of heroin self-acquisition. However, this combination **Her/Mor** vaccine still resulted in more significant heroin-induced nociceptive protection than **Mor** alone despite the substantially reduced antibody titers, strongly suggesting that raising a sufficient concentration of anti-heroin and anti-6-AM antibodies is required for protection against heroin abuse. Furthermore, the reduction in total antibody response suggests that co-vaccination with these two opioid haptens compromises the immune response towards both haptens (Stowe et al. 2011).

18.5.2 Multivalent Haptens Targeting Multiple Drugs

A successful targeted drug of abuse vaccine, able to fully and specifically sequester the desired drug, may still prove inadequate to prevent drug user relapse due to ready availability of related drugs. It is therefore worthy to pursue the development of vaccines that sequester multiple related drugs of abuse.

Heroin and oxycodone are current opioid vaccine targets which to date exhibit limited cross-reactivity in their antibody responses. Pravetoni investigated the potential of co-vaccination using oxycodone and morphine haptens **OXY(Gly)**$_4$ (Pravetoni et al. 2012b, 2013, 2014a, 2014b) and **M(Gly)**$_4$ (Raleigh et al. 2013) that had previously been shown to elicit protective effects against their respective opioids in multiple animal models (Pravetoni et al. 2012c) (Fig. 18.17). The divalent vaccine elicited significantly higher titers towards each opioid than the individual vaccines. Furthermore, a greater increase in serum retention was observed for both 6-AM and oxycodone by the divalent vaccine than either monovalent vaccine independently, although vaccination with **M(Gly)**$_4$ resulted in the lowest brain concen-

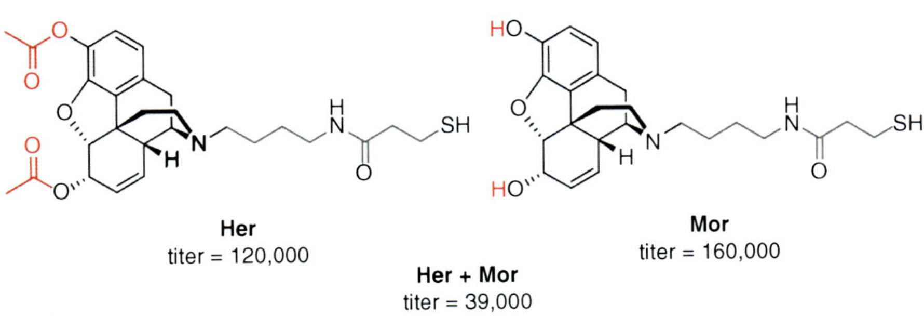

Fig. 18.16 Janda's co-vaccination of heroin and morphine haptens (Stowe et al. 2011)

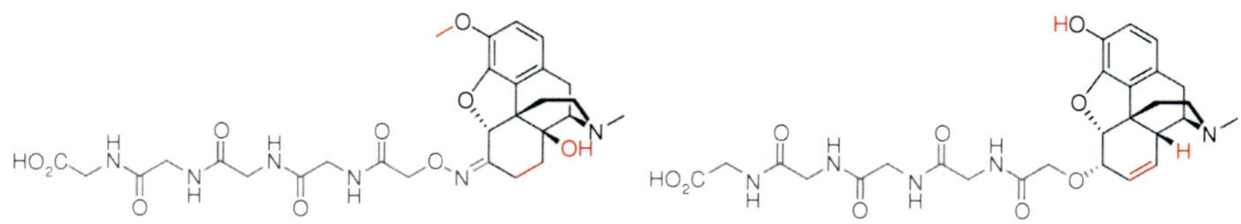

OXY(Gly)$_4$
titer (M(Gly)$_4$) = 18,000
titer (OXY(Gly)$_4$) = 100,000

M(Gly)$_4$
titer (M(Gly)$_4$) = 140,000
titer (OXY(Gly)$_4$) = 29,000

OXY(Gly)$_4$ + M(Gly)$_4$
titer (M(Gly)$_4$) = 330,000
titer (OXY(Gly)$_4$) = 240,000

Fig. 18.17 Pravetoni's investigation of a bivalent oxycodone–morphine vaccine (Pravetoni et al. 2012c)

trations of morphine. One caveat in interpreting these results is that the total amount of conjugate administered for the divalent vaccine is double than for the monovalent vaccines, which is likely partially responsible for the raised titers and increased behavioral effects. Furthermore, unconjugated KLH was added to the monovalent vaccine to keep the total protein injected constant. In the case of a bivalent nicotine vaccine, this has been shown to result in significant reduction in both ELISA titer and drug serum retention, likely due to immune system diversion towards the highly immunogenic protein (de Villiers et al. 2013). Furthermore, although ELISA data demonstrates that a limited proportion of the antibodies bind to both haptens, this may not be the case for the soluble opioids. Overall, however, this study does suggest that co-vaccination with multiple haptens targeting different opioids can be an effective strategy.

18.5.3 Multivalent Haptens Targeting One Drug

To date, all drugs of abuse vaccines promising enough to have advanced to the clinic have subsequently failed, predominantly due to a high variability of the immune response between individuals (Cornuz et al. 2008; Hatsukami et al. 2005, 2011; Martell et al. 2005, 2009; Kosten and Biegel 2002; Haney et al. 2010). One proposed explanation for this disparity is that the immune system of different individuals will respond differently to the same hapten, each ultimately favoring a slightly different and pharmacologically distinct antibody epitope, thus resulting in the observed variable responses to the parent drug (Keyler et al. 2008; Cornish et al. 2013; de Villiers et al. 2013). Since each epitope has the potential to stimulate a subpopulation of B cells, it has therefore been postulated that co-vaccination using multiple haptens displaying alternative presentations of the same drug may provide a more uniform response throughout a population.

This strategy has been attempted for nicotine, initially using two racemic haptens, **(±)-6-CMU** and **(±)-3'-AmNIC**; these haptens were shown to result in the stimulation of distinct B cell populations, and when co-vaccinated, higher anti-nicotine antibody concentrations were observed with a greater potential for binding nicotine in the bloodstream (Keyler et al. 2008), the effect maintained at a range of doses (Cornish et al. 2013) (Fig. 18.18). The same trend was seen when comparing a trivalent vaccine, containing the original two haptens and a third immunologically distinct enantiopure nicotine immunogen, **1'-SNic** (Pravetoni et al. 2012a), to a dose-matched monovalent **(±)-3'-AmNic** vaccine (de Villiers et al. 2013). Both examples demonstrated that there was no correlation between the concentrations of antibodies against the individual haptens and the total antibody titers produced by the combination vaccines. Furthermore, more high responders were observed in the trivalent compared with the monovalent group, consistent with the stimulation of independent B cell populations, and fewer low responders were observed. Coupling this with the additive, noncompetitive effect of co-vaccination suggests that this strategy could decrease the likelihood of a low immune response in individuals, the primary reason for failure of previous nicotine vaccines in the clinic (Cornuz et al. 2008; Hatsukami et al. 2005, 2011).

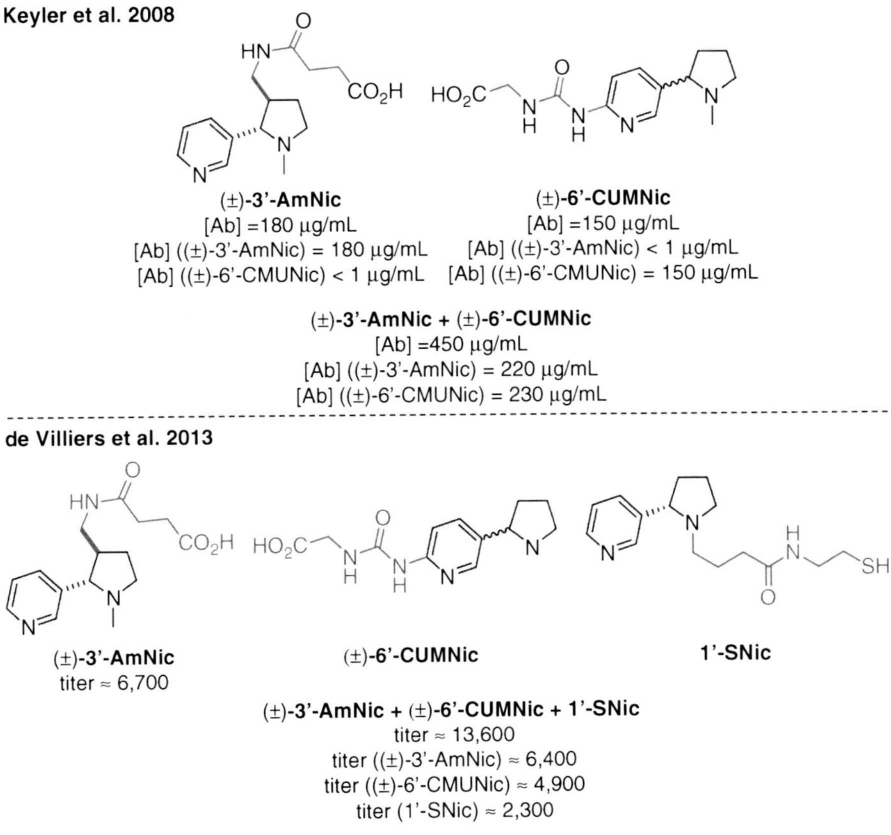

Fig. 18.18 Pentel's investigation of bivalent and trivalent vaccinations using nicotine haptens (Keyler et al. 2008; Cornish et al. 2013; Pravetoni et al. 2012a; de Villiers et al. 2013)

Although this strategy has only been used thus far against nicotine vaccines, it has the potential to work against other drugs of abuse given the availability of structurally distinct haptens for cocaine, methamphetamine, and heroin/morphine and should be a general focus of investigation by the vaccine research community.

18.6 Affinity Enhancement

18.6.1 Decreasing Structural Flexibility

While methamphetamine and nicotine are small, stable drugs, with limited metabolism in vivo, their simple and flexible structures pose a new challenge: reduced potential for high binding affinities due to the entropic penalty of binding a flexible molecule in a specific conformation (Chang et al. 2007). Constraining flexible haptens in a low-energy conformation reduces the quantity of attainable conformations, narrowing the antibody heterogeneity towards a population that has increased target affinity. It must be noted, however, that constraint will only elicit antibodies efficacious against the target drug when the conformation selected is attainable by the drug and is biologically relevant.

Janda has attempted to use this strategy against methamphetamine, designing **MH2** as a constrained mimic of a low-energy conformation, with retention of the basic amine as a likely important pharmacophore/epitope for antibody binding and with the linker projecting away from the epitope for optimal recognition (Moreno et al. 2011) (Fig. 18.19). In comparison with unconstrained hapten **MH6**, higher-affinity antibodies were generated in mice. However, repetition of this work in rats using a different vaccination schedule yielded a vastly different result, with **MH2** giving substantially poorer antibody affinities at comparable concentrations; unsurprisingly only **MH6** showed a decrease in locomotor activity (Miller et al. 2013).

A similar disparity was observed when attempting to apply conformational restraint to nicotine haptens (Fig. 18.20), with two low-energy constrained haptens **CNI** and **CNA** directly compared with unconstrained hapten **NIC** (Meijler et al.

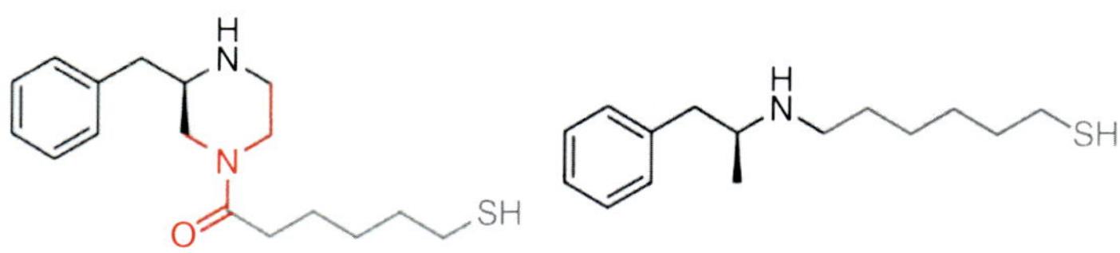

	MH2	**MH6**
Moreno et al. 2011	K_d = 82 nM [Ab] = 45 µg/mL	K_d = 130 nM [Ab] = 110 µg/mL
Miller et al. 2013	K_d = 2,200 nM [Ab] = 290 µg/mL	K_d = 30 nM [Ab] = 270 µg/mL

Fig. 18.19 Janda's comparison of constrained and non-constrained methamphetamine haptens (Moreno et al. 2011; Miller et al. 2013)

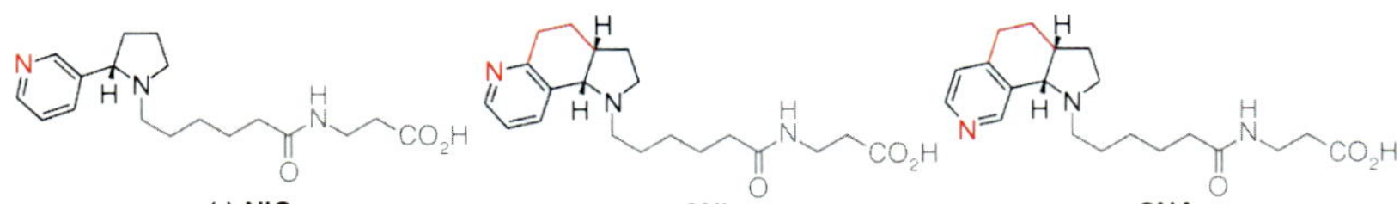

	(-)-NIC	CNI	CNA
Meijler et al. 2003	K_d = 1,700 nM	K_d = 600 nM	K_d = 1,000 nM
	(±)-NIC		
Moreno et al. 2012	K_d = 3.1 nM [Ab] = 56 μg/mL	K_d = 3,300 nM [Ab] = 330 μg/mL	

Fig. 18.20 Janda's comparison of constrained and non-constrained nicotine haptens (Meijler et al. 2003; Moreno et al. 2012)

2003; Moreno et al. 2012). A small increase in antibody affinity was observed for both the constrained haptens in an initial study in mice (Meijler et al. 2003), but again a second study in rats with a different adjuvant and schedule resulted in radically lower antibody affinities for **CNI** when compared with **(±)-NIC**, with higher concentrations (using serum from the top 35 % of responders) (Moreno et al. 2012). However, surprisingly in the latter case, **CNI** and not **NIC** showed an effect in two behavioral assays. This may partially be a result of the higher antibody concentration, which is known to be a key factor in generating an effective immune response, but there is likely to be additional unmeasured variables producing the observed effects, such as the selectivity of the resulting antibodies for nicotine over cotinine.

The disparity of the data between studies for these two sets of haptens exemplifies the problems when analyzing drugs of abuse vaccines. Even comparison within the same study can result in significantly different results upon modification of the vaccine components, schedule, and changing species. This latter variable is particularly crucial, as unsuccessful translation to humans was responsible for previous failures of vaccines in the clinic that had shown good protection in preclinical work.

18.6.2 Hapten Halogenation

Fluorination is frequently used in medicinal chemistry to enhance the binding of a ligand to its target. While fluorine and hydrogen are considered isosteric, resulting in minimal structural perturbation, fluorine has increased hydrophobicity and the potential to participate in weak halogen bonding, often resulting in a strengthened interaction (Gómez-Nuñez et al. 2008; Müller et al. 2007). Application to hapten design should theoretically allow a stronger interaction to occur between the hapten and both the T cell and B cell receptors, promoting a stronger immune response. This hydrogen–fluorine substitution has shown potential in the enhancement of immune recognition (Gómez-Nuñez et al. 2008) and has successfully increased the antigenicity of an sTn hapten (Yang et al. 2010). This strategy may be especially useful for methamphetamine and nicotine haptens since these drugs have a much more poorly defined epitope than cocaine or the opioids. However, it is primarily the interaction with TCRs that needs to be strengthened as modulation of binding to

BCRs would confer selectivity of the corresponding antibodies towards the fluorinated derivative over the target drug, and as yet, these immune cell interactions cannot be rationally differentiated in the hapten design.

Janda applied halogenation to cocaine hapten **SNC**; monofluorination in **GNF** appeared to slightly decrease antibody affinity and increase concentration (Cai et al. 2013a) (Fig. 18.21), as was seen for fluorination of the carbohydrate in MUC1 peptide (Hoffmann-Röder et al. 2010). The reduction in antibody affinity for the target cocaine is likely due to the absence of the fluorine, but the increase in antibody concentration may stem from the increased affinity for TCRs. Further additions to the series only complicated the structure–activity relationship, demonstrating the difficulty of rational design in this field. Trifluoromethyl hapten **GNCF** elicited a reduced antibody concentration, albeit with similar affinity, but the introduction of chlorine in **GNCl** resulted in a substantial loss in antibody affinity for cocaine. Although this effect has been observed elsewhere in data for a chlorinated sTn hapten (Wang and Guo 2011), these results are difficult to rationalize in terms of traditional steric or electronic considerations. A fourth hapten that contained a pentafluoroaryl group was designed but was found to be hydrolytically unstable due to the increased electrophilicity of the adjacent amide.

Fluorination of cocaine resulted in a slight elevation in antibody concentration, albeit at the slight detriment of the affinity. Further investigation may proceed to identify key locations in drugs of abuse haptens that could benefit from an increase in affinity through fluorination.

18.7 Stability Enhancement

As shown in Fig. 18.2, heroin, cocaine, nicotine, and methamphetamine are all metabolized in vivo and have active metabolites that need to be considered when designing the structure of the hapten. However, heroin and cocaine pose additional problems in that both are prone to nonenzymatic ester hydrolysis, rapidly converting to 6-AM and benzoyl ecgonine, respectively. Vaccines derived from these drugs have been found to be unstable during hapten-protein conjugate synthesis, vaccine preparation and storage, and following administration. Stabilization of these esters is therefore an important consideration in hapten design, both in terms of the epitope that the vaccine will display to the immune system and practical considerations of synthesis and desired shelf-life.

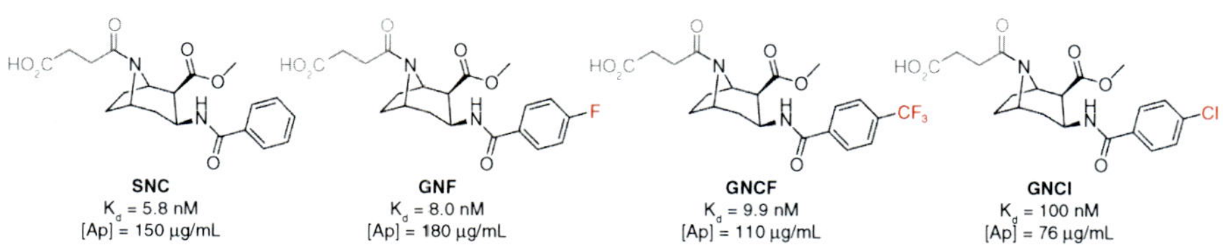

Fig. 18.21 Janda's investigation of hapten halogenation (Cai et al. 2013a)

18.7.1 Heroin

As discussed previously, heroin has a complex metabolism profile; the parent compound is pharmacologically inactive, with the psychoactive metabolites released upon the hydrolysis of the labile esters (Umans and Inturrisi 1981; Inturrisi et al. 1983; Selley et al. 2001) (Fig. 18.2). However, this does not discount heroin from being an important target for immunopharmacotherapy. Heroin's low polarity allows rapid BBB penetration, faster than both 6-AM and morphine (Seleman et al. 2014). Given that antibodies cannot themselves cross the BBB, it may be important to rapidly sequester the non-metabolized heroin itself before it can enter the brain. Once sequestered, the ester hydrolysis should also proceed at a slower rate, allowing the antibody to function effectively.

Replacement of the labile esters of heroin is one strategy to attempt to improve the immune response to the parent compound(s) and generate a vaccine that has greater stability. A strategy to stabilize the more labile phenol ester was pursued by Janda, giving **3-AcNH-Her** (Bremer and Janda 2012) (Fig. 18.22a). However, the resulting antibodies had lower affinity for heroin and especially 6-AM when compared with those elicited by **Her**, perhaps unsurprising given the lack of a 6-AM-like epitope. Data has previously suggested that it is crucial to elicit antibodies against 6-AM to obtain a protective effect against heroin administration (Fig. 18.3), and therefore stabilization of the C3 ester may be a detrimental strategy.

Stabilization of *both* esters by Alving to give **DiAmHap** resulted in antibodies that had unwanted selective affinity for the hapten over the targets, evidenced through exclusively preferential binding of the antibodies elicited to the **DiAmHap** antigen over the soluble drug targets (Matyas et al. 2014) (Fig. 18.22b). The subset of antibodies that could bind **MorHap** showed comparable affinity for heroin and 6-AM, with poorer affinity for morphine, but the overall immune response conferred poor inhibition of heroin-induced antinociception. Rice offered an alternative stabilization, using ketones rather than amides, giving **DiPrOxyHap** and **6-PrOxyHap** (Li et al. 2014) (Fig. 18.22c). Ketones are typically avoided in therapeutics as they can result in toxicity due to nonspecific covalent modification of proteins. **DiPrOxyHap**, like **DiAmHap**, appeared to confer high antibody selectivity to the hapten over the target drugs, although this effect appeared to be reduced in the case of **6-PrOxyHap**. Again, poor inhibition of heroin-induced antinociception protection was observed for both haptens. However, the limited protection observed against heroin administration cannot necessarily be attributed to bioisosteric replacement of the esters, as the alkene present in the C ring of heroin was also saturated in these haptens, which would be expected to alter the conformation of the molecule.

18.7.2 Cocaine

Strategic considerations for the stabilization of cocaine are far less complicated than for heroin. There are fewer active metabolites involved, with the primary active species being the drug itself, and thus, stabilization of the parent is a simple and

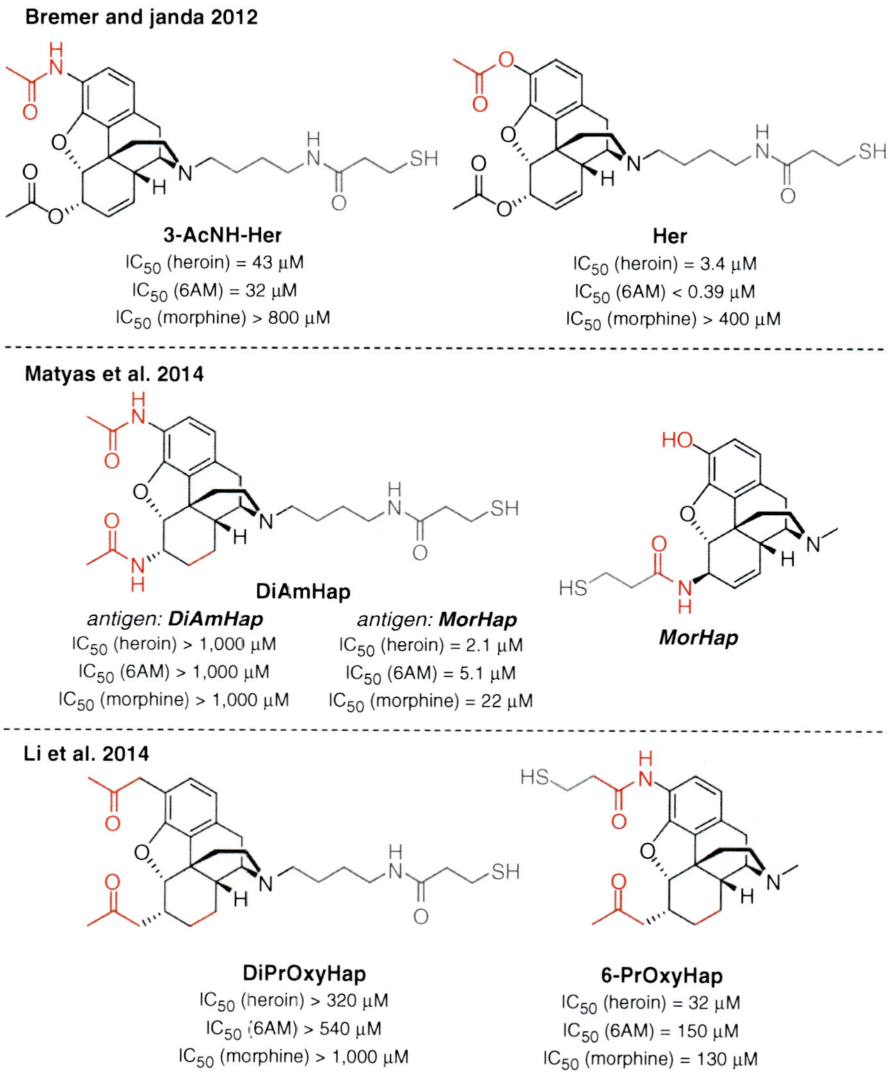

Fig. 18.22 Janda, Alving, and Rice's stabilized heroin haptens (Bremer and Janda 2012; Matyas et al. 2014; Li et al. 2014)

obvious target in this case. However, here it is crucial to understand the mechanism of instability. It has been demonstrated that the C2 ester is much more labile than the C3 ester despite its greater inherent chemical stability, resulting from bridgehead nitrogen-promoted hydrolysis (Li et al. 1999) (Fig. 18.23). Furthermore, although benzoyl ecgonine is believed to be a nonpsychoactive metabolite, it has greater plasma exposure than cocaine. Thus, an immune response that differentiates between cocaine and benzoyl ecgonine is an important goal in this area of research.

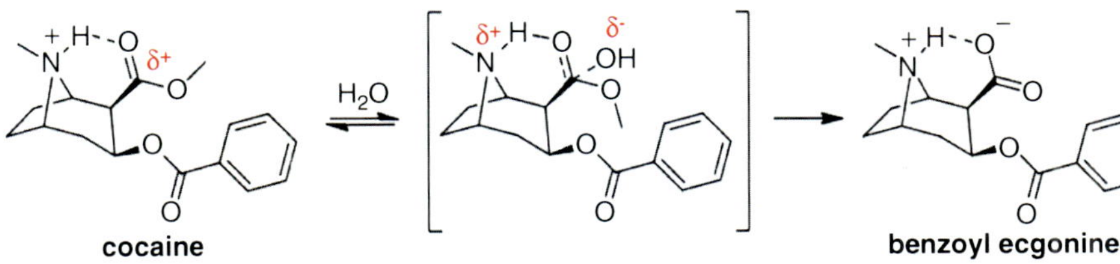

Fig. 18.23 Bridgehead nitrogen-promoted hydrolysis of cocaine to benzoyl ecgonine (Li et al. 1999)

The first cocaine vaccine to show efficacy in vivo utilized Janda's **GNC** hapten, protecting rats against cocaine self-administration relapse (Fig. 18.24) (Carrera et al. 1995; Carrera et al. 2000). However, the unstabilized C2 ester would still be expected to undergo the amine-promoted hydrolysis, resulting in an unpredictable loss of the hapten from the carrier. Stabilization of this ester was therefore proposed to likely increase the observed immune response. Bioisosteric replacement of both esters with amides in hapten **GND** did indeed elicit antibodies that gave longer-lasting protection, albeit only directly comparing to passive immunization of a monoclonal antibody raised against **GNC** (Carrera et al. 2001). However, **GND** proved challenging to synthesize (Sakurai et al. 1996), and thus, the more synthetically accessible **GNE** was designed, with the modification of only the labile C2 ester (Cai et al. 2013b). In direct comparison with **GNC**, **GNE** showed enhanced antibody concentration (123 μg/mL *versus* 48 μg/mL), likely resulting from the observed increase in conjugate stability (Cai et al. 2013c). However, with the increase in antibody concentration came a more significant decrease in affinity, suggesting that the amide is not a perfect bioisostere of the ester. It must also be considered that linking off the C2 ester is likely to generate antibodies that have limited selectivity for cocaine over benzoyl ecgonine.

The importance of C2 stabilization was further exemplified by Janda through direct comparison of bridgehead nitrogen-linked haptens **GNNA** and **GNNS** (Cai et al. 2013c). Both retain the bridgehead amine, but **GNNA** has a stable alternative to the C2 ester, again in the form of an amide. The amide in **GNNA** again resulted in marginally increased concentration and reduced antibody affinity compared with the ester in **GNNS** (3.59 nM, 73 μg/mL for **GNE** compared with 2.05 nM, 65 μg/mL for **GNC**), weakly paralleling the results seen with **GNE** and **GNC**. Again, the presence of the amide slightly impacts on the antibody affinity as would be expected. However, hydrolysis of **GNNS** would produce a benzoyl ecgonine epitope, rather than loss from the carrier protein as would be seen for **GNC**. Without either behavioral data or affinity to benzoyl ecgonine, it is difficult to assess the true impact of replacement of these ester replacement strategies.

An alternative approach to stabilizing the C2 ester is through derivatization of the bridgehead nitrogen to remove its basicity, sacrificing a potential interaction with the antibody but enabling retention of the ester, which appeared to be important in maintaining binding affinity. Fox designed **SNC**, which allowed stable linkage through the bridgehead, and elicited antibodies that reduced the brain concentration of cocaine (Fox et al. 1996) (Fig. 18.25). This hapten showed great

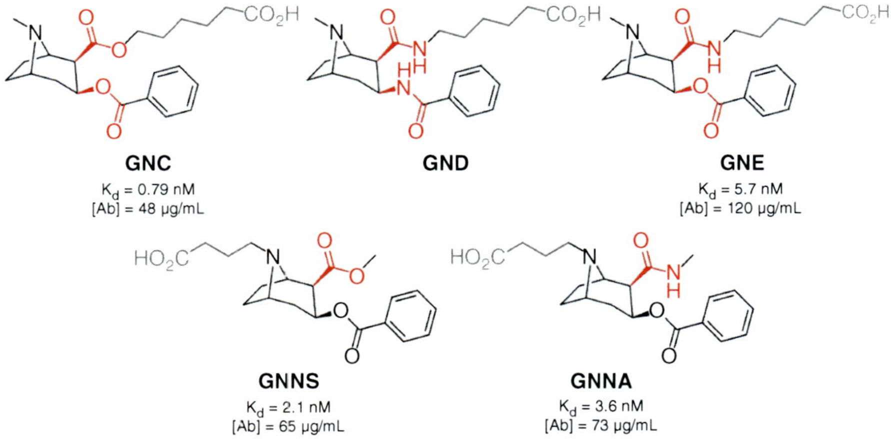

Fig. 18.24 Janda's investigation of C2-linked and bridgehead nitrogen-linked stabilized cocaine haptens (Cai et al. 2013c)

Fig. 18.25 Fox's stabilized cocaine hapten (Fox et al. 1996)

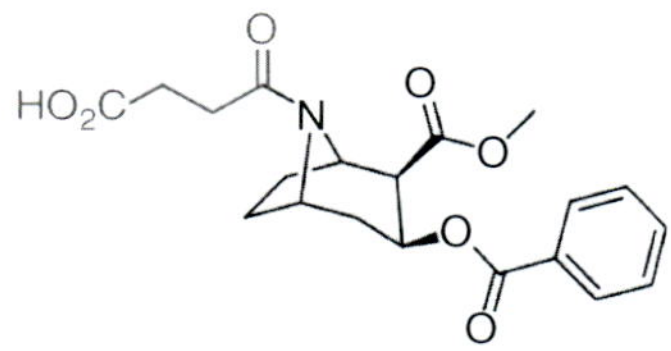

promise, and advanced to clinical trials, but unfortunately the response was highly variable between individuals (Kosten and Biegel 2002; Martell et al. 2005, 2009; Haney et al. 2010).

Orson investigated whether retention of the amine without concomitant C2 ester lability was possible (Ramakrishnan et al. 2014) (Fig. 18.26). **BNC** and **HNC**, two of the three haptens designed, had their methyl ester hydrolyzed during synthesis, and the resulting antibodies generated unsurprisingly bound benzoyl ecgonine with higher affinity than cocaine. The third hapten, **SBNC**, was reported to show no hydrolysis, and the resulting antibodies displayed binding to cocaine but no appreciable binding to benzoyl ecgonine, suggesting that it is possible to preserve both the bridgehead amine and the C2 ester in a stable cocaine hapten. The **SBNC** hapten was directly compared with amide-linked **SNC**; the antibodies raised against **SNC** showed no differentiation between binding to **SNC** and **SBNC**. However, the **SBNC**-raised serum was harder to compete off with cocaine when bound to the **SNC** hapten than the **SBNC** antigen, suggesting that **SBNC** elicited antibodies that have a higher affinity for cocaine. Additional data would be required for this to be more conclusive, but retention of the bridgehead amine does appear to have a positive impact on antibody selectivity. Although the origin of the stabilization of the C2 ester in this case is hard to rationalize, this suggests that exploration of further design features that would allow retention of the C2 ester may be fruitful. The best

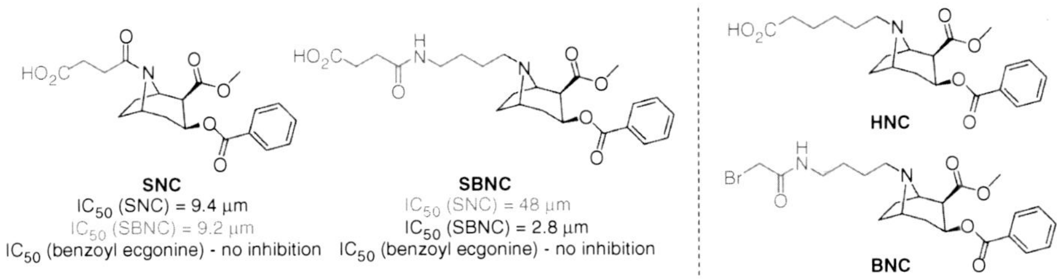

Fig. 18.26 Orson's stabilized cocaine haptens (Ramakrishnan et al. 2014)

approach based on these studies may be to attempt to retain the bridgehead amine but reduce its basicity through the use of proximal electron-withdrawing substituents in the linker.

18.8 Hapten Clustering

It has been shown that attaching a sufficient number of copies of the hapten to the carrier protein (known as the copy number or hapten density) is crucial to generating a good immune response, with a generally observed increase in immune response and specificity as the hapten density increases (Marco et al. 1995). This is especially true for non-opioid drugs, which have much smaller epitopes and hence have reduced potential to generate a high-affinity interaction (Pravetoni et al. 2012c). However, the opportunities for conjugation of the hapten to the carrier are fully dependent on the sequence of the protein. Thus, the maximum copy number is limited to the number of intrinsic surface-exposed lysine or glutamate/aspartate residues, and the haptenation pattern/decoration is dependent on the tertiary structure.

In the field of carbohydrate vaccines, haptens are often designed as clusters to mimic the natural arrangement on cancer cells and promote B cell receptor cross-linking, a requirement for the activation of B cells and antibody production (Peri 2013; Buskas et al. 2009).

Janda theorized that clustering using an appended multivalent scaffold linker could also provide a method to increase the theoretical maximum number of copies of a hapten on the surface of the protein, and this, plus the clustering effect itself, should result in an increase in BCR cross-linking (Collins and Janda 2014). In the initial trials, **triAM1**, a hapten cluster of **AM1** joined to an adamantane scaffold, elicited a substantially poorer immune response than the comparable monovalent vaccine, which could be explained at least in part on the significantly lower hapten density achieved for **triAM1** (Fig. 18.27a). However, significantly greater antibody binding was observed to **triAM1** than **AM1**, suggesting inefficient antibody recognition of the monomer. The second-generation approach used the peptidic linker strategy described in Sect. 18.3.3, inserting a diglycine unit into the trivalent scaffold. **TriAM1(Gly)$_2$** obtained a significantly improved response and binding selectivity, although still with a slightly lower antibody affinity and concentration than

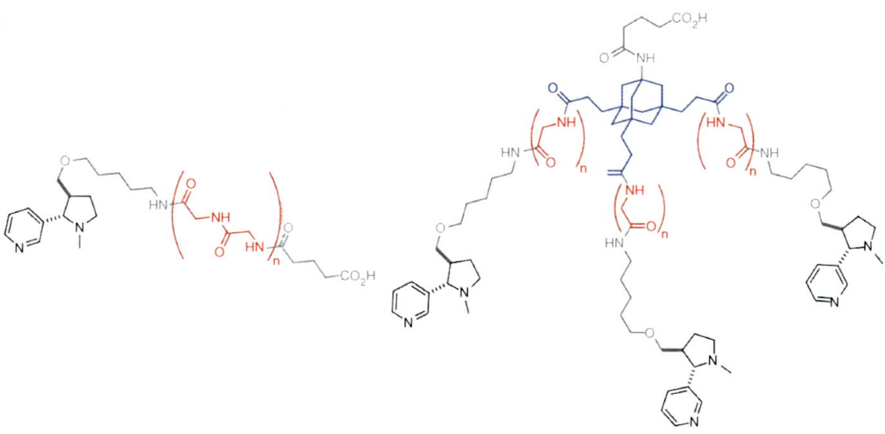

n = 0

(±)-AM1
titer ((±)-AM1) = 34,000
titer ((±)-triAM1) = 45,000
hapten denstiy = 11

(±)-triAM1
titer ((±)-triAM1) = 7,800
titer ((±)-triAM1) = 32,000
hapten denstiy = 2.8

n = 2

(±)-AM1(Gly)$_2$
K_d = 82 nM
[Ab] = 82 μg/mL
titer ((±)-AM1(Gly)$_2$) = 65,000
titer ((±)-triAM1(Gly)2) = 84,000
hapten denstiy = 5.8

(±)-triAM1(Gly)$_2$
K_d = 160 nM
[Ab] = 38 μg/mL
titer ((±)-AM1(Gly)$_2$) = 64,000
titer ((±)-triAM1(Gly)2) = 140,000
hapten denstiy = 2.0

Fig. 18.27 Janda's investigation of a nicotine hapten cluster (Collins and Janda 2014)

the comparable monovalent vaccine **AM1(Gly)$_2$** (Fig. 18.27b), likely due to the lower hapten density. This multivalent scaffold strategy appears to have potential to increase the anti-drug immune response, with general applicability. However, there are two main limitations in this specific case, namely, the greater synthetic complexity and increased difficulty of hapten conjugation, which present practical hurdles that will need to be addressed before it is a viable approach.

An alternative approach by Sanderson using a peptidic vaccine allowed facile conjugation of multiple copies of the hapten using a facile synthetic approach, *via* peptide coupling (Duryee et al. 2009) (Fig. 18.28). However, the bivalent hapten showed an inferior antibody concentration (as measured by competitive ELISA) and decreased stimulation CD4$^+$ T cells. Although further analysis of antibody responses wasn't carried out, this likely parallels the observations for the **triAM1** hapten in generating an immune response against the dimer rather than the monomeric hapten. Therefore, the use of increased spacing between the haptens would likely increase the chance of success.

18.9 Enantiopurity

Heroin/morphine, cocaine, and nicotine are all taken in an enantiopure form, whereas methamphetamine can contain small amounts of the less active (-)-stereoisomer, which has a pharmacodynamic profile less favorable for

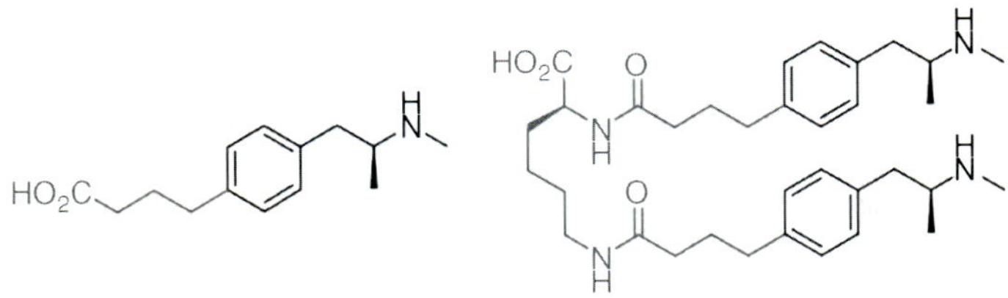

Fig. 18.28 Sanderson's investigation of a methamphetamine hapten cluster (Duryee et al. 2009)

Fig. 18.29 Janda's comparison of enantiopure nicotine haptens (Lockner et al. 2015)

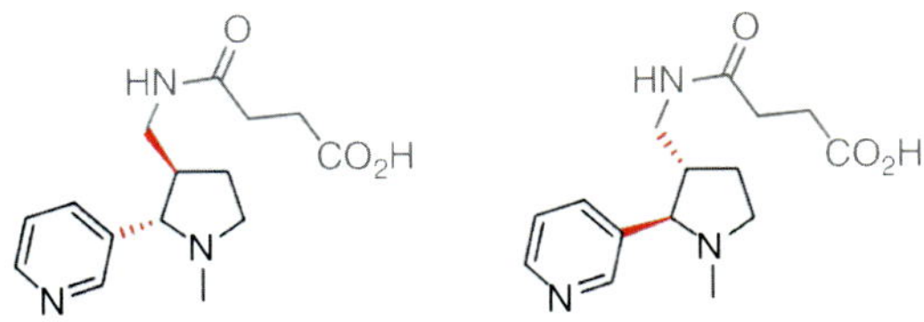

addiction (Mendelson et al. 2006; Kuczenski et al. 1995). It has been known for almost a century that the immune system can differentiate between enantiomers of the same hapten (Landsteiner and van der Scheer 1928), and therefore, vaccination with an enantiopure hapten will likely result in a more effective immune response directed only at the relevant stereoisomer.

Where synthetically accessible, the majority of haptens assessed in the literature contain the correct stereochemistry to obtain an immune response directed towards the biologically relevant target. However, there are many cases of racemic haptens being utilized, including both nicotine haptens **(±)-3'-EstNic** and **(±)-3'-AmNic** that were used in clinical trials. This resulted from the ready availability of a racemic *trans*-2,3-substituted synthetic precursor. Janda therefore investigated the potential for an increase in immune response upon vaccination using each enantiopure stereoisomer (Fig. 18.29) (Lockner et al. 2015). The hapten with the matched 2' stereochemistry to nicotine, **(-)-3'-AmNic**, showed a significant increase in antibody concentration but a decrease in affinity for nicotine when compared with antibodies elicited by the alternative enantiomer **(+)-3'-AmNic**. This is surprising, as nicotine would at first glance be expected to bind with higher affinity to antibodies raised using an epitope that retained the natural 2' stereochemistry. One potential explanation for this is that linker introduction at the 3' position proximal to the pyridine and pyrrolidine ring junction may result in significant perturbation of the natural conformation, leading to antibodies that bind to an epitope that is not representative of nicotine. This theory is consistent with a mAb raised against **3'-EstNic** having drastically different binding modes for nicotine and the hapten (Tars et al. 2012). Furthermore, the disparity in antibody

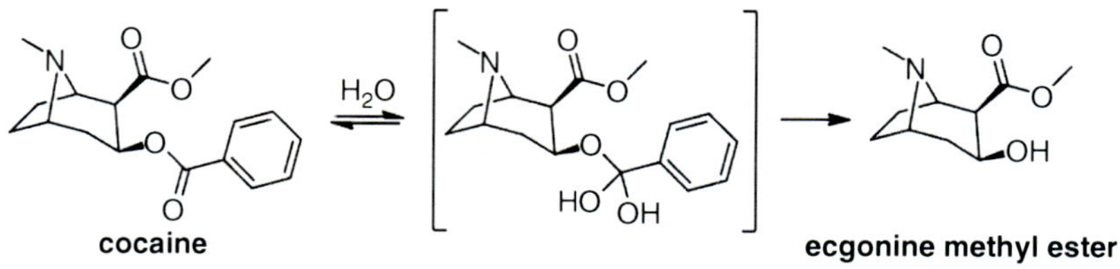

Fig. 18.30 Mechanism of cocaine hydrolysis (Zheng and Zhan 2008)

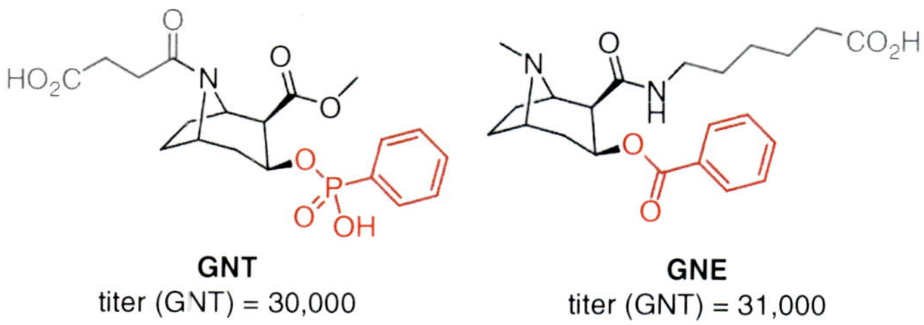

Fig. 18.31 Janda's investigation into anti-cocaine catalytic antibody design (Cai et al. 2013b)

concentration elicited by the two haptens is also surprising and suggests that there is a difference in either processing or display, resulting in either reduced T cell help or B cell recognition. There was little cross-reactivity between the two sets of antibodies, suggesting that distinct subpopulations of B cells were produced. This study clearly demonstrates that the stereochemistry of the hapten influences the immune response and that efforts should be made to investigate the effects of individual enantiomers.

18.10 Active Catalytic Vaccine

Antibodies for the majority of drugs of abuse vaccines have a defined binding potential: the combination of the binding affinity and concentration will define the maximum binding capacity. An alternative approach uses catalytic antibodies, designed to specifically catalyze the hydrolysis of the target drug by transition state stabilization. Catalytic antibodies would theoretically remove much higher concentrations of a drug from circulation than the standard stoichiometric sequestering antibody approach. This strategy has mainly been applied to the production of monoclonal antibodies (Chandrakumar et al. 1993; Landry et al. 1993), but application to active vaccination is also viable. In the case of cocaine, this strategy involves catalysis of the hydrolysis of the benzoyl ester to nonpsychoactive ecgonine methyl ester (Fig. 18.30).

Janda has explored active vaccination against cocaine using **GNT**, designed to contain phenylphosphonate as a transition state mimic of the hydrolyzing benzoic ester (Cai et al. 2013b, Fig. 18.31). This hapten was able to elicit comparable antibody titers to **GNE** and reduced cocaine-induced psychomotor stimulation, albeit not as substantially as **GNE**. However, upon further cocaine challenges, the protective effect diminished, resulting from covalent modification of the antibodies by cocaine. Thus, although this approach may eventually garner improved protection against cocaine administration, further investigation is required to bring this to fruition.

References

Agard NJ, Prescher JA, Bertozzi CR. A strain-promoted [3+2] azide–alkyne cycloaddition for covalent modification of biomolecules in living systems. J Am Chem Soc. 2004;126(46):15046–7. doi:10.1021/ja044996f.

Ambre J, Ruo TI, Nelson J, Belknap S. Urinary excretion of cocaine, benzoylecgonine, and ecgonine methyl ester in humans. J Anal Toxicol. 1988;12(6):301–6. doi:10.1093/jat/12.6.301.

Andrews NJ, Waight PA, George RC, Slack MPE, Miller E. Impact and effectiveness of 23-valent pneumococcal polysaccharide vaccine against invasive pneumococcal disease in the elderly in England and wales. Vaccine. 2012;30(48):6802–8. doi:10.1016/j.vaccine.2012.09.019.

Barceloux DG. Amphetamine and methamphetamine. In: Medical toxicology of drug abuse. Hoboken, NJ, USA: John Wiley & Sons, Inc.; 2012. p. 1–56. doi:10.1002/9781118105955.ch1.

Berzofsky JA, Schechter AN. The concepts of crossreactivity and specificity in immunology. Mol Immunol. 1981;18(8):751–63. doi:10.1016/0161-5890(81)90067-5.

Bremer PT, Janda KD. Investigating the effects of a hydrolytically stable hapten and a Th1 adjuvant on heroin vaccine performance. J Med Chem. 2012;55(23):10776–80. doi:10.1021/jm301262z.

Brust JCM. Chapter 5 – cocaine. In: Brust JCM, editor. Neurological aspects of substance abuse. 2nd ed. Philadelphia: Butterworth-Heinemann; 2004. p. 139–99. doi:10.1016/B978-0-7506-7313-6.50009-X.

Buskas T, Thompson P, Boons G-J. Immunotherapy for cancer: synthetic carbohydrate-based vaccines. Chem Commun. 2009;36:5335–49.

Byrnes-Blake KA, Carroll FI, Abraham P, Owens SM. Generation of anti-(+)methamphetamine antibodies is not impeded by (+)methamphetamine administration during active immunization of rats. Int Immunopharmacol. 2001;1(2):329–38.

Cai X, Tsuchikama K, Janda KD. Modulating cocaine vaccine potency through hapten fluorination. J Am Chem Soc. 2013a;135(8):2971–4. doi:10.1021/ja400356g.

Cai X, Whitfield T, Hixon MS, Grant Y, Koob GF, Janda KD. Probing active cocaine vaccination performance through catalytic and noncatalytic hapten design. J Med Chem. 2013b;56(9):3701–9. doi:10.1021/jm400228w.

Cai X, Whitfield T, Moreno AY, Grant Y, Hixon MS, Koob GF, Janda KD. Probing the effects of hapten stability on cocaine vaccine immunogenicity. Mol Pharm. 2013c;10(11):4176–84. doi:10.1021/mp400214w.

Carrera MRA, Ashley JA, Parsons LH, Wirsching P, Koob GF, Janda KD. Suppression of psychoactive effects of cocaine by active immunization. Nature. 1995;378(6558):727–30.

Carrera MRA, Ashley JA, Zhou B, Wirsching P, Koob GF, Janda KD. Cocaine vaccines: antibody protection against relapse in a rat model. Proc Natl Acad Sci. 2000;97(11):6202–6. doi:10.1073/pnas.97.11.6202.

Carrera MRA, Ashley JA, Wirsching P, Koob GF, Janda KD. A second-generation vaccine protects against the psychoactive effects of cocaine. Proc Natl Acad Sci U S A. 2001;98(4):1988–92. doi:10.1073/pnas.98.4.1988.

Carroll FI, Blough BE, Pidaparthi RR, Abraham P, Gong PK, Deng L, Huang X, Gunnell M, Lay JO, Peterson EC, Owens SM. Synthesis of mercapto-(+)-methamphetamine haptens and their use for obtaining improved epitope density on (+)-methamphetamine conjugate vaccines. J Med Chem. 2011;54(14):5221–8. doi:10.1021/jm2004943.

Cerny EH, Lévy R, Mauel J, Mpandi M, Mutter M, Henzelin-Nkubana C, Patiny L, Tuchscherer G, Cerny T. Preclinical development of a vaccine 'against smoking'. Onkologie. 2002;25(5):406–11.

Chandrakumar NS, Carron CP, Meyer DM, Beardsley PM, Nash SA, Tam LL, Rafferty M. Phenylphosphonate monoester analogs of cocaine. Potential haptens for the generation of catalytic antibodies. Bioorg Med Chem Lett. 1993;3(2):309–12. doi:10.1016/S0960-894X(01)80899-4.

Chang C-eA, Chen W, Gilson MK. Ligand configurational entropy and protein binding. Proc Natl Acad Sci. 2007;104(5):1534–9. doi:10.1073/pnas.0610494104.

Collins KC, Janda KD. Investigating hapten clustering as a strategy to enhance vaccines against drugs of abuse. Bioconjug Chem. 2014;25(3):593–600. doi:10.1021/bc500016k.

Collins KC, Schlosburg JE, Lockner JW, Bremer PT, Ellis BA, Janda KD. Lipid tucaresol as an adjuvant for methamphetamine vaccine development. Chem Commun. 2014;50(31):4079–81. doi:10.1039/c4cc00682h.

Cook CE, Jeffcoat AR, Hill JM, Pugh DE, Patetta PK, Sadler BM, White WR, Perez-Reyes M. Pharmacokinetics of methamphetamine self-administered to human subjects by smoking S-(+)-methamphetamine hydrochloride. Drug Metab Dispos. 1993;21(4):717–23.

Cornish KE, de Villiers SHL, Pravetoni M, Pentel PR. Immunogenicity of individual vaccine components in a bivalent nicotine vaccine differ according to vaccine formulation and administration conditions. PLoS One. 2013;8(12), e82557. doi:10.1371/journal.pone.0082557.

Cornuz J, Zwahlen S, Jungi WF, Osterwalder J, Klingler K, van Melle G, Bangala Y, Guessous I, Müller P, Willers J, Maurer P, Bachmann MF, Cerny T. A vaccine against nicotine for smoking cessation: a randomized controlled trial. PLoS One. 2008;3(6), e2547.

de Villiers SHL, Lindblom N, Kalayanov G, Gordon S, Malmerfelt A, Johansson AM, Svensson TH. Active immunization against nicotine suppresses nicotine-induced dopamine release in the rat nucleus accumbens shell. Respiration. 2002;69(3):247–53.

de Villiers SHL, Lindblom N, Kalayanov G, Gordon S, Baraznenok I, Malmerfelt A, Marcus MM, Johansson AM, Svensson TH. Nicotine hapten structure, antibody selectivity and effect relationships: results from a nicotine vaccine screening procedure. Vaccine. 2010;28(10):2161–8. doi:10.1016/j.vaccine.2009.12.051.

de Villiers SHL, Cornish KE, Troska AJ, Pravetoni M, Pentel PR. Increased efficacy of a trivalent nicotine vaccine compared to a dose-matched monovalent vaccine when formulated with alum. Vaccine. 2013;31(52):6185–93. doi:10.1016/j.vaccine.2013.10.051.

DeTar DF, Silverstein R. Reactions of carbodiimides. I. The mechanisms of the reactions of acetic acid with dicyclohexylcarbodiimide1,2. J Am Chem Soc. 1966;88(5):1013–9. doi:10.1021/ja00957a027.

Duncan RJS, Weston PD, Wrigglesworth R. A new reagent which may be used to introduce sulfhydryl groups into proteins, and its use in the preparation of conjugates for immunoassay. Anal Biochem. 1983;132(1):68–73. doi:10.1016/0003-2697(83)90426-8.

Duryee MJ, Bevins RA, Reichel CM, Murray JE, Dong Y, Thiele GM, Sanderson SD. Immune responses to methamphetamine by active immunization with peptide-based, molecular adjuvant-containing vaccines. Vaccine. 2009;27(22):2981–8.

Dwoskin LP, Teng L, Buxton ST, Crooks PA. (S)-(−)-cotinine, the major brain metabolite of nicotine, stimulates nicotinic receptors to evoke [3H]dopamine release from rat striatal slices in a calcium-dependent manner. J Pharmacol Exp Ther. 1999;288(3):905–11.

Fontaine SD, Reid R, Robinson L, Ashley GW, Santi DV. Long-term stabilization of maleimide–thiol conjugates. Bioconjug Chem. 2014;26(1):145–52. doi:10.1021/bc5005262.

Fox BS, Kantak KM, Edwards MA, Black KM, Bollinger BK, Botka AJ, French TL, Thompson TL, Schad VC, Greenstein JL, Gefter ML, Exley MA, Swain PA, Briner TJ. Efficacy of a therapeutic cocaine vaccine in rodent models. Nat Med. 1996;2(10):1129–32.

Gómez-Nuñez M, Haro KJ, Dao T, Chau D, Won A, Escobar-Alvarez S, Zakhaleva V, Korontsvit T, Gin DY, Scheinberg DA. Non-natural and photo-reactive amino acids as biochemical probes of immune function. PLoS One. 2008;3(12), e3938.

Grandjean C, Boutonnier A, Guerreiro C, Fournier J-M, Mulard LA. On the preparation of carbohydrate–protein conjugates using the traceless Staudinger ligation. J Org Chem. 2005;70(18):7123–32. doi:10.1021/jo0505472.

Haney M, Gunderson EW, Jiang H, Collins ED, Foltin RW. Cocaine-specific antibodies blunt the subjective effects of smoked cocaine in humans. Biol Psychiatry. 2010;67(1):59–65. doi:10.1016/j.biopsych.2009.08.031.

Hatsukami DK, Grillo M, Pentel PR, Oncken C, Bliss R. Safety of cotinine in humans: physiologic, subjective, and cognitive effects. Pharmacol Biochem Behav. 1997;57(4):643–50. doi:10.1016/S0091-3057(97)80001-9.

Hatsukami DK, Rennard S, Jorenby D, Fiore M, Koopmeiners J, de Vos A, Horwith G, Pentel PR. Safety and immunogenicity of a nicotine conjugate vaccine in current smokers. Clin Pharmacol Ther. 2005;78(5):456–67. doi:10.1016/j.clpt.2005.08.007.

Hatsukami DK, Jorenby DE, Gonzales D, Rigotti NA, Glover ED, Oncken CA, Tashkin DP, Reus VI, Akhavain RC, Fahim REF, Kessler PD, Niknian M, Kalnik MW, Rennard SI. Immunogenicity and smoking-cessation outcomes for a novel nicotine immunotherapeutic. Clin Pharmacol Ther. 2011;89(3):392–9.

Hieda Y, Keyler DE, Vandevoort JT, Kane JK, Ross CA, Raphael DE, Niedbalas RS, Pentel PR. Active immunization alters the plasma nicotine concentration in rats. J Pharmacol Exp Ther. 1997;283(3):1076–81.

Hieda Y, Keyler DE, Vandevoort JT, Niedbalas RS, Raphael DE, Ross CA, Pentel PR. Immunization of rats reduces nicotine distribution to brain. Psychopharmacology (Berl). 1999;143(2):150–7.

Hieda Y, Keyler DE, Ennifar S, Fattom A, Pentel PR. Vaccination against nicotine during continued nicotine administration in rats: immunogenicity of the vaccine and effects on nicotine distribution to brain. Int J Immunopharmacol. 2000;22(10):809–19. doi:10.1016/S0192-0561(00)00042-4.

Hoffmann-Röder A, Kaiser A, Wagner S, Gaidzik N, Kowalczyk D, Westerlind U, Gerlitzki B, Schmitt E, Kunz H. Synthetic antitumor vaccines from tetanus toxoid conjugates of MUC1 glycopeptides with the thomsen–friedenreich antigen and a fluorine-substituted analogue. Angew Chem Int Ed. 2010;49(45):8498–503. doi:10.1002/anie.201003810.

Hukkanen J, Jacob P, Benowitz NL. Metabolism and disposition kinetics of nicotine. Pharmacol Rev. 2005;57(1):79–115. doi:10.1124/pr.57.1.3.

Inturrisi CE, Schultz M, Shin S, Umans JG, Angel L, Simon EJ. Evidence from opiate binding studies that heroin acts through its metabolites. Life Sci. 1983;33:773–6. doi:10.1016/0024-3205(83)90616-1.

Isomura S, Wirsching P, Janda KD. An immunotherapeutic program for the treatment of nicotine addiction: hapten design and synthesis. J Org Chem. 2001;66(12):4115–21. doi:10.1021/jo001442w.

Janda KD, Treweek JB. Vaccines targeting drugs of abuse: is the glass half-empty or half-full? Nat Rev Immunol. 2012;12(1):67–72.

Jeffcoat AR, Perez-Reyes M, Hill JM, Sadler BM, Cook CE. Cocaine disposition in humans after intravenous injection, nasal insufflation (snorting), or smoking. Drug Metab Dispos. 1989;17(2):153–9.

Jufer RA, Wstadik A, Walsh SL, Levine BS, Cone EJ. Elimination of cocaine and metabolites in plasma, saliva, and urine following repeated oral administration to human volunteers. J Anal Toxicol. 2000;24(7):467–77. doi:10.1093/jat/24.7.467.

Keenan RM, Hatsukami DK, Pentel PR, Thompson TN, Grillo MA. Pharmacodynamic effects of cotinine in abstinent cigarette smokers. Clin Pharmacol Ther. 1994;55(5):581–90. doi:10.1038/clpt.1994.72.

Keyler DE, Roiko SA, Earley CA, Murtaugh MP, Pentel PR. Enhanced immunogenicity of a bivalent nicotine vaccine. Int Immunopharmacol. 2008;8(11):1589–94.

Kim Pei L, Smith MT. The antinociceptive potencies of oxycodone, noroxycodone and morphine after intracerebroventricular administration to rats. Life Sci. 1994;54(17):1229–36. doi:10.1016/0024-3205(94)00849-3.

Kolbrich EA, Barnes AJ, Gorelick DA, Boyd SJ, Cone EJ, Huestis MA. Major and minor metabolites of cocaine in human plasma following controlled subcutaneous cocaine administration. J Anal Toxicol. 2006;30(8):501–10. doi:10.1093/jat/30.8.501.

Kosten TR, Biegel D. Therapeutic vaccines for substance dependence. Expert Rev Vaccines. 2002;1(3):365–71. doi:10.1586/14760584.1.3.365.

Kubler-Kielb J, Liu T-Y, Mocca C, Majadly F, Robbins JB, Schneerson R. Additional conjugation methods and immunogenicity of bacillus anthracis poly-γ-d-glutamic acid-protein conjugates. Infect Immun. 2006;74(8):4744–9. doi:10.1128/iai.00315-06.

Kuczenski R, Segal DS, Cho AK, Melega W. Hippocampus norepinephrine, caudate dopamine and serotonin, and behavioral responses to the stereoisomers of amphetamine and methamphetamine. J Neurosci. 1995;15(2):1308–17.

Lalovic B, Kharasch E, Hoffer C, Risler L, Liu-Chen L-Y, Shen DD. Pharmacokinetics and pharmacodynamics of oral oxycodone in healthy human subjects: Role of circulating active metabolites. Clin Pharmacol Ther. 2006;79(5):461–79. doi:10.1016/j.clpt.2006.01.009.

Landry D, Zhao K, Yang G, Glickman M, Georgiadis T. Antibody-catalyzed degradation of cocaine. Science. 1993;259(5103):1899–901. doi:10.1126/science.8456315.

Landsteiner K, van der Scheer J. Serological differentiation of steric isomers. J Exp Med. 1928;48(3):315–20. doi:10.1084/jem.48.3.315.

Langman RE. The specificity of immunological reactions. Mol Immunol. 2000;37(10):555–61. doi:10.1016/S0161-5890(00)00083-3.

Langone JJ, Gjika HB, Van Vunakis H. Nicotine and its metabolites. Radioimmunoassays for nicotine and cotinine. Biochemistry. 1973;12(24):5025–30.

LeSage MG, Pentel PR. Vaccines and drug-specific antibodies. In: Stolerman I, editor. Encyclopedia of psychopharmacology. Berlin/Heidelberg: Springer; 2010. p. 1355–7. doi:10.1007/978-3-540-68706-1_356.

Li P, Zhao K, Deng S, Landry DW. Nonenzymatic hydrolysis of cocaine via intramolecular acid catalysis. Helv Chim Acta. 1999;82(1):85–9. doi:10.1002/(SICI)1522-2675(19990113)82:1<85::AID-HLCA85>3.0.CO;2-Q.

Li F, Cheng K, Antoline JFG, Iyer MR, Matyas GR, Torres OB, Jalah R, Beck Z, Alving CR, Parrish DA, Deschamps JR, Jacobson AE, Rice KC. Synthesis and immunological effects of heroin vaccines. Org Biomol Chem. 2014;12:7211. doi:10.1039/C4OB01053A.

Lockner JW, Lively JM, Collins KC, Vendruscolo JCM, Azar MR, Janda KD. A conjugate vaccine using enantiopure hapten imparts superior nicotine-binding capacity. J Med Chem. 2015;58:1005–11. doi:10.1021/jm501625j.

Marco M-P, Gee S, Hammock BD. Immunochemical techniques for environmental analysis II. Antibody production and immunoassay development. TrAC-Trends Anal Chem. 1995;14(8):415–25. doi:10.1016/0165-9936(95)90920-I.

Martell BA, Mitchell E, Poling J, Gonsai K, Kosten TR. Vaccine pharmacotherapy for the treatment of cocaine dependence. Biol Psychiatry. 2005;58(2):158–64. doi:10.1016/j.biopsych.2005.04.032.

Martell BA, Orson FM, Poling J, Mitchell E, Rossen RD, Tracie G, Kosten TR. Cocaine vaccine for the treatment of cocaine dependence in methadone-maintained patients: a randomized, double-blind, placebo-controlled efficacy trial. Arch Gen Psychiatry. 2009;66(10):1116–23. doi:10.1001/archgenpsychiatry.2009.128.

Matsushita M, Hoffman TZ, Ashley JA, Zhou B, Wirsching P, Janda KD. Cocaine catalytic antibodies: the primary importance of linker effects. Bioorg Med Chem Lett. 2001;11(2):87–90. doi:10.1016/S0960-894X(00)00659-4.

Matyas GR, Rice KC, Cheng K, Li F, Antoline JFG, Iyer MR, Jacobson AE, Mayorov AV, Beck Z, Torres OB, Alving CR. Facial recognition of heroin vaccine opiates: type 1 cross-reactivities of antibodies induced by hydrolytically stable haptenic surrogates of heroin, 6-acetylmorphine, and morphine. Vaccine. 2014;32(13):1473–9. doi:10.1016/j.vaccine.2014.01.028.

Maurer P, Jennings GT, Willers J, Rohner F, Lindman Y, Roubicek K, Renner WA, Müller P, Bachmann MF. A therapeutic vaccine for nicotine dependence: preclinical efficacy, and phase I safety and immunogenicity. Eur J Immunol. 2005;35(7):2031–40. doi:10.1002/eji.200526285.

McCance EF, Price LH, Kosten TR, Jatlow PI. Cocaethylene: pharmacology, physiology and behavioral effects in humans. J Pharmacol Exp Ther. 1995;274(1):215–23.

Meijler MM, Matsushita M, Altobell LJ, Wirsching P, Janda KD. A new strategy for improved nicotine vaccines using conformationally constrained haptens. J Am Chem Soc. 2003;125(24):7164–5. doi:10.1021/ja034805t.

Mendelson J, Uemura N, Harris D, Nath RP, Fernandez E, Jacob P, Everhart ET, Jones RT. Human pharmacology of the methamphetamine stereoisomers. Clin Pharmacol Ther. 2006;80(4):403–20. doi:10.1016/j.clpt.2006.06.013.

Miller ML, Moreno AY, Aarde SM, Creehan KM, Vandewater SA, Vaillancourt BD, Wright Jr MJ, Janda KD, Taffe MA. A methamphetamine vaccine attenuates methamphetamine-induced disruptions in thermoregulation and activity in rats. Biol Psychiatry. 2013;73(8):721–8. doi:10.1016/j.biopsych.2012.09.010.

Moreno AY, Azar MR, Warren NA, Dickerson TJ, Koob GF, Janda KD. A critical evaluation of a nicotine vaccine within a self-administration behavioral model. Mol Pharm. 2010;7(2):431–41. doi:10.1021/mp900213u.

Moreno AY, Mayorov AV, Janda KD. Impact of distinct chemical structures for the development of a methamphetamine vaccine. J Am Chem Soc. 2011;133(17):6587–95. doi:10.1021/ja108807j.

Moreno AY, Azar MR, Koob GF, Janda KD. Probing the protective effects of a conformationally constrained nicotine vaccine. Vaccine. 2012;30(47):6665–70. doi:10.1016/j.vaccine.2012.08.064.

Morishima HO, Whittington RA, Iso A, Cooper TB. The comparative toxicity of cocaine and its metabolites in conscious rats free. Anaesthesiology. 1999;90(6):1684–90. doi: 0000542-199906000-00025.

Müller K, Faeh C, Diederich F. Fluorine in pharmaceuticals: looking beyond intuition. Science. 2007;317(5846):1881–6. doi:10.1126/science.1131943.

Nowak MA. Immune responses against multiple epitopes: a theory for immunodominance and antigenic variation. Semin Virol. 1996;7(1):83–92. doi:10.1006/smvy.1996.0010.

Oliver JL, Pashmi G, Barnett P, Mettens P, Biemans R, Monteyne P, Palmantier R, Gallagher T, Ramaya S, Wonnacott S. Development of an anti-cotinine vaccine to potentiate nicotine-based smoking cessation strategies. Vaccine. 2007;25(42):7354–62.

Orson FM, Wang R, Brimijoin S, Kinsey BM, Singh RA, Ramakrishnan M, Wang HY, Kosten TR. The future potential for cocaine vaccines. Expert Opin Biol Ther. 2014;14(9):1271–83. doi :10.1517/14712598.2014.920319.

Osborne R, Thompson P, Joel S, Trew D, Patel N, Slevin M. The analgesic activity of morphine-6-glucuronide. Br J Clin Pharmacol. 1992;34(2):130–8.

Pentel PR, Malin DH, Ennifar S, Hieda Y, Keyler DE, Lake JR, Milstein JR, Basham LE, Coy RT, Moon JWD, Naso R, Fattom A. A nicotine conjugate vaccine reduces nicotine distribution to brain and attenuates its behavioral and cardiovascular effects in rats. Pharmacol Biochem Behav. 2000;65(1):191–8.

Perez-Reyes M, White WR, McDonald SA, Hill JM, Jeffcoat AR, Cook CE. Clinical effects of methamphetamine vapor inhalation. Life Sci. 1991;49(13):953–9. doi:10.1016/0024-3205(91)90078-P.

Peri F. Clustered carbohydrates in synthetic vaccines. Chem Soc Rev. 2013;42(11):4543–56. doi:10.1039/c2cs35422e.

Pöyhiä R, Seppälä T, Olkkola KT, Kalso E. The pharmacokinetics and metabolism of oxycodone after intramuscular and oral administration to healthy subjects. Br J Clin Pharmacol. 1992;33(6):617–21.

Pravetoni M, Keyler DE, Raleigh MD, Harris AC, LeSage MG, Mattson CK, Pettersson S, Pentel PR. Vaccination against nicotine alters the distribution of nicotine delivered via cigarette smoke inhalation to rats. Biochem Pharmacol. 2011;81(9):1164–70. doi:10.1016/j.bcp.2011.02.004.

Pravetoni M, Keyler DE, Pidaparthi RR, Carroll FI, Runyon SP, Murtaugh MP, Earley CA, Pentel PR. Structurally distinct nicotine immunogens elicit antibodies with non-overlapping specificities. Biochem Pharmacol. 2012a;83(4):543–50.

Pravetoni M, Le Naour M, Harmon TM, Tucker AM, Portoghese PS, Pentel PR. An oxycodone conjugate vaccine elicits drug-specific antibodies that reduce oxycodone distribution to brain and hot-plate analgesia. J Pharmacol Exp Ther. 2012b;341(1):225–32. doi:10.1124/jpet.111.189506.

Pravetoni M, Raleigh MD, Le Naour M, Tucker AM, Harmon TM, Jones JM, Birnbaum AK, Portoghese PS, Pentel PR. Co-administration of morphine and oxycodone vaccines reduces the distribution of 6-monoacetylmorphine and oxycodone to brain in rats. Vaccine. 2012c;30(31):4617–24. doi:10.1016/j.vaccine.2012.04.101.

Pravetoni M, Le Naour M, Tucker AM, Harmon TM, Hawley TM, Portoghese PS, Pentel PR. Reduced antinociception of opioids in rats and mice by vaccination with immunogens containing oxycodone and hydrocodone haptens. J Med Chem. 2013;56(3):915–23. doi:10.1021/jm3013745.

Pravetoni M, Pentel PR, Potter DN, Chartoff EH, Tally L, LeSage MG. Effects of an oxycodone conjugate vaccine on oxycodone self-administration and oxycodone-induced brain gene expression in rats. PLoS One. 2014a;9(7), e101807. doi:10.1371/journal.pone.0101807.

Pravetoni M, Vervacke JS, Distefano MD, Tucker AM, Laudenbach M, Pentel PR. Effect of currently approved carriers and adjuvants on the pre-clinical efficacy of a conjugate vaccine against oxycodone in mice and rats. PLoS One. 2014b;9(5), e96547. doi:10.1371/journal.pone.0096547.

Pryde DC, Jones LH, Gervais DP, Stead DR, Blakemore DC, Selby MD, Brown AD, Coe JW, Badland M, Beal DM, Glen R, Wharton Y, Miller GJ, White P, Zhang N, Benoit M, Robertson K, Merson JR, Davis HL, McCluskie MJ. Selection of a novel anti-nicotine vaccine: influence of antigen design on antibody function in mice. PLoS One. 2013;8(10), e76557.

Raleigh MD, Pravetoni M, Harris AC, Birnbaum AK, Pentel PR. Selective effects of a morphine conjugate vaccine on heroin and metabolite distribution and heroin-induced behaviors in rats. J Pharmacol Exp Ther. 2013;344(2):397–406. doi:10.1124/jpet.112.201194.

Ramakrishnan M, Kinsey BM, Singh RA, Kosten TR, Orson FM. Hapten optimization for cocaine vaccine with improved cocaine recognition. Chem Biol Drug Des. 2014;84(3):354–63. doi:10.1111/cbdd.12326.

Rook E, Huitema AR, van den Brink W, van Ree J, Beijnen J. Population pharmacokinetics of heroin and its major metabolites. Clin Pharmacokinet. 2006a;45(4):401–17. doi:10.2165/00003088-200645040-00005.

Rook EJ, Van Ree JM, Van Den Brink W, Hillebrand MJX, Huitema ADR, Hendriks VM, Beijnen JH. Pharmacokinetics and pharmacodynamics of high doses of pharmaceutically prepared heroin, by intravenous or by inhalation route in opioid-dependent patients. Basic Clin Pharmacol. 2006b;98(1):86–96. doi:10.1111/j.1742-7843.2006.pto_233.x.

Rostovtsev VV, Green LG, Fokin VV, Sharpless KB. A stepwise huisgen cycloaddition process: copper(I)-catalyzed regioselective "ligation" of azides and terminal alkynes. Angew Chem Int Ed. 2002;41(14):2596–9. doi:10.1002/1521-3773(20020715)41:14<2596::AID-ANIE2596>3.0.CO;2-4.

Sakurai M, Wirsching P, Janda KD. Design and synthesis of a cocaine-diamide hapten for vaccine development. Tetrahedron Lett. 1996;37(31):5479–82. doi:10.1016/0040-4039(96)01170-7.

Schep LJ, Slaughter RJ, Beasley DMG. The clinical toxicology of metamfetamine. Clin Toxicol. 2010;48(7):675–94. doi:10.3109/15563650.2010.516752.

Schlosburg JE, Vendruscolo LF, Bremer PT, Lockner JW, Wade CL, Nunes AAK, Stowe GN, Edwards S, Janda KD, Koob GF. Dynamic vaccine blocks relapse to compulsive intake of heroin. Proc Natl Acad Sci U S A. 2013;110(22):9036–41. doi:10.1073/pnas.1219159110.

Schneerson R, Kubler-Kielb J, Liu T-Y, Dai Z-D, Leppla SH, Yergey A, Backlund P, Shiloach J, Majadly F, Robbins JB. Poly(γ-d-glutamic acid) protein conjugates induce IgG antibodies in mice to the capsule of bacillus anthracis: a potential addition to the anthrax vaccine. Proc Natl Acad Sci. 2003;100(15):8945–50. doi:10.1073/pnas.1633512100.

Schramm W, Craig PA, Smith RH, Berger GE. Cocaine and benzoylecgonine in saliva, serum, and urine. Clin Chem. 1993;39(3):481–7.

Seleman M, Chapy H, Cisternino S, Courtin C, Smirnova M, Schlatter J, Chiadmi F, Scherrmann J-M, Noble F, Marie-Claire C. Impact of P-glycoprotein at the blood-brain barrier on the uptake of heroin and its main metabolites: behavioral effects and consequences on the transcriptional responses and reinforcing properties. Psychopharmacology (Berl). 2014;231(16):3139–49. doi:10.1007/s00213-014-3490-9.

Selley DE, Cao C-C, Sexton T, Schwegel JA, Martin TJ, Childers SR. μ Opioid receptor-mediated G-protein activation by heroin metabolites: evidence for greater efficacy of

6-monoacetylmorphine compared with morphine. Biochem Pharmacol. 2001;62(4):447–55. doi:10.1016/S0006-2952(01)00689-X.

Shen XY, Kosten TA, Lopez AY, Kinsey BM, Kosten TR, Orson FM. A vaccine against methamphetamine attenuates its behavioral effects in mice. Drug Alcohol Depen. 2013;129(1-2):41–8. doi:10.1016/j.drugalcdep.2012.09.007.

Skibinski DAG, Baudner BC, Singh M, O'Hagan DT. Combination vaccines. J Global Infect Dis. 2011;3(1):63–72.

Skopp G, Ganssmann B, Cone EJ, Aderjan R. Plasma concentrations of heroin and morphine-related metabolites after intranasal and intramuscular administration. J Anal Toxicol. 1997;21(2):105–11. doi:10.1093/jat/21.2.105.

Stowe GN, Schlosburg JE, Vendruscolo LF, Edwards S, Misra KK, Schulteis G, Zakhari JS, Koob GF, Janda KD. Developing a vaccine against multiple psychoactive targets: a case study of heroin. CNS Neurol Disord Drug Targets. 2011;10(8):865–75.

Tars K, Kotelovica S, Lipowsky G, Bauer M, Beerli RR, Bachmann MF, Maurer P. Different binding modes of free and carrier-protein-coupled nicotine in a human monoclonal antibody. J Mol Biol. 2012;415(1):118–27. doi:10.1016/j.jmb.2011.10.042.

Tietze LF, Arlt M, Beller M, Gl üsenkamp K-H, Jähde E, Rajewsky MF. Anticancer agents, 15. Squaric acid diethyl ester: a new coupling reagent for the formation of drug biopolymer conjugates. Synthesis of squaric acid ester amides and diamides. Chem Ber. 1991;124(5):1215–21. doi:10.1002/cber.19911240539.

Tornøe CW, Christensen C, Meldal M. Peptidotriazoles on solid phase: [1,2,3]-triazoles by regiospecific copper(I)-catalyzed 1,3-dipolar cycloadditions of terminal alkynes to azides. J Org Chem. 2002;67(9):3057–64. doi:10.1021/jo011148j.

Ulrich S, Boturyn D, Marra A, Renaudet O, Dumy P. Oxime ligation: a chemoselective click-type reaction for accessing multifunctional biomolecular constructs. Chem Eur J. 2014;20(1):34–41. doi:10.1002/chem.201302426.

Umans JG, Inturrisi CE. Pharmacodynamics of subcutaneously administered diacetylmorphine, 6-acetylmorphine and morphine in mice. J Pharmacol Exp Ther. 1981;218(2):409–15.

Wagena EJ, de Vos A, Horwith G, van Schayck CP. The immunogenicity and safety of a nicotine vaccine in smokers and nonsmokers: results of a randomized, placebo-controlled phase 1/2 trial. Nicotine Tob Res. 2008;10(1):213–8. doi:10.1080/14622200701704921.

Wang Q, Guo Z. Synthetic and immunological studies of sTn derivatives carrying substituted phenylacetylsialic acids as cancer vaccine candidate. ACS Med Chem Lett. 2011;2(5):373–8. doi:10.1021/ml100313d.

Yang F, Zheng X-J, Huo C-X, Wang Y, Zhang Y, Ye X-S. Enhancement of the immunogenicity of synthetic carbohydrate vaccines by chemical modifications of STn antigen. ACS Chem Biol. 2010;6(3):252–9. doi:10.1021/cb100287q.

Yuki D, Kikuchi A, Miura N, Kakehi A, Onozawa M. Good relationship between saliva cotinine kinetics and plasma cotinine kinetics after smoking one cigarette. Regul Toxicol Pharm. 2013;67(2):240–5. doi:10.1016/j.yrtph.2013.08.002.

Zheng F, Zhan C-G. Structure-and-mechanism-based design and discovery of therapeutics for cocaine overdose and addiction. Org Biomol Chem. 2008;6(5):836–43. doi:10.1039/B716268E.

Chapter 19
B Cell Mechanisms Underlying Vaccine Efficacy Against Drugs of Abuse

Marco Pravetoni

Abbreviations

APC	Antigen-presenting cells
ASC	Antibody-secreting cells
BCR	B cell receptor
GC	Germinal center
IL	Interleukin
PBMC	Peripheral blood mononuclear cells
swIg	Switched immunoglobulin B cells
T_{fH}	T follicular helper cells
MHC	Major histocompatibility complex

19.1 Vaccines for Chronic Noncommunicable Diseases

Vaccines against infectious diseases have been the most effective intervention introduced in medical practice and have had a significant impact on global public health and economics (Rappuoli et al. 2014). Among commercially available vaccines, immunogens consisting of bacterial polysaccharides conjugated to carrier proteins have been successfully used to fight many deadly infectious agents including *H. influenza* type B or various meningococcal and pneumococcal strains (Rappuoli et al. 2014). Other conjugate

M. Pravetoni, PhD
Departments of Medicine and Pharmacology, University of Minnesota Medical School, Minneapolis, MN, USA

Department of Medicine, Minneapolis Medical Research Foundation, Minneapolis, MN, USA
e-mail: prave001@umn.edu

I.D. Montoya (ed.), *Biologics to Treat Substance Use Disorders: Vaccines, Monoclonal Antibodies, and Enzymes*, DOI 10.1007/978-3-319-23150-1_19

vaccine candidates are currently under development to target saccharides expressed on the surface of a variety of microorganisms, the human immunodeficiency virus (HIV), or cancer-associated carbohydrate antigens (Astronomo and Burton 2010). A wealth of animal and clinical data indicates that vaccines are safe and suggests that future use may be extended to a variety of nontraditional targets, including noncommunicable diseases.

According to the Center for Disease Control and Prevention (CDC) and the World Health Organization (WHO), the current leading causes of death are cancer, tobacco and opioid addiction, and cardiovascular, neurodegenerative, and metabolic diseases (Wide-ranging OnLine Data for Epidemiologic Research (WONDER) 2014). Therapies are available for some of these chronic noncommunicable diseases; however, their use is somewhat limited by cost (e.g., therapeutic monoclonal antibodies for cancer), suboptimal efficacy, or administrative hurdles (e.g., methadone or buprenorphine therapy for opioid addiction). In contrast, no therapies are yet commercially available for neurodegenerative diseases such as Alzheimer's, or for the treatment of cocaine and methamphetamine dependence. Vaccines may offer a promising strategy to treat drug addiction, cancer, Alzheimer's, or other noncommunicable chronic diseases. However, as discussed in this chapter and book, compared to infectious diseases, the development of vaccines against these diseases presents unique challenges.

In contrast to toxoids, protein subunits, or virus-like particles included in infectious disease vaccines, small molecules are poor immunogens and evade recognition from the immune system. Indeed, drugs of abuse do not elicit an immune response because of their low molecular weight (e.g., nicotine $\approx$ 162 Da and oxycodone $\approx$ 315 Da). Similarly, cancer-associated mucin-type O-glycans derived from the monosaccharide Tn antigen, an N-acetylgalactosamine upregulated in the majority of malignant breast tumors, elicit either no or weak immune responses due to their small size (Tn antigen MW $\approx$ 310 Da).

Small molecules lack the necessary signaling required to stimulate T cells and are thereby often referred to as "T cell-independent antigens" or antigens that "do not break B cell tolerance". To elicit an immune response against drugs of abuse, immunogens consist of drug-derived haptens (B cell epitope) chemically bound to larger foreign immunogenic structures (T cell epitope) that stimulate T cell-dependent B cell activation to generate antibodies against drugs of abuse (Figure 19.1 provides an example of a conjugate immunogen containing an oxycodone-based hapten). As described in details in previous chapters (4, 16, and 18), addiction vaccines elicit drug-specific antibodies that bind drug in serum, decrease drug distribution to the brain, and block drug-induced behaviors. Translation of therapeutic vaccines against drugs of abuse has been slow because clinical efficacy (e.g., smoking cessation or abstinence from cocaine use) was only met in the subset (~30 %) of immunized human subjects with the highest drug-specific antibody levels (Cornuz et al. 2008; Hatsukami et al. 2011; Martell et al. 2009).

This is not a limitation of addiction vaccines *per se*, but it appears to generalize to other conjugate immunogens against small molecules. Synthetic glycan-based haptens are conjugated to carrier proteins to elicit antibodies that bind carbohydrates expressed on cancer cells, which then elicit antibody-dependent cell toxicity or complement-dependent cytotoxicity (Astronomo and Burton 2010). Similar to nicotine and cocaine vaccines, in a clinical trial of the sialyl Tn hapten conjugated to KLH, an increase in

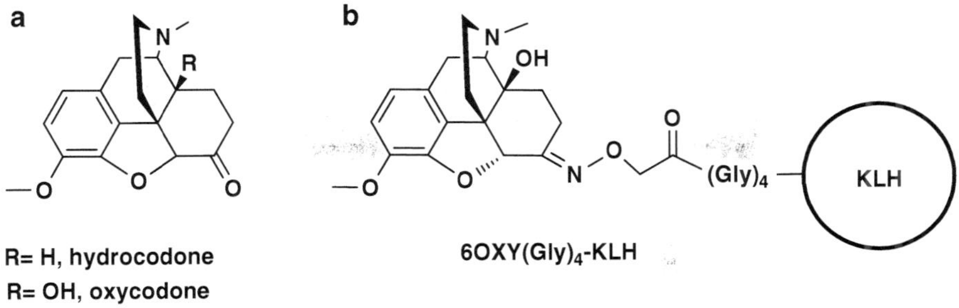

Fig. 19.1 Therapeutic vaccines for drug addiction elicit an adaptive immune response against drugs of abuse. The composition of the vaccine is critical for recognition by antigen-presenting cells (APC) and activation of antigen-specific B and T cells. (**a**) Drug targets, shown oxycodone and hydrocodone structures. (**b**) A conjugate immunogen is composed of (i) a hapten derivatized from the structure of the targeted drug of abuse, which represents the B cell epitope that binds hapten-specific B cells that will proliferate and mature into antibody-secreting and memory B cells; (ii) a larger immunogenic structure, called carrier, which activates carrier-specific $CD4^+$ helper T cells by providing T cell epitopes (carrier proteins are digested by APCs, either macrophages or B cells, and presented to $CD4^+$ T cells as smaller peptides bound to MHCII); and (iii) the conjugate is packaged in an adjuvant to increase its immunogenicity and provide an injectable formulation. The figure shows an oxycodone-based hapten containing a tetraglycine linker at the C6 position ($6OXY(Gly)_4$) conjugated to the keyhole limpet hemocyanin (KLH) carrier protein

overall survival against metastatic breast cancer was observed only in vaccinated subjects developing high levels of Tn-specific serum antibodies (Ibrahim et al. 2013).

The mechanism(s) underlying individual variability in the magnitude of hapten-specific serum antibody responses is not well understood because, in comparison to protein-based infectious diseases vaccines, less is known about B cell responses specific for drugs of abuse or other clinically relevant small molecules (e.g., Tn antigen). To design better vaccines, it is important to understand the mechanisms underlying vaccine efficacy against the targeted drug and the observed variability across immunized subjects. Currently, it is not fully understood whether the large portion of nonresponders may be due to vaccine design, disease heterogeneity, or specific interactions between the vaccine's components and the host immune system. The following sections will discuss concepts and proposed models that are based on current knowledge of B cells specific for known model antigens. As a *cautionary note*, a broad and general perspective on B cell biology that is relevant to the development of addiction vaccines will be provided.

19.2 Concepts of B Cell Biology

19.2.1 Cellular Biology and B Cell Phenotypes

Bone marrow produces immature lymphocyte precursors of B cells, whereas T cells are produced in the thymus (McHeyzer-Williams and McHeyzer-Williams 2005). Prior to immunization, the host immune system contains millions of naïve

B cells circulating through the spleen and lymph nodes via the bloodstream. Each naïve B cell expresses a transmembrane form of antibody (immunoglobulin or Ig) called the B cell receptor (BCR) that is *unique* to each cell (Pape et al. 2011; Taylor et al. 2012a). The presence of a functional BCR defines a B cell identity. To enable adaptive immune responses against infections, vaccination, or the variety of antigens that individuals may encounter during a lifetime, the naïve (i.e., pre-immunization or in unimmunized subjects) B cell pool requires a large BCR repertoire. In mammals, BCR diversity is established through rearrangement of immunoglobulin heavy and light chain V, D, and J gene segments, a process known as V(D)J recombination (Tonegawa 1983). In addition to V(D)J recombination, other mechanisms contribute to the highly diverse BCR repertoire, such as addition or subtraction of nucleotides at gene segment junctions. Both B and T cells are main players in humoral adaptive immune responses to infections and vaccines. Yet B cells are the only immune cell type capable of generating antibodies against antigens, including drugs of abuse.

19.2.2 B Cell Ontogeny

In mammals, B cells are derived from two lineages, B-1 and B-2, and their commitment to either is based on complex processes (Scholz et al. 2014). It is not clear the extent to which B cells derive from a common precursor cell type and evolve into separate lineages driven by antigen selection, or alternatively originate from distinct precursors. The B-1 cell lineage has been well characterized in mice, whereas its relevance to the human immune system is less understood. In contrast, the B-2 lineage has been studied in depth in both mice and humans. In mice, prenatal production of the B-1 lymphocytes occurs in the liver, while the B-2 lineage emerges from the bone marrow in adults, and its is responsible for the generation of B cell pools found in the lymph nodes and spleen (Scholz et al. 2014). The characteristics of B-2 cell development and rearrangement of the immunoglobulin variable regions in mice provide a close preclinical model of human B cell and BCR processes.

19.2.3 Overview of T Cell-Dependent B Cell Generation of Antibodies Against Antigens

After immunization with the antigen of interest, T cell-dependent B cell activation largely occurs within secondary lymphoid organs in the germinal center (GC) (McHeyzer-Williams and McHeyzer-Williams 2005). The GC-dependent T cell-dependent B cell activation is a critical aspect of the adaptive immune response to generate mature switched immunoglobulin memory B cells and antibody-secreting plasma B cells, which are B cell types essential for the generation of long-term high-affinity antibody responses against antigens and responding to booster vaccine injections (McHeyzer-Williams and McHeyzer-Williams 2005).

Shortly after immunization (i.e., 3–7 days), within secondary lymphoid organs, proliferating antigen-specific B cells move toward the B/T cell border, a specific anatomical area of B and T cell interaction, and migrate deeper into follicles to form GC (McHeyzer-Williams and McHeyzer-Williams 2005). Germinal centers are dynamic hot spots where T cell-dependent B cell activation, somatic hypermutation, and affinity maturation processes occur (Victora and Nussenzweig 2012). The formation of GC involves coordinated interaction between activated antigen-specific B and T cells in the presence of a professional antigen-presenting cell (APC) displaying the major histocompatibility complex II (MHCII) receptor. In the GC, antigen-specific B cells interact with a subset of $CD4^+$ T cells, known as T follicular helper cells (T_{fH}), which specialize in sustaining B cell maturation (McHeyzer-Williams et al. 2012; Crotty 2011). $CD4^+$ T cells promote GC B cell activation by a variety of signaling mechanisms that include either direct interaction through membrane receptors (e.g., CD40) or secretion of interleukins (e.g., IL-4) and other soluble molecules (Victora and Nussenzweig 2012).

Within the GC, antigen-specific B cells go through affinity maturation to become either switched immunoglobulin (swIg) memory B cells carrying specialized immunoglobulins (e.g., IgG, IgA, or IgE) or long-lived antibody-secreting plasma B cells (Taylor et al. 2012a). Both GC-dependent B cell maturation and T_{fH} activation are dependent upon a complex transcriptional program involving balanced activity of a variety of downstream signals (McHeyzer-Williams et al. 2012; Crotty 2011). These pathways include the signal transducers and activators of transcription (STAT), the transcription factors B cell 6 lymphoma protein (bcl-6) and B lymphocyte-induced maturation protein 1 (blimp-1) (McHeyzer-Williams et al. 2012; Crotty 2011). Affinity maturation is a complex process that involves somatic hypermutation, class switch recombination, and clonal selection (Victora and Nussenzweig 2012). Somatic hypermutation, which is characterized by high mutations rates in B cells, involves the key effector activation-induced deaminase (AID) which introduces mutations in the variable regions of the V(D)J gene segments, to modify the binding affinity of the BCR (Maul and Gearhart 2010). Somatic hypermutation is critical to increase the diversity of the BCR within the B cell repertoire and generate immunoglobulins with high affinity for the target antigen. Similarly, class switch recombination is instrumental in generating B cells that switched their immunoglobulin from the low-affinity IgM, or IgD, to the more specialized IgG, IgA, and IgE. After the occurrence of somatic hypermutation and class switch recombination events, B cells will compete for the antigen and other resources through clonal selection. Only the antigen-specific B cell clones that have the highest affinity for the antigen will survive (McHeyzer-Williams and McHeyzer-Williams 2005; Victora and Nussenzweig 2012; McHeyzer-Williams et al. 2012).

19.3 B Cells Specific for Drugs of Abuse Haptens and Addiction Vaccines

In the field of addiction vaccines, limited information is available in regard to B and T cell responses to immunization. Most studies have focused on vaccine development and screening of the most effective vaccines for their ability to elicit antibodies, their effect on drug distribution to the serum and to the brain compartments, and their efficacy in preventing various drug-induced behaviors. As detailed in this book, these studies have focused on the role of hapten and conjugation chemistry, use of novel adjuvants and carriers, and new delivery platforms including nanoparticles or liposomes or synthetic materials. This wealth of literature provides an in-depth understanding of how vaccine components contribute to elicit the antibody response required for vaccine efficacy against drugs of abuse but provides only clues about the adaptive immune response underlying vaccine efficacy. Vaccine development will benefit from complementary studies aimed at understanding the molecular and cellular mechanisms underlying effective and long-lasting immunization against drugs of abuse.

In regard to adaptive immune responses to addiction vaccines, many questions remain unanswered. For instance, it is not clear whether the number of the B cells specific for a drug-based hapten or the number of carrier-specific T cells present prior to immunization determines the quantity and quality of the antibody response to vaccination. Recent studies have developed strategies to study B cells specific for drug-based haptens and showed that a greater population size of polyclonal hapten-specific B cells correlates to increased vaccine ability to induce drug-specific antibodies and their efficacy in preventing oxycodone distribution to the brain and its behavioral effects in mice. These novel analytical tools and data support screening new vaccine formulations for their ability to activate specific subsets of naïve B and T cells or to target critical aspects of the immune response.

19.3.1 T Cell-Dependent B Cell Responses to Haptens and Conjugate Vaccines

Addiction vaccines consist of drug-derived haptens chemically bound to larger foreign immunogenic structures that stimulate T cell-dependent B cell activation to generate antibodies against drugs of abuse (Fig. 19.1). The physical and chemical structure of the conjugate immunogen (i.e., the vaccine) is crucial for the coordinated activation of B and T cells, in the presence of APC. As shown in Fig. 19.1, a conjugate vaccine is composed of (1) a hapten derived from the structure of the targeted drug of abuse, which represents the B cell epitope that binds hapten-specific B cells that, in turn, will proliferate and mature into memory and antibody-secreting plasma B cells; (2) a larger immunogenic structure, called a carrier, which activates carrier-specific $CD4^+$ helper T cells by providing T cell epitopes in the form of smaller peptide sequences presented by MHCII receptors on APC; and (3) an adjuvant that enhances immunogenicity of the conjugate through various mechanisms.

After immunization, haptens can directly bind to the BCR and activate hapten-specific B cells. However, the generation of antibodies against the drug-based hapten and free drug requires T cell-dependent B cell activation involving professional APC that display surface MHCII receptors, including macrophages, dendritic cells, and B cells. After immunization, macrophages and dendritic cells uptake the conjugate in a nonselective manner or carry the whole immunogen to the draining lymph node for processing. Alternatively, the antigen passively drains to the lymph nodes through the lymphatic system. After internalization, APC digest the carrier protein to shorter peptides, which are displayed on their MHCII receptors. Peptide presentation on MHCII receptors is necessary for engagement of $CD4^+$ T helper cells. MHCII presentation by either B cells or other APC will engage T cell help through recognition by T cell receptors (TCR) specific for the peptide sequence derived from the carrier protein. MHCII-dependent activation of naïve T cells specific for peptides derived from carrier proteins promotes their differentiation into mature effector T cells including antigen-specific $CD4^+$ T helper (T_H) cells. $CD4^+$ T_H cells can be further subdivided in T_H1 or T_H2 cells, which activate either the cellular (e.g., antigen-specific $CD8^+$ T cells or NK cells) or the humoral (i.e., B cells and antibodies) branch of the adaptive immune response, respectively. This is of particular importance for understanding the mechanisms underlying vaccine efficacy since most adjuvants are characterized by their ability to activate the T_H1, T_H2, or T_H1/T_H2 (for details on adjuvants, see Chap. 16). For example, alum is a known T_H2 adjuvant while complete Freund's adjuvant (CFA) activates a mixed T_H1/T_H2 response. Activated antigen-specific $CD4^+$ T_H cells support hapten-specific B cell clonal expansion and maturation by direct interaction through membrane receptors, such as CD40:CD40L, or by soluble molecules such as interleukins (e.g., IL-4, IL-6, and IL-21) and other inducible costimulatory signals (e.g., ICOS:ICOSL). Supported by T_{fH} cells, activated B cells will then go through expansion, maturation, and differentiation in various B cell phenotypes including swIg memory B cells displaying high-affinity BCR or antibody-secreting B cells capable of secreting high-affinity switched immunoglobulins, such as IgG, specific for drugs of abuse. The next paragraphs will cover in detail the initiation and progression of hapten-specific B cell responses to conjugate vaccines for drug addiction.

19.3.2 *Proposed Mechanisms of Hapten-Specific B Cell Responses to Immunization*

Among the polyclonal naïve B cell population, very few B cells display a BCR with high affinity for the hapten of interest. After immunization with drug hapten-protein conjugates, successful activation and maturation of B cells that recognize the vaccine will generate high-affinity antibodies against the target drug. In secondary lymphoid organs, such as the spleen and lymph nodes, hapten-specific naïve B cells expressing surface immunoglobulins, which recognize and bind the vaccine, undergo activation and proliferation with the help of $CD4^+$ T cells. Based on studies of protein-based antigens, we know that these processes generate (1) short-lived antibody-secreting B cells, (2) GC-independent differentiation in low-affinity IgM^+ memory B cells, and (3) GC B cells (Fig. 19.2) (Taylor et al. 2012a). Germinal center B cells then mature into either long-lived antibody-secreting B cells (ASC or plasma cells) that maintain serum immunoglobulin levels or long-lived memory B cells which will switch their Ig constant region from IgM to IgG, IgA, or IgE while acquiring somatic mutations in their variable region (i.e., swIg B cells) (McHeyzer-Williams and McHeyzer-Williams 2005; Maul and Gearhart 2010; Tarlinton 2008). Long-lived antibody-secreting and memory B cells will then transit and reside to the bone marrow (i.e., homing). After subsequent boost immunizations, the IgM^+ or swIg memory B cell subsets respond to the antigen challenge and generate more antibody-secreting B cells, which boost the amount of antigen-specific serum antibodies (Taylor et al. 2012a). Depending upon the timing of the secondary antigen challenge, memory B cells may form more IgM^+ or swIg memory B cells and also GC B cells (Taylor et al. 2012a). These models are likely to apply to hapten-specific B cells elicited by addiction vaccine; however, their validity still remains to be tested.

In subjects immunized against infectious diseases, exposure to the infectious agent (e.g., the hepatitis B virus) will activate antigen-specific memory B cells and induce an antigen-specific antibody response that will contain the infection.

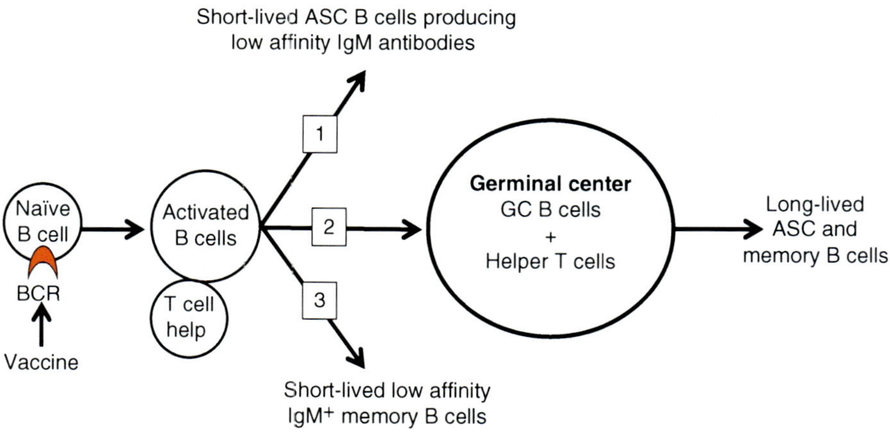

Fig. 19.2 T cell-dependent B cell activation. After immunization with conjugate immunogens, successful activation of naïve hapten-specific B cells is required for the generation of antibody-secreting cells (ASC) and the production of antibodies against the target drug. In the spleen and lymph nodes, naïve B cells expressing a BCR specific for the hapten will undergo activation and clonal expansion with the help of $CD4^+$ T cells. This initial critical event will lead to the generation of (1) short-lived ASC B cells, (2) GC B cells and (3) low-affinity IgM^+ memory B cells. In the GC, hapten-specific B cells mature into either long-lived ASC or swIg memory B cells

In contrast, in subjects immunized with vaccines for drug addiction, subsequent exposure to drugs of abuse, lacking T cell epitopes, is not sufficient to boost memory B cells and induce differentiation in antibody-secreting B cells. In fact, to maintain drug-specific antibody responses is necessary to administer boost immunizations with hapten-carrier conjugate immunogens. Current animal and human studies of addiction vaccines have employed immunization protocols that involved multiple repeated immunizations to rapidly achieve the required high antibody titers required to counteract plasma concentrations of drugs. Clinical trials of vaccines for nicotine and cocaine involved immunization regimens of 3–5 monthly doses followed by booster injections every 2 or 6 months to preserve serum anti-drug antibody levels (Cornuz et al. 2008; Hatsukami et al. 2011; Martell et al. 2009). Similar immunization regimens, involving repeated immunizations every few weeks with hapten-protein conjugates, have also been used to generate antibody responses against tumor-associated carbohydrate and peptide small antigens and peptide derived from Alzheimer's pathological proteins, which are also known as weak immunogens. The rationale for this approach has been that to curb addiction, an aggressive immunization protocol may elicit a fast and robust anti-drug antibody response that would rapidly block the reinforcing effects of drugs from the initiation of treatment.

Future evaluation of new addiction vaccines may include screening of different vaccination schedules (e.g., longer time intervals between immunizations) with the goal of achieving long-term antibody and memory responses. Future studies may also test the challenging hypothesis of generating high-affinity swIg memory B cells that would recognize unconjugated drugs of abuse, so that exposure to drug would boost a protective drug-specific antibody response. Tracking the hapten-specific B cell population will provide data to support analysis of antibody quantity and quality. For instance, B cell analysis may be performed prior to immunization when antibodies are not yet present or shortly after immunization when antibody levels are below the detection threshold of current assays. Alternatively, B cells may be measured in subjects long after the antibody response waned to determine whether vaccine formulations or immunization protocols elicited long-lived memory B cells.

19.4 A Novel Method to Detect Antigen-Specific B Cells

In contrast to other components of the immune system (e.g., T cells), analysis of antigen-specific B cells has been limited by the lack of methods to detect very scarce B cells displaying BCR specific for a given antigen (i.e., antigen-specific B cells). Most studies relied on the use of transgenic mice carrying mutations in their BCR to track antigen-specific B cells. A recent technology allows detection and analysis of very low numbers of antigen-specific B cells present in the whole B cell repertoire (Pape et al. 2011). This method has high resolution permitting detection of antigen-specific B cells in a naïve or unimmunized mouse. In the original report, the authors tracked B cells specific for the fluorescent protein phycoerythrin (PE) in naïve and immunized mice (Pape et al. 2011). To isolate PE-specific B cells, the whole B cell repertoire from pooled lymph nodes and spleen was first incubated with PE, and then B cells bound to PE were isolated by means of anti-PE magnetic beads, using separation columns in a magnetic field (Pape et al. 2011). After this enrichment step, PE-specific B cells were identified by means of flow cytometry and further characterized for their surface markers. This analysis allows the counting of individual antigen-specific B cells and determines whether they are IgM^{high} memory B cells, memory B cells carrying isotype-switched immunoglobulin such as IgG or IgA, GC B cells displaying the GL7 surface marker, or antibody-secreting plasma B cells displaying high levels of immunoglobulin. The use of fluorescent antigen-based magnetic enrichment paired to flow cytometry showed that within the ~2 × 10^8 nucleated cells from the spleen and lymph nodes in a naïve mouse, only ~20,000 B cells were specific for PE (Pape et al. 2011), ~7000 for allophycocyanin, ~4000 for chicken ovalbumin (OVA), and even fewer for the enzyme glucose-6-phosphate isomerase (GPI). This method to detect antigen-specific B cells in unimmunized subjects has now been applied to study B cell memory formation, autoimmunity, and development of addiction vaccines (Pape et al. 2011; Taylor et al. 2012b, c, 2014).

19.4.1 Analysis of Hapten-Specific B Cells

The fluorescent antigen-based magnetic enrichment strategy paired to flow cytometry analysis has been recently adapted to study hapten-specific B cells before and after immunization with vaccines against drugs of abuse. As described in detail in Sects. 19.4.2 and 19.4.3, this strategy consists of two consecutive steps: magnetic enrichment of hapten-specific B cells and multiparameter flow cytometry analysis of hapten-specific B cell subsets. This analysis can be easily performed in wild-type and genetically modified mice (Pravetoni et al. 2014; Taylor et al. 2014). Although strain differences must be taken in account for proper experimental design, this method is not strain- or species-specific because it depends exclusively on the ability of B cells to bind the hapten or antigen of interest and on the availability of flow cytometry reagents. For instance, it is not currently feasible to perform this analysis in rats because critical reagents to identify rat B cell surface markers are missing. However, this method has been currently applied to analyze human peripheral blood mononuclear cells (PBMC, Pravetoni, unpublished). The most complete set of antibodies for characterization of lymphocytes are directed toward mouse, human, and nonhuman primate markers.

19.4.2 Method I: Magnetic Enrichment of Hapten-Specific B Cells

First, peripheral lymph nodes, spleen, or blood samples are processed into a single-cell suspension that includes a fraction of the whole B cell repertoire. Then, B cells are incubated with the hapten of interest (Figure 19.3 shows an

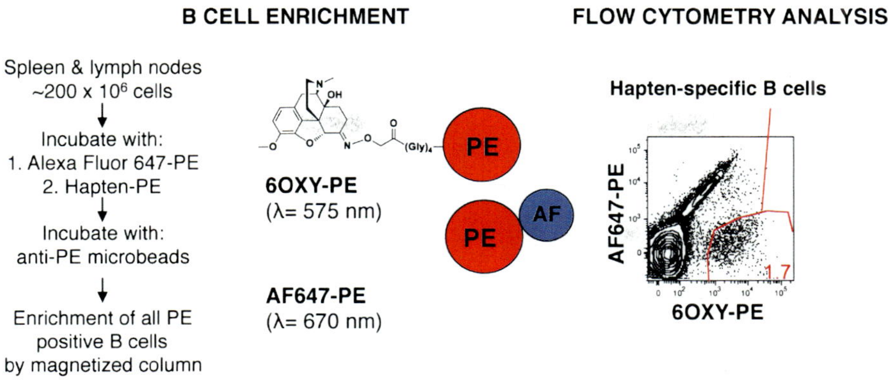

Fig. 19.3 Enrichment strategy to analyze hapten-specific B cells. The whole B cell repertoire, from individual mouse peripheral lymph nodes and spleen, is first incubated with a decoy reagent consisting of PE-AF647 followed by incubation with the hapten-PE (shown 6OXY-PE). All B cells binding the AF647-PE or the hapten-PE detection decoy reagent are positively isolated using anti-PE antibody-conjugated magnetic beads and magnetic columns. Using flow cytometry, it is possible to identify hapten-specific B cells from PE-specific B cells because the AF647-PE conjugate fluorescences at a different wavelength than PE

oxycodone-based hapten, 6OXY) conjugated to the red-phycoerythrin (PE) fluorescent protein and with a decoy reagent consisting of an additional fluorochrome, Alexa Fluor (AF) 647, conjugated directly to PE. Using anti-PE magnetic microbeads and magnetic columns, all B cells that recognized the hapten and PE are positively isolated (i.e., enrichment as shown in Fig. 19.3). Using flow cytometry, 6OXY-specific B cells are separated from B cells that recognize PE because the PE-AF conjugate fluoresces at a wavelength different than PE alone (λ, Fig. 19.3). Once 6OXY-specific B cells are identified (Fig. 19.3), they are further characterized by the use of antibodies specific for B cell markers conjugated to additional fluorochromes.

19.4.3 Method II: Multiparameter Flow Cytometry Analysis of Hapten-Specific B Cells

In order to perform analysis of antigen-specific B cells, a commercially available flow cytometer that permits multiparameter acquisition is needed. For instance, the procedures discussed in this chapter used a four-laser flow cytometer that allows analysis of up to 16 colors. After collection of raw data by flow cytometry, B cells are analyzed by standard commercial software (e.g., FlowJo, FlowJo LLC, Ashland, OR) using a specific analysis generally described as "gating strategy," because it involves the application of flow cytometry gates to define specific B cell population characterized by specific sets of non-B and B cell markers as described below and shown in Fig. 19.4.

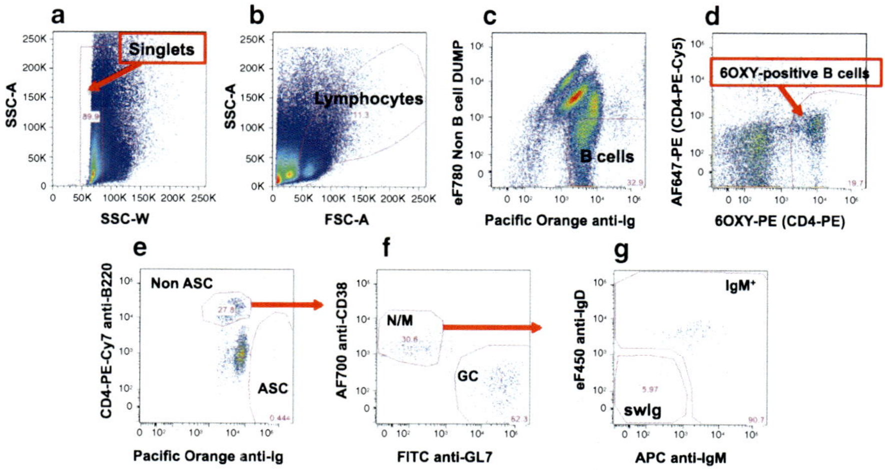

Fig. 19.4 B cell gating strategy of 6OXY-specific B cells in a representative dot plot from a mouse immunized with the 6OXY-KLH immunogen. (**a**) Singlet gating to remove any cells that have aggregated. (**b**) Total lymphocytes. (**c**) Total B cells expressing immunoglobulin (Ig^{high}) but not the following non-B cell markers: CD90.2 (T cells), Gr-1 (neutrophils), CD11.c (dendritic cells), and F4/80 (macrophages). (**d**) To differentiate between 6OXY-specific B cells from PE-binding B cells, B cells were further identified using the AF647-PE decoy. (**e**) Hapten-specific B cells were classified as either B220^{high} non-ASC B cells or Ig^{high} ASC B cells. (**f**) Hapten-specific B220^{high} non-ASC B cells were further identified as GL7^{high} germinal center (GC) or CD38^{high} naïve/memory (N/M). (**g**) Naïve/memory B cells were then identified as IgM^{high} or IgM^{neg}/IgD^{neg} swIg B cells

First using a standard gating procedure (forward-scattered light, or FSC, vs side-scattered light, or SSC), single cells are separated from cell aggregates (see Fig. 19.4, panel a). Within the single-cell gate, lymphocytes are identified from residual non-lymphocytes or dead cells (Fig. 19.4, panel b). Once lymphocytes are identified, they are further identified as either B cells expressing intracellular immunoglobulin or non-B cells expressing surface markers for T cells (CD90.2), neutrophils (Gr-1), dendritic cells (CD11.c), and macrophages (F4/80) as shown in Fig. 19.4, panel c. At this stage, B cells that bound the 6OXY hapten or the PE carrier are differentiated based on the fluorescence of the decoy reagent AF647-PE, which fluorescences at a wavelength of 670 nm compared to the PE alone at 575 nm.

Within the population of B cells that bound the 6OXY hapten, actual 6OXY-specific B cells are identified as either non-antibody-secreting cells (non-ASC) expressing high levels of B220^{high} or antibody-secreting cells (ASC) expressing high levels of intracellular immunoglobulin (Ig^{high}). The use of multiple gating and B cell markers ensure that analysis of B cells is accurate and does not include "contaminant or residual cells". For instance, B220^{mid} Ig^{mid} FC-binding cells may appear soon often immunization (Fig. 19.4, panel e), but they are not B cells (Bell and Gray 2003) and are not included in further analysis. Once B220^{high} non-ASC 6OXY-specific B cells are identified, these cells are classified as CD38^{neg} GL7^{high} GC B cells or GL7^{neg} CD38^{high} naïve and memory B cells. Then, the CD38^{high} B cell population is characterized as B cells expressing either high levels of IgM (IgM^{high} B cells) or high-affinity swIg B cells (Pape et al. 2011; Taylor et al. 2014). Limited markers are available to differentiate between GL7^{neg} CD38^{high} naïve and memory B cells; therefore, it is critical to include in the experimental design both naïve and immunized mice so that naïve and memory B cells can be compared before and after immunization.

In general, when assessing the contribution of hapten-specific B cells to vaccine responses, it is important to include several controls in the experimental design. For instance, analysis of B cells should be performed in naïve mice or mice exposed to the vehicle or the adjuvant alone to determine background or baseline numbers of hapten-specific B cells. Analysis of vaccine-induced hapten-specific B cells should be performed in mice immunized with either the unconjugated carrier or the hapten-carrier conjugate to ensure that B cell responses are specific to the hapten. To further assess the specificity of this procedure, B cells are preincubated in the presence of the free drug, hapten, or conjugate to inhibit binding of the hapten-PE reagent (Taylor et al. 2014). Alternative negative controls may include magnetic enrichment of B cells in the presence of PE alone or in the absence of anti-PE microbeads.

19.5 Hapten-Specific B Cells Are Markers of Vaccine Efficacy Against Prescription Opioids

As described in Chapter 1, the prescription opioids oxycodone, hydrocodone, and oxymorphone are among the most commonly abused drugs in the USA (National Survey on Drug Use and Health: National Findings 2010; Oxymorphone abuse: a growing threat nationwide 2011; Epidemic: responding to America's prescription drug abuse crisis 2011). The Center for Disease Control and Prevention estimated that ~2.1 million of people abused prescription opioids in 2012 and that prescription opioids accounted for ~17,000 overdose deaths (Wide-ranging OnLine Data for Epidemiologic Research (WONDER) 2014).

To develop a vaccine that targets prescription opioids, a series of immunogens containing oxycodone- and hydrocodone-based haptens has been synthesized (Pravetoni et al. 2013). These haptens were derived from the C6 and the C8 positions on the morphinan structure and conjugated to the keyhole limpet hemocyanin (KLH) carrier protein to study the effects of hapten design and bioconjugation chemistry on vaccine efficacy. Haptens were conjugated to proteins through a tetraglycine linker by an amide bond obtained through carbodiimide chemistry or by thioether linkage obtained through maleimide chemistry (Fig. 19.5).

Despite the closely related structures, a C6-derivatized oxycodone-based hapten (6OXY) conjugated through a tetraglycine linker to KLH was more effective than immunogens containing C6- and C8-derivatized hydrocodone-based haptens in blocking both oxycodone and hydrocodone distributions to the brain and their behavioral effects in mice and rats (Pravetoni et al. 2013). Specifically, the 6OXY-KLH immunogen was superior to the other immunogens

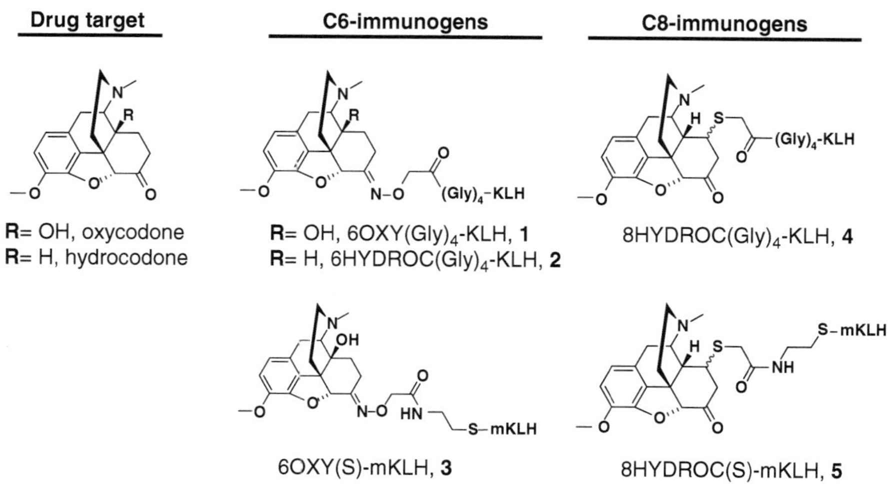

Fig. 19.5 Development of a series of conjugate immunogens to target prescription opioids. A series of haptens were synthesized from the oxycodone and the hydrocodone structures. The oxycodone, hydrocodone, and codeinone pharmacophores were functionalized at the C6 and C8 positions of the morphinan structure to attach a tetraglycine linker with free C-term or a thiol group (-SH). Using different coupling chemistry approaches, haptens were attached to carriers and evaluated in mice and rats for efficacy against oxycodone and hydrocodone

in terms of its selectivity and efficacy in blocking acute distribution to the brain of oxycodone and hydrocodone after intravenous and subcutaneous administration (Pravetoni et al. 2013). Also, compared to the other immunogens, immunization with the 6OXY-KLH conjugate increased protein binding of both oxycodone and hydrocodone in sera of immunized rats and was effective in blocking oxycodone and hydrocodone antinociception (Pravetoni et al. 2013). In follow-up studies, the 6OXY-KLH conjugate was also effective in preventing acquisition of intravenous oxycodone self-administration in rats, a model of human drug dependence (Pravetoni et al. 2014). As discussed in Sect. 19.6, structurally related haptens derived from oxycodone and hydrocodone provided model antigens to study the relevance of B cells to addiction vaccine efficacy. As discussed in Sects. 19.7 and 19.8, model oxycodone conjugates were also used to study the role of hapten-specific B cells in immunization studies involving different vaccine formulations in various mouse strains.

19.6 Hapten Design Affects Activation of Naïve B Cells

Despite closely related structures and equivalent haptenization ratio, a hapten based on the derivatization of oxycodone at the C6 position (6OXY) generated higher levels of serum antibodies that bound both oxycodone and hydrocodone, while a similar hapten based on derivatization of hydrocodone at the C8 position

(8HYDROC) was less effective (Fig. 19.6). The observed differences in the ability of generating drug-specific serum antibody titers translated in different efficacy in blocking oxycodone distribution to the brain (Fig. 19.6). From all these studies focusing on the evaluation of *in vivo* vaccine efficacy against oxycodone pharmacokinetics and behavioral effects, it was concluded that the 8HYDROC-KLH conjugate was a poor immunogen in contrast to the promising candidate 6OXY-KLH immunogen.

Structurally similar oxycodone haptens and conjugate immunogens have provided excellent models to test the extent to which the naïve B cell repertoire contributes to vaccine efficacy. Using the fluorescent-antigen enrichment method and flow cytometry analysis, it was found that a higher number of naïve and activated hapten-specific B cells were associated with greater vaccine efficacy in mice (Taylor et al. 2014). As a potential future application, this approach may be important for the development of screening assays predictive of vaccine efficacy against drugs of abuse or other small molecules associated with chronic diseases (e.g., cancer). Such screening assays may speed vaccine discovery or support patient stratification in clinical trials or provide basis for personalized medicine.

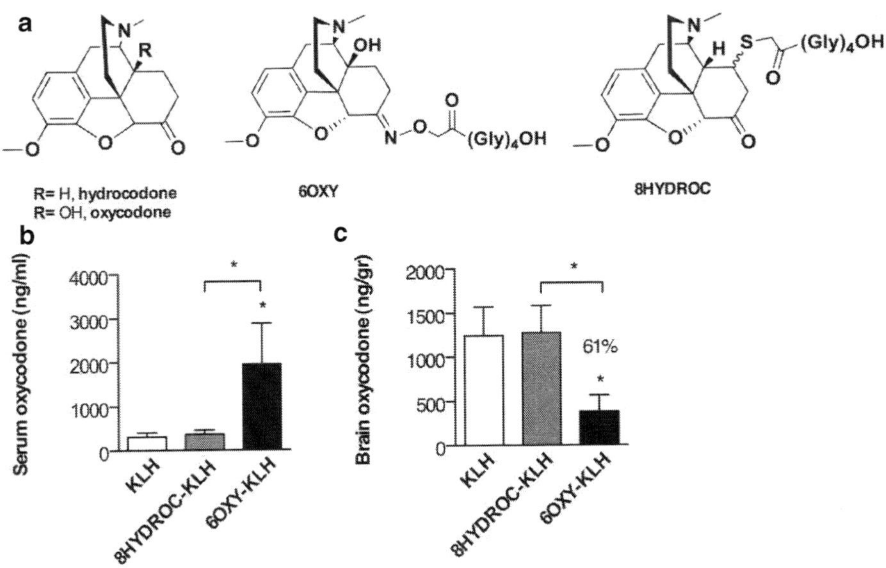

Fig. 19.6 Hapten structure determines vaccine efficacy in preventing oxycodone distribution to the brain in mice. (**a**) Target drugs and haptens. Oxycodone distribution to the (**b**) serum and (**c**) brain in mice vaccinated with either 6OXY-KLH, 8HYDROC-KLH, or unconjugated KLH at 30 min after s.c. administration of 2.25 mg/kg oxycodone (n=5–6 mice each group). In previous studies, the 6OXY-KLH immunogen was more effective than 8HYDROC-KLH in blocking oxycodone distribution to the brain in rats and preventing oxycodone behavioral effects in both mice and rats. Statistical symbols: * p<0.05 from unconjugated KLH control or brackets to indicate between-group differences

19.6.1 Naïve Hapten-Specific B Cells Prior to Immunization

Antigen-based enrichment paired to flow cytometry was used to test the extent to which the presence of hapten-specific naïve B cells in the pre-immunization repertoire predicted the increased efficacy of conjugate immunogens containing structurally related derived from oxycodone and hydrocodone (Pravetoni et al. 2013). This study tested the main hypothesis that the number or the affinity of naïve B cells specific for the 6OXY and the 8HYDROC haptens may determine the efficacy of 6OXY-KLH and 8HYDROC-KLH against oxycodone. In a first experiment, samples consisting of pooled peripheral lymph nodes and spleens from individual BALB/c mice were enriched for either 6OXY-PE or 8HYDROC-PE, to detect both 6OXY- and 8HYDROC-specific B cells within each subject. The number of 6OXY- and 8HYDROC-specific B cells, including both non-ASC and ASC, was nearly identical (Pravetoni et al. 2013). This data suggested that the majority of B cells may be able to bind both haptens or that 6OXY- and 8HYDROC-specific B cell populations coexist within the naïve B cell repertoire and cannot be distinguished using enrichment alone. However, the authors further hypothesized that vaccine efficacy may be due to the naïve B cells having greater affinity for the target drug or hapten rather than the numbers of naïve hapten-specific B cells. For instance, the interaction between hapten, or conjugate immunogen, and BCR or antibodies may have been influenced by structural differences between oxycodone and hydrocodone or between their respective immunogens. As shown in Fig. 19.6a, the structures of oxycodone and hydrocodone differ at the C14 position, which may affect BCR or antibody affinity for binding the free hapten or the conjugate immunogen.

The analysis of the affinity of naïve B cells for haptens and immunogens revealed that naïve B cells preferentially bound 6OXY over 8HYDROC. Individual samples were preincubated with increasing concentrations of free oxycodone, hapten, or each respective conjugate immunogen prior to enrichment. Preincubation with free oxycodone, 6OXY hapten or 6OXY conjugated to the chicken ovalbumin (OVA) carrier protein, reduced the % of recovered 6OXY-specific B cells compared to saline controls (Pravetoni et al. 2013). Using this approach, it was shown that 6OXY-specific B cells have relative higher affinity for the 6OXY hapten and for the target drug oxycodone compared to the lower binding of 8HYDROC-specific B cells. Interestingly, only 10 % of the 6OXY-specific B cells bound 8HYDROC-OVA or a control immunogen containing a nicotine hapten, and 10 % of the 8HYDROC-specific B cells bound 6OXY-OVA, suggesting that these two B cell populations minimally cross-react or overlap with each other. The affinity of hapten-specific B cells for free drug, hapten, and immunogens may explain differences in efficacy between the two conjugate immunogens. Using the mean % of hapten-specific B cells that bound free drug or the conjugated immunogens, and the individual numbers of hapten-specific naïve B cells found in naïve mice, it was possible to calculate the individual numbers of naïve B cells with high affinity for each respective hapten (Fig. 19.7a). The presence of higher numbers of 6OXY-specific naïve B cells may explain the greater efficacy of the 6OXY-KLH immunogen compared to the less effective 8HYDROC-KLH in preventing oxycodone distribution and behavioral effects.

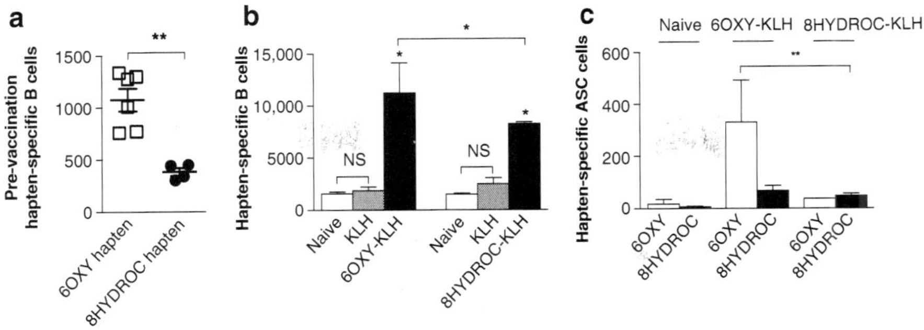

Fig. 19.7 The number of pre- and post-immunization hapten-specific B cells underlies efficacy of structurally related conjugate immunogens. (**a**) The number of hapten-specific naïve B cells (including B220^{high} non-ASC and Ig^{high} ASC B cells) in peripheral lymph nodes and spleen samples enriched for 6OXY-PE or 8HYDROC-PE conjugates in naïve mice. Data shown include hapten-specific B cells with higher affinity for each respective hapten. (**b**) The number of 6OXY-specific and 8HYDROC-specific B cells (including B220^{high} non-ASC and Ig^{high} ASC) before and 14 days after immunization with 6OXY-KLH, 8HYDROC-KLH, or unconjugated KLH. c) The number of 6OXY- and 8HYDROC-specific Ig^{high} ASC B cells in mice immunized with the 6OXY-KLH or the 8HYDROC-KLH immunogen. In this study, individual mouse samples were split and enriched with either 6OXY-PE or 8HYDROC-PE to perform within-subject analysis. Statistical symbols: * $p<0.05$, ** $p<0.01$ from control group or brackets to indicate between-group differences

These data must be interpreted carefully because the authors studied only two haptens based on the structures of oxycodone and hydrocodone. More studies are required to extend these findings to other drugs of abuse or other addiction vaccines. For instance, B cells also distinguish between structurally related nicotine-based haptens and the frequency of early-activated hapten-specific B cell subsets predicts efficacy of nicotine against nicotine dependence (Laudenbach et al. 2015b).

Overall the described study showed that naïve B cells differentiate between structurally related haptens and preferentially bind the most effective hapten. These data support the hypothesis that distinct hapten-specific naïve B cell subsets may coexist within the pre-immunization repertoire. Also, only naïve B cells with the highest affinity for haptens, free drug, or conjugate immunogens responded to immunization, suggesting that BCR affinity for antigen determines the extent to which hapten-specific naïve B cells respond to vaccination and generate drug-specific serum antibodies. These data indicated that structural differences between free drugs (e.g., oxycodone and hydrocodone) or between their respective haptens affect interaction with BCR or antibodies. For example, the hydroxyl group at the C14 position of oxycodone may affect binding for BCR or antibody by providing additional electrostatic attractions. The presence of a hydroxyl group may have also influenced the three-dimensional structure of the hapten and its proximity to the carrier protein by increasing affinity for BCR or antibodies, which may explain the superior efficacy of 6OXY-KLH over 8HYDROC-KLH. However, it has been found that oxycodone-based haptens performed better than hydrocodone-based haptens (Pravetoni et al. 2013). As discussed in Chapter X, other studies highlight the importance of hapten and linker design to generate effective drug-specific serum antibodies that block drug distribution to the brain and drug-induced behaviors (Cai et al. 2013; Pryde et al. 2013; Pravetoni et al. 2012).

19.6.2 Early Activated Hapten-Specific B Cells After Immunization

A practical limitation of studying vaccine immunogenicity is the considerable time delay for the appearance of drug-specific antibodies after immunization. For oxycodone vaccines, no serum antibody titers were detectable by ELISA within 14 days after vaccination. Thus, the authors tested whether hapten-specific B cells would provide earlier evidence of vaccine efficacy between 0 and 14 days after a first immunization. Indeed, shortly after vaccination, the more effective oxycodone vaccine elicited more hapten-specific B cells than the less effective immunogen or controls (Fig. 19.7b, c). These findings suggest that hapten-specific B cells are early markers predictive of vaccine efficacy, which provide an effective means for assessing early stages of vaccine clinical trials or monitoring how patients respond to vaccination.

Using the antigen-based enrichment strategy, it was possible to detect hapten-specific B cells as soon as 3 days after immunization with either 6OXY-KLH or 8HYDROC-KLH. At 14 days after vaccination, the numbers of 6OXY- and 8HYDROC-specific B cells in mice vaccinated with either 6OXY-KLH or 8HYDROC-KLH were significantly higher than in naïve mice or in the control group immunized with unconjugated KLH carrier protein (Fig. 19.7b). More importantly, it was possible to detect a difference in the numbers of hapten-specific B cells between mice immunized with either the 6OXY-KLH or the 8HYDROC-KLH immunogen.

At 14 days after immunization, the numbers of hapten-specific antibody-secreting B cells were significantly higher in mice immunized with the 6OXY-KLH than the 8HYDROC-KLH (Fig. 19.7c). At 14 days after the first vaccination, the analysis of oxycodone-specific serum antibody titers by ELISA was not reliable. In these experiments, analysis of B cells soon after immunization provided evidence of vaccine success or failure much earlier than serum antibody responses.

The lead immunogen 6OXY-KLH selectively induced 6OXY-specific B cell subsets within the polyclonal response 14 days after the first immunization. In naïve mice, it was found that most of 6OXY-specific and 8HYDROC-specific B cells consisted of the $CD38^{+}$ $GL7^{-}$ IgM^{high} phenotype, which is characteristic of naïve and memory B cells prior to vaccination. Immunization with 6OXY-KLH induced selective expansion of the $CD38^{+}$ $GL7^{-}$ IgM^{high} and the $CD38^{-}$ $GL7^{+}$ GC 6OXY-specific B cell subsets, but not 8HYDROC-specific B cells. These data indicate that immunization with 6OXY-KLH effectively induced proliferation of memory B cells and germinal center B cells in the peripheral lymph nodes and spleen, which may provide early immune correlates of successful vaccination against drugs of abuse.

However, to establish long-lived adaptive immune responses, vaccines are required to stimulate production of swIg B cells (Pape et al. 2011). These high-affinity, antigen-primed memory B cells can be distinguished from $CD38^+$ $GL7^-$ IgM^{high} or "unswitched" memory B cells because they switched their immunoglobulin isotype from IgM or D to IgG, IgA, or IgE (Taylor et al. 2012a). A single immunization with 6OXY-KLH was sufficient to induce a sizeable population of swIg B cells within the 6OXY-specific B cell population.

These data showed that the naïve B cell repertoire contains both 6OXY- and 8HYDROC-specific B cells and that immunization with either 6OXY-KLH or 8HYDROC-KLH elicits independent proliferation of each respective hapten-specific B cell subset. The more effective 6OXY-KLH induced stronger hapten-specific B cell responses than 8HYDROC-KLH. Immunization with 6OXY-KLH induced selective activation of 6OXY-specific germinal center B cells. Activation of GC-dependent processes is crucial for achieving long-lived high-affinity antibody-secreting and memory B cells. It will be important to compare existing and novel addiction vaccines for their ability of inducing germinal center formation and long-lived plasma or memory B cells.

In this first study, B cell analysis was performed in mouse peripheral lymph nodes and spleens, as in the original report (Pape et al. 2011). In clinical studies, it will be possible to analyze human PBMC from subjects before and after vaccination. Using this approach, it will be possible to predict the best candidate vaccines or to identify the subjects that will likely respond to vaccination. Analysis of hapten-specific B cell subsets may provide predictive markers for the development of vaccines that target specific B cell populations (Pauli et al. 2011). For example, hapten-specific B cells may be isolated by fluorescent-assisted cell sorting (FACS) and analyzed for V(D)J mutations (Sundling et al. 2012), single-nucleotide polymorphisms associated with immune responses, predictive markers of vaccine efficacy (Koff et al. 2013), or isolation of monoclonal antibodies (Wilson and Andrews 2012).

19.7 Different Vaccine Formulations Differentially Activate B Cells

As discussed earlier (Chapter X), several groups have studied the relevance of optimizing carrier and adjuvant. A recent study reported the effect of conjugating an oxycodone-based hapten to various carriers and the effect of different adjuvants on the generation of oxycodone-specific serum antibodies and their efficacy in blocking oxycodone brain distribution and oxycodone-induced behavior (Pravetoni et al. 2014). These studies were supported by the analysis of hapten-specific B cells after vaccination.

A lead oxycodone-based hapten (6OXY) was conjugated to the tetanus toxoid (TT), a TT-derived peptide previously shown as an effective carrier for hapten conjugate immunogens (Schellenberger et al. 2012), the native KLH decamer (nKLH), and the GMP grade KLH dimer (dKLH). The immunogenicity and efficacy of these conjugate immunogens were tested in mice and rats using the model Freund's adjuvant or the clinically approved alum and monophosphoryl lipid A (MPLA) adjuvants, administered through s.c. or i.p. route of injection. As described in Chapter X, alum is an adjuvant known for inducing Th_2 responses, while the recently approved MPLA is a Toll-like receptor 4 (TLR4) agonist that induces robust Th_1 activation.

In this study, 6OXY conjugated to TT or dKLH dimer was as effective as the previously characterized 6OXY conjugated to the nKLH decamer in mice and rats. Instead, 6OXY conjugated to a TT-derived peptide was not as effective as conjugates consisting of protein carriers. Vaccination s.c. with conjugate immunogens absorbed on alum adjuvant provided similar protection to immunization i.p. with Freund's adjuvant in mouse and rats. In contrast, immunization with 6OXY-nKLH using alum s.c. was more effective in inducing oxycodone-specific serum antibody titers than using MPLA by either the s.c. or i.p routes. Additionally, combining alum with MPLA did not produce a significant increase in the efficacy of 6OXY-nKLH relative to alum alone.

The MPLA adjuvant, alone or in combination with alum, did not stimulate higher serum IgG antibody levels than alum alone in mice vaccinated with an oxycodone vaccine (Pravetoni et al. 2014). Instead, MPLA improved the efficacy of a heroin vaccine that used TT as a carrier (Matyas et al. 2013). As detailed in Chapter X, adjuvants may have species- and strain-dependent efficacy and also different effects on vaccines containing haptens of different design. Similar vaccine-specific discrepancies in the effects of adjuvants were reported using the Th_1 adjuvant CpG mixed with alum. A mixture of CpG (B class ODN) and alum increased the immunogenicity of a nicotine vaccine compared to alum in mice and nonhuman primates (McCluskie et al. 2013). In contrast, CpG (B class ODN 1826) mixed with alum was no more effective than alum alone in mice vaccinated with a heroin conjugate vaccine (Bremer and Janda 2012). A follow-up study from the same group showed that a phosphorothioated CpG ODN 1826 mixed with alum was significantly more effective than alum in mice vaccinated with the same heroin vaccine (Bremer et al. 2014). Compared to CpG composed of oligonucleotides containing native phosphodiester bonds between base pairs, the addition of a nuclease-resistant phosphorothioated backbone provided a more stable and effective CpG formulation that enhanced vaccine efficacy (Bremer et al. 2014).

Various adjuvants or adjuvant combinations are commercially available, and it is often challenging to compare efficacy across studies or species. For instance, alum is often a safe first-choice adjuvant to test vaccines in humans because its effects are consistent across species and strains. Specifically, the efficacy of the 6OXY-nKLH, 6OXY-dKLH, and 6OXY-TT conjugates administered in alum adjuvant was conserved in Holtzman rats and mice of the BALB/c, C57Bl/6, C57BL/1-ScSnJ, and C57BL/1-ScNJ strains (Pravetoni et al. 2014). These data suggested that TT, nKLH, and dKLH carriers provide consistent vaccine immunogenicity and efficacy across species and strains and via different routes of administration, while adjuvant formulations may need to be tailored to individual immunogens or patient populations.

To test the extent to which the observed MPLA lack of adjuvanting effects were specific to the nKLH carrier or generalized to other carriers, the authors compared the effect of MPLA versus alum adjuvant on the immunogenicity of 6OXY-TT. As expected, immunization with 6OXY-TT in MPLA s.c. failed to elicit higher oxycodone-specific IgG titers than alum adjuvant (Fig. 19.8, panel a). Consistently, immunization with 6OXY-TT in alum tended to produce higher TT-specific serum antibody titers compared to MPLA (Fig. 19.8). The different effects of the alum and MPLA adjuvants were supported by evidence that alum adjuvant was more effective in stimulating 6OXY-specific Ig^{high} ASC B cells than MPLA in immunized mice (Fig. 19.8, panel c). Additionally, a higher number of 6OXY-specific Ig^{high} ASC B cells correlated to increased oxycodone-specific serum IgG antibodies (Fig. 19.8, panel c).

These data were consistent with the notion that different hapten, carrier, and adjuvants affect T cell-dependent B cell activation and the generation of drug-specific serum antibodies. In fact, in mice vaccinated with 6OXY-TT in MPLA, the reduced number of hapten-specific ASC B cells reflected the observed lower oxycodone-specific serum IgG antibody titers compared to alum. These data suggested that analysis of hapten-specific ASC B cells provides an additional benchmark for improving vaccine design.

19.8 Hapten-Specific B Cells Are Markers of Vaccine Efficacy in Different Genetic Backgrounds

In vaccine development, it is informative and often recommended by the Food and Drug Administration (FDA) to compare the efficacy of novel vaccines in various strains or species. Hapten-specific B cell analysis is effectively performed in various mouse strains, including genetically modified mice (Pravetoni et al. 2014).

The molecular mechanism(s) underlying vaccine efficacy against drugs of abuse is still largely unknown. Among other B cell surface markers, Toll-like receptors (TLR) modulate adaptive immune responses against a variety of pathogens or xenobiotics (O'Neill et al. 2009). Recent evidence shows that TLR4 binds opioids and tricyclic antidepressant and that TLR4 signaling may be modulated by nicotine and ketamine (Chen et al. 2009; Franchi et al. 2012; Hutchinson et al. 2010a, b, c; Wang et al. 2012). Based on this evidence, it has been hypothesized that TLR4 may also modulate B cell responses to haptens structurally similar to drugs of abuse. Toll-like receptor 4 gene polymorphisms or TLR4 expression on B cells predict immune responses to TLR4 agonists and vaccines in mice (Tsukamoto et al. 2013) and humans (Grondahl-Yli-Hannuksela et al. 2012; Kimman et al. 2008; Schroder and Schumann 2005). It is possible that human subjects with certain mutations in the TLR4 or expressing lower levels of TLR4 on B cells are more likely to respond poorly to an opioid vaccine.

A recent study explored the contribution of TLR4 signaling to the efficacy of oxycodone vaccines using TLR4-deficient ($TRL4^{-/-}$) mice and tested the relevance of hapten-specific B cells to vaccine efficacy in different genetic backgrounds. The immunogenicity of the 6OXY-nKLH conjugate in alum was

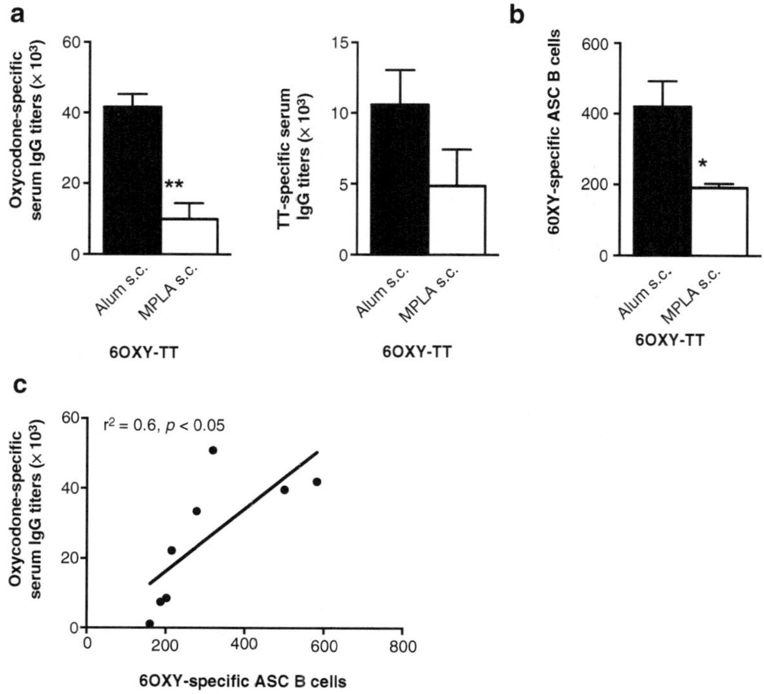

Fig. 19.8 The number of hapten-specific antibody-secreting B cells provides an immune correlate of vaccine efficacy. (**a**) Oxycodone-specific and TT-specific serum IgG antibody titers in mice immunized s.c. with 6OXY-TT in alum or MPLA adjuvants. (**b**) The number of 6OXY-specific ASC B cells in mice immunized s.c. with 6OXY-TT adsorbed on either alum or MPL. (**c**) Relationship between oxycodone-specific serum IgG antibody titers and 6OXY-specific ASC B cells including all subjects immunized with 6OXY-TT. Statistical symbols: * $p<0.05$ and ** $p<0.01$ between groups

evaluated in C57Bl/10ScNJ TRL4$^{-/-}$mice versus C57Bl/6 J and C57Bl/10ScSnJ wild-type (wt) controls. The authors found a significant effect of genotype and time on oxycodone-specific serum antibody titers, suggesting that host genetic background may affect responses to immunization with opioid vaccines. At 6 and 9 weeks after the first immunization, TLR4$^{-/-}$mice showed lower oxycodone-specific serum antibody titers than their C57Bl/10ScSnJ wt controls (Fig. 19.9a). Five weeks after the last immunization, TLR4$^{-/-}$mice showed a significant reduction in 6OXY-specific Ig^{high} ASC B cells compared to C57Bl/10ScSnJ wild-type control mice (Fig. 19.9b).

These data suggested that modulation of the TLR4 signaling pathway may be required for T cell-dependent B cell activation in response to oxycodone vaccines. Given that TLR4 can bind opioids (Wang et al. 2012), it is tempting to speculate that TLR4 may also mediate B cell responses to opioid-based haptens. However, an alternative interpretation is that TLR4 modulate immune responses

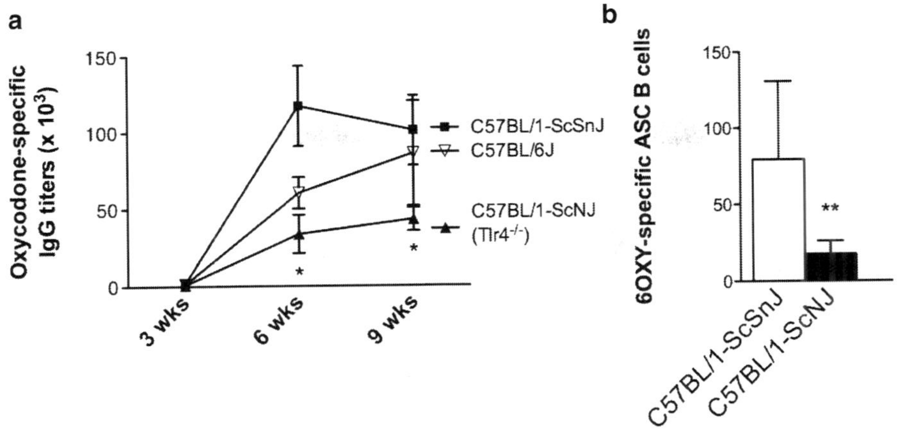

Fig. 19.9 Host genetics affects immunogenicity of a vaccine against oxycodone. The immunogenicity of 6OXY-nKLH was reduced in C57Bl/10ScNJ TRL4$^{-/-}$mice versus C57Bl/10ScSnJ wild-type controls. (**a**) Oxycodone-specific serum IgG antibody titers in mice vaccinated s.c. with 6OXY-nKLH in alum adjuvant. (**b**) The number of 6OXY-specific antibody-secreting B cells in C57Bl/10ScNJ TRL4$^{-/-}$and C57Bl/10ScSnJ wild-type mice immunized s.c. with 6OXY-nKLH in alum. Statistical symbols: * $p<0.05$ and **$p<0.01$ compared to C57Bl/10ScSnJ wild-type control mice

to KLH or TT. Interpretation of experiments involving the use of constitutional knockout mice is complicated by the presence of compensatory mechanisms or by the genetic background of the parent strain (Picciotto and Wickman 1998). Based upon these findings, it is possible that subjects with certain mutations in the TLR4 gene, or lower expression of TLR4 on B cells, may be less likely to respond to an oxycodone vaccine. More studies are needed to establish a clear link between TLR and addiction vaccines. Analysis of TLR polymorphisms in human PBMC may provide novel biomarkers to assess the efficacy of addiction vaccines.

19.9 The Frequency of Naïve and Early Activated Hapten-Specific B Cell Subsets Accounts for Individual Variability in Vaccine Efficacy Against Drugs of Abuse

Recent preclinical studies showed that the individual variability in the size of the polyclonal naïve and early-activated hapten-specific B cell subsets in the spleen and blood correlates to post-vaccination serum antibody levels and the magnitude of vaccine efficacy against drugs of abuse (Laudenbach et al. 2015a, b). Furthermore, CD4^{+} T cell-dependent B cell activation is required for vaccine efficacy and the number of carrier-specific CD4^{+} T cells prior to immunization correlates with subsequent vaccine efficacy against oxycodone in mice (Laudenbach et al. 2015a).

This study provided evidence that a large population of naïve and early-activated hapten-specific B cells, in the presence of an adequate number of carrier-specific CD4+ T cells, is required for successful T cell-dependent B cell activation and vaccine efficacy against drugs of abuse. Hence, these findings suggested that individual variability in the frequency of vaccine-specific B and T cells, prior and shortly after immunization, may account for individual responses to addiction vaccines and may provide immune correlates predictive of vaccine clinical efficacy (Laudenbach et al. 2015a, b). This study also showed that flow cytometry paired with antigen-based magnetic enrichment allows the analysis of the hapten-specific B cell repertoire in small volumes of mouse blood (Laudenbach et al. 2015a). Translation of this approach to human blood may support clinical evaluation of new addiction vaccines and the development of screening tests to identify patients that will likely respond to vaccination.

19.10 New Technologies or Materials Enhance B and T Cell Responses to Conjugate Vaccines Against Drugs of Abuse

New strategies to increase T cell-dependent B cell activation are critical for increasing the efficacy of addiction vaccines. As detailed in this book, new technologies or materials may enable us to create novel platforms for delivery of optimized haptens and immunogens to B and T cells. As described in Chapter X, a new generation of synthetic carriers consisting of DNA scaffolds combined with proteins may provide an appealing approach to increase induction of memory B cell responses to immunization. As described in Chapter X, another promising approach under development is the use of nanoparticles composed of polymers covalently bound to nicotine haptens and adjuvants, which contain a universal peptide to stimulate robust memory CD4+ T cell responses and nicotine-specific serum IgG antibody titers (Fraser et al. 2014).

19.11 Conclusions

Analysis of B and T cells should be incorporated in rational vaccine design and screening of new vaccines. The frequency of naïve and early-activated hapten-specific B cell subsets, and also carrier-specific CD4+ T cells, provides a biomarker predictive of post-immunization anti-drug antibody levels and vaccine efficacy against drugs of abuse. Analysis of the hapten-specific B cell and carrier-specific CD4+ T cell populations may speed vaccine discovery by screening the lead haptens that best bind B cells or the most effective novel carriers that best activate T cell help. In the clinic, screening the frequency of hapten-specific B cell subsets in human PBMC prior to immunization may identify patients that will likely benefit from vaccine therapy or may provide individualized selection criteria for choosing the best vaccination strategy for each patient. Further studies are needed to gain a better understanding of the cellular and molecular mechanisms underlying T cell-dependent B cell responses to conjugate vaccines and to appreciate their role in vaccine design. Studying the basic immunology underlying addiction vaccine efficacy may aid the development of novel mechanism-based strategies to increase the overall efficacy of vaccines against drugs of abuse.

References

Astronomo RD, Burton DR. Carbohydrate vaccines: developing sweet solutions to sticky situations? Nat Rev Drug Discov. 2010;9:308–24.

Bell J, Gray D. Antigen-capturing cells can masquerade as memory B cells. J Exp Med. 2003;197:1233–44.

Bremer PT, Janda KD. Investigating the effects of a hydrolytically stable hapten and a Th1 adjuvant on heroin vaccine performance. J Med Chem. 2012;55:10776–80.

Bremer PT, Schlosburg JE, Lively JM, Janda KD. Injection route and TLR9 agonist addition significantly impact heroin vaccine efficacy. Mol Pharm. 2014;11:1075–80.

Cai X, Whitfield T, Moreno AY, Grant Y, Hixon MS, Koob GF, Janda KD. Probing the effects of hapten stability on cocaine vaccine immunogenicity. Mol Pharm. 2013;10(11):4176–84.

Chen TL, Chang CC, Lin YL, Ueng YF, Chen RM. Signal-transducing mechanisms of ketamine-caused inhibition of interleukin-1 beta gene expression in lipopolysaccharide-stimulated murine macrophage-like Raw 264.7 cells. Toxicol Appl Pharmacol. 2009;240:15–25.

Cornuz J, Zwahlen S, Jungi WF, Osterwalder J, Klingler K, van Melle G, Bangala Y, Guessous I, Muller P, Willers J, Maurer P, Bachmann MF, Cerny T. A vaccine against nicotine for smoking cessation: a randomized controlled trial. PLoS One. 2008;3:e2547.

Crotty S. Follicular helper CD4 T cells (TFH). Annu Rev Immunol. 2011;29:621–63.

Epidemic: responding to America's prescription drug abuse crisis; 2011.

Franchi S, Moretti S, Castelli M, Lattuada D, Scavullo C, Panerai AE, Sacerdote P. Mu opioid receptor activation modulates Toll like receptor 4 in murine macrophages. Brain Behav Immun. 2012;26:480–8.

Fraser CC, Altreuter DH, Ilyinskii P, Pittet L, LaMothe RA, Keegan M, Johnston L, Kishimoto TK. Generation of a universal CD4 memory T cell recall peptide effective in humans, mice and non-human primates. Vaccine. 2014;32:2896–903.

Grondahl-Yli-Hannuksela K, Vuononvirta J, Barkoff AM, Viander M, Van Der Meeren O, Mertsola J, He Q. Gene polymorphism in toll-like receptor 4: effect on antibody production and persistence after acellular pertussis vaccination during adolescence. J Infect Dis. 2012;205:1214–9.

Hatsukami DK, Jorenby DE, Gonzales D, Rigotti NA, Glover ED, Oncken CA, Tashkin DP, Reus VI, Akhavain RC, Fahim RE, Kessler PD, Niknian M, Kalnik MW, Rennard SI. Immunogenicity and smoking-cessation outcomes for a novel nicotine immunotherapeutic. Clin Pharmacol Ther. 2011;89:392–9.

Hutchinson MR, Lewis SS, Coats BD, Rezvani N, Zhang Y, Wieseler JL, Somogyi AA, Yin H, Maier SF, Rice KC, Watkins LR. Possible involvement of toll-like receptor 4/myeloid differentiation factor-2 activity of opioid inactive isomers causes spinal proinflammation and related behavioral consequences. Neuroscience. 2010a;167:880–93.

Hutchinson MR, Loram LC, Zhang Y, Shridhar M, Rezvani N, Berkelhammer D, Phipps S, Foster PS, Landgraf K, Falke JJ, Rice KC, Maier SF, Yin H, Watkins LR. Evidence that tricyclic small molecules may possess toll-like receptor and myeloid differentiation protein 2 activity. Neuroscience. 2010b;168:551–63.

Hutchinson MR, Zhang Y, Shridhar M, Evans JH, Buchanan MM, Zhao TX, Slivka PF, Coats BD, Rezvani N, Wieseler J, Hughes TS, Landgraf KE, Chan S, Fong S, Phipps S, Falke JJ, Leinwand LA, Maier SF, Yin H, Rice KC, Watkins LR. Evidence that opioids may have toll-like receptor 4 and MD-2 effects. Brain Behav Immun. 2010c;24:83–95.

Ibrahim NK, Murray JL, Zhou D, Mittendorf EA, Sample D, Tautchin M, Miles D. Survival Advantage in Patients with Metastatic Breast Cancer Receiving Endocrine Therapy plus Sialyl Tn-KLH Vaccine: Post Hoc Analysis of a Large Randomized Trial. J Cancer 2013;4:577–584.

Kimman TG, Banus S, Reijmerink N, Reimerink J, Stelma FF, Koppelman GH, Thijs C, Postma DS, Kerkhof M. Association of interacting genes in the toll-like receptor signaling pathway and the antibody response to pertussis vaccination. PLoS One. 2008;3:e3665.

Koff WC, Burton DR, Johnson PR, Walker BD, King CR, Nabel GJ, Ahmed R, Bhan MK, Plotkin SA. Accelerating next-generation vaccine development for global disease prevention. Science. 2013;340:1232910.

Laudenbach M, Vervacke JS, Distefano MD, Titcombe PJ, Mueller DL, Tubo NJ, Griffith TS, Pravetoni M. The frequency of naïve and early-activated hapten-specific B cell subsets dictates the efficacy of a therapeutic vaccine against prescription opioid abuse. J Immunol. 2015a Jun 15;194(12):5926-36.

Laudenbach M, Tucker AM, Runyon SP, Carroll FI, Pravetoni M. Vaccine. 2015b Sep 24. pii: S0264-410X(15)01273-6. doi: 10.1016/j.vaccine.2015.09.015.

Martell BA, Orson FM, Poling J, Mitchell E, Rossen RD, Gardner T, Kosten TR. Cocaine vaccine for the treatment of cocaine dependence in methadone-maintained patients: a randomized, double-blind, placebo-controlled efficacy trial. Arch Gen Psychiatry. 2009;66:1116–23.

Martin S. Naradikian, Jean L. Scholz, Michael A. Oropallo, and Michael P. Cancro. Chapter: Understanding B Cell Biology. In Book: Drugs Targeting B-Cells in Autoimmune Diseases. Chapter: Understanding B Cell Biology Martin S. Naradikian, Jean L. Scholz, Michael A. Oropallo, and Michael P. Cancro In: Drugs targeting B-cells in autoimmune diseases. Basel: Springer Ed; 2014.

Matyas GR, Mayorov AV, Rice KC, Jacobson AE, Cheng K, Iyer MR, Li F, Beck Z, Janda KD, Alving CR. Liposomes containing monophosphoryl lipid A: a potent adjuvant system for inducing antibodies to heroin hapten analogs. Vaccine. 2013;31(26):2804–10.

Maul RW, Gearhart PJ. AID and somatic hypermutation. Adv Immunol. 2010;105:159–91.

McCluskie MJ, Pryde DC, Gervais DP, Stead DR, Zhang N, Benoit M, Robertson K, Kim IJ, Tharmanathan T, Merson JR, Davis HL. Enhancing immunogenicity of a 3′aminomethylnicotine-DT-conjugate anti-nicotine vaccine with CpG adjuvant in mice and non-human primates. Int Immunopharmacol. 2013;16:50–6.

McHeyzer-Williams LJ, McHeyzer-Williams MG. Antigen-specific memory B cell development. Annu Rev Immunol. 2005;23:487–513.

McHeyzer-Williams M, Okitsu S, Wang N, McHeyzer-Williams L. Molecular programming of B cell memory. Nat Rev Immunol. 2012;12:24–34.

National Survey on Drug Use and Health: National Findings. 2010. http://www.oas.samhsa.gov/nsduh/2k8nsduh/2k8Results.cfm.

O'Neill LA, Bryant CE, Doyle SL. Therapeutic targeting of Toll-like receptors for infectious and inflammatory diseases and cancer. Pharmacol Rev. 2009;61:177–97.

Oxymorphone Abuse: A Growing Threat Nationwide. U.S. department of justice ews report 000011 May 19, 2011.

Pape KA, Taylor JJ, Maul RW, Gearhart PJ, Jenkins MK. Different B cell populations mediate early and late memory during an endogenous immune response. Science. 2011;331:1203–7.

Pauli NT, Henry Dunand CJ, Wilson PC. Exploiting human memory B cell heterogeneity for improved vaccine efficacy. Front Immunol. 2011;2:77.

Picciotto MR, Wickman K. Using knockout and transgenic mice to study neurophysiology and behavior. Physiol Rev. 1998;78:1131–63.

Pravetoni M, Keyler DE, Pidaparthi RR, Carroll FI, Runyon SP, Murtaugh MP, Earley CA, Pentel PR. Structurally distinct nicotine immunogens elicit antibodies with non-overlapping specificities. Biochem Pharmacol. 2012;83:543–50.

Pravetoni M, Le Naour M, Tucker AM, Harmon TM, Hawley TM, Portoghese PS, Pentel PR. Reduced antinociception of opioids in rats and mice by vaccination with immunogens containing oxycodone and hydrocodone haptens. J Med Chem. 2013;56:915–23.

Pravetoni M, Vervacke JS, Distefano MD, Tucker AM, Laudenbach M, Pentel PR. Effect of currently approved carriers and adjuvants on the Pre-clinical efficacy of a conjugate vaccine against oxycodone in mice and rats. PLoS One. 2014;9:e96547.

Pravetoni M, Pentel PR, Potter DN, Chartoff EH, Tally L, Lesage MG. Effects of an oxycodone conjugate vaccine on oxycodone self-administration and oxycodone-induced brain gene expression in rats. PLoS One. 2014;9(7):e101807.

Pryde DC, Jones LH, Gervais DP, Stead DR, Blakemore DC, Selby MD, Brown AD, Coe JW, Badland M, Beal DM, Glen R, Wharton Y, Miller GJ, White P, Zhang N, Benoit M, Robertson K, Merson JR, Davis HL, McCluskie MJ. Selection of a novel anti-nicotine vaccine: influence of antigen design on antibody function in mice. PLoS One. 2013;8:e76557.

Rappuoli R, Pizza M, Del Giudice G, De Gregorio E. Vaccines, new opportunities for a new society. Proc Natl Acad Sci U S A. 2014 Aug 26;111(34):12288-93.

Schellenberger MT, Grova N, Farinelle S, Willieme S, Revets D, Muller CP. Immunogenicity of a promiscuous T cell epitope peptide based conjugate vaccine against benzo[a]pyrene: redirecting antibodies to the hapten. PLoS One. 2012;7:e38329.

Schroder NW, Schumann RR. Single nucleotide polymorphisms of Toll-like receptors and susceptibility to infectious disease. Lancet Infect Dis. 2005;5:156–64.

Sundling C, Phad G, Douagi I, Navis M, Karlsson Hedestam GB. Isolation of antibody V(D)J sequences from single cell sorted rhesus macaque B cells. J Immunol Methods. 2012;386:85–93.

Tarlinton DM. Evolution in miniature: selection, survival and distribution of antigen reactive cells in the germinal centre. Immunol Cell Biol. 2008;86:133–8.

Taylor JJ, Jenkins MK, Pape KA. Heterogeneity in the differentiation and function of memory B cells. Trends Immunol. 2012a;33:590–7.

Taylor JJ, Martinez RJ, Titcombe PJ, Barsness LO, Thomas SR, Zhang N, Katzman SD, Jenkins MK, Mueller DL. Deletion and anergy of polyclonal B cells specific for ubiquitous membrane-bound self-antigen. J Exp Med. 2012b;209:2065–77.

Taylor JJ, Pape KA, Jenkins MK. A germinal center-independent pathway generates unswitched memory B cells early in the primary response. J Exp Med. 2012c;209:597–606.

Taylor JJ, Laudenbach M, Tucker AM, Jenkins MK, Pravetoni M. Hapten-specific naive B cells are biomarkers of vaccine efficacy against drugs of abuse. J Immunol Methods. 2014; 405:74–86.

Tonegawa S. Somatic generation of antibody diversity. Nature. 1983;302:575–81.

Tsukamoto H, Fukudome K, Takao S, Tsuneyoshi N, Ohta S, Nagai Y, Ihara H, Miyake K, Ikeda Y, Kimoto M. Reduced surface expression of TLR4 by a V254I point mutation accounts for the low lipopolysaccharide responder phenotype of BALB/c B cells. J Immunol. 2013;190:195–204.

Victora GD, Nussenzweig MC. Germinal centers. Annu Rev Immunol. 2012;30:429–57.

Wang X, Loram LC, Ramos K, de Jesus AJ, Thomas J, Cheng K, Reddy A, Somogyi AA, Hutchinson MR, Watkins LR, Yin H. Morphine activates neuroinflammation in a manner parallel to endotoxin. Proc Natl Acad Sci U S A. 2012;109:6325–30.

Wide-ranging OnLine Data for Epidemiologic Research (WONDER); 2014.

Wilson PC, Andrews SF. Tools to therapeutically harness the human antibody response. Nat Rev Immunol. 2012;12:709–19.

Part V
Practical Considerations

Chapter 20
Practical Considerations for the Development of Vaccines Against Drugs of Abuse

Oscar B. Torres, Carl R. Alving, Arthur E. Jacobson, Kenner C. Rice, and Gary R. Matyas

20.1 Hapten Design

Drugs of abuse are small molecules that typically do not induce an antibody response following injection or inhalation. To induce antibodies against small molecules, structural surrogates of the molecules, which were named "haptens" by Karl Landsteiner, must be coupled to immunogenic proteins, called "carriers" (Landsteiner and Jacobs 1935). For drugs of abuse vaccines, these structural surrogates are typically drug-linker adducts, in which the linker has a terminal functional group that forms a covalent bond with the carrier (Hermanson 2008). We believe that the hapten should be sufficiently stable to ensure the fidelity of the antibody against the target drug. The hapten must be stable during (1) the conjugation reaction, (2) formulation with the adjuvant, (3) storage of the vaccine, (4) shipment of the vaccine vials; and (5) after injection of the vaccine. Unstable hapten would be expected to generate antibody subpopulations that may not be pharmacologically

O.B. Torres
Laboratory of Adjuvant and Antigen Research, US Military HIV Research Program, Walter Reed Army Institute of Research, 503 Robert Grant Avenue, Silver Spring, MD 20910, USA

U.S. Military HIV Research Program, Henry M. Jackson Foundation for the Advancement of Military Medicine, 6720A Rockledge Drive, Bethesda, MD 20817, USA

C.R. Alving • G.R. Matyas, PhD (✉)
Laboratory of Adjuvant and Antigen Research, US Military HIV Research Program, Walter Reed Army Institute of Research, 503 Robert Grant Avenue, Silver Spring, MD 20910, USA
e-mail: gmatyas@hivresearch.org

A.E. Jacobson • K.C. Rice
Drug Design and Synthesis Section, Molecular Targets and Medications Discovery Branch, Department of Health and Human Services, National Institute on Drug Abuse, National Institutes of Health, 9800 Medical Drive, Bethesda, MD 20892, USA

National Institute on Alcohol Abuse and Alcoholism, National Institutes of Health, 9800 Medical Drive, Bethesda, MD 20892, USA

I.D. Montoya (ed.), *Biologics to Treat Substance Use Disorders: Vaccines, Monoclonal Antibodies, and Enzymes*, DOI 10.1007/978-3-319-23150-1_20

relevant (i.e., reactivity to a degradation product that is not active or cannot cross the blood–brain barrier). Hapten that require tedious resolution of enantiomers or diastereomers are also not recommended due to poor yield and a high cost of synthesis. The overall synthetic yield for hapten should be sufficient to make it economically feasible for vaccine manufacture.

When designing a hapten, the point of attachment of the linker should be carefully considered, since conjugation of these drug surrogates to a carrier protein restricts their freedom of motion in aqueous milieu. Consequently, the drug's three-dimensional structure bifurcates into two immunologically defined "faces." The "front face" constitutes the framework that is exposed to the immune system, which is the portion of the hapten that is oriented away from the linker. The "back face" is the sterically immunological inaccessible moieties near the conjugation site. We have used this concept of facial recognition by the immune system to explain the antibody specificity and cross-reactivity of heroin/morphine haptens (Matyas et al. 2014).

Among the drugs of abuse, heroin is particularly challenging because it is rapidly hydrolyzed in vivo to its psychoactive metabolites, 6-acetylmorphine (6AM) and morphine, and glycosylated to morphine-3-glucuronide (M3G) and morphine-6-glucuronide (M6G) (Fig. 20.1) (Stowe et al. 2011a). Based on the sequential nature of the hydrolysis, half-life, and lipophilicity of heroin's metabolites, the vaccine against heroin must induce antibodies that sequester not only heroin but also 6AM and morphine. Furthermore, the antibodies should exhibit reduced cross-reactivity with opiates used as clinical therapeutics (Fig. 20.2a) and should not cross-react with medications that are used to treat heroin overdose (naloxone and nalorphine) and addiction (naltrexone, methadone, and buprenorphine) (Fig. 20.2b).

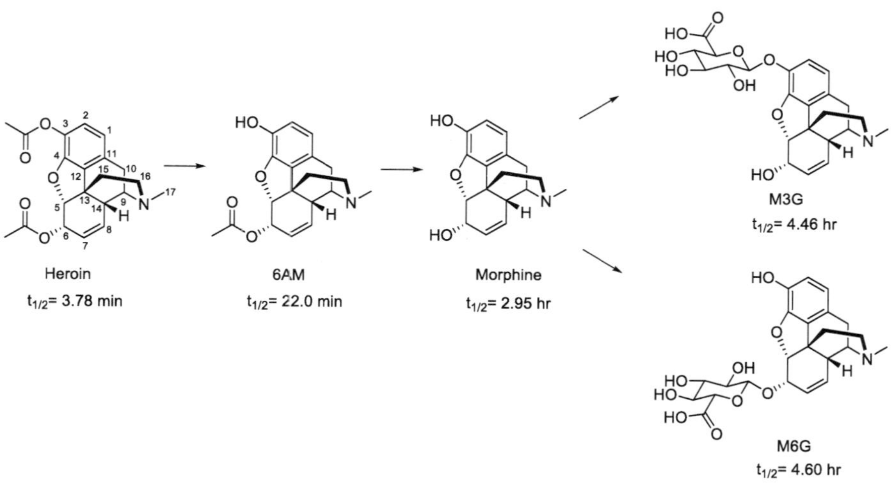

Fig. 20.1 Metabolites of heroin and half-lives in plasma that need to be considered in the design of heroin vaccines

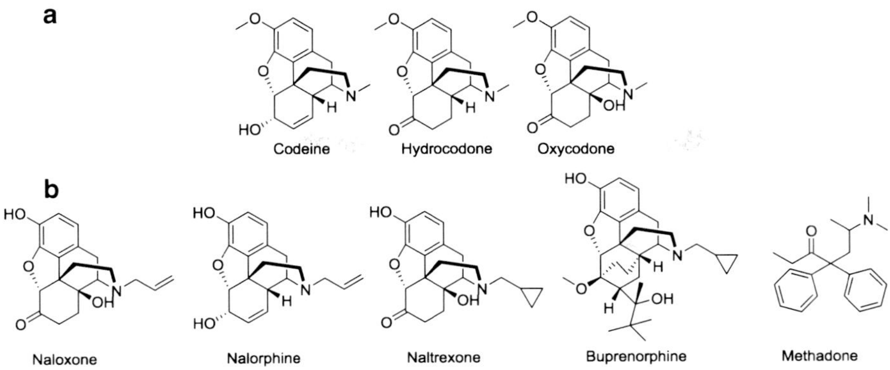

Fig. 20.2 Clinically used opiates that are related to heroin. (**a**) Structural analogs of heroin. (**b**) Pharmaceutical medications used in the treatment of heroin addiction and overdose

We have attached the linker to positions C3 and C6 and the bridge nitrogen of heroin/morphine surrogates in our efforts to develop a heroin vaccine (Fig. 20.3) (Matyas et al. 2013, 2014; Li et al. 2014). For attachment at the C3 position, 6-PrOxyHap was selected and synthesized with a thiol-amide linker at the C3 position (Fig. 20.3a). It contains a 2-oxopropyl group at C6 as a stable mimic of 6AM (Li et al. 2014). Immunization with 6-PrOxyHap conjugated to tetanus toxoid (TT) produced high titer antibody responses that cross-reacted with 6AM, heroin, morphine, and codeine. 6-PrOxyHap presented the C6 and bridge nitrogen portion of opiate structure as the front face to the immune system, while the immune system was unable to recognize the C3 linker attachment point or back face. Consequently, the induced antibodies have a subsite that binds to the 2-oxopropyl group that can also accommodate the acetyl group of 6AM and heroin and the hydroxyl group of morphine and codeine. Since there is no recognition of the C3 by the antibodies induced by 6-PrOxyHap, the C3 methyl ether of codeine and the acetyl of heroin do not inhibit binding. C3 linkers were also tested by Spector et al. and Koida et al., who observed cross-reactivity with codeine and morphine (Spector and Parker 1970; Koida et al. 1974a). Although 6-PrOxyHap induced high titer antibodies with the expected cross-reactivity to other opiates, the ability of heroin to effectively inhibit pain in antinociception assays of 6-PrOxyHap immunized mice was only partially blunted (Li et al. 2014). This suggests that C3 may not be the optimal linkage site for a vaccine against heroin or that the 2-oxopropyl group at C6 is not an adequate substitute of the C6 acetyl of heroin and 6AM.

Numerous investigators have used C6-linked haptens (Wainer et al. 1973; Koida et al. 1974b; Bonese et al. 1974; Akbarzadeh et al. 1999, 2009; Farhangi et al. 2012; Anton and Leff 2006; Li et al. 2011). We developed a hapten called MorHap that contains a thiol-amide linker at the C6 of morphine (Fig. 20.3b) (Matyas et al. 2013, 2014). Mice immunized with MorHap-TT conjugates exhibited high titer antibodies and reduced antinociceptive effects caused by injection of heroin. Using the strategies described in this chapter, we have effectively abolished the antinociceptive

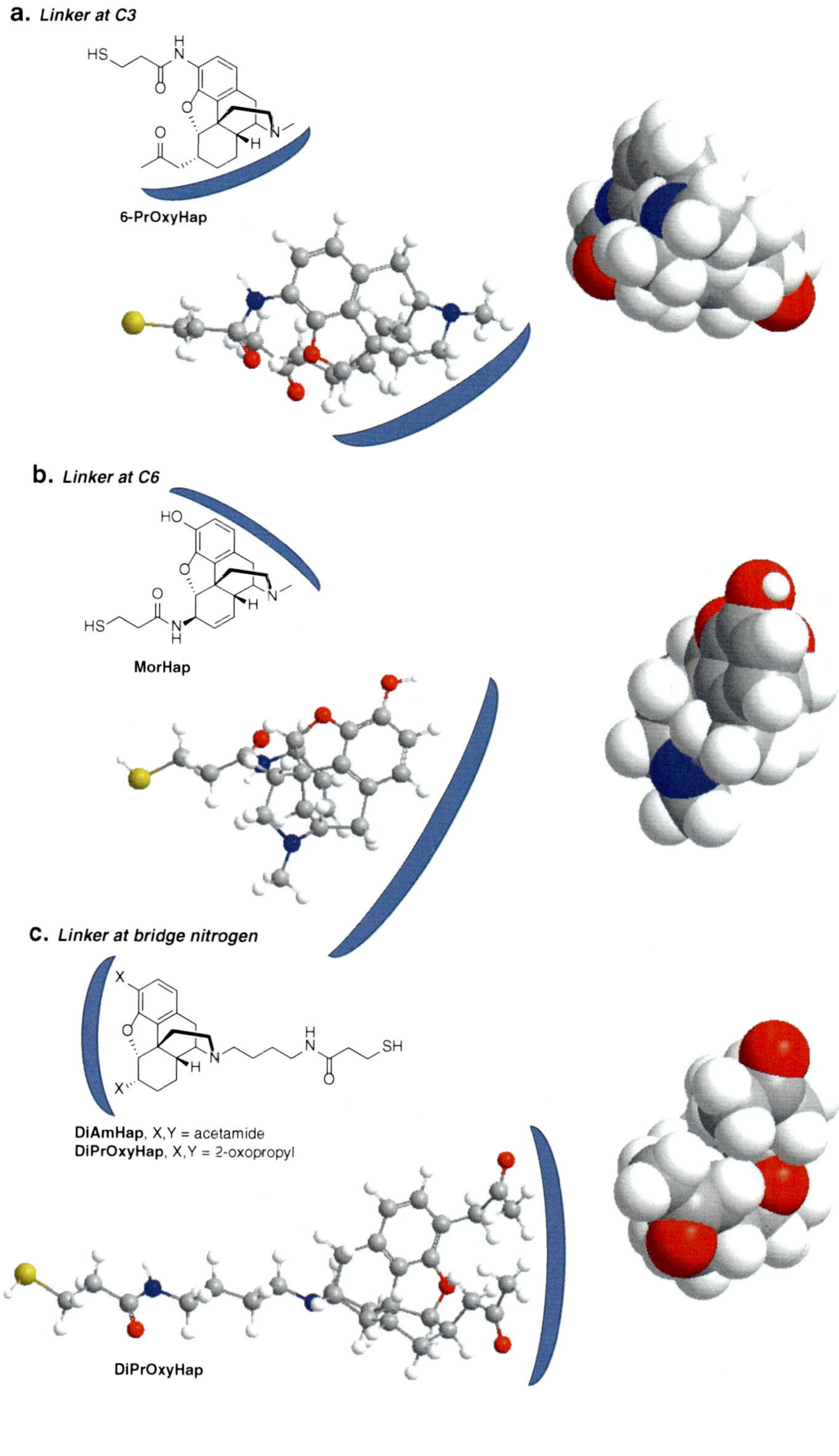
a. Linker at C3
6-PrOxyHap
b. Linker at C6
MorHap
c. Linker at bridge nitrogen
DiAmHap, X,Y = acetamide
DiPrOxyHap, X,Y = 2-oxopropyl
DiPrOxyHap

effects due to heroin challenge (Jalah et al., 2015). Competitive ELISA showed MorHap-induced antibodies that cross-reacted with 6AM and morphine but very poorly cross-reacted with heroin (Matyas et al. 2014). The antibodies also did not cross-react with codeine (Matyas et al., unpublished). Since MorHap is linked at the C6 position (back face), the C3 and bridge nitrogen (front face) are presented to the immune system. The cross-reactivity of the induced antibodies with 6AM and morphine is undoubtedly due to the binding to the C3 hydroxyl and the bridge nitrogen. Heroin contains a C3 acetyl group and codeine a C3 methyl ether which cannot be accommodated in the C3 hydroxyl subsite of the MorHap-induced antibodies.

Bridge nitrogen-linked haptens of morphine also have been investigated and induced antibodies that were specific for morphine (Morris et al. 1975; Findlay et al. 1981; Usagawa et al. 1993). In an effort to synthesize a stable hapten that would induce antibodies that cross-react with heroin, we synthesized two bridge nitrogen-linked haptens, DiPrOxyHap and DiAmHap (Fig. 20.3c) (Matyas et al. 2014; Li et al. 2014). DiPrOxyHap contains a 2-oxopropyl group at both the C3 and C6 positions, whereas DiAmHap contains an amido group at both the C3 and C6 positions. Attachment of the linker to the bridge nitrogen presented the C3 and C6 groups (front face) to the immune system, whereas the bridge nitrogen (back face) was not presented. Immunization with DiPrOxyHap or DiAmHap conjugated to TT induced very high antibody titers in mice and partially reduced the antinociceptive effects from heroin challenge. Antibodies induced by DiPrOxyHap cross-reacted with heroin and 6AM, but not with morphine or codeine (Li et al. 2014). However, the cross-reactivities with heroin and 6AM were only observed at higher concentrations in competitive ELISA suggesting that the binding to heroin and 6AM was lower affinity. Heroin, 6AM, or morphine did not inhibit the binding of DiAmHap-induced antibodies to DiAmHap-BSA-coated ELISA plates (Matyas et al. 2014). Subsequent competitive ELISA of DiAmHap-induced antibodies demonstrated that heroin, 6AM, and morphine inhibited the binding of the antibodies to MorHap-BSA-coated ELISA plates. This suggests that the binding affinity of the DiAmHap-induced antibodies to DiAmHap is very high and that the cross-reactivity to heroin, 6AM and morphine, although present, is low affinity.

We have demonstrated that by using the concept of facial recognition, it is possible to understand the antibody specificities obtained following immunization with stable heroin/morphine haptens containing linkers at different positions. Based on these observations, it may be possible to use the concept of facial recognition to design a hapten that would be expected to induce antibodies of a desired specificity. This concept is not only applicable to the design of a heroin vaccine but may also be useful for the design of other substance abuse vaccines or other hapten-based vaccines.

Fig. 20.3 Relevant hapten–protein conjugates that we have used as potential heroin vaccines. The blue arcs denote the front face. The space-filling models were created in ChemBio3D Ultra with a minimized energy calculation. They are oriented with the linker pointing back into the page, and the front face is forward depicting the portion seen by the antibody (coming straight down). The ball-and-stick models are rotated 90° counterclockwise from the space-filling models (**a**) Linker at C3. (**b**) Linker at C6. (**c**) Linker at bridge nitrogen

20.2 Hapten–Protein Conjugates

Congruent with hapten design, the carrier protein must be selected at the onset of the development process because the immunological potency of a given hapten–protein conjugate may not be translatable to other carriers. *What are the "practical" characteristics of an ideal carrier protein*? The ideal carrier protein for vaccines against drugs of abuse (1) must be safe for human use, (2) should generate reproducible hapten–protein conjugates of consistent hapten density, (3) can be characterized using established analytical methods, and (4) should have acceptable yield of the hapten–protein conjugate. Since assessment of vaccine efficacy utilizes animals or human volunteers which give variable responses, immunization without quantitative analysis of the hapten–protein conjugates can lead to unpredictable and greatly irregular responses. This section will address the intricate relationships of hapten design and carrier proteins and how these relationships determine the reproducibility and yield of the hapten–protein conjugates.

20.2.1 Carrier Proteins

What are the attributes of an ideal carrier for a conjugate vaccine, particularly a substance abuse vaccine?

1. The carrier should be a homogenous, nonaggregated protein that can be characterized by analytical techniques.
2. It should be readily able to be produced under current Good Manufacturing Practices to allow for human use.
3. It should be reproduced by recombinant molecular biology methods or isolated from nonvertebrate sources to eliminate concerns of adventitious agents.
4. It should be safe for human use, inducing no adverse reactions following immunization and, if possible, should be beneficial to the recipient.
5. It should be highly immunogenic to all recipients without genetic restrictions and should induce potent immune responses following the initial immunization.
6. It should not induce cross-reactive immune responses to normal recipient molecules, including proteins, lipids, carbohydrates, DNA, etc.
7. Preexisting immunity should not negatively impact the immune response to the conjugate.
8. A previous record of clinical use would be very beneficial to ensure the above criteria.

The five carriers that have been used for licensed polysaccharide conjugate vaccines are diphtheria toxoid (DT), a genetically modified cross-reacting material of diphtheria toxin (CRM_{197}), tetanus toxoid (TT), meningococcal outer membrane complex (OMPC), and *Hemophilus influenza* protein D (Knuf et al. 2011; Pichichero

2013; Tontini et al. 2013). These carriers have been extensively studied and are safe for human use, including babies and children. These polysaccharide conjugate vaccines are very different than substance abuse vaccines, since polysaccharide conjugate vaccines contain large oligosaccharides conjugated to the carrier protein and are not single small molecule hapten-based vaccines. Nevertheless, the safety profiles of the carrier protein and its ability to induce potent T-cell-dependent antibody response should be readily applicable to substance abuse vaccines. OMPC induced high levels of antibody following primary immunization, which further increased after the second dose, but failed to further increase with further boosts (Einhorn et al. 1986; Weinberg et al. 1987). Since substance abuse vaccines are expected to need continuing boosts to maintain antibody levels, OMPC may not be suitable as a carrier. Both TT and DT are formaldehyde treated to detoxify the tetanus toxin and diphtheria toxin, respectively (Knuf et al. 2011; Pichichero 2013). In addition to being carriers in conjugate vaccines, they are the antigens in the licensed tetanus and diphtheria vaccines, respectively, which are potent and safe (Barkin et al. 1985). CRM_{197} is a detoxified mutant of DT (Malito et al. 2012). Although there are a few exceptions, preexisting immunity to TT, DT, or CRM_{197} does not appear to have a significant negative impact on the potency or efficacy of the polysaccharide vaccines (Pichichero 2013; Pollabauer et al. 2009; Borrow et al. 2011; Pobre et al. 2014). These carrier proteins meet all of the above-listed criteria for substance vaccine carriers. TT, DT, and CRM_{197} have been used as carriers for preclinical studies for substance abuse vaccines and have generally induce potent immune responses (Matyas et al. 2013, 2014; Li et al. 2014; Anton and Leff 2006; Moreno et al. 2010; McCluskie et al. 2013; Pravetoni et al. 2014) establishing them as acceptable protein carriers.

Other carriers, such as bovine serum albumin (BSA), keyhole limpet hemocyanin (KLH), recombinant cholera toxin B, disrupted adenovirus serotype 5 (Ad5) proteins or hexons, and recombinant *Pseudomonas aeruginosa* exoprotein A (rEPA), have been used as carriers for substance abuse vaccines (Alving et al. 2014). Among these carriers, BSA has been used extensively in preclinical studies involving drugs of abuse. BSA, a 66 kDa protein, is an attractive carrier for vaccine development because it (1) contains 30–35 surface lysines amenable for conjugation (Hermanson 2008), (2) has high aqueous solubility, (3) is commercially available in acceptable purity, and (4) is relatively cheap. In 2009 and 2012, a team of Iranian scientists, who used 6SM-BSA to vaccinate morphine addicts, reported successful clinical trials (Akbarzadeh et al. 2009; Farhangi et al. 2012). However, BSA is not suitable for human vaccines in the United States or Europe due to the risk of prions and other adventitious agents associated with bovine products.

KLH has been extensively studied in human clinical trials as a carrier for therapeutic cancer vaccines (Curigliano et al. 2006; Kantele et al. 2011). It is isolated from the hemolymph of the inedible mollusk, *Megathura crenulata*, also known as giant keyhole limpets. It is a cylindrical, copper-containing molecule responsible for oxygen transportation (Swaminathan et al. 2014). KLH is a mixture of two isoforms, both of which are didecamers, consisting of 400 kDa glycoproteins (Swerdlow et al. 1996; Gatsogiannis and Markl 2009). It contains ~2000 lysines allowing for easy conjugation of haptens (Hermanson 2008). However, it has a tendency to precipitate and aggregate. Due to the large molecular weight of the particle, it is very difficult to quantify the haptens conjugated to the carrier. The tendency of KLH to precipitate and aggregate makes it difficult to handle and characterize in a vialed vaccine. Recently, monomers or dimers of KLH have been produced using recombinant technology and may eliminate some of the disadvantages of the high molecular weight KLH, but the recombinant KLH may be less immunogenic (Lebrec et al. 2014). Nevertheless, the use of KLH as a carrier for preclinical studies of they vaccines has successfully demonstrated the principal that substance vaccines can have efficacy against substances of abuse. Its use as a carrier protein on the clinical path for licensure remains unclear due to the source, its tendency to aggregate, and the inability to determine the number of haptens attached.

The B subunit of the cholera toxin has been tested as a carrier for a candidate cocaine vaccine in human clinical trials through a phase III efficacy trial, where it failed to have efficacy in cocaine addicts (Martell et al. 2009; Haney et al. 2010; Kosten et al. 2002, 2014a). Cholera toxin is produced by *Vibrio cholera* (Spangler 1992). It is the causative agent of cholera in which the secreted toxin binds to the intestinal epithelial cells resulting in the production of cyclic AMP and the subsequent excessive secretion of fluid. The B subunit of cholera toxin is a pentamer of 11 kDa protein. Each monomer binds to the ganglioside GM1. The pentamer binding results in a very high, nearly irreversible, binding to the cell surface, and it has been reported to have modest adjuvant activity, binding to both dendritic cells and lymphocytes and causing activation (Isomura et al. 2005; Luci et al. 2006; Hou et al. 2014). The binding site for GM1 contains lysine as a critical residue for GM1 recognition (Merritt et al. 1994). It is important that these lysines are not used to conjugate the substance abuse hapten, but it is difficult to control the conjugation to lysines during the conjugation process. This may represent one of the reasons why the cocaine vaccine was not efficacious. The cholera toxin B subunit has been used in numerous clinical trials with a good safety record (Martell et al. 2009; Haney et al. 2010; Kosten et al. 2002, 2014a; Sun et al. 2010) and represents a potential carrier protein for substance abuse vaccines if lysine conjugation is not used for attachment of the hapten.

Disrupted and partially purified adenovirus serotype 5 (Ad5) proteins or capsids have been used as carriers for experimental cocaine and nicotine vaccines (Koob et al. 2011; Hicks et al. 2011; Wee et al. 2012; Maoz et al. 2013; Rosenberg et al. 2013; De et al. 2013; Hicks et al. 2014). They elicited potent antibody titers, which block the effects of cocaine and nicotine. There are a number of concerns related to the use of Ad5 as a carrier. First, the partially purified proteins and capsids are mixture of proteins, which makes it very difficult to reproducibly manufacture the hapten conjugated vaccine and very difficult to quantify the number of haptens per carrier molecule. In addition, the use of carbodiimide coupling chemistry would be expected to lead to cross-linking of the proteins in the formulation, further making it difficult to quantify the number of conjugated haptens. The rationale of selecting a pulmonary virus as a carrier for vaccines of drugs of abuse that are typically taken by the respiratory route is intriguing, allowing for the development of a mucosal antibody response which will potentially block the drug from entering the bloodstream. However, it is noted that in 2008, an HIV vaccine trial that used Ad5 as vector was halted due to futility (Buchbinder et al. 2008; McElrath et al. 2008; Robb 2008). The HIV vaccine did not prevent HIV infection and had an increased incidence of HIV infection rates in male participants who received vaccine compared to placebo. Analysis indicated that preexisting immunity to Ad5 was one of the factors that was associated with increased HIV infection rates (Buchbinder et al. 2008; Cheng et al. 2012). Further analysis indicated that preexisting Ad5 immunity significantly reduced the immune response to Ad5 vaccines (Cheng et al. 2012). The net effect of these studies is that Ad5 has been replaced by other Ad vectors, such as Ad26, which do not naturally infect humans.

Pseudomonas aeruginosa exoprotein A (rEPA) contains a single amino acid deletion of glutamic acid at position 553 of exotoxin A (Lukac et al. 1988). Similar to CRM_{197}, the deletion effectively blocks the toxic ribosyltransferase activity. It is a 67 kDa protein that has been used in clinical trials as a carrier for polysaccharide vaccines (Passwell et al. 2010; Thiem et al. 2011; Rondini et al. 2011; Szu et al. 2014), but to date, there is no licensed vaccine that uses rEPA as a carrier. However, it has also been tested in clinical trials as a carrier for a nicotine vaccine (NicVAX®) by Nabi Biopharmaceuticals (Hatsukami et al. 2011; Hoogsteder et al. 2012, 2014). Vaccination with NicVAX® gave promising results through phase II trials, but in 2011, Nabi Biopharmaceuticals announced that the phase III trials failed to achieve its primary endpoint and that there was no statistical difference between the treated and placebo groups (NicVAX® phase III trial result. 2015). Conjugate vaccines based on rEPA are well tolerated with generally good safety profiles in humans. However, given the failure of NicVAX® and the lack of licensure of any other conjugate vaccine utilizing rEPA, the utility of rEPA as a carrier for substance abuse vaccines remains questionable.

What is the preferred carrier for substance abuse vaccines? Based on the criteria listed at the beginning of this section, the preferred carrier proteins would be TT and CRM_{197}. Both have been extensively used in licensed polysaccharide-based conjugate vaccines and have an excellent safety profile. The downside to TT is that it is formaldehyde treated, which reduces the number of surface lysines available for conjugation. However, this allows for increased spacing among the attached haptens on the surface. We believe that the best strategy is to test multiple carriers at different hapten densities to the select the best carrier for a given hapten.

20.2.2 Conjugation Chemistry

Azo coupling (Matsushita et al. 1974; Matsukura et al. 1975; Castro et al. 1980, 1985a, b), photoactivatable cross-linking (Ettinger et al. 1997), carbodiimide-mediated conjugation, imine formation (Beike et al. 1999), thioalkylation using halogenated compounds (Ramakrishnan et al. 2014), and maleimide–thiol chemistry (Matyas et al. 2014; Stowe et al. 2011b; Pravetoni et al. 2012a; Moreno et al. 2011; Carroll et al. 2011) have been used for the preparation of hapten–protein conjugates. Azo coupling involves in situ generation of hapten-diazonium species, which react rapidly with tyrosine, histidine, and lysine residues of proteins (Tabachnick and Sobotka 1959), and the aminophenyl hapten precursor itself. The fast kinetics of "self-conjugation" may result in poor reproducibility of the coupling reactions and the harsh conditions (alkaline pH, 0 °C) used for coupling may also denature the carrier.

In the photoactivatable cross-linking approach, aryl azide is attached to the surface lysines of the carrier protein and generates nitrenes when exposed to UV light (250–350 nm). Nitrenes are highly reactive and can react in multiple ways with the hapten or the proteins, such as addition to double bonds, insertion into C-H and N-H, and ring expansion followed by nucleophilic attack (Gilchrist and Charles 1969; Sinz 2006). Because nitrene reactions give a multitude of possible products, the hapten–protein conjugates may not be precisely reproduced. Exposure of the carrier to UV may also damage key epitopes. In addition, this approach may be difficult to scale up for the production of a vaccine.

Carbodiimide chemistry, which involves the formation of an amide bond between an activated acid and amine (Hoare and Koshland 1966), is a popular conjugation strategy in vaccines against drugs of abuse. In this strategy, a carboxylic acid moiety is synthesized into the haptenic surrogate and reacted with surface lysines. Since the carboxylic acid itself is present in proteins (i.e., aspartic and glutamic acids), intermolecular amide bond formation that results in insoluble oligomers can also take place. In addition, carbodiimide chemistry is not compatible for some haptens possessing a primary or secondary amine, as in the case of amphetamine.

Imine formation uses a homobifunctional linker that possesses carbonyl groups at both ends (DeCaprio et al. 1987). The surface lysines of the protein are allowed to react with the linker, and the resulting intermediate is conjugated with an amino hapten. Like carbodiimide-mediated conjugation, imine formation is prone to intramolecular oligomerization. Thioalkylation using halogenated compounds involves cysteine and a halogenated hapten as the reacting partners. However, this strategy is not frequently used because thiols in proteins are predominantly in an oxidized state and cysteine residues are less abundant in proteins (Stephanopoulos and Francis 2011). The maleimide–thiol chemistry (Smyth et al. 1964) employs a heterobifunctional linker with N-hydroxysuccinimide (NHS) and maleimide at its ends for coupling to surface lysines and thiols, respectively. In contrast to carbodiimide, a thiol is attached on the framework of the molecule to obtain the surrogate hapten. As the maleimide–thiol chemistry does not produce oligomerization (Hermanson 2008), the yield of the protein conjugates could be solely assessed in terms of hydrophobicity of the hapten–protein conjugates. For these reasons, we believe that the maleimide–thiol chemistry is the optimal coupling strategy. In addition, Fontaine et al. have recently reported a method to stabilize maleimide–thiol conjugates in vivo through ring opening of the succinimide moiety (Fontaine et al. 2015).

20.2.3 Hapten Density and Conjugate Yield

Hapten density, defined as the number of haptens covalently attached at the surface of a carrier molecule, is pivotal to vaccine efficacy. The effect of hapten density on the immunological properties of small molecule hapten–protein conjugates was elegantly demonstrated from the works of Klaus et al. (Klaus and Cross 1974a, b; Klaus and Mitchell 1974). Klaus et al. showed that dinitrophenyl (DNP)-BSA conjugates with hapten densities of less than 30 induced a modest primary response, an IgM to IgG switch, and concomitant hapten-specific memory, while highly substituted conjugates with hapten density of 50 elicited a dose-dependent primary IgM response, little IgG antibody, and little or no memory. The immunogenicity of small molecule–protein conjugates of dopamine (DA), 2,4-dichlorophenoxyacetic acid (2,4-D), and atrazine (AT) was also reported to be dependent on the hapten density. Malaitsev et al. reported that DA-BSA conjugates with hapten density of 6–14 produced the optimal immune response (Malaitsev and Azhipa 1993). On the other hand, DA-BSA with low hapten density (4) and higher hapten density (18–22) yielded lower antibody titers. Boro et al. showed that a significantly higher titer was obtained from 2,4-D-BSA conjugates with a hapten density of 20 relative to higher density (31) and lower density (2–9) conjugates of 2,4-D-BSA conjugates (Boro et al. 2009). Rajesh et al. demonstrated that atrazine–protein conjugates with hapten density of 15–30 evoke higher antibody titer with moderate antibody affinities (Rajesh et al. 2013). Adamczyk et al. argued that a lower hapten density conjugate induced a slower immune response but often led to an antibody with a higher affinity, while a high hapten density conjugate resulted in an IgM response which exceeded that of IgG and produced antibodies of lower affinity (Adamczyk et al. 1996). Pryde et al. and Carroll et al. also reported the effect of hapten density on the efficacy of vaccines against drugs of abuse. Pryde et al. showed that hapten density is correlated to the functional efficacy of anti-nicotine vaccines (Pryde et al. 2013). In general, nicotine–DT conjugates with a hapten density of <9 induced either low-titer or low-affinity antibodies, while hapten densities of 13–19 generated antibodies that retained nicotine in the plasma. Carroll et al. demonstrated that active immunization of METH-BSA conjugates with hapten density of 5 and 12 hapten densities generated IgG responses in 10 % and 90 % of the mice respondents, respectively (Carroll et al. 2011). The findings of Carroll et al. infer that responses would be less variable if optimal hapten density conjugates were used. Overall, these studies indicated the importance of hapten density on vaccine efficacy and demonstrate that the optimal density must be determined for each given hapten and carrier.

Using maleimide–thiol chemistry, we were able to synthesize hapten–protein conjugates with reproducible hapten densities (Torres et al. 2014). Recently, we demonstrated that hapten density (1) can be controlled using appropriate conjugation protocols and stoichiometry, (2) is a determinant of protein yield for MorHap-BSA conjugates, and (3) is crucial to ELISA absorbance as the plate coating antigen. We further investigated if the optimized procedure is applicable to

TT. Different hapten density profiles were observed for BSA and TT conjugates (Fig. 20.4). These results could be explained by the difference in size between BSA and TT. By trinitrobenzenesulfonic acid (TNBS) assay, the surface lysines of TT (~27–35) and BSA (~30–35) are comparable. The size of TT (152 kDa) is more than twice the size of BSA (66 kDa), and consequently, the "effective concentration" of surface amines would be relatively lower in TT. The protein yield profile for MorHap-BSA and MorHap-TT conjugates showed that hapten density determines the yield of the reaction (Fig. 20.5). BSA with a MorHap density of 34 exhibited the lowest yield, while TT and BSA conjugates with 22–24 MorHap attached gave quantitative yields.

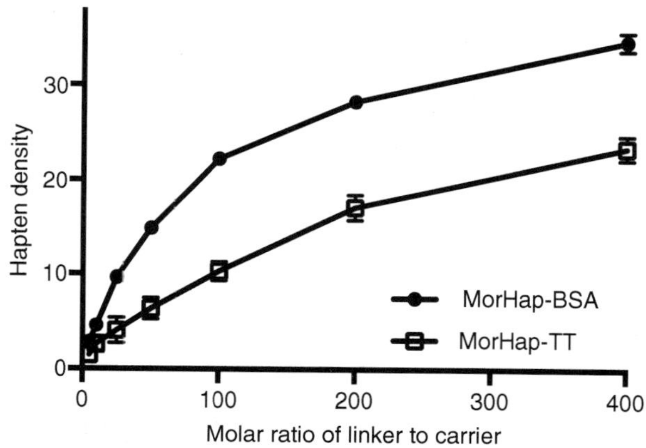

Fig. 20.4 Effect of linker ratios on hapten density of MorHap conjugates. BSA and TT were treated with varying molar ratios of the SM-$(PEG)_2$. Excess linker was removed by spin desalting column. The maleimide-BSA and maleimide-TT were reacted with 100-fold excess of MorHap. Excess hapten was removed by dialysis. Hapten density was determined using MALDI-TOF MS

Fig. 20.5 Effect of linker ratios on protein yield of MorHap conjugates. BSA and TT were treated with varying molar ratios of the SM-$(PEG)_2$. Excess linker was removed by spin desalting column. The maleimide-BSA and maleimide-TT were reacted with 100-fold excess of MorHap. Excess hapten was removed by dialysis. Protein yield was measured by BCA

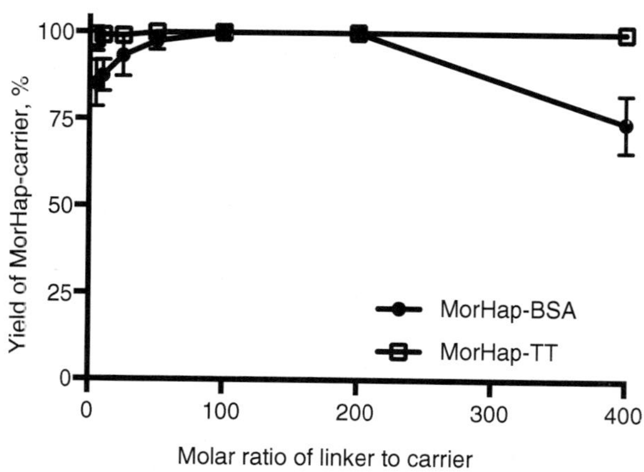

Is the optimized procedure applicable to other haptens? We further tested our optimized procedure by coupling a more hydrophobic hapten, 6-PrOxyHap, to BSA, TT, and KLH. 6-PrOxyHap is a suitable model hapten to assess protein yield because most haptenic surrogates used for vaccines against drugs of abuse have high hydrophobicity. As anticipated the hapten profiles between BSA and TT were different (Fig. 20.6). The determination of hapten density of KLH conjugates was a formidable task as we were not able to accurately measure the molecular weight of 6-PrOxyHap-KLH conjugates by MALDI-TOF MS. Several groups have also reported the same challenge (Stowe et al. 2011b; Pravetoni et al. 2012b). Comparable hapten densities were observed for MorHap-BSA and 6-PrOxyHap-BSA as well as for MorHap-TT and 6-PrOxyHap-TT conjugates using the same coupling ratios. The yields of 6-PrOxyHap conjugates were significantly reduced relative to MorHap conjugates (Fig. 20.7). For example, 6-PrOxyHap-BSA and MorHap-BSA with ~34 haptens have 5 % and 74 % yields, respectively. Although 6-PrOxyHap-KLH conjugates have a higher yield as compared to 6-PrOxyHap-BSA and 6-PrOxyHap-TT conjugates, it is difficult to assess their conjugation advantage without the information on hapten density. Whether the high yield is due to lower hapten density or the ability of hapten–KLH conjugate to maintain high aqueous solubility is difficult to determine. Based on these findings, one can infer that KLH and BSA conjugates have different hapten densities even though they were treated with the same [linker]/[protein] molar ratios. Collectively, these results suggest that the stoichiometry of the reacting partners and the nature of the carrier protein mediate hapten density. Furthermore, protein yield is highly dependent on hapten density and hydrophobicity of the hapten.

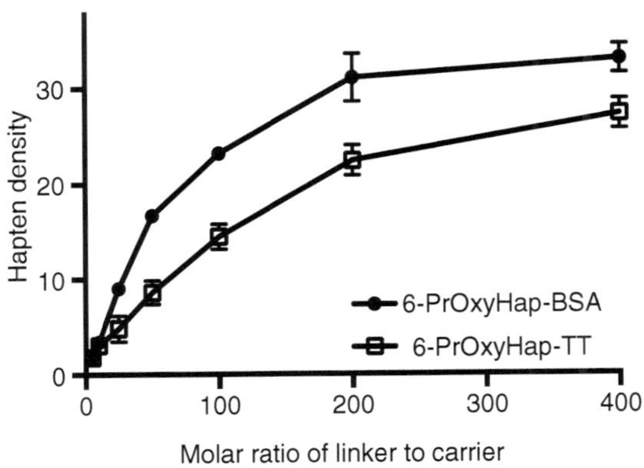

Fig. 20.6 Effect of linker ratios on hapten density of 6-PrOxyHap conjugates. BSA, TT and KLH were treated with varying molar ratios of the SM-$(PEG)_2$. Excess linker was removed by spin desalting column. The maleimide-BSA, maleimide-TT, and maleimide-KLH were reacted with 100-fold excess of 6-PrOxyHap. Excess hapten was removed by dialysis. Hapten density was determined using MALDI-TOF MS. The hapten density of 6-PrOxyHap-KLH could not be accurately assessed by MALDI-TOF MS and is consequently not shown

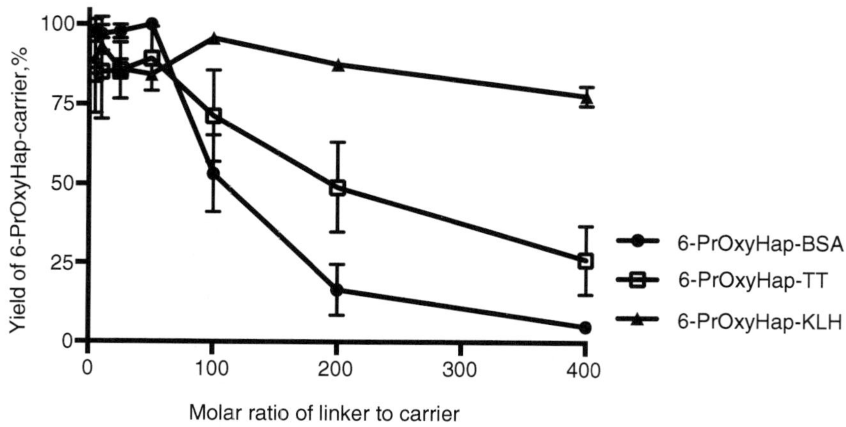

Fig. 20.7 Effect of linker ratios on protein yield of 6-PrOxyHap conjugates. BSA, TT, and KLH were treated with varying molar ratios of the SM-(PEG)$_2$. Excess linker was removed by spin desalting column. The maleimide-BSA, maleimide-TT, and maleimide-KLH were reacted with 100-fold excess of 6-PrOxyHap. Excess hapten was removed by dialysis. Protein yield was measured by BCA

20.2.4 Linker

The linker moiety in the hapten–linker–carrier complex can affect the immunological as well as the practical aspects of a vaccine formulation. The linker directly influences the presentation of the hapten to the immune system. A long linker can generate antibodies which have a deep binding site for the hapten and the target drug (Lim et al. 1998; Larsen et al. 2001; Celikel et al. 2009) as compared to a short linker which generates antibodies that bind the hapten near the surface of the antibody binding site (Pozharski et al. 2005). The linker can also impact the protein yield of the conjugate due to the hydrophobicity of the linker.

The nature and length of the linker must be considered during the design of the hapten–protein conjugate because the linker itself can serve as an additional antigenic determinant. Bridge effect or the co-recognition of the linker during antibody generation has been reported (Franek 1987). For heroin vaccines, aliphatic (Wainer et al. 1973; Koida et al. 1974b; Bonese et al. 1974; Akbarzadeh et al. 1999, 2009; Farhangi et al. 2012; Anton and Leff 2006; Li et al. 2011; Morris et al. 1975; Findlay et al. 1981; Usagawa et al. 1993; Beike et al. 1999), aromatic (Spector et al. 1973; Gross et al. 1974), and polyethylene glycol (PEG)-based (Matyas et al. 2013, 2014; Li et al. 2014) linkers have been used. We do not recommend the use of aromatic linker as they may induce antibodies with promiscuous binding sites for aromatic ligands (James et al. 2003). Although aliphatic linkers do not contain functional groups, Gorris et al. showed that long, aliphatic chains can be recognized by antibodies (Gorris et al. 2011). In fact, Gorris et al. have exploited the bridge effect to enhance the affinity of the antibodies to 2,4-dinitrophenol (2,4-DNP) and demonstrated that the affinity of the antibodies for 2,4-DNP increased with increasing linker length. We were not able to obtain hapten–TT conjugates with a high hapten density (i.e., 30–35) using aliphatic linkers due to the poor aqueous solubility of the resulting hapten–TT conjugates.

PEG-based molecules are attractive linkers for conjugating haptens to carriers because: (1) They have low immunogenicity (Schellekens et al. 2013) and PEG-based materials have been used as drug delivery agents (Gombotz and Pettit 1995). (2) They are hydrophilic molecules and thereby increase the solubility of the hapten–protein conjugate. The synthesis of conjugates with high hapten density, even when the hapten itself is hydrophobic, is feasible. There have been reports also that hydrophilic linkers better display the hapten to the immune system than hydrophobic linkers (Nara et al. 2008; Mercader et al. 2008). In addition, PEG linkers have been shown to improve hapten presentation at bilayer interfaces (Ahlers et al. 1992; Leckband et al. 1995; Jung et al. 2008). (3) SM $(PEG)_n$ series linkers with varying chain length are commercially available (Information on SM(PEG)n crosslinking reagents. 2015). Since NHS and maleimide moieties are already present in the linker, the synthesis, providing reproducible hapten–carrier conjugates using maleimide–thiol chemistry, becomes facile and economical (Torres et al. 2014).

What is the optimal nature and length of the linker for the drug hapten–protein conjugates? To address this problem, Pryde et al. synthesized nicotine hapten, H7, appended to 12 linkers of varying lipophilicity, hydrophilicity, and flexibility (Pryde et al. 2013). Surprisingly, none of the 12 linkers gave a better functional response to the hapten. It is difficult to dissect the "linker effect," if there is any, because H7-DT conjugates of different hapten densities were compared. As discussed *vide supra*, hapten density affects the immunogenicity of conjugates. A systematic approach to assess "linker effect" would be a rigorous head-to-head comparison of hapten–protein conjugates with similar hapten densities. In our opinion, there is an optimal PEG linker length that would generate a superior immune response. However, this should be determined empirically once the lead hapten design has been identified.

20.2.5 Choosing the Lead Hapten–Protein Conjugate

The commercial feasibility of a vaccine formulation depends heavily on the (1) hapten design, (2) carrier protein, and (3) resulting hapten–protein conjugate. (1) The hapten design must strike a balance among immunogenicity, stability, and yield of hapten–carrier conjugate. Inadequate presentation of the hapten will lead to low-titer and low-affinity antibodies and unwarranted cross-reactivity. Labile haptens will compromise the reproducibility and potency of the vaccine. Highly hydrophobic haptens will result in low yields of the hapten–protein conjugates that would make them difficult to characterize. (2) Safety, cost, and the ability to induce potent antibody responses are the major concerns for choosing the carrier. Proven immunologically potent protein carriers that are already present in FDA licensed vaccines should be selected to avoid unanticipated safety issues during clinical trials. (3) The resulting hapten–protein conjugates should utilize simple conjugation schemes that result in acceptable yield, and the conjugates should be easily characterized using routine analytical methods, such as MALDI-TOF MS, chemical assays, and liquid chromatography. Finally, hapten density should be measured as one of the "quality control tests" for vaccine release to ensure batch-to-batch consistency of the vaccine formulation.

20.3 Adjuvants

Substance abuse vaccines require that the vaccine induce antibodies of both high titer and high affinity and that the antibodies must be of long duration. In general, both the haptens and the protein carriers, by themselves, are poorly immunogenic. Consequently, an adjuvant is required to stimulate the immune response to the hapten, and the proper selection of the adjuvant is critical to the development of the vaccine to substances of abuse (Alving et al. 2014). While aluminum salts have been widely utilized worldwide as an adjuvant in numerous licensed vaccines against a variety of diseases (Brito et al. 2013; Brito and O'Hagan 2014; Oleszycka and Lavelle 2014; Powell et al. 2015), the limited experience with human responses to aluminum salt-adjuvanted vaccines for drugs of abuse suggests that the immune responses may be too low in magnitude and duration for the development of a successful vaccine (Alving et al. 2014; Martell et al. 2009; Hatsukami et al. 2011; Cornuz et al. 2008; Kosten et al. 2014b). An adjuvant or combination of adjuvants that is safe and potent for enhancing both the magnitude and durability of the immune response is therefore needed. It also should be easily available, easily manufactured, and cost-effective. Although many potential experimental adjuvants have been proposed, our approach has been to utilize generic adjuvant formulations that would mimic or enhance the compositions, safety, and efficacy properties of adjuvants present in licensed vaccines. In our experience, the adjuvants that are present in licensed proprietary vaccines generally can be reproduced in generic forms with considerable freedom to operate regarding intellectual property.

Adjuvants in licensed vaccines: As described by Alving et al. (Alving et al. 2014), there are only six types of adjuvants in licensed vaccines:

- Aluminum salts are the most commonly used adjuvants (Brito et al. 2013; Brito and O'Hagan 2014; Oleszycka and Lavelle 2014; Powell et al. 2015; Baylor et al. 2002).
- Virosomes (Crucell) are derived from influenza virus and contain the surface hemagglutinin and neuraminidase proteins to which natural and synthetic phospholipids are added to form a liposome-based formulation (Felnerova et al. 2004).
- Oil-in-water emulsions. Three stable emulsions, MF59 (Novartis), AS03 (GlaxoSmithKline), and AF03 (Sanofi Pasteur), are used as adjuvants in vaccines for influenza in Europe (MF59), Spain (AF03) and the United States (AS03).

- Monophosphoryl lipid A adsorbed to an aluminum salt (GlaxoSmithKline), also known as AS04 (Alving et al. 2012a).
- Liposomes containing MPLA and QS 21 saponin (GlaxoSmithKline) (license approval pending) is also known as AS01 (Alving et al. 2012a, b).
- CpG oligodeoxynucleotide adsorbed to aluminum salt is a constituent of HEPLISAV™ hepatitis B vaccine that is pending approval for licensing (Dynavax hepatitis B vaccine information. 2014).

Based on the summary above, and in general, single adjuvants alone, such as aluminum hydroxide or monophosphoryl lipid A (MPLA), are less stimulatory in humans for the induction of antibodies than combinations of adjuvants. Consequently, combinations of adjuvants may be required in humans for substance abuse vaccines.

Adjuvants used in animal studies of substance abuse vaccines: There are numerous recent reviews of adjuvants (Brito et al. 2013; Brito and O'Hagan 2014; Alving et al. 2012b), including detailed reviews of aluminum-based adjuvants (Alving et al. 2014; Oleszycka and Lavelle 2014; Powell et al. 2015; Janda and Treweek 2012). We have recently reviewed the adjuvants used in animal studies for substance abuse vaccines (Alving et al. 2014), and we will not review them again in detail here. Briefly, the most frequently used adjuvant was aluminum salts of various forms. A number of other studies used adjuvants that are experimental, such as flagellum (Lockner et al. 2015), Pam_3CAG (Lockner et al. 2013), and C5a agonist peptide (Sanderson et al. 2003), or adjuvants that cannot be used in humans, such as Freund's adjuvant, Imject® Alum, and Sigma Adjuvant System (Alving et al. 2014). Generally, the results of comparative adjuvant studies in rodents and rabbits are not predictive of the performance of a given adjuvant in humans (Alving 2002; Kenney and Edelman 2003; Mestas and Hughes 2004; Sesardic et al. 2007; Davis 2008; Rao et al. 2011; Vaure and Liu 2014). For example, aluminum salts are very potent adjuvants in mice and rabbits but are considered relatively weak adjuvants for some antigens in humans (Alving et al. 2014; McElrath et al. 2008; Baylor et al. 2002; Mbow et al. 2010). We recently conducted a series of comparative adjuvant studies in animals of anthrax protective antigen. Our goal was to develop an improved anthrax vaccine. The licensed anthrax vaccine is a culture supernatant that is predominately protective antigen adsorbed with aluminum hydroxide (Wright et al. 2010). It requires a five dose immunization series in the first 18 months and yearly boosters to maintain efficacy in humans (Approval Letter for BioThrax®. 2015). We compared protective antigen adjuvanted with Alhydrogel® to different adjuvant formulations in mice (Matyas et al. 2004; Shivachandra et al. 2006; Peachman et al. 2006), New Zealand White rabbits (Peachman et al. 2012), and Dutch-belted rabbits (Li et al. 2009). Following three immunizations, Alhydrogel®-protective antigen vaccination always induced very high-titer protective antigen-binding antibodies, lethal toxin (protective antigen + lethal factor) neutralizing antibodies in mice and rabbits, and 100 % efficacy against Ames strain spore challenge in rabbits. The other adjuvants tested equaled that of Alhydrogel® in efficacy but either did not reach or just reached the binding and lethal toxin neutralizing antibody titers induced by Alhydrogel®. Only when the studies were transitioned to nonhuman primates were the antibody binding and neutralizing titers induced by Alhydrogel® surpassed by liposomes containing MPLA [L(MPLA)] (Rao et al. 2011). Efficacy from spore challenge was 100 % for all of the adjuvants studied in the nonhuman primates. Efficacy in rabbits and nonhuman primates was achieved with only three doses of aluminum hydroxide-adjuvanted protective antigen, in contrast to humans, which require five immunizations in 18 months. This suggests that aluminum is a relatively weak adjuvant for protective antigen in humans. Recent reviews have summarized the other studies that demonstrate the inability of animal studies to predict vaccine efficacy in humans (Alving 2002; Davis 2008). Mestas and Hughes reviewed significant differences in the immunology of mice and humans that may partially explain these observations (Mestas and Hughes 2004). This does not mean that animal studies should not be used in the development pathway for human vaccines. They are a critical element for vaccine development. For example, if a substance abuse hapten fails to induce antibodies that cross-react with drug of abuse in mouse or rat studies, it is likely that a similar result will be seen in humans and the hapten should not move to human clinical trials. We recommend caution when comparing adjuvants in animals to predict vaccine performance in humans and recommend using adjuvants that have a history of inducing high titer antibodies and are safe in humans as the best approach to ensure efficacy in humans.

How do adjuvants function? Recent advances in the understanding of both innate immunity and adaptive immunity have been instrumental in the understanding of adjuvant function. The innate immune system has a family of pattern recognition receptors (PRR) which it uses to recognize foreign molecules that are present in bacteria, viruses, parasites, and fungi (for reviews, see Brown et al. (2011), Kagan and Barton (2015), Brubaker et al. (2015), and Motta et al. (2015)). One example of PRR is Toll-like receptors (TLR). Many adjuvants stimulate one of the ten known TLRs, including LPS (MPLA) for TLR4, CpG for TLR9, and TLR5 for flagellin (Maisonneuve et al. 2014). The TLRs are located on various cell types, but many are located on phagocytic cells including dendritic cells and macrophages. They are stimulated by the adjuvant, phagocytize the antigen, and move to the draining lymph node, where the antigen is presented to the T and B cells for the induction of the adaptive immune response. There are significant differences between rodents and humans with regard to expression of certain TLR on different cells at different levels, recognition motifs (such as CpG), and signaling pathways (Davis 2008; Vaure and Liu 2014; Brubaker et al. 2015), which can explain some of the observed differences in the potency of adjuvant between rodents and humans.

The function of adjuvants can be separated into two categories, immune stimulators and delivery vehicles (Brito et al. 2013; Alving et al. 2012b). Many have both functions or are a combination of components that produce both functions. Examples include aluminum-based adjuvants that among their functions are the stimulation of phagocyte cell uptake and activation, and they also serve as a depot to permit prolonged stimulation of the immune response (Brito et al. 2013; Oleszycka and Lavelle 2014; Powell et al. 2015). L(MPLA) contains MPLA, which activates phagocytic cells via TLR4 signaling and other mechanisms (Alving 2002; Alving and Rao 2008; Gavin et al. 2006), and phospholipid vesicles of the liposomes, which serves as a vehicle and depot for the presentation of antigen. Further mechanisms by which adjuvants stimulate the immune response have been reviewed (Brito et al. 2013; Brito and O'Hagan 2014; Powell et al. 2015; Gavin et al. 2006).

One further factor that must be considered when selecting an adjuvant is the interaction of the antigen with the adjuvant. Vaccines are formulated with the antigen and adjuvant together. For substance abuse vaccines, there is an interaction among the carrier, hapten, adjuvant, and adjuvant vehicle. For example, our candidate heroin vaccine (Matyas et al. 2014) contains tetanus toxoid, MorHap, MPLA, and liposomes (phospholipid-cholesterol vesicles). The fatty acids of MPLA are inserted in the phospholipid–cholesterol bilayer (Alving 2002; Alving and Rao 2008). MorHap is covalently attached to tetanus toxoid (TT). Since MorHap tends to be hydrophobic and the MorHap-TT conjugate is water soluble, it is unclear if the MorHap is pointing perpendicular to the TT surface or if it is folded back along the surface. When the MorHap-TT is mixed with the liposomal MPLA, the MorHap-TT binds to the liposomes, but the nature of the interaction among them is unclear. Liposomal MPLA is a very potent adjuvant for MorHap-TT, which implies that the MorHap-TT binding does not interfere with the MPLA's ability to function as an adjuvant. If the MorHap conjugate were replaced by other haptens that have different solubilities or chemical functional groups, the interaction of the conjugated hapten would be expected to be altered with the TT surface, and the hapten–TT may interact differently with the liposomal MPLA resulting in altered immune responses. We compared several different heroin/morphine candidate haptens and observed varying antibody titers and apparent affinities (Matyas et al. 2013; Li et al. 2014). The unpredictable nature of the interaction of the antigen with adjuvant is a complicating factor in accounting for differences in the performance of adjuvants within a species/strain when comparing different hapten–carriers among laboratories and further justifies the need for animal studies prior to clinical trials.

What is the best adjuvant for substance abuse vaccine? This is a difficult question because there may not be a single adjuvant that is best for all substance abuse vaccines. As stated above, the vaccines vary by the carrier, the linker, and the hapten. The linker and hapten may have different levels of hydrophilicity or hydrophobicity among the various substance abuse vaccines and, consequently, may require different adjuvants. Our approach has been to select the adjuvants or closely related adjuvants that have previously shown clinical potency and safety and test them with the hapten–carriers in animals. If they induce both high-titer antibodies that cross-react with the drug of abuse and have efficacy against the drug of abuse, we believe that they can be transitioned to human clinical trials, where they would be expected to induce high-titer and durable antibodies. Based on our experience, we have selected L(MPLA) as our adjuvant of choice. It has an excellent safety profile and has been used in many phase I–II clinical trials (Alving 2002). Furthermore, except for lacking QS21, L(MPLA) has similar components to AS01b and AS01e, which is expected to be licensed as part of a malaria vaccine.

20.4 Summary

There are many factors that must be considered in the development of a substance abuse vaccine. These include hapten design, cross-reactivity of the induced antibodies, carrier protein selection, conjugation chemistry, linker selection, hapten density, and adjuvant selection. Additional factors that should be considered include long-term stability of the formulation, cost of manufacture, and methods to characterize the vialed vaccine. Some of the risks associated with these factors can be mitigated by the selection of those components that have been demonstrated to be safe and immunologically potent in humans.

Acknowledgments This work was supported through a Cooperative Agreement Award (no. W81XWH-07-2-067) between the Henry M. Jackson Foundation for the Advancement of Military Medicine and the U.S. Army Medical Research and Materiel Command (MRMC). The work was partially supported by an Avant Garde award to GRM from the National Institute on Drug Abuse (NIH grant no. 1DP1DA034787-01). The work of AEJ and KCR was supported by the NIH Intramural Research Programs of the National Institute on Drug Abuse and the National Institute of Alcohol Abuse and Alcoholism, NIH, DHHS. Research was conducted in compliance with the Animal Welfare Act and other federal statutes and regulations relating to animals and experiments involving animals and adhered to principles stated in the Guide for the Care and Use of Laboratory Animals, NRC Publication, 1996 edition. The views expressed in this article are those of the authors and do not necessarily reflect the official policy of the Department of the Army, Department of Defense, or NIH, or the U.S. Government.

References

Adamczyk M, Gebler JC, Mattingly PG. Characterization of protein-hapten conjugates. 2. Electrospray mass spectrometry of bovine serum albumin-hapten conjugates. Bioconjug Chem. 1996;7:475–81.

Ahlers M, Grainger DW, Herron JN, Lim K, Ringsdorf H, Salesse C. Quenching of fluorescein-conjugated lipids by antibodies. Quantitative recognition and binding of lipid-bound haptens in biomembrane models, formation of two-dimensional protein domains and molecular dynamics simulations. Biophys J. 1992;63:823–38.

Akbarzadeh A, Mehraby M, Zarbakhsh M, Farzaneh H. Design and synthesis of a morphine-6-succinyl-bovine serum albumin hapten for vaccine development. Biotechnol Appl Biochem. 1999;30(Pt 2):139–46.

Akbarzadeh A, Norouzian D, Farhangi A, Mehrabi M, Chiani M, Zare D, Saffari Z, Mortazavi M, Nikdel A. Immunotherapy of 347 volunteer outpatient morphine addicts by human therapeutic morphine vaccine in Kermanshah province of Iran. J Pharmacol Toxicol. 2009;4:30–5.

Alving CR. Design and selection of vaccine adjuvants: animal models and human trials. Vaccine. 2002;20 Suppl 3:S56–64.

Alving CR, Rao M. Lipid A and liposomes containing lipid A as antigens and adjuvants. Vaccine. 2008;26:3036–45.

Alving CR, Rao M, Steers NJ, Matyas GR, Mayorov AV. Liposomes containing lipid A: an effective, safe, generic adjuvant system for synthetic vaccines. Expert Rev Vaccines. 2012a;11:733–44.

Alving CR, Peachman KK, Rao M, Reed SG. Adjuvants for human vaccines. Curr Opin Immunol. 2012b;24:310–5.

Alving CR, Matyas GR, Torres O, Jalah R, Beck Z. Adjuvants for vaccines to drugs of abuse and addiction. Vaccine. 2014;32:5382–9.

Anton B, Leff P. A novel bivalent morphine/heroin vaccine that prevents relapse to heroin addiction in rodents. Vaccine. 2006;24:3232–40.

Approval Letter for BioThrax®. http://www.fda.gov/BiologicsBloodVaccines/Vaccines/ApprovedProducts/ucm304758.html. Accessed on 19 Mar 2015.

Barkin RM, Pichichero ME, Samuelson JS, Barkin SZ. Pediatric diphtheria and tetanus toxoids vaccine: clinical and immunologic response when administered as the primary series. J Pediatr. 1985;106:779–81.

Baylor NW, Egan W, Richman P. Aluminum salts in vaccines--US perspective. Vaccine. 2002;20 Suppl 3:S18–23.

Beike J, Blaschke G, Mertz A, Kohler H, Brinkmann B. A specific immunoassay for the determination of morphine and its glucuronides in human blood. Int J Legal Med. 1999;112:8–14.

Bonese KF, Wainer BH, Fitch FW, Rothberg RM, Schuster CR. Changes in heroin self-administration by a rhesus monkey after morphine immunisation. Nature. 1974;252:708–10.

Boro RC, Singh KV, Suri CR. Characterization of hapten-protein conjugates: antibody generation and immunoassay development for chlorophenoxyacetic acid pesticides. J AOAC Int. 2009;92:1773–9.

Borrow R, Dagan R, Zepp F, Hallander H, Poolman J. Glycoconjugate vaccines and immune interactions, and implications for vaccination schedules. Expert Rev Vaccines. 2011;10:1621–31.

Brito LA, O'Hagan DT. Designing and building the next generation of improved vaccine adjuvants. J Control Release. 2014;190:563–79.

Brito LA, Malyala P, O'Hagan DT. Vaccine adjuvant formulations: a pharmaceutical perspective. Semin Immunol. 2013;25:130–45.

Brown J, Wang H, Hajishengallis GN, Martin M. TLR-signaling networks: an integration of adaptor molecules, kinases, and cross-talk. J Dent Res. 2011;90:417–27.

Brubaker SW, Bonham KS, Zanoni I, Kagan JC. Innate immune pattern recognition: a cell biological perspective. Annu Rev Immunol. 2015;33:257–90.

Buchbinder SP, Mehrotra DV, Duerr A, Fitzgerald DW, Mogg R, Li D, Gilbert PB, Lama JR, Marmor M, Del Rio C, McElrath MJ, Casimiro DR, Gottesdiener KM, Chodakewitz JA, Corey L, Robertson MN. Efficacy assessment of a cell-mediated immunity HIV-1 vaccine (the Step Study): a double-blind, randomised, placebo-controlled, test-of-concept trial. Lancet. 2008;372:1881–93.

Carroll FI, Blough BE, Pidaparthi RR, Abraham P, Gong PK, Deng L, Huang X, Gunnell M, Lay Jr JO, Peterson EC, Owens SM. Synthesis of mercapto-(+)-methamphetamine haptens and their use for obtaining improved epitope density on (+)-methamphetamine conjugate vaccines. J Med Chem. 2011;54:5221–8.

Castro A, Monji N, Ali H, Yi JM, Bowman ER, McKennis Jr H. Nicotine antibodies: comparison of ligand specificities of antibodies produced against two nicotine conjugates. Eur J Biochem. 1980;104:331–40.

Castro A, Monji N, Ali H, Bowman ER, McKennis H. Characterization of antibodies to nicotine. Biochem Arch. 1985a;1:173–83.

Castro A, McKennis H, Monji N, Bowman ER. "Semi-rigid" and "flexible" linkage in antibody production for determination of nicotine. Biochem Arch. 1985b;1:205–14.

Celikel R, Peterson EC, Owens SM, Varughese KI. Crystal structures of a therapeutic single chain antibody in complex with two drugs of abuse-Methamphetamine and 3,4-methylenedioxymeth amphetamine. Protein Sci. 2009;18:2336–45.

Cheng C, Wang L, Gall JG, Nason M, Schwartz RM, McElrath MJ, DeRosa SC, Hural J, Corey L, Buchbinder SP, Nabel GJ. Decreased pre-existing Ad5 capsid and Ad35 neutralizing antibodies increase HIV-1 infection risk in the Step trial independent of vaccination. PLoS One. 2012;7:e33969.

Cornuz J, Zwahlen S, Jungi WF, Osterwalder J, Klingler K, van Melle G, Bangala Y, Guessous I, Muller P, Willers J, Maurer P, Bachmann MF, Cerny T. A vaccine against nicotine for smoking cessation: a randomized controlled trial. PLoS One. 2008;3:e2547.

Curigliano G, Spitaleri G, Pietri E, Rescigno M, de Braud F, Cardillo A, Munzone E, Rocca A, Bonizzi G, Brichard V, Orlando L, Goldhirsch A. Breast cancer vaccines: a clinical reality or fairy tale? Ann Oncol. 2006;17:750–62.

Davis HL. Novel vaccines and adjuvant systems: the utility of animal models for predicting immunogenicity in humans. Hum Vaccin. 2008;4:246–50.

De BP, Pagovich OE, Hicks MJ, Rosenberg JB, Moreno AY, Janda KD, Koob GF, Worgall S, Kaminsky SM, Sondhi D, Crystal RG. Disrupted adenovirus-based vaccines against small addictive molecules circumvent anti-adenovirus immunity. Hum Gene Ther. 2013;24:58–66.

DeCaprio AP, Jackowski SJ, Regan KA. Mechanism of formation and quantitation of imines, pyrroles, and stable nonpyrrole adducts in 2,5-hexanedione-treated protein. Mol Pharmacol. 1987;32:542–8.

Dynavax hepatitis B vaccine information. http://www.dynavax.com/hepatitis_bv.html. Accessed on 7 Dec 2014.

Einhorn MS, Weinberg GA, Anderson EL, Granoff PD, Granoff DM. Immunogenicity in infants of Haemophilus influenzae type B polysaccharide in a conjugate vaccine with Neisseria meningitidis outer-membrane protein. Lancet. 1986;2:299–302.

Ettinger RH, Ettinger WF, Harless WE. Active immunization with cocaine-protein conjugate attenuates cocaine effects. Pharmacol Biochem Behav. 1997;58:215–20.

Farhangi A, Akbarzadeh A, Mehrabi M, Chiani M, Saffari Z, Mortazavi M, Ghassemi S. Immunotherapy of 436 morphine addicts by therapeutic morphine vaccine in Kerman province (I.R. Iran). J Vaccin Vaccination. 2012;3:117.

Felnerova D, Viret JF, Gluck R, Moser C. Liposomes and virosomes as delivery systems for antigens, nucleic acids and drugs. Curr Opin Biotechnol. 2004;15:518–29.

Findlay JW, Butz RF, Jones EC. Relationships between immunogen structure and antisera specificity in the narcotic alkaloid series. Clin Chem. 1981;27:1524–35.

Fontaine SD, Reid R, Robinson L, Ashley GW, Santi DV. Long-term stabilization of maleimide-thiol conjugates. Bioconjug Chem. 2015;26:145–52.

Franek M. Structural aspects of steroid-antibody specificity. J Steroid Biochem. 1987;28:95–108.

Gatsogiannis C, Markl J. Keyhole limpet hemocyanin: 9-A CryoEM structure and molecular model of the KLH1 didecamer reveal the interfaces and intricate topology of the 160 functional units. J Mol Biol. 2009;385:963–83.

Gavin AL, Hoebe K, Duong B, Ota T, Martin C, Beutler B, Nemazee D. Adjuvant-enhanced antibody responses in the absence of toll-like receptor signaling. Science. 2006;314:1936–8.

Gilchrist TL, Charles RW. Carbenes, nitrenes, and arynes, studies in modern chemistry. London: Nelson; 1969.

Gombotz WR, Pettit DK. Biodegradable polymers for protein and peptide drug delivery. Bioconjug Chem. 1995;6:332–51.

Gorris HH, Bade S, Rockendorf N, Franek M, Frey A. Pushing antibody-based labeling systems to higher sensitivity by linker-assisted affinity enhancement. Bioconjug Chem. 2011;22:1619–24.

Gross SJ, Grant JD, Wong SR, Schuster R. Critical antigenic determinants for production of antibody to distinguish morphine from heroin, codeine and dextromethorphan. Immunochemistry. 1974;11:453–6.

Haney M, Gunderson EW, Jiang H, Collins ED, Foltin RW. Cocaine-specific antibodies blunt the subjective effects of smoked cocaine in humans. Biol Psychiatry. 2010;67:59–65.

Hatsukami DK, Jorenby DE, Gonzales D, Rigotti NA, Glover ED, Oncken CA, Tashkin DP, Reus VI, Akhavain RC, Fahim RE, Kessler PD, Niknian M, Kalnik MW, Rennard SI. Immunogenicity and smoking-cessation outcomes for a novel nicotine immunotherapeutic. Clin Pharmacol Ther. 2011;89:392–9.

Hermanson GT. Bioconjugation techniques. 2nd ed. San Diego: Elsevier Inc.; 2008.

Hicks MJ, De BP, Rosenberg JB, Davidson JT, Moreno AY, Janda KD, Wee S, Koob GF, Hackett NR, Kaminsky SM, Worgall S, Toth M, Mezey JG, Crystal RG. Cocaine analog coupled to disrupted adenovirus: a vaccine strategy to evoke high-titer immunity against addictive drugs. Mol Ther. 2011;19:612–9.

Hicks MJ, Kaminsky SM, De BP, Rosenberg JB, Evans SM, Foltin RW, Andrenyak DM, Moody DE, Koob GF, Janda KD, Ricart Arbona RJ, Lepherd ML, Crystal RG. Fate of systemically administered cocaine in nonhuman primates treated with the dAd5GNE anticocaine vaccine. Hum Gene Ther Clin Dev. 2014;25:40–9.

Hoare DG, Koshland DE. A procedure for selective modification of carboxyl groups in proteins. J Am Chem Soc. 1966;88:2057.

Hoogsteder PH, Kotz D, van Spiegel PI, Viechtbauer W, Brauer R, Kessler PD, Kalnik MW, Fahim RE, van Schayck OC. The efficacy and safety of a nicotine conjugate vaccine (NicVAX(R)) or placebo co-administered with varenicline (Champix(R)) for smoking cessation: study protocol of a phase IIb, double blind, randomized, placebo controlled trial. BMC Public Health. 2012;12:1052.

Hoogsteder PH, Kotz D, van Spiegel PI, Viechtbauer W, van Schayck OC. Efficacy of the nicotine vaccine 3′-AmNic-rEPA (NicVAX) co-administered with varenicline and counselling for smoking cessation: a randomized placebo-controlled trial. Addiction. 2014;109:1252–9.

Hou J, Liu Y, Hsi J, Wang H, Tao R, Shao Y. Cholera toxin B subunit acts as a potent systemic adjuvant for HIV-1 DNA vaccination intramuscularly in mice. Hum Vaccin Immunother. 2014;10:1274–83.

Information on SM(PEG)n crosslinking reagents. http://www.lifetechnologies.com/order/catalog/product/22102. Accessed on 23 Mar 2015.

Isomura I, Yasuda Y, Tsujimura K, Takahashi T, Tochikubo K, Morita A. Recombinant cholera toxin B subunit activates dendritic cells and enhances antitumor immunity. Microbiol Immunol. 2005;49:79–87.

James LC, Roversi P, Tawfik DS. Antibody multispecificity mediated by conformational diversity. Science. 2003;299:1362–7.

Janda KD, Treweek JB. Vaccines targeting drugs of abuse: is the glass half-empty or half-full? Nat Rev Immunol. 2012;12:67–72.

Jalah R, Torres OB, Mayorov AV, Li F, Antoline JFG, Jacobson AE, Rice KC, Deschamps JR, Beck Z, Alving CR, Matyas GR. Efficacy, but not antibody titer or affinity, of a heroin hapten conjugate vaccine correlates with increasing hapten densities on tetanus toxoid, but not on CRM197 carriers. Bioconjugate Chem. 2015;26:1041–53.

Jung H, Yang T, Lasagna MD, Shi J, Reinhart GD, Cremer PS. Impact of hapten presentation on antibody binding at lipid membrane interfaces. Biophys J. 2008;94:3094–103.

Kagan JC, Barton GM. Emerging principles governing signal transduction by pattern-recognition receptors. Cold Spring Harb Perspect Biol. 2015;7:a016253

Kantele A, Hakkinen MP, Zivny J, Elson CO, Mestecky J, Kantele JM. Humoral immune response to keyhole limpet haemocyanin, the protein carrier in cancer vaccines. Clin Dev Immunol. 2011;2011:614383.

Kenney RT, Edelman R. Survey of human-use adjuvants. Expert Rev Vaccines. 2003;2:167–88.

Klaus GG, Cross AM. The influence of epitope density on the immunological properties of hapten-protein conjugates. I. Characteristics of the immune response to hapten-coupled albumen with varying epitope density. Cell Immunol. 1974a;14:226–41.

Klaus GG, Cross AM. The influence of epitope density on the immunological properties of hapten-protein conjugates. III. Induction of hapten-specific tolerance by heavily and lightly hapten-substituted serum albumin. Scand J Immunol. 1974b;3:797–808.

Klaus GG, Mitchell GF. The influence of epitope density on the immunological properties of hapten-protein conjugates. II. The in vivo and in vitro metabolism of heavily and lightly conjugated protein. Immunology. 1974;27:699–710.

Knuf M, Kowalzik F, Kieninger D. Comparative effects of carrier proteins on vaccine-induced immune response. Vaccine. 2011;29:4881–90.

Koida M, Takahashi M, Kaneto H. The morphine 3-glucuronide directed antibody: its immunological specificity and possible use for radioimmunoassay of morphine in urine. Jpn J Pharmacol. 1974a;24:707–14.

Koida M, Takahashi M, Muraoka S, Kaneto H. Antibodies to BSA conjugates of morphine derivatives: strict dependency of the immunological specificity on the hapten structure. Jpn J Pharmacol. 1974b;24:165–7.

Koob G, Hicks MJ, Wee S, Rosenberg JB, De BP, Kaminsky SM, Moreno A, Janda KD, Crystal RG. Anti-cocaine vaccine based on coupling a cocaine analog to a disrupted adenovirus. CNS Neurol Disord Drug Targets. 2011;10:899–904.

Kosten TR, Rosen M, Bond J, Settles M, Roberts JS, Shields J, Jack L, Fox B. Human therapeutic cocaine vaccine: safety and immunogenicity. Vaccine. 2002;20:1196–204.

Kosten TR, Domingo CB, Shorter D, Orson F, Green C, Somoza E, Sekerka R, Levin FR, Mariani JJ, Stitzer M, Tompkins DA, Rotrosen J, Thakkar V, Smoak B, Kampman K. Vaccine for cocaine dependence: a randomized double-blind placebo-controlled efficacy trial. Drug Alcohol Depend. 2014a;140:42–7.

Kosten T, Domingo C, Orson F, Kinsey B. Vaccines against stimulants: cocaine and MA. Br J Clin Pharmacol. 2014b;77:368–74.

Landsteiner K, Jacobs J. Studies on the sensitization of animals with simple chemical compounds. J Exp Med. 1935;61:643–56.

Larsen NA, Zhou B, Heine A, Wirsching P, Janda KD, Wilson IA. Crystal structure of a cocaine-binding antibody. J Mol Biol. 2001;311:9–15.

Lebrec H, Hock MB, Sundsmo JS, Mytych DT, Chow H, Carlock LL, Joubert MK, Reindel J, Zhou L, Bussiere JL. T-cell-dependent antibody responses in the rat: forms and sources of keyhole limpet hemocyanin matter. J Immunotoxicol. 2014;11:213–21.

Leckband DE, Kuhl T, Wang HK, Herron J, Muller W, Ringsdorf H. 4-4-20 anti-fluorescyl IgG Fab' recognition of membrane bound hapten: direct evidence for the role of protein and interfacial structure. Biochemistry. 1995;34:11467–78.

Li Q, Peachman KK, Sower L, Leppla SH, Shivachandra SB, Matyas GR, Peterson JW, Alving CR, Rao M, Rao VB. Anthrax LFn-PA hybrid antigens: biochemistry, immunogenicity, and protection against lethal ames spore challenge in rabbits. Open Vaccine J. 2009;2:92–9.

Li QQ, Luo YX, Sun CY, Xue YX, Zhu WL, Shi HS, Zhai HF, Shi J, Lu L. A morphine/heroin vaccine with new hapten design attenuates behavioral effects in rats. J Neurochem. 2011;119:1271–81.

Li F, Cheng K, Antoline JF, Iyer MR, Matyas GR, Torres OB, Jalah R, Beck Z, Alving CR, Parrish DA, Deschamps JR, Jacobson AE, Rice KC. Synthesis and immunological effects of heroin vaccines. Org Biomol Chem. 2014;12:7211–32.

Lim K, Owens SM, Arnold L, Sacchettini JC, Linthicum DS. Crystal structure of monoclonal 6B5 Fab complexed with phencyclidine. J Biol Chem. 1998;273:28576–82.

Lockner JW, Ho SO, McCague KC, Chiang SM, Do TQ, Fujii G, Janda KD. Enhancing nicotine vaccine immunogenicity with liposomes. Bioorg Med Chem Lett. 2013;23:975–8.

Lockner JW, Eubanks LM, Choi JL, Lively JM, Schlosburg JE, Collins KC, Globisch D, Rosenfeld-Gunn RJ, Wilson IA, Janda KD. Flagellin as carrier and adjuvant in cocaine vaccine development. Mol Pharm. 2015;12:653–62.

Luci C, Hervouet C, Rousseau D, Holmgren J, Czerkinsky C, Anjuere F. Dendritic cell-mediated induction of mucosal cytotoxic responses following intravaginal immunization with the nontoxic B subunit of cholera toxin. J Immunol. 2006;176:2749–57.

Lukac M, Pier GB, Collier RJ. Toxoid of Pseudomonas aeruginosa exotoxin A generated by deletion of an active-site residue. Infect Immun. 1988;56:3095–8.

Maisonneuve C, Bertholet S, Philpott DJ, De Gregorio E. Unleashing the potential of NOD- and Toll-like agonists as vaccine adjuvants. Proc Natl Acad Sci U S A. 2014;111:12294–9.

Malaitsev VV, Azhipa O. The effect of epitope density on the immunogenic properties of hapten-protein conjugates. Biull Eksp Biol Med. 1993;115:645–6.

Malito E, Bursulaya B, Chen C, Lo Surdo P, Picchianti M, Balducci E, Biancucci M, Brock A, Berti F, Bottomley MJ, Nissum M, Costantino P, Rappuoli R, Spraggon G. Structural basis for lack of toxicity of the diphtheria toxin mutant CRM197. Proc Natl Acad Sci U S A. 2012;109:5229–34.

Maoz A, Hicks MJ, Vallabhjosula S, Synan M, Kothari PJ, Dyke JP, Ballon DJ, Kaminsky SM, De BP, Rosenberg JB, Martinez D, Koob GF, Janda KD, Crystal RG. Adenovirus capsid-based anti-cocaine vaccine prevents cocaine from binding to the nonhuman primate CNS dopamine transporter. Neuropsychopharmacology. 2013;38:2170–8.

Martell BA, Orson FM, Poling J, Mitchell E, Rossen RD, Gardner T, Kosten TR. Cocaine vaccine for the treatment of cocaine dependence in methadone-maintained patients: a randomized, double-blind, placebo-controlled efficacy trial. Arch Gen Psychiatry. 2009;66:1116–23.

Matsukura S, Sakamoto N, Imura H, Matsuyama H, Tamada T, Ishiguro T, Muranaka H. Radioimmunoassay of nicotine. Biochem Biophys Res Commun. 1975;64:574–80.

Matsushita H, Noguchi M, Tamaki E. Conjugate of bovine serum albumin with nicotine. Biochem Biophys Res Commun. 1974;57:1006–10.

Matyas GR, Friedlander AM, Glenn GM, Little S, Yu J, Alving CR. Needle-free skin patch vaccination method for anthrax. Infect Immun. 2004;72:1181–3.

Matyas GR, Mayorov AV, Rice KC, Jacobson AE, Cheng K, Iyer MR, Li F, Beck Z, Janda KD, Alving CR. Liposomes containing monophosphoryl lipid A: a potent adjuvant system for inducing antibodies to heroin hapten analogs. Vaccine. 2013;31:2804–10.

Matyas GR, Rice KC, Cheng K, Li F, Antoline JF, Iyer MR, Jacobson AE, Mayorov AV, Beck Z, Torres OB, Alving CR. Facial recognition of heroin vaccine opiates: type 1 cross-reactivities of antibodies induced by hydrolytically stable haptenic surrogates of heroin, 6-acetylmorphine, and morphine. Vaccine. 2014;32:1473–9.

Mbow ML, De Gregorio E, Valiante NM, Rappuoli R. New adjuvants for human vaccines. Curr Opin Immunol. 2010;22:411–6.

McCluskie MJ, Pryde DC, Gervais DP, Stead DR, Zhang N, Benoit M, Robertson K, Kim IJ, Tharmanathan T, Merson JR, Davis HL. Enhancing immunogenicity of a 3′aminomethylnicotine-DT-conjugate anti-nicotine vaccine with CpG adjuvant in mice and non-human primates. Int Immunopharmacol. 2013;16:50–6.

McElrath MJ, De Rosa SC, Moodie Z, Dubey S, Kierstead L, Janes H, Defawe OD, Carter DK, Hural J, Akondy R, Buchbinder SP, Robertson MN, Mehrotra DV, Self SG, Corey L, Shiver JW, Casimiro DR. HIV-1 vaccine-induced immunity in the test-of-concept Step Study: a case-cohort analysis. Lancet. 2008;372:1894–905.

Mercader JV, Suarez-Pantaleon C, Agullo C, Abad-Somovilla A, Abad-Fuentes A. Hapten synthesis and monoclonal antibody-based immunoassay development for detection of the fungicide trifloxystrobin. J Agric Food Chem. 2008;56:2581–8.

Merritt EA, Sarfaty S, van den Akker F, L'Hoir C, Martial JA, Hol WG. Crystal structure of cholera toxin B-pentamer bound to receptor GM1 pentasaccharide. Protein Sci. 1994;3:166–75.

Mestas J, Hughes CC. Of mice and not men: differences between mouse and human immunology. J Immunol. 2004;172:2731–8.

Moreno AY, Azar MR, Warren NA, Dickerson TJ, Koob GF, Janda KD. A critical evaluation of a nicotine vaccine within a self-administration behavioral model. Mol Pharm. 2010;7:431–41.

Moreno AY, Mayorov AV, Janda KD. Impact of distinct chemical structures for the development of a methamphetamine vaccine. J Am Chem Soc. 2011;133:6587–95.

Morris BA, Robinson JD, Piall E, Aherne GW, Marks V. Proceedings: development of a radioimmunoassay for morphine having minimal cross-reactivity with codeine. J Endocrinol. 1975;64:6P–7.

Motta V, Soares F, Sun T, Philpott DJ. NOD-like receptors: versatile cytosolic sentinels. Physiol Rev. 2015;95:149–78.

Nara S, Tripathi V, Chaube SK, Rangari K, Singh H, Kariya KP, Shrivastav TG. Influence of hydrophobic and hydrophilic spacer-containing enzyme conjugates on functional parameters of steroid immunoassay. Anal Biochem. 2008;373:18–25.

NicVAX® Phase III trial result. http://phx.corporate-ir.net/phoenix.zhtml?c=100445&p=irol-newsArticle&ID=1350155&highlight=. Accessed 19 Mar 2015.

Oleszycka E, Lavelle EC. Immunomodulatory properties of the vaccine adjuvant alum. Curr Opin Immunol. 2014;28:1–5.

Passwell JH, Ashkenzi S, Banet-Levi Y, Ramon-Saraf R, Farzam N, Lerner-Geva L, Even-Nir H, Yerushalmi B, Chu C, Shiloach J, Robbins JB, Schneerson R. Age-related efficacy of Shigella O-specific polysaccharide conjugates in 1-4-year-old Israeli children. Vaccine. 2010;28:2231–5.

Peachman KK, Rao M, Alving CR, Burge R, Leppla SH, Rao VB, Matyas GR. Correlation between lethal toxin-neutralizing antibody titers and protection from intranasal challenge with

Bacillus anthracis Ames strain spores in mice after transcutaneous immunization with recombinant anthrax protective antigen. Infect Immun. 2006;74:794–7.

Peachman KK, Li Q, Matyas GR, Shivachandra SB, Lovchik J, Lyons RC, Alving CR, Rao VB, Rao M. Anthrax vaccine antigen-adjuvant formulations completely protect New Zealand white rabbits against challenge with Bacillus anthracis Ames strain spores. Clin Vaccine Immunol. 2012;19:11–6.

Pichichero ME. Protein carriers of conjugate vaccines: characteristics, development, and clinical trials. Hum Vaccin Immunother. 2013;9:2505–23.

Pobre K, Tashani M, Ridda I, Rashid H, Wong M, Booy R. Carrier priming or suppression: understanding carrier priming enhancement of anti-polysaccharide antibody response to conjugate vaccines. Vaccine. 2014;32:1423–30.

Pollabauer EM, Petermann R, Ehrlich HJ. The influence of carrier protein on the immunogenicity of simultaneously administered conjugate vaccines in infants. Vaccine. 2009;27:1674–9.

Powell BS, Andrianov AK, Fusco PC. Polyionic vaccine adjuvants: another look at aluminum salts and polyelectrolytes. Clin Exp Vaccine Res. 2015;4:23–45.

Pozharski E, Moulin A, Hewagama A, Shanafelt AB, Petsko GA, Ringe D. Diversity in hapten recognition: structural study of an anti-cocaine antibody M82G2. J Mol Biol. 2005;349:570–82.

Pravetoni M, Keyler DE, Pidaparthi RR, Carroll FI, Runyon SP, Murtaugh MP, Earley CA, Pentel PR. Structurally distinct nicotine immunogens elicit antibodies with non-overlapping specificities. Biochem Pharmacol. 2012a;83:543–50.

Pravetoni M, Raleigh MD, Le Naour M, Tucker AM, Harmon TM, Jones JM, Birnbaum AK, Portoghese PS, Pentel PR. Co-administration of morphine and oxycodone vaccines reduces the distribution of 6-monoacetylmorphine and oxycodone to brain in rats. Vaccine. 2012b;30:4617–24.

Pravetoni M, Vervacke JS, Distefano MD, Tucker AM, Laudenbach M, Pentel PR. Effect of currently approved carriers and adjuvants on the pre-clinical efficacy of a conjugate vaccine against oxycodone in mice and rats. PLoS One. 2014;9:e96547.

Pryde DC, Jones LH, Gervais DP, Stead DR, Blakemore DC, Selby MD, Brown AD, Coe JW, Badland M, Beal DM, Glen R, Wharton Y, Miller GJ, White P, Zhang N, Benoit M, Robertson K, Merson JR, Davis HL, McCluskie MJ. Selection of a novel anti-nicotine vaccine: influence of antigen design on antibody function in mice. PLoS One. 2013;8:e76557.

Rajesh K, Rana KV, Suri CR. Characterization of hapten-protein conjugates: antibody generation and immunoassay development for pesticides monitoring. Bionanoscience. 2013;3:137–44.

Ramakrishnan M, Kinsey BM, Singh RA, Kosten TR, Orson FM. Hapten optimization for cocaine vaccine with improved cocaine recognition. Chem Biol Drug Des. 2014;84:354–63.

Rao M, Peachman KK, Li Q, Matyas GR, Shivachandra SB, Borschel R, Morthole VI, Fernandez-Prada C, Alving CR, Rao VB. Highly effective generic adjuvant systems for orphan or poverty-related vaccines. Vaccine. 2011;29:873–7.

Robb ML. Failure of the Merck HIV vaccine: an uncertain step forward. Lancet. 2008;372:1857–8.

Rondini S, Micoli F, Lanzilao L, Hale C, Saul AJ, Martin LB. Evaluation of the immunogenicity and biological activity of the Citrobacter freundii Vi-CRM197 conjugate as a vaccine for Salmonella enterica serovar Typhi. Clin Vaccine Immunol. 2011;18:460–8.

Rosenberg JB, De BP, Hicks MJ, Janda KD, Kaminsky SM, Worgall S, Crystal RG. Suppression of nicotine-induced pathophysiology by an adenovirus hexon-based antinicotine vaccine. Hum Gene Ther. 2013;24:595–603.

Sanderson SD, Cheruku SR, Padmanilayam MP, Vennerstrom JL, Thiele GM, Palmatier MI, Bevins RA. Immunization to nicotine with a peptide-based vaccine composed of a conformationally biased agonist of C5a as a molecular adjuvant. Int Immunopharmacol. 2003;3:137–46.

Schellekens H, Hennink WE, Brinks V. The immunogenicity of polyethylene glycol: facts and fiction. Pharm Res. 2013;30:1729–34.

Sesardic D, Rijpkema S, Patel BP. New adjuvants: EU regulatory developments. Expert Rev Vaccines. 2007;6:849–61.

Shivachandra SB, Rao M, Janosi L, Sathaliyawala T, Matyas GR, Alving CR, Leppla SH, Rao VB. In vitro binding of anthrax protective antigen on bacteriophage T4 capsid surface through Hoc-capsid interactions: a strategy for efficient display of large full-length proteins. Virology. 2006;345:190–8.

Sinz A. Chemical cross-linking and mass spectrometry to map three-dimensional protein structures and protein-protein interactions. Mass Spectrom Rev. 2006;25:663–82.

Smyth DG, Blumenfeld OO, Konigsberg W. Reactions of N-ethylmaleimide with peptides and amino acids. Biochem J. 1964;91:589–95.

Spangler BD. Structure and function of cholera toxin and the related Escherichia coli heat-labile enterotoxin. Microbiol Rev. 1992;56:622–47.

Spector S, Parker CW. Morphine: radioimmunoassay. Science. 1970;168:1347–8.

Spector S, Berkowitz B, Flynn EJ, Peskar B. Antibodies to morphine, barbiturates, and serotonin. Pharmacol Rev. 1973;25:281–91.

Stephanopoulos N, Francis MB. Choosing an effective protein bioconjugation strategy. Nat Chem Biol. 2011;7:876–84.

Stowe GN, Schlosburg JE, Vendruscolo LF, Edwards S, Misra KK, Schulteis G, Zakhari JS, Koob GF, Janda KD. Developing a vaccine against multiple psychoactive targets: a case study of heroin. CNS Neurol Disord Drug Targets. 2011a;10:865–75.

Stowe GN, Vendruscolo LF, Edwards S, Schlosburg JE, Misra KK, Schulteis G, Mayorov AV, Zakhari JS, Koob GF, Janda KD. A vaccine strategy that induces protective immunity against heroin. J Med Chem. 2011b;54:5195–204.

Sun JB, Czerkinsky C, Holmgren J. Mucosally induced immunological tolerance, regulatory T cells and the adjuvant effect by cholera toxin B subunit. Scand J Immunol. 2010;71:1–11.

Swaminathan A, Lucas RM, Dear K, McMichael AJ. Keyhole limpet haemocyanin – a model antigen for human immunotoxicological studies. Br J Clin Pharmacol. 2014;78:1135–42.

Swerdlow RD, Ebert RF, Lee P, Bonaventura C, Miller KI. Keyhole limpet hemocyanin: structural and functional characterization of two different subunits and multimers. Comp Biochem Physiol B Biochem Mol Biol. 1996;113:537–48.

Szu SC, Lin KF, Hunt S, Chu C, Thinh ND. Phase I clinical trial of O-acetylated pectin conjugate, a plant polysaccharide based typhoid vaccine. Vaccine. 2014;32:2618–22.

Tabachnick M, Sobotka H. Azoproteins. I. Spectrophotometric studies of amino acid azo derivatives. J Biol Chem. 1959;234:1726–30.

Thiem VD, Lin FY, Canh do G, Son NH, Anh DD, Mao ND, Chu C, Hunt SW, Robbins JB, Schneerson R, Szu SC. The Vi conjugate typhoid vaccine is safe, elicits protective levels of IgG anti-Vi, and is compatible with routine infant vaccines. Clin Vaccine Immunol. 2011;18:730–5.

Tontini M, Berti F, Romano MR, Proietti D, Zambonelli C, Bottomley MJ, De Gregorio E, Del Giudice G, Rappuoli R, Costantino P, Brogioni G, Balocchi C, Biancucci M, Malito E. Comparison of CRM197, diphtheria toxoid and tetanus toxoid as protein carriers for meningococcal glycoconjugate vaccines. Vaccine. 2013;31:4827–33.

Torres OB, Jalah R, Rice KC, Li F, Antoline JF, Iyer MR, Jacobson AE, Boutaghou MN, Alving CR, Matyas GR. Characterization and optimization of heroin hapten-BSA conjugates: method development for the synthesis of reproducible hapten-based vaccines. Anal Bioanal Chem. 2014;406:5927–37.

Usagawa T, Itoh Y, Hifumi E, Takeyasu A, Nakahara Y, Uda T. Characterization of morphine-specific monoclonal antibodies showing minimal cross-reactivity with codeine. J Immunol Methods. 1993;157:143–8.

Vaure C, Liu Y. A comparative review of toll-like receptor 4 expression and functionality in different animal species. Front Immunol. 2014;5:316.

Wainer BH, Fitch FW, Fried J, Rothberg RM. A measurement of the specificities of antibodies to morphine-6-succinyl-BSA by competitive inhibition of 14 C-morphine binding. J Immunol. 1973;110:667–73.

Wee S, Hicks MJ, De BP, Rosenberg JB, Moreno AY, Kaminsky SM, Janda KD, Crystal RG, Koob GF. Novel cocaine vaccine linked to a disrupted adenovirus gene transfer vector blocks cocaine psychostimulant and reinforcing effects. Neuropsychopharmacology. 2012;37:1083–91.

Weinberg GA, Einhorn MS, Lenoir AA, Granoff PD, Granoff DM. Immunologic priming to capsular polysaccharide in infants immunized with Haemophilus influenzae type b polysaccharide-Neisseria meningitidis outer membrane protein conjugate vaccine. J Pediatr. 1987;111:22–7.

Wright JG, Quinn CP, Shadomy S, Messonnier N. Use of anthrax vaccine in the United States: recommendations of the Advisory Committee on Immunization Practices (ACIP), 2009. MMWR Recomm Rep. 2010;59:1–30.

Chapter 21
Ethical Considerations of Biologics to Treat Substance Use Disorders

Ivan D. Montoya

21.1 Clinical Studies of SUDs

Clinical studies must adhere to the seven ethical principles of conducting research in humans. They include value, validity, fair subject selection, favorable risk/benefit ratio, independent review, informed consent, and respect for enrolled participants (Grady 2004). Applying these principles to biologics to treat SUDs is of paramount relevance given the uncertainties of the risk and benefits of this approach, the potential of a large exposition to the biologic due to the high prevalence of drug use, and the vulnerabilities associated with having an SUD.

Participants in clinical studies of SUDs can be classified as "treatment seekers" or "nontreatment seekers." The latter group can be "drug naïve" or "drug exposed," depending on the exposure to the substance of abuse. Studies of the abuse liability of new chemical entities and those to evaluate the interaction of potentially therapeutic compounds with drugs of abuse are typically conducted in individuals who have used the target drug of abuse and are not seeking treatment. An ethical challenge is the potential appeal to individuals with SUDs of participating in these studies because they may receive the drug of abuse as part of the experiment. Given the relevance of this issue, practice guidelines for drug self-administration studies have been developed (Adler 1995; Almond 1992; Mendelson 1991; Kleber 1989).

A critical ethical issue in clinical studies is the validity of the data. One of the concerns in SUD studies is the surge of professional research subjects, which may be due to the increase of clinical trials and the access of protocol information in clinicaltrials.gov. These subjects may misrepresent themselves in order to meet the study inclusion/exclusion criteria and provide unreliable information during the study. To prevent the admission of these subjects, some clinical trials of SUDs

I.D. Montoya, MD, MPH
Division of Therapeutics and Medical Consequences of Drug Abuse, National Institute on Drug Abuse, Bethesda, MD, USA
e-mail: imontoya@mail.nih.gov

I.D. Montoya (ed.), *Biologics to Treat Substance Use Disorders: Vaccines, Monoclonal Antibodies, and Enzymes*, DOI 10.1007/978-3-319-23150-1_21

require a positive urine sample for the drug of abuse, which can be perceived as coercion. Furthermore, when SUD individuals are under the effect of a psychoactive drug, the voluntary nature of the consent, understanding of the research methods and risks/benefits, and the validity of the collected information may also be questionable. Methods, including data repositories of study subjects, are being developed to detect and prevent the admission of professional subjects in clinical trials and, therefore avoid the need of requiring positive urine toxicology tests for study admission.

Clinical studies usually provide compensation to study subjects, especially when there is little or no direct benefit. Subjects are generally compensated for their time, effort, and discomfort associated with participating in the study. Compensation of subjects with active SUDs should be carefully designed. It should prevent the use of the money to buy drugs and the risk to overdose. Often, compensation is in the form of vouchers, paying to third parties on their behalf, or in small amounts.

21.2 Clinical Studies of Biologics

Biologics have shown enormous public health benefit and they are making a significant impact in many areas of medicine such as oncology, rheumatology, dermatology, neurology, and psychiatry, including SUDs. However, there is some controversy about their use, even for those conditions such as measles for which their efficacy is widely established. The general public sometimes is concerned about the potential side effects of biologics and the perception of disturbing the natural order by modifying the natural defenses (i.e., vaccines and monoclonal antibodies) or the natural drug metabolism (i.e., enzymes). Moreover, the compulsory vaccination of children against some infectious diseases and the claim of adverse effects have created some resistance and a negative attitude toward the use of vaccines (Grady 2004). The reality is that all biologics have risks and benefits and there are important ethical considerations to keep in mind when they are administered to a few individuals for therapeutic purposes or to a large number of people for prophylaxis.

Biologics are complex and "large" molecules that do not cross the blood–brain barrier and thus have no CNS effects. Their main mechanism of action for SUDs is a pharmacokinetic antagonism in which the biologic precludes the access of drugs of abuse to the brain and thus prevents the reinforcing effects on this organ. Biologics target the molecule responsible for the SUD peripherally and change its metabolism, distribution, or clearance. Therefore, biologics are highly specific against a target drug of abuse and have limited side effects.

Biologics being investigated for SUDs include vaccines, monoclonal antibodies, and enzymes. Vaccines induce the production of antibodies by the immune system of the host. Monoclonal antibodies are produced by external methods. Both types of antibodies are expected to sequester the drug of abuse in serum. Enzymes are produced by multiple and complex methods with the goal of accelerating the degradation of the drug of abuse in serum, before it reaches the brain.

Biologics may be useful to treat SUDs because they prevent the effects of drugs of abuse on the brain reward systems. Studies have shown that biologics reduce the amount of drug that reaches the brain and the expected outcome is a reduction of the drug self-administration. The expectation is that biologics attenuate the rewarding effects of drugs of abuse and help to prevent drug use relapse. Biologics could also be used as antidotes for drug overdose and, eventually, to prevent the onset and progression of SUDs, and to prevent the access to the brain of the fetus when pregnant mothers use drugs.

One of the best methods to predict the risks and benefits of therapeutic products to humans is with a thorough evaluation in animals using preclinical models. Unfortunately, animal testing not always predicts the safety and efficacy in humans of the tested compound. This is particularly relevant in the study of biologics and especially for SUDs. Therefore, the clinical evaluation of biologics for SUDs inherently has a high degree of uncertainty, which poses special ethical issues (Kantak 2003; Katsnelson 2004).

The biologic products investigated for SUDs include vaccines against nicotine, cocaine, methamphetamine, and opioids; monoclonal antibodies against nicotine, cocaine, methamphetamine, and phencyclidine; and enzymes against cocaine. Of these products, vaccines to treat nicotine and cocaine addiction, monoclonal antibodies to treat methamphetamine addiction, and enzymes to treat cocaine addiction and intoxication have been investigated in humans. The fact that these products have been clinically evaluated indicates that the research protocols have been reviewed and approved by Institutional Review Boards (IRBs) and/or ethics committees and reviewed and authorized by the FDA. Therefore, it is expected that the products tested in humans offer an acceptable risk/benefit to study participants and have the potential to be safe and effective approaches to facilitate abstinence, reduce drug use, or prevent drug use relapse.

Regulatory agencies treat biologics differently than regular medications because of their complex chemical structures and susceptibility to variation during manufacturing. In some cases, the FDA decides whether new products are biologic or non-biologic on a case-by-case basis. To test a biologic in humans, the FDA requires an Investigational New Drug (IND) application in effect. The IND must contain adequate information about the product to determine if it is reasonably safe to be evaluated in humans. The IND should include the product's chemistry, manufacturing methods, pharmacologic effects, and mechanism of action as well as its absorption, distribution, metabolism, and excretion. Additionally, for vaccines, the FDA requires an assessment of their immunogenicity. The IND application should also include the plan of future clinical studies and any new study should be submitted as an amendment to the FDA. At any time in the process, the FDA can place the study on hold when the risk is greater than the benefit of a biologic.

The IRBs play a key role in ensuring that a biologic is not only medically safe but also ethically acceptable to be evaluated in humans. IRBs are expected to review the IND application and should have all the safety information to make an informed decision about approving the administration of a biologic to humans. The IRB has the authority to disapprove a study even when the IND is in effect but not the other way around. Investigators are not allowed to run the protocol and administered the biologic subjects when the FDA has place the study on clinical hold.

Typically, the clinical development of biologics involves three phases. Phase I involves the administration of the biologic for the first time in humans. Usually, the investigators evaluate the safety, pharmacology, and, in the case of vaccines, immunogenicity. Depending on the aims, these studies may be conducted in healthy volunteers with or without SUDs. In general, there are few ethical concerns of conducting phase I studies of biologics in individuals with the respective SUD unless there is another contraindication. It is considered that healthy volunteers without SUD will not derive benefit from the biologic and the risk–benefit profile of the product is acceptable for ethical purposes (Kingham et al. 2014).

Phase II and III trials are controlled studies that evaluate the safety and efficacy of the biologic usually in a large sample of patients with the respective SUD. Phase II studies further the knowledge about the safety and efficacy (including immunogenicity for vaccines) of the product. Phase III are usually pivotal studies to determine the efficacy and are required for registration with the FDA. These studies generally include placebo controls. However, they may not be justified when an effective treatment is available and withholding treatment would expose patients to unnecessary risk. This may be the case of biologics to treat opioids and nicotine dependence, for which FDA-approved medications are available and the use of active controls receiving treatment as usual may be an alternative to the placebo control group.

It may be conceivable that the "animal rule" could apply to biologics. This rule addresses serious or life-threatening conditions caused by exposure to lethal or permanently disabling toxic biological, chemical, radiological, or nuclear substances and for which human efficacy studies are unethical and infeasible. In theory, a biologic such as a monoclonal antibody or an enzyme to treat a life-threatening illicit drug overdose could be approved by the FDA following this rule. Possibly, clinical studies may be conducted during the post-marketing phase to confirm the clinical benefit.

One of the most critical challenges in the development of biologics to treat SUDs is the selection of endpoints that are clinically meaningful and acceptable to the FDA for the approval of the product. Currently, the only acceptable endpoint by the FDA for clinical trials of pharmacotherapies for SUDs is drug use abstinence. However, this endpoint is practically unattainable. Therefore, there is a concern about the appropriateness of enrolling patients in clinical trials of SUDs when the studies are unlikely to provide the results that will support an FDA approval of the biologic. Efforts are being made by NIDA and multiple investigators to develop alternate endpoints that can be accepted by the FDA (Kiluk et al. 2014; Carroll et al. 2014).

21.3 Vaccines

The notion of a vaccine against drugs of abuse was first described in 1974 in a study in monkeys that showed that after morphine immunization, they showed a reduction in heroin self-administration (Bonese et al. 1974). Vaccines induce the production of antibodies by the immune system. The mechanism of vaccines for drug addiction is based on a pharmacokinetic antagonism in which the antigen–antibody complex is a large-size molecule that cannot cross the blood–brain barrier and prevent the access of the drug to the brain. Thus, vaccines do not have psychoactive effects and are expected to prevent the reinforcing effects of the drug and extinguish the cycle of addiction. In the case of SUDs, vaccines induce the production of antibodies specifically against the drug of abuse. Vaccines against nicotine, cocaine, methamphetamine, and opioids are being investigated. Of these, vaccines to treat nicotine and cocaine dependence have been tested in humans (Montoya 2008).

One of the main requirements for vaccines to be effective is that vaccinated individuals have an immune system that is capable of generating the respective antidrug antibodies. For this reason, immunosuppressed individuals, such as those with advanced AIDS or malnutrition, may not be good candidates for vaccination. This is relevant because these conditions are frequently observed among individuals with SUDs. Therefore, antidrug vaccines may have a limited applicability for SUD individuals with those conditions and it may be necessary to exclude them from participation in clinical trials.

Of the potential unintended consequences of vaccines is the limited access to the brain of the drug of abuse, which may result in increasing drug use to compensate. Vaccinated individuals may try to overcome the pharmacokinetic antagonism and present the peripheral effects of drug overdose. Moreover, when the effect of the vaccine is decreasing and the antibody titers are lower, the vaccinated individual may also be at risk of overdose because the amount of antibodies is not enough to prevent the access of the drug to the brain. This is particularly relevant among individuals with opioid dependence who were able to reduce or stop their opioid use and developed lower tolerance to the brain effects of opioids. Therefore, it is critical to inform individuals with SUDs who participate in clinical trials about the risks of compensatory drug use, the development of tolerance, and the possibility of drug overdose.

A potential application of an antidrug vaccine is to treat individuals with SUDs who have been detoxified, are about to be released from prison, and are motivated to remain abstinent. A vaccine, in this case, could be used as a tool for relapse prevention. This approach is similar to the relapse prevention treatment with depot naltrexone for opioid-dependent individuals before they are released from prison, which has shown encouraging results (Lee et al. 2015). In these cases, patients should be instructed that they must refrain from using drugs when they are release from prison because of the risk of drug overdose, as it was mentioned before.

One of the risks of antidrug vaccines is the precipitation or exacerbation of drug use craving due to the blockade of the access of the drug to the brain. As a result, clinical studies with vaccines and concomitant anti-craving medications may be necessary. In this case, the anti-craving medications may carry additional risks. Therefore, clinical investigators need to consider the risks and benefits of the combined investigational treatments and carefully communicate them to patients. Human laboratory studies of craving, which provide SUD individuals the drug of abuse, may reduce cravings but undermine the individual's ability to consider the risks of participation or become motivated to seek treatment. It is important to remind the study participant that if any time during the study he/she becomes interested in receiving drug abuse treatment, the participation in the study will need to be stopped and support/referral to a treatment program will be provided (Carter and Hall 2013). In general, the treatment with biologics should always include psychosocial support to help patients with the craving and other clinical manifestation of the SUD (Ashcroft and Franey 2004; Wolters et al. 2014a, b; Hall et al. 2004).

Given that the current biologics are specific for a single drug of abuse, it is possible that some treated individuals switch to use another type of drug. For example, patients treated with a heroin vaccine may switch to a different type of opioid such as oxycodone. It is also possible that a patient treated with a cocaine vaccine may switch to use another stimulant such as amphetamines. It is important, therefore, for research ethics committees and IRB to consider the risks that study subjects or patients may increase their drug of abuse or acquire a new form of drug addiction (Ashcroft and Franey 2004). Currently, investigators are evaluating polyvalent vaccines that may be effective for more than one drug of abuse (Pravetoni et al. 2012, 2013).

Treatment with antidrug vaccines can produce antidrug antibodies that can be detected in blood and may raise ethical concerns about privacy, social stigma, and discrimination. This unwanted disclosure may have social or occupational implications that need to be addressed with persons receiving this type of treatment (Ashcroft and Franey 2004). Another potential risk of vaccines is the induction of allergic reactions or anaphylaxis. In this case, the consent form should warn participants of this risk and research programs should have the necessary tools to treat an anaphylactic shock.

One of the potential applications of biologics, more specifically vaccines, is the prevention of the neurobehavioral effects of drugs of abuse. As such, vaccines could be prescribed to prevent the initiation of drug use or the progression from drug use to addiction. These potential indications have not yet been evaluated and it is unlikely that they will be because of the methodological complexity of this type of research. If these indications were demonstrated, there is a concern about their administration without consent to individuals who may be at risk of developing drug addiction or in whom a drug addiction has a significantly higher clinical risk (Ashcroft and Franey 2004; Hasman and Holm 2004). However, for now, this is more a hypothetical than a real concern that may be addressed if or when clinical studies are developed.

Drug abuse is frequently associated with HIV infection, and comorbid SUD and HIV infection are clinically complex. Some investigators are proposing vaccines to treat both HIV infection and SUD (more details at http://projectreporter.nih.gov PI: Gary Matyas, Grant ID: 5DP1DA034787-03). Although an anti HIV–SUD vaccine appears interesting, clinical research on HIV infection involves additional ethical issues. They include first-in-human testing of potentially ineffective or harmful interventions, the presence of immunodeficiency, the medical and psychosocial consequences of each disorder, the expectations and access to potentially efficacious therapies in the early stages of clinical testing, and, sometimes, the involvement of communities and advocacy groups in the design and conduct of clinical trials. Moreover, there is controversy about how to move compounds from bench to bedside and whether the first trial participants should be the sickest-first (oncology) or the healthiest-first (pharmacology) model. It may be especially challenging to accurately communicate in the consent form all the risks and benefits of a biologic for HIV and SUD because of the uncertain and complex risk/benefit (Lo and Grady 2013; Henderson 2015; Garner et al. 2014; Sugarman et al. 2014; Bailey and Sugarman 2013). Currently, anti HIV–SUD vaccines are more a concept than a reality. If they become available, investigators will need to address the added ethical complexities of conducting SUD and HIV clinical research.

The negative results of the phase III trial of anti-cocaine and nicotine vaccines conducted to date suggest that a number of major technical challenges need to be overcome before vaccines are approved for clinical use. A significant challenge of antidrug vaccines is the unpredictability of antibody levels in vaccinated patients and the relationship between those levels and vaccine efficacy. Another challenge is the availability of endpoints that can meet regulatory approval for this type of treatment approach. Furthermore, given that nicotine replacement therapy, bupropion, and varenicline are approved by the FDA for nicotine dependence, anti-nicotine vaccines are expected to demonstrate better efficacy than those medications (Hall and Gartner 2011).

A significant clinical benefit of antidrug vaccines is that they can produce acceptable levels of antibodies after a schedule of injections is administered days or weeks apart. Therefore, these vaccines have long-lasting effects and do not require daily dosing. This is particularly relevant for the treatment of SUDs because of the low treatment adherence of this population and a long-acting formulation will improve the chances of treatment success (Hall et al. 2004).

It has been reported that about two thirds of patients with SUDs have other psychiatric disorders. The fact that biologics do not have effects on the brain makes them good candidates for the treatment of SUDs in patients with comorbid psychiatric disorders because they unlikely affect the outcome of the comorbidities. Also, because biologics have no abuse liability, there is no risk that SUD patients will became addicted to biologics, which is not the case for some pharmacotherapies for SUDs. Therefore, biologics can be a safe alternative for individuals with SUD and comorbid psychiatric disorders, without the risk of acquiring a new drug addiction.

Because of the great success of prophylactic vaccines for infectious diseases, the public in general could have the misconception that an antidrug vaccine is the panacea that will solve the drug abuse problem. In fact, often, subjects recruited for antidrug vaccine clinical trials have high expectations of their efficacy and can be rapidly frustrated when they do not improve right away. Therefore, it is important that anti-addiction vaccine trials provide an adequate and comprehensive educational scheme for the participants as well as the general public (Young et al. 2012). It is important to ensure that clinical trial participants and, hopefully, patients fully understand the risks and benefits of biologics and seek this therapeutic approach with the sincere intention to stop drug use.

21.4 Monoclonal Antibodies

There is no doubt that the discovery of monoclonal antibodies (MAbs) revolutionized immunology and the treatment of many clinical conditions, including SUDs. Recent advances have facilitated the development of techniques for preparing monoclonal antibodies, which have had a major impact on their rapid expansion, increased specificity, and number of potential applications. Monoclonal antibodies are being investigated as anti-inflammatory, antitumor, for passive immunization, and treatment of SUDs. Specifically, anti-SUD MAbs may be indicated to treat the actual addictive disorder (similar to vaccines) or drug overdose (Owens et al. 2011; Pitas et al. 2006).

One of the biggest advantages of MAbs is that the immune system of the host is circumvented and the antibodies can be administered in the amounts necessary to prevent the access of the drug of abuse to the brain. Therefore, MAbs to some extent eliminate the unpredictability of the production of antibodies, which is inherent to vaccines. On the other hand, MAbs are foreign proteins and cannot only produce anaphylaxis but also be rejected by the immune system by the production of antibodies against the MAbs. While clinical protocols can be more precise on the dose of the MAb, they cannot ignore the potential rate of elimination by the MAbs, which can be unpredictable. This can be an important issue when determining the risks/benefits of MAbs.

A major challenge in the development of mAbs is the choice of species for preclinical studies that can accurately predict their safety when they are administered to humans. Due to the high target and species specificity of mAbs, the use of rodents may not be appropriate, and sometimes, the only relevant species is a nonhuman primate (Chapman et al. 2009). Moreover, preclinical testing is challenging because MAbs are proteins with complex structures and can undergo posttranslational modifications such as glycosylation, and the preclinical evaluation should include an assessment of immunotoxicity and immunogenicity. Unwanted side effects of antibodies may be a consequence of cross-reactivity, i.e., unwanted binding to molecular structures similar to the original epitope. Therefore, unwanted immunogenicity associated with mAb products can be a problem when designing clinical trials because they may result in adverse effects and reduction in clinical efficacy (Liedert et al. 2007; Chapman et al. 2010; Food and Drug Administration 2015; Lynch et al. 2009; Schneider 2008a, b; Chapman et al. 2012; Glassy and Gupta 2014; Roberts et al. 2013).

Currently, a phase I clinical trial of ch-mAb7F9, a monoclonal antibody against methamphetamine, was recently completed and is registered in clinicaltrials.gov (NCT01603147). The primary objective was to determine the safety and tolerability of single, ascending intravenous doses of ch-mAb7F9 in healthy subjects. Each subject received a single dose of ch-mAb7F9 or placebo (saline). The trial accepted males and females 18–50 years of age. Female subjects were required to have non-childbearing potential or use a secure method of contraception because of the unknown risks of the mAb on the fetus. Study applicants who were males had to avoid getting a woman pregnant or donate sperm for 90 days after the last dose given the unknown teratogenicity of the antibodies. Subjects were excluded if they had a history of treatment with a monoclonal antibody in the past year to avoid a potential cross-reactivity. Also, applicants with history of severe allergy were excluded given the high risk of anaphylaxis in this population. Given the hepatic metabolism and renal excretion of the mAb, applicants with liver or kidney problems or taking medications that can affect those organs were excluded. Other exclusion criteria were routinary and can be consulted in the website.

In principle, the ethical requirements for clinical trials of mAbs are not different from the general requirements and regulatory framework of other potential therapeutics. The identification of a safety problem might not necessarily mean that a mAb is not suitable for the treatment of a particular disease. Specific measures like adequate safety endpoints can be implemented that might nevertheless allow for a relatively safe administration of such drugs to patients (Schneider 2008a, b). Similar to vaccines, MAbs for drug addictions do not require a daily dose, which represents an advantage in the treatment of SUDs because they improve the chances of treatment success (Hall et al. 2004).

21.5 Enzymes

Highly efficient enzymes can bind and degrade cocaine in the bloodstream at a very high rate and are investigated for the treatment of SUDs and drug intoxications. These enzymes act directly on the cocaine molecule itself to rapidly degrade it before it gets into the brain. This approach has shown promise in preclinical studies. Studies in humans suggest that enzymes are safe and have no risk of drug interactions or abuse liability (Gorelick 2008; Narasimhan et al. 2012). The enzymes that have tested in humans are a butyrylcholinesterase (BchE) and a cocaine esterase. Their mechanism of action is similar but the investigated clinical indications are different. BchE has been evaluated for the treatment of cocaine dependence (www.clinicaltrials.gov NCT01887366) and a cocaine esterase for the treatment of cocaine overdose (NCT01846481).

One of the risks of the administration of BchE to humans is the off-target hydrolysis of acetylcholine. To solve this issue, a computational modeling approach identified a variant of BchE that hydrolyzes acetylcholine less efficiently. Another risk is the presence of BchE in β-amyloid plaques in patients with Alzheimer's disease, which has also been technically circumvented (Murthy et al. 2015). Unfortunately, as a result of the highly elaborated production of this enzyme, the cost of its production is high and it is expected that, if approved by the FDA, the cost to patients will also be high. This may be an important limitation in terms of access to all populations.

BchE's rapid enzyme action causes a sharp rise in plasma levels of two cocaine metabolites: benzoic acid (BA) and ecgonine methyl ester (EME), which is a smooth muscle relaxant that is mildly hypotensive and weakly rewarding. A recent report suggests that a single administration of a high cocaine dose (that could be lethal) after the administration of the enzyme did not affect blood pressure and the animals survived (Murthy et al. 2015). The hypotension associated to EME does not seem a significant risk factor. However, clinically, it is possible that a cocaine user who takes very large amounts in an effort to compensate the accelerated cocaine metabolism by the enzyme may suffer toxicity from the sudden increase of EME and BA. So, it may be worthwhile to describe this risk in the consent form to potential study participants.

Clinical studies of a recombinant human serum albumin (HSA)-mutated BchE (TV-1380) have focused on facilitating cocaine abstinence in cocaine-dependent subjects. Subjects assigned to TV-1380 150 or 300 mg were administered one intramuscular injection once weekly over 12 weeks (NCT01887366). The protocol included male and female subjects aged 18–60 years old who were seeking treatment. To avoid enrolling professional subjects, study applicants had to meet criteria for cocaine dependence and provide at least one urine sample positive for cocaine during the 2-week screening period. Applicants were excluded if they had liver function problems or allergy to BchE, human serum albumin (HSA), or any other component of the formulation. The protocol excluded individuals who have been exposed to organophosphates within 60 days preceding screening because they can irreversibly inactivate acetylcholinesterase. Women of childbearing potential who did not practice an acceptable method of birth control and pregnant or nursing women were excluded because of the potential risk of teratogenicity.

The cocaine esterase is isolated from bacteria that grow in the soil surrounding coca plants. It hydrolyzes cocaine faster than the natural enzyme and to release ecgonine methyl ester and benzoic acid. This enzyme is under evaluation in a phase II clinical trial for cocaine overdose treatment. The protocol includes males and females between 21 and 50 years of age. To prevent the risk of congenital anomalies, males have to agree to refrain from sperm donations for the entire duration of the study and for at least 90 days after the last dose of study drug and males with childbearing potential must agree to use a contraception barrier for at least 28 days after the last dose of study medication. Females also have to agree to avoid becoming pregnant during the study. In addition, subjects should not have clinically significant history of cardiac disease and QTcF greater than or equal to 450 for male subjects and 470 for female subjects as measure and history of clinically significant severe anaphylactic reactions (Fang et al. 2014; Meyer et al. 2014; Nasser et al. 2014).

The clinical trials of these two enzymes have served to provide a good idea to investigators, IRBs, and regulatory agencies of the ethics committees of the risks and benefits of this approach. Hopefully, studies will demonstrate that enzymes are safe and effective for the treatment of SUDs and drug overdose and that benefits clearly outweigh any possible risks.

21.6 Biosimilars

The regulatory approval of traditional generic drug products depends, in part, on the determination that the active substance of the generic is structurally the same as and bioequivalent to the reference product. Generic versions of biologically derived products pose complex regulatory and ethical issues. Manufacturers of generic products are now seeking approval of follow-on versions of a number of biologics and it has become necessary to address their ethics and regulatory approval (Kingham and Lietzan 2008).

The Patient Protection and Affordable Care Act amended the Public Health Service Act and the Biologics Price Competition and Innovation Act created a pathway for abbreviated licensure of products that are biosimilar to an FDA-licensed biologic product. FDA requires that the licensed biosimilar meet their rigorous standards of safety and efficacy and that the public can rely on the biosimilar product just as they would the reference product (Food and Drug Administration 2015). IRBs are expected to review clinical protocols with biosimilars and may use the respective FDA guidelines to assess the risk/benefit of testing a new generic biologic product.

21.7 Conclusion

Clinical research is based on the understanding that the risks to study participants are ethically and morally acceptable given the potential benefits of the tested intervention. These risks are justified only when the studies are conducted with the best possible scientific methods. Even if a clinical trial is ethically justified, society is getting short changed if the science is inadequate (Kleber 1989). So far, biologics appear safe for SUDs but the efficacy has not been established. New and more potent biologics are being developed which hopefully will improve their efficacy without additional risks. Bioethicists, IRBs, and regulatory agencies will likely find new ethical challenges with the new biologics. Hopefully, those challenges will be resolved and biologics will be approved by the FDA for SUDs and become part of the therapeutic armamentarium to curtail this important public health problem.

References

Adler MW. Human subject issues in drug abuse research. College on problems of drug dependence. Drug Alcohol Depend. 1995;37:167–75.

Almond B. Drug use and abuse: the ethical issues. Ciba Found Symp. 1992;166:277–83.

Ashcroft RE, Franey C. Further ethical and social issues in using a cocaine vaccine: response to Hall and Carter. J Med Ethics. 2004;30:341–3.

Bailey TC, Sugarman J. Social justice and HIV vaccine research in the age of pre-exposure prophylaxis and treatment as prevention. Curr HIV Res. 2013;11:473–80.

Bonese KF, Wainer BH, Fitch FW, Rothberg RM, Schuster CR. Changes in heroin self-administration by a rhesus monkey after morphine immunisation. Nature. 1974;252:708–10.

Carroll KM, Kiluk BD, Nich C, DeVito EE, Decker S, LaPaglia D, et al. Toward empirical identification of a clinically meaningful indicator of treatment outcome: features of candidate indicators and evaluation of sensitivity to treatment effects and relationship to one year follow up cocaine use outcomes. Drug Alcohol Depend. 2014;137:3–19.

Carter A, Hall W. Ethical implications of research on craving. Addict Behav. 2013;38:1593–9.

Chapman K, Pullen N, Coney L, Dempster M, Andrews L, Bajramovic J, et al. Preclinical development of monoclonal antibodies: considerations for the use of non-human primates. MAbs. 2009;1:505–16.

Chapman KL, Andrews L, Bajramovic JJ, Baldrick P, Black LE, Bowman CJ, et al. The design of chronic toxicology studies of monoclonal antibodies: implications for the reduction in use of non-human primates. Regul Toxicol Pharmacol. 2012;62:347–54.

Chapman KL, Pullen N, Andrews L, Ragan I. The future of non-human primate use in mAb development. Drug Discov Today. 2010;15:235–42.

Cohen PJ. Immunization for prevention and treatment of cocaine abuse: legal and ethical implications. Drug Alcohol Depend. 1997;48:167–74.

Fang L, Chow KM, Hou S, Xue L, Chen X, Rodgers DW, et al. Rational design, preparation, and characterization of a therapeutic enzyme mutant with improved stability and function for cocaine detoxification. ACS Chem Biol. 2014;9:1764–72.

Food and Drug Administration. Biosimilars. 2015. http://www.fda.gov/Drugs/GuidanceComplianceRegulatoryInformation/Guidances/ucm290967.htm

Garner SA, Anude CJ, Adams E, Dawson L. Ethical considerations in HIV prevention and vaccine research in resource-limited settings. J Acquir Immune Defic Syndr. 2014;67:77–83.

Glassy MC, Gupta R. Technical and ethical limitations in making human monoclonal antibodies (an overview). Methods Mol Biol. 2014;1060:9–36.

Gorelick DA. Pharmacokinetic approaches to treatment of drug addiction. Expert Rev Clin Pharmacol. 2008;1:277–90.

Grady C. Ethics of vaccine research. Nat Immunol. 2004;5:465–8.

Hall W, Carter L, Morley KI. Neuroscience research on the addictions: a prospectus for future ethical and policy analysis. Addict Behav. 2004;29:1481–95.

Hall W, Gartner C. Ethical and policy issues in using vaccines to treat and prevent cocaine and nicotine dependence. Curr Opin Psychiatry. 2011;24:191–6.

Hasman A, Holm S. Nicotine conjugate vaccine: is there a right to a smoking future? J Med Ethics. 2004;30:344–5.

Henderson GE. The ethics of HIV "cure" research: what can we learn from consent forms? AIDS Res Hum Retroviruses. 2015;31:56–63.

Kantak KM. Vaccines against drugs of abuse: a viable treatment option? Drugs. 2003;63:341–52.

Katsnelson A. Ethical quagmire awaits vaccine for cocaine addiction. Nat Med. 2004;10:1007.

Kiluk BD, Nich C, Witkiewitz K, Babuscio TA, Carroll KM. What happens in treatment doesn't stay in treatment: cocaine abstinence during treatment is associated with fewer problems at follow-up. J Consult Clin Psychol. 2014;82:619–27.

Kingham R, Klasa G, Hessler Carver K. Key regulatory guidelines for the development of biologics in the United States and Europe. In: Wang W, Singh M, editors. Biological drug products: development and strategies. 1st ed. Hoboken, New Jersey: John Wiley & Sons, Inc.; 2014.

Kingham RF, Lietzan E. Current regulatory and legal considerations for follow-on biologics. Clin Pharmacol Ther. 2008;84:633–5.

Kleber HD. Drug abuse liability testing: human subject issues. NIDA Res Monogr. 1989;92:341–56.

Lee JD, Friedmann PD, Boney TY, Hoskinson Jr RA, McDonald R, Gordon M, et al. Extended-release naltrexone to prevent relapse among opioid dependent, criminal justice system involved adults: rationale and design of a randomized controlled effectiveness trial. Contemp Clin Trials. 2015;41:110–7.

Liedert B, Bassus S, Schneider CK, Kalinke U, Lower J. Safety of phase I clinical trials with monoclonal antibodies in Germany—the regulatory requirements viewed in the aftermath of the TGN1412 disaster. Int J Clin Pharmacol Ther. 2007;45:1–9.

Lo B, Grady C. Ethical considerations in HIV cure research: points to consider. Curr Opin HIV AIDS. 2013;8:243–9.

Lynch CM, Hart BW, Grewal IS. Practical considerations for nonclinical safety evaluation of therapeutic monoclonal antibodies. MAbs. 2009;1:2–11.

Mendelson JH. Protection of participants and experimental design in clinical abuse liability testing. Br J Addict. 1991;86:1543–8.

Meyer MR, Schutz A, Maurer HH. Contribution of human esterases to the metabolism of selected drugs of abuse. Toxicol Lett. 2014;232:159–66.

Montoya I. Immunotherapies for drug addictions. Adicciones. 2008;20:111–5.

Murthy V, Geng L, Gao Y, Zhang B, Miller JD, Reyes S, et al. Reward and toxicity of cocaine metabolites generated by cocaine hydrolase. Cell Mol Neurobiol. 2015;35(6):819–26.

Narasimhan D, Woods JH, Sunahara RK. Bacterial cocaine esterase: a protein-based therapy for cocaine overdose and addiction. Future Med Chem. 2012;4:137–50.

Nasser AF, Fudala PJ, Zheng B, Liu Y, Heidbreder C. A randomized, double-blind, placebo-controlled trial of RBP-8000 in cocaine abusers: pharmacokinetic profile of rbp-8000 and cocaine and effects of RBP-8000 on cocaine-induced physiological effects. J Addict Dis. 2014;33:289–302.

Owens SM, Atchley WT, Hambuchen MD, Peterson EC, Gentry WB. Monoclonal antibodies as pharmacokinetic antagonists for the treatment of (+)-methamphetamine addiction. CNS Neurol Disord Drug Targets. 2011;10:892–8.

Pitas G, Laurenzana EM, Williams DK, Owens SM, Gentry WB. Anti-phencyclidine monoclonal antibody binding capacity is not the only determinant of effectiveness, disproving the concept that antibody capacity is easily surmounted. Drug Metab Dispos. 2006;34:906–12.

Pravetoni M, Le NM, Tucker AM, Harmon TM, Hawley TM, Portoghese PS, et al. Reduced antinociception of opioids in rats and mice by vaccination with immunogens containing oxycodone and hydrocodone haptens. J Med Chem. 2013;56:915–23.

Pravetoni M, Raleigh MD, Le NM, Tucker AM, Harmon TM, Jones JM, et al. Co-administration of morphine and oxycodone vaccines reduces the distribution of 6-monoacetylmorphine and oxycodone to brain in rats. Vaccine. 2012;30:4617–24.

Roberts SA, Andrews PA, Blanset D, Flagella KM, Gorovits B, Lynch CM, et al. Considerations for the nonclinical safety evaluation of antibody drug conjugates for oncology. Regul Toxicol Pharmacol. 2013;67:382–91.

Schneider CK. First-in-human trials with therapeutic proteins: regulatory rethink? Expert Rev Clin Pharmacol. 2008a;1:327–31.

Schneider CK. Monoclonal antibodies – regulatory challenges. Curr Pharm Biotechnol. 2008b;9:431–8.

Sugarman J, Rose SM, Metzger D. Ethical issues in HIV prevention research with people who inject drugs. Clin Trials. 2014;11:239–45.

Wolters A, de Wert G, van Schayck O, Horstman K. Vaccination against smoking: an annotated agenda for debate. A review of scientific journals, 2001-13. Addiction. 2014a;109:1268–73.

Wolters A, de Wert G, van Schayck O, Horstman K. Constructing a trial as a personal lifestyle change project: participants' experiences in a clinical study for nicotine vaccination. Soc Sci Med. 2014b;104:116–23.

Young MJ, Sisti DA, Rimon-Greenspan H, Schwartz JL, Caplan AL. Immune to addiction: the ethical dimensions of vaccines against substance abuse. Nat Immunol. 2012;13:521–4.

Index

A

Acetylcholine (ACh), 10, 155, 191–192, 331
Acyl loop back doors, BChE, 190–192
Addiction pharmacotherapy
  cocaine esterase (CocE)
    dose-response analysis, 158
    double mutant (DM), 158–159
    polyethylene glycol groups, 159
    principles of reinforcement theory, 157
    self-administration, 157
  cocaine hydrolases (CocH), 159–161
  toxic effects, 157
Addiction vaccines, B cells specific
  responses to immunization, 373–375
  T cell-dependent B cell responses, 372–373
Adenovirus-based anti-nicotine vaccine HexonAM1, 241–242
Adenovirus-based vaccines. *See also* Disrupted adenovirus vaccine (dAd5GNE)
  adenovirus-based anti-nicotine vaccine HexonAM1, 241–242
  anti-adenovirus immunity, dAd5GNE efficacy, 237
  capsid, immunogenic properties, 231
  cystic fibrosis transmembrane conductance regulator (CFTR) coding, 230–231
  dAd5GNE
    CNS protection and redistribution of cocaine, 237–238
    design, 234–236
    immune response, 236–237
    protection in binge drug use, 239
    reductions in cocaine self-administration, 240
    suppression of cocaine-induced behavior, 238–239
  gene transfer vector, 230–231
  hapten-carrier addictive molecule vaccines, 232–233
  potential of, 242
  safety, 240–241
  for substance use disorders, 233–234
  therapeutics, 230–231
Adenovirus serotype 5 (Ad5) proteins, 404–405
Adjuvant-incorporated ID nicotine vaccination, 316–317
Adjuvants. *See also* Cytokines; Hapten–protein conjugates
  aluminum salts, 412, 413
  in animal studies, 413–414
  categories, 414–415
  CpG TLR-agonist, 19
  encapsulation in nanoparticles (SVP), 260
  function, 414–415
  haptens and protein carriers, 412
  in licensed vaccines, 412–413
  monophosphoryl lipid A (MPLA), 413
  MorHap-TT conjugate, 415
  nanoparticle design, selection and development
    antigen exposure, 258
    AS04, TLR agonist-based composition, 258
    cytokine production
    dendritic cells (DC), 258
    imiquimod, 259
    immune responses, 259
    inflammatory cytokine induction in vitro, 260–261

I.D. Montoya (ed.), *Biologics to Treat Substance Use Disorders: Vaccines, Monoclonal Antibodies, and Enzymes*, DOI 10.1007/978-3-319-23150-1

Adjuvants. *See also* Cytokines; Hapten–protein conjugates (*cont.*)
micro- and nanocarriers, 259
pattern recognition receptors (PRRs), 258
polylactide-co-glycolide (PLGA), 258
PRR ligand, 259
rapid infiltration, 261–262
systemic inflammatory cytokines production (*see* Cytokines)
TLRs, 258–259
phospholipid–cholesterol bilayer, 415
for substance abuse vaccines, 415
alum, 297–298
antigens and immunogenic epitopes attachment, 299
ASO3 and ASO4, 298
bacterial flagellin, 299
combinations, 300–301
costimulatory pathways, 296–297
CpG oligonucleotides, 299
D2-D3 hypervariable flagellin domains, 300
entolimod, 299–300
formulation complexities, 302
humanized mice (HM), 301–302
MF59, 298
protein vaccines, 296
Th1-biased response, 299
tetanus toxoid (TT), 415
Affinity enhancement, hapten design
hapten halogenation, 349–350
structural flexibility, 348–349
AIDSVAX® protein, 78
AlbuBChE (recombinant human serum albumin-fused CocH1), 206–207
Albu-CocH, 206–207
Albu-CocH1, 206–207
Alum, 297–298
Aluminum salts, adjuvants, 412, 413
ALVAC-AIDSVAX vaccine, 81
Amino-acid mutations to stabilize oligomer structure, 215–217
Animal rule, biologics, 428
Anti-addiction vaccine, hapten design. *See* Hapten design for anti-addiction vaccine development
Antibody-targeted epitope, 81–82
Anti-cocaine, 85
antibodies, 26
IgG, 30
immunity, 232
monoclonal antibodies
action of, 109
blood-brain barrier, 113
catalytic antibodies, 112
chemical antagonism, 110
cocaethylene, 113–114
cocaine, 113
environment-induced cocaine-seeking behavior, 110
Fab fragments, 111–112
human addicts/abusers, 116
murine and human/chimeric, 110–111
pharmacokinetic antagonism, 110
pharmacokinetics, 112–113
rehabilitation facilities, 109
self-administration, 114–116
toxic effects, 114
use of, 109
vaccine, 27
Antidrug vaccines, 167, 233, 429–431
Antigen ovalbumin (OVA), 286, 314
Antigens and immunogenic epitopes attachment, 299
Antigen-specific B cells detection
fluorescent antigen-based magnetic enrichment, 376
hapten-specific B cells, analysis, 376
magnetic enrichment, 376–377
multiparameter flow cytometry analysis, 377–379
phycoerythrin (PE), 375–376
transgenic mice, 375
unimmunized mouse, 375
Anti-HIV immunogens, 85
Anti-METH chimeric mAb7F9
administration, 136–137
clinical safety, 137
clinical testing, 139
design and development, 135–136
duration, 136, 137
ECG, 137
ELISA, 137
HACA, 137
human phase, 136, 137
pharmacokinetic parameters, 137
physical examinations, 137
physiological recycling, 137–138
predicted serum mAb concentrations, 138–139
properties, 137
treatment, 139
Anti-METH monoclonal antibodies (anti-METH mAb)
action mechanism

effects, METH brain concentrations, 123, 124
locomotor activity, 124
measurement, 124
reduction, 124
volume of distribution, human, 123
advantages and disadvantages, 122
clinical testing, 121
duration of action, 125
high-affinity METH binding sites, 121
mAb7F9 (*see* Methamphetamine (METH))
and MCV, 122
medications and preclinical testing
haptens usage, 131, 132
K_d value, 127
large-scale production, 127–128
mAb6H4, 128–130
MCV, 128
MO10, 132
mouse antiserum, 128
non-amphetamine-like stimulant drugs, 132
pretreatment model, 129–130
rats, 130–131
serum concentrations, 129, 131
protective effects, 121
reduction, 121–122
Anti-nicotine
antibodies, 9, 271–273
HexonAM1, 241–242
induction, 269, 272
Anti-SUD MAbs, 432
Anti-V1V2 Abs, 80
ASO3 and ASO4, 298
A199S/S287G/A328W/Y332G mutant
activity validation, 204
AlbuBChE, 206–207
Albu-CocH, 206–207
Albu-CocH1, 206–207
catalytic efficiency, 204
in cocaine addiction treatment, 206–207
CocH1, 206
HSA-fused form, 206
human BChE, 204
human serum albumin (HSA), 206
inhibition rate constants, 207
time-dependent radiometric data, 204
TV-1380, 206–207
Atrazine–protein conjugates, 407
Azo coupling, 405–406

B
Bacterial cocaine esterase
active sites, 150
cellular characterization, 151
double mutant (DM) CocE
administration, 153
capacity, 152
effects, 153
elimination, 153
hydrolyze norcocaine and cocaethylene, 153
peptide degradation, 155
proteolysis, 153
rats, 151
repeated doses effects, 153, 154
rhesus monkeys, 153–155
human BChE, 151
in vivo function, 151
isolated and purified, 150
molecular dynamics simulations, 151
Rhodococcus bacterium, 150
B cell mechanisms
antigen-specific B cells detection
analysis, 376
magnetic enrichment, 376–377
multiparameter flow cytometry analysis, 377–379
B cell receptor (BCR), 370
cellular biology and phenotypes, 369–370
conjugate vaccines against drugs of abuse, 390
drugs of abuse haptens and addiction vaccines
responses to immunization, 373–375
T cell-dependent B cell responses, 372–373
hapten design (*see* Naïve B cells activation)
immature lymphocyte precursors of, 369–370
individual variability in vaccine efficacy, 389–390
ontogeny, 370
oxycodone-based hapten (6OXY), 385–387
T cell-dependent B cell generation, 370–371
vaccine efficacy (*see* hapten-specific B cells)
vaccine formulations, 385–387
V(D)J recombination, 370
BChE. *See* Butyrylcholinesterase (BChE)
Benzoylecgonine (BE), 26, 111, 187, 236

Biodegradable polymeric particles, 251
Biologics
  animal rule, 428
  antibodies production, 426
  controversy, 426
  Institutional Review Boards (IRBs), 427
  Investigational New Drug (IND) application, 427
  methamphetamine addiction treatment, 427
  nicotine and cocaine addiction treatment, 427
  pharmacokinetic antagonism, 426
  pharmacotherapies for SUDs, 428
  phases, 428
  preclinical models, 427
  public health benefit, 426
  regulatory agencies, 427
  SUDs treatment, 427
Biosimilars, 435
bNAbs. *See* Broadly neutralizing monoclonal antibodies (bNAbs)
Bovine serum albumin (BSA), 28, 232, 403
Broadly neutralizing monoclonal antibodies (bNAbs), 83, 87
B subunit, cholera toxin, 404
Bupropion, 1, 8, 431
Butyrylcholinesterase (BChE). *See also* Cocaine hydrolase (CocH)
  active site, 186–192
  cocaine metabolism, 187
  ecgonine methyl ester (EME), 187–188
  in human serum, 187–189
  native enzymes, 188
  positron emission tomography (PET) visualization, 188–189
  pseudocholinesterase, 188–189
  structure, 189–190, 191
  substrate binding, 188
  wild-type, 188

C
Carbodiimide
  conjugation chemistry, 405–406
  coupling chemistry, 404
Chemokines, NAFL treatment, 315–316
Chinese hamster ovary (CHO) cells, 111, 135, 214
Cholera toxin B (CTB), 2, 28, 29, 84–85, 232, 403
Classical force field, transition-state modeling and simulation, 198–199
Cocaethylene
  anti-cocaine mAbs effect, 113–114
  and norcocaine, catalytic activities, 210–211
Cocaine, 113
  anti-cocaine antibodies, 26
  brain disorders, 25
  cardiovascular system, 25–26
  CBT, 33
  drug abuse, 33
  drug-related ED visits, 25
  drug target consideration, 330–331
  esterase, 434
  group sex participation, 97
  hydrolysis
    acylation and deacylation stages, 195–196
    A328W/Y332A and A328W/Y332G mutants, 192–193
    catalytic activity, 193
    chemical reaction pathway, 194–195, 196
    cocaine methyl ester group, 192
    ES binding process, 193
    MD simulations, 192
    potential of mean force (PMF) simulations, 193
    prereactive ES complex, 193–194
    relative free energy barriers, 194
    substrate binding, 192
    targeted molecular dynamics (TMD), 193–194
  immunotherapies, 27–29, 93
  inactive metabolites, 26, 33
  intravenous route, 27
  linker composition, 340–341
  linker introduction, structure modification, 333–334
  myocardial infarction, 26
  optimal pharmacotherapeutic interventions, 26
  "priming effect", 33
  SAMHSA, 25
  stability enhancement, 351–355
  TA-CD vaccinations, 29–33
  transporter-based antagonist, 27
  underwent diagnostic angiography, 26
  UNODC, 25
  vaccine-induced antibodies, 26
  vaccines, 3
    Ab levels, 75
    bioethical, legal and policy issues, 76–77
    cholera toxin B-based vaccines, 75–76
    CNS protection, 75

high-risk sexual behavior, 89–90
IgG antibody levels, 76
ImmuLogic product, 75
immunogens, 81
medicinal intervention, 90–91
molecular interactions, 88–89
TA-CD vaccine, 76
Cocaine esterase (CocE)
addiction pharmacotherapy
dose-response analysis, 158
double mutant (DM), 158–159
polyethylene glycol groups, 159
principles of einforcement theory, 157
self-administration, 157
bacterial (*see* Bacterial cocaine esterase)
in brain, 212–213
Cocaine hydrolase (CocH)
BChE, 172, 173
BChE vector
animals, 176
cholinergic neurotransmission, 175
cocaine docking and catalysis, 175–176
cocaine reward, 177, 178
human, 176–177
overdose, 175
reduction, brain access, 175
reinstatement model, 176–177
threapy, 175
butyrylcholinesterase, 187–189
chemical reaction pathway, 194–195
enzyme treatments, rats, 173
hdAD, 173
human, 173
from human BChE
A199S/S287G/A328W/Y332G mutant, 204–207
catalytic activities against cocaethylene and norcocaine, 210–211
CocH2 and CocH3, 207–209
effectiveness, computational prediction, 211–213
investigation, 213
IND application, 183
iso-OMPA, 173
liver, 174–175
muscle, 174
PEGylation, 173
prechemical reaction process, 192–194
protein engineering and biological half-life
amino-acid mutations to stabilize oligomer structure, 215–217
fusion proteins, 217
posttranslational modifications and pegylation, 214–215
standards, manufacturing process, 183
tissue tropism, 174
Cocaine pharmacotherapies
abuse liability, 147–148
active and passive immunization, 161
addiction (*see* Addiction pharmacotherapy)
advantages, 162
alkaloid, 145
behavioral measures, 148–149
behavioral therapies, 162–163
characterization, enzymatic therapy
bacterial cocaine esterase, 150–155
chemical structure, cocaine, 149, 150
human butyrylcholinesterase, 155–157
native butyrylcholinesterase activity, 149–150
consumption, 145
evaluation, humans, 161
in vivo evaluation, 148
toxic effects
body and brain, 146
cardiac-related complications, 146
hyperthermia, 146
myocardial infarction, 146
overdose, 146–147
recommended treatment, 146
sympathomimetic, 146
vasoconstrictive, 146
vaccine and gene transfer, 162
CocE. *See* Cocaine esterase (CocE)
CocH. *See* Cocaine hydrolase (CocH)
CocH2 and CocH3, improved catalytic efficiency
AChE and BChE, molar concentrations, 208
advanced viral gene transfer vector (AAV-VIP-mCocH), 209
amino-acid mutations, 207–208
anti-aggression and anti-obesity effects, 209
catalytic efficiency, 209
cholinergic synapses, 208
cocaine-induced hyperactivity, 208
CocH2 and CocH3, 208
convulsions and lethality, 208
E12-4/CocH2, 207
gene therapy for cocaine abuse, 209
human BChE (hBChE)-based, 209
lentiviral vector, 207
mouse neuromuscular junction, 208
plasma cocaine hydrolase activity, 209
prophylaxis, 208
stable CHO-S cell line, 207

CocH2 and CocH3, improved catalytic efficiency (*cont.*)
in vitro and in vivo testing, 208–209
wide-type human BChE, 208
CocH1-based gene therapy, 206
Computational enzyme redesign
amino-acid mutations, 195, 197
A328W/Y332A/A328W/Y332G mutant, 197
classical force field, 198–199
free energy perturbation on rate-determining transition state (FEP-TS), 199–201
QM/MM and QM/MM-FE calculations, 197–198
systematic virtual screening, 201–203
Conditioned place preference (CPP), 71
Congenital anomalies and enzymes, 434
Conjugation chemistry, hapten–protein conjugates
azo coupling, 405–406
carbodiimide chemistry, 406
imine formation, 406
photoactivatable cross-linking approach, 406
Conjugation method, heptan design
bromide-derivatized haptens, 344
direct amide bond formation, 343
functionality, 342–343
hapten–protein conjugation, 343
maleimide-containing activated carboxylic acid, 343
protein lysine residues, 343
reverse amide bond formation, 343–344
squaric acid diamides production, 344
thiol-containing hapten, 343
Conventional adjuvants, skin vaccination, 312–313
Coupling ratios, 409
CRM_{197}, 402–403
Cross-reacting material of diphtheria toxin (CRM_{197}), 402–403
Cytokines
antigen-containing SVP, 266–267
focused local, 264–265
nanoparticle-encapsulated R848, 262
nanoparticle-encapsulated *vs.* free R848, 264
serum concentrations, 266
SVP-encapsulated, 264
SVP-R848, 265–266
systemic inflammatory, 265–266

D
dAd5GNE. *See* Disrupted adenovirus vaccine (dAd5GNE)
Damage associated molecule patterns (DAMPs), 315
DAMPs. *See* Damage associated molecule patterns (DAMPs)
D2-D3 hypervariable flagellin domains, 300
Dinitrophenyl (DNP)-BSA conjugates, 407
Diphtheria-tetanus-pertussis (DTaP), 85–86
Diphtheria toxoid (DT), 252, 402–403
Disrupted adenovirus vaccine (dAd5GNE)
CNS protection and redistribution of cocaine, 237–238
cocaine-induced behavior, suppression, 238–239
cocaine self-administration reductions, 240
design, 234–236
dose escalation, 237
formulation buffer, 236
immune response, 236–237
protection in binge drug use, 239
DNA nanostructures, vaccines design. *See also* DNA-tetrahedron-SA platform, nicotine vaccines
biocompatible, 283
biodegradable polymer micro- or nanoparticles, 281
biomedical applications, 281, 282–283
DNA-nanoscaffolded vaccines, 286–287
immune stimulatory activity
DNAse I and III defects, 285
internalized CpG DNA, 284
macrophages and dendritic cells, 285
microbial DNA, 284
myeloid differentiation primary response 88 (MYD88)-mediated signaling pathway, 284
PAMPs, 284
sterile inflammation, 284
stimulator of interferon genes (STINGs), 284
systemic lupus erythematosus (SLE), 285
long-lived plasma cells (LLPCs), 280
memory B cells, 280
representative, 282–283
self-assembly, 282–283
toll-like receptor (TLR) ligands, 281
vaccine efficacy, 280
DNA-tetrahedron-SA platform, nicotine vaccines

antigen and adjuvants, co-delivery, 287
immunogenicity, 287–288
innate stimulatory effect, 288
modular optimizations, 289
nicotine-KLH (Nic-KLH) conjugates, 289
nicotine-SA conjugate, 287
nicotine-specific antibody response, 289
pharmacokinetics, 287–288
soluble Nic-SA-CpG conjugates, 289
structural features, 287–288
types, 287–288
Drug exposed, 425
Drug naïve, 425
Drug target consideration, hapten design
cocaine, 330–331
heroin, 328–330
methamphetamine, 331
nicotine, 331
oxycodone, 330

E

Ecgonine methyl ester (EME), 2, 27, 111, 187, 330, 358
Electrostatic potential (ESP), QM/MM method, 198
ELISA. *See* Enzyme-linked immunosorbent assay (ELISA)
Enantiopurity, hapten design
antibodies binding affinity, 357–358
cross-reactivity, 358
linker introduction, 357
methamphetamine, 356–357
nicotine haptens, 357
Entolimod, 68, 299–300
Enzyme-linked immunosorbent assay (ELISA), 68, 137, 356
Enzymes. *See also* Cocaine hydrolase (CocH)
benzoic acid (BA) and ecgonine methyl ester (EME), 433–434
butyrylcholinesterase (BchE), 433
cocaine esterase, 434
congenital anomalies, 434
and drug intoxications, 433
viral gene transfer (*see* Viral gene transfer, enzymes)
EPD. *See* Epidermal powder delivery (EPD)
Epidermal powder delivery (EPD), 320–321
Epitopes
antibody-targeted, 81–82
dominant mouse T-cell, 268
HIV protein immunogens, 83
memory, 268
vaccines, 83–84
Ethical considerations, SUD
biologics, 426–428
biosimilars, 435
clinical studies, 425–426
enzymes, 433–434
monoclonal antibodies, 432–433
vaccines (*see* Vaccines)

F

Fab fragments, 111–112
Feasibility and translation
cessation *vs.* relapse prevention, 58
drug switching, 58
preexisting antibodies, 58–59
treatment, 58
vaccine components, 58
Fisher's exact test, 17
Free energy perturbation on rate-determining transition state (FEP-TS)
amino-acid residue, 200
catalytic efficiency, 201
enzymatic reactions, 200
Gibbs free energy change, 200
rate-determining transition states, 199–200
Freund's adjuvant elicited nic · IgG, 14
Fusion proteins, 217

G

GMP grade KLH dimer (dKLH), 385–386
G-quadruplexes and i-motifs, 283

H

HACA. *See* Human anti-chimeric antibodies (HACA)
Hapten(s)
clustering, 355–356
halogenation, 349–350
selection, 257–258
Hapten-carrier addictive molecule vaccines
anti-cocaine immunity, 232
anti-methamphetamine antibody titers, 232
bovine serum albumin (BSA), 232
cholera toxin B, 232
heroin self-administration behavior, 232
keyhole limpet hemocyanin (KLH), 232
Nic002, 233

Hapten-carrier addictive molecule vaccines (*cont.*)
  nicotine addiction treatment, 233
  NicVax, phase III clinical trials, 233
  Pseudomonas aeruginosa recombinant exoprotein, 233
Hapten design for anti-addiction vaccine development
  active catalytic vaccine, 358–359
  clustering, 355–357
  conjugation method, 342–344
  drug target consideration
    cocaine, 330–331
    heroin, 328–330
    methamphetamine, 331
    nicotine, 331
    oxycodone, 330
  enantiopurity, 356–358
  hapten halogenation, 349–350
  immunopharmacotherapy, drugs of abuse targets, 327–328
  linker
    cocaine, 333–334, 340–341
    heroin, 332–333
    methamphetamine, 337
    nicotine, 334–337, 338–340
    oxycodone, 333
    peptidic linkers, 341–342
  multivalent haptens targeting
    multiple drugs, 345–346
    multiple species, 344–345
    one drug, 346–348
  stability enhancement
    cocaine, 351–355
    heroin, 351–352
  structural flexibility, 348–349
Hapten–KLH conjugate, 409
Hapten–protein conjugates. *See also* Vaccines against drugs of abuse
  carrier proteins
    adenovirus serotype 5 (Ad5) proteins, 404–405
    bovine serum albumin (BSA), 403
    B subunit, cholera toxin, 404
    CRM_{197}, 402–403
    human use, 403
    immunization, 403
    keyhole limpet hemocyanin (KLH), 403–404
    licensed polysaccharide conjugate vaccines, 402
    nicotine vaccine, 405
    polysaccharide conjugate vaccines, 403
    Pseudomonas aeruginosa exoprotein A (rEPA), 405
    substance abuse vaccines, 403, 405
    T-cell-dependent antibody response, 403
  conjugation chemistry
    azo coupling, 405–406
    carbodiimide chemistry, 406
    imine formation, 406
    photoactivatable cross-linking approach, 406
  hapten density and conjugate yield
    atrazine–protein conjugates, 407
    coupling ratios, 409
    definition, 407
    dinitrophenyl (DNP)-BSA conjugates, 407
    hapten–KLH conjugate, 409
    maleimide–thiol chemistry, 407–408
    METH-BSA conjugates, active immunization, 407
    MorHap conjugates, 407–408
    nicotine–DT conjugates, 407
    6-PrOxyHap conjugates, 409–410
    trinitrobenzenesulfonic acid (TNBS) assay, 408
    vaccines efficacy, 407
  hapten–protein conjugate, 411–412
  linker, 410–411
Hapten-specific B cells
  and addiction vaccines
    antigen-specific serum antibodies, 374
    booster injections, 375
    boost immunizations, 375
    hapten-carrier conjugate immunogens, 375
    high-affinity antibodies, 373–374
    high-affinity swIg memory B cells, 375
    T cell-dependent B cell activation, 374
    T cell-dependent B cell responses, 372–373
    weak immunogens, 375
  analysis, 376
  magnetic enrichment of, 376–377
  markers of vaccine efficacy
    in genetic backgrounds, 387–389
    prescription opioids, 379–380
  multiparameter flow cytometry analysis, 377–379
  naïve and early activated, frequency of, 389–390
HCV infection, 97
Helper-dependent adenoviral vector (hdAD), 170–173, 177, 178

Hemophilus influenza protein D, 402–403
Heroin vaccine
adjuvant, 49
carrier and hapten density, 48
drug target consideration, 328–330
efficacy
and metabolite pharmacokinetics, 51–53
morphine-associated behaviors in animals, 53–54
opioid doses, 51
immunogenicity
affinity and specificity, 49
antibody concentration, 49–50
opioid administration, 50
linker introduction, structure modification, 332–333
linker structure, 48
and morphine haptens, 329–330
opioid scaffold and linker position, 45–48
stability enhancement, 351–352
HexonAM1-vaccinated mice, 242
Highly active antiretroviral therapy (HAART), 86, 94
HIV-1-associated neurocognitive disorder (HAND), 88, 89
HIV vaccine trials
acquisition, 78–79
AIDSVAX® protein immunogen boosts, 78
ALVAC canarypox prime-AIDSVAX recombinant protein, 79
efforts, 81
high-risk sexual behavior, 89–90
human immune, 79–81
medicinal intervention, 90–91
medicinal prototypes, 85
molecular interactions, 88–89
non-HIV vaccines, 77
prevention, 86
primary evidence in humans, 87
RV144 trial, 78
STEP study, 78
vaccination/vaccine coadministration, 85–86
VaxGen trial, 78
viral subunit vaccines, 77–78
HSA-fused form A199S/S287G/A328W/Y332G mutant, 206
Human anti-chimeric antibodies (HACA), 137
Human brain microvascular endothelial cells, 88–89
Humanized mice (HM), 301–302
Human serum albumin (HSA), 162, 206, 434
huPBL-SCID mouse, 88

I
ICMVs. *See* Interbilayer-cross-linked multilamellar lipid vesicles (ICMVs)
Imine formation, conjugation chemistry, 406
Immunogenic skin vaccination
antigen-presenting cells (APCs), 311
dermal dendritic cells (DCs), 311
epidermal Langerhans cells (LCs), 311
hepatitis B vaccine (NCT02186977), 312
immune responses, 312
keyhole limpet hemocyanin (KLH), 312
in muscular tissue, 312
scarification, 311
smallpox vaccine, 311
stratum corneum (SC), 311
tuberculosis vaccine (MVA85A, NCT01954563), 312
vaccination routes, 311
Indoleamine-2, 3-dioxygenase (IDO), 285
Institutional Review Boards (IRBs), 427
Integrated immunologic design
lymph nodes (LNs), 256–257
mimic key recognition features, 256
Interbilayer-cross-linked multilamellar lipid vesicles (ICMVs), 281
Intradermal (ID) immunization
BCG vaccine, 318
ID adapter, 318–319
ID microinjection system, 319
microneedle (MN)-based device, 318–319
needle-free injection system, 319
rabies vaccine, 318
tuberculin for tuberculosis (TB), 318
Investigational New Drug (IND) application, 427

K
Keyhole limpet hemocyanin (KLH), 27, 28, 68
carrier proteins, 403–404
hapten-carrier addictive molecule vaccines, 232
immunogenic skin vaccination, 312
native KLH decamer (nKLH), 385–386
NIC-KLH vaccine, 11

L

Laser vaccine adjuvant (LVA), 314
Lesion-free skin vaccination
  BCG vaccine induced minimal local reactions, 320
  epidermal powder delivery (EPD), 320–321
  handheld laser- or MN-based EPD device, 321–322
  lipopolysaccharide (LPS) delivery, 320
  LPS/CpG adjuvant, local reactogenicity, 320–321
  microchannels (MC), 320
  micro-injuries, 320
  NicAb titer, 321
  powder nicotine vaccines, 321
  skin injury, 320
  skin morphology, 319–320
  transdermal vaccine delivery, 320
Licensed polysaccharide conjugate vaccines, 402
Licensed vaccines, 77, 412–413
Linker composition
  B cell receptors (BCRs), 338
  cocaine, 340–341
  nicotine, 338–340
  peptidic linkers, 341–342
Linker introduction, structure modification
  antibody binding, 332
  cocaine, 333–334
  heroin, 332–333
  methamphetamine, 337
  nicotine
    brain concentrations, 336
    comparison, 336
    competitive ELISA data, 336
    conjugation, 335
    high-affinity antibodies, 334
    immunogenicity, 337
    pyrrolidine amine, 334–335
    pyrrolidine nitrogen-linked nicotine vaccine, 335–336
  oxycodone, 333
  sites for, 332
Liposomes, 251
Long-lived plasma cells (LLPCs), 280
LVA. *See* Laser vaccine adjuvant (LVA)

M

mAb4G9, 132–133
Maleimide–thiol chemistry, 407–408
MCP-1 expression, 88
MCV. *See* METH-conjugate vaccine (MCV)
Memory epitopes, 268
Methamphetamine (METH)
  addictive drug, 120
  advantages, addiction therapy, 120, 121, 427
  anti-METH mAb (*see* Anti-METH monoclonal antibodies (anti-METH mAb))
  anti-METH polyclonal antibodies, 121
  CNS effects, 120, 139
  control, 121
  drug target consideration, 331
  in vivo elimination processes
    ch-mAb7F9 and METH $t_{1/2}$ values, 126
    maintaining functional capacity, 126
    regeneration, antibody binding capacity, 126, 127
  large doses, 139
  linker introduction, structure modification, 337
  mAb7F9 capacity
    doses, 133, 134
    elevations, 134–135
    higher doses, 135
    human, 134
    locomotor activity, 135
    and mAb4G9, 132–133
    male Sprague-Dawley rats, 134
    safety, 134
    treatment regimen, 133
  MCV, 121
  mechanisms of action, 120
  treatment, 139
Methamphetamine (MA) abuse
  administration, 68–69
  animal studies, 72–73
  antibody titers and affinity, 69–70
  anti-MA antibodies, 72
  behavior and physiology, 65–66
  construction, 67–68
  functional tests, 70–71
  immunotherapy
    advantages, 66–67
    hypothetical mechanism, 67
    and pharmacotherapy, 66
  monoclonal antibodies, 72
  problem of, 65
  SMA-KLH preparation, 71
  SMA-TT vaccine, 72
  stereotypic effects, 72
  TLR4/TLR5 adjuvants, 71–72
METH-BSA conjugates, active immunization, 407

METH-conjugate vaccine (MCV), 121, 122, 128
MF59, 298, 313
Micro-inflammation zones, NAFL, 315
Monoclonal antibodies (MAbs), 9
 adverse effect, 108
 FDA clinical trial, 108
 heavy- and light-chain immunoglobulin constant, 107
 "humanized", 108
 human sequences, 107
 mouse B-cell hybridomas, 107
 SUD
  advantages, 432
  anti-SUD MAbs, 432
  challenge, 432
  ethical requirements, 433
  phase, 432–433
  preclinical testing, 432
 therapeutic, 108
 use of, 107
Monoclonal anti-HIV neutralizing antibody, 87
Monophosphoryl lipid A (MPL), 68
MorHap conjugates, 407–408
MorHap-TT conjugate, 415
Mouse PK model, 20
Multivalent haptens targeting
 multiple drugs, 345–346
 multiple species, 344–345
 one drug, 346–348
Multivalent opioid vaccines, 56–57
Myeloid differentiation primary response 88 (MYD88)-mediated signaling pathway, 284
Myocardial infarction (MI) and cocaine intake, 26, 146

N

NAFL. *See* Non-ablative fractional laser (NAFL)
Naïve B cells activation
 conjugate immunogens, 381
 drug-specific serum antibody titers, 381
 flow cytometry analysis, 381
 fluorescent-antigen enrichment method, 381
 haptenization ratio, 380–381
 hapten-specific
  after immunization, 384–385
  pre-immunization, 382–384
 oxycodone haptens, 381
Nanoparticle-based nicotine vaccine
 advantages, 251
 antigens and adjuvants, encapsulation, 251
 in clinical development, 252–253
 long-term smoking cessation, 250
 nanoparticle-based vaccine development, 254–255
 nanoparticle design (*see* Nanoparticle design)
 preclinical and clinical literature, 250
 synthetic vaccine particles (SVP), 251
 VLPs, 253–254
Nanoparticle design
 adjuvant selection and development, 258–267
 design criteria, 255–256
 hapten selection, 257–258
 integrated immunologic design, 256–257
 T helper peptide development, 267–269
Native KLH decamer (nKLH), 385–386
Natural human butyrylcholinesterase (BChE), 112
Natural oligonucleotide sequences, 260
Networks
 cocaine-HIV vaccine, 91
 comorbidities, 91–92
 general population, 94
 HIV/AIDS, 91
 individual behavior, 92–94
 middle-aged African-American women, 91
 nonmedical prescription opioid, 95–98
 speedballers/cocaine injectors, 95
NIC7–CRM candidate vaccine variants, 253
NIC7-DT developers, 252–253
Nic12 experiments, 13, 14
NIC-KLH vaccine, 11
Nicotine
 and cocaine addiction treatment, 427
 drug target consideration, 331
 hapten–protein conjugates, 405
 linker composition, 338–340
 linker introduction, structure modification, 334–337
 patches, 1
 vaccine, 3, 252
Nicotine addiction
 Abs with abstinence rates
  dose-response and affinity-response, 11–15
  preclinical experiments, 11
 cigarette smoking, 249
 Cytos NicQβ program, 21
 immune response, 21

Nicotine addiction (*cont.*)
Nabi NicVAX program, 21–22
NicVAX phase III studies, 15–17
Post hoc analyses, 22
second-generation vaccines
NIC7-001, 19–21
SEL-068, 18
Selecta Biosciences and Pfizer, 18
skin vaccination against (*see* Skin vaccination against nicotine addiction)
smoking-cessation therapeutics, 8
therapeutic vaccines
animal models, 8
clinical progress and late-stage failure, 8–9
early clinical success (phase I and II), 10
independent academic research laboratories, 8
late-stage clinical setbacks, 11
mechanism of action, 10
tobacco smoking, 7
Nicotine–DT conjugates, 407
Nicotine-specific Abs, 10
Nicotine-specific mAbs, 11
NicQβ analogue, 20
NicVAX
non-particulate nicotine vaccines, 252
phase IIb study, 10
phase III clinic trials, 11
phase III studies, 16
NMDA receptor, 89
Non-ablative fractional laser (NAFL)
chemokines, 315–316
micro-inflammation zones, 315
skin vaccination against nicotine addiction, 315–316
Non-HIV scaffold, 83–84
Non-human primates (NHP), 18, 153, 232, 236, 237, 252, 271
Non-immunogenic nicotine analog, 241
Nontreatment seekers, 425
Nuclease-resistant CpG sequences, 260

O
OMPC. *See* Outer membrane protein complex (OMPC)
Opioid addiction
candidate heroin/oxycodone vaccines, 59
challenges, 41–44
history of, 39–40
mechanism of action, 38–39
pharmacotherapies, 59
vaccine strategy, 37–38
Opioid vaccines
antagonist therapy, 57
medication noncompliance, 57
nonaddictive and well-tolerated alternative, 57
pharmacotherapies, 57
regulation, 57
treatment modalities, 58
Outer membrane protein complex (OMPC), 296
OVA. *See* Antigen ovalbumin (OVA)
6OXY. *See* Oxycodone-based hapten (6OXY)
Oxycodone
drug target consideration, hapten design, 330
linker introduction, structure modification, 333
vaccines, 56
Oxycodone-based hapten (6OXY), 385–387

P
Pathogen-associated molecular pattern (PAMP) molecules, 281
Patient Protection and Affordable Care Act, 435
People who inject drugs (PWID), 95, 98
Peptidic linkers, 341–342
Pfizer Vaccines Research group, 19
Pharmacotherapy
cocaine addiction (*see* Cocaine pharmacotherapies)
hapten design for anti-addiction vaccine, 327–328
methamphetamine (MA) abuse, 66
opioid addiction, 57, 59
Phase III intent-to-treat (ITT) population, 16
Photoactivatable cross-linking approach, conjugation chemistry, 406
Phycoerythrin (PE), 375–376
Plasma cholinesterase, BChE, 188–189
Polyclonal nicotine-specific IgGs, 14
Polysaccharide conjugate vaccines, carrier proteins, 403
Polysubstance abuse, 3
Polyvalent vaccines, 430
Posttranslational modifications and pegylation, human BChE, 214–215
Post-vaccine Ab level, 15
Powder nicotine vaccines, 321

PRAD. *See* Proline-rich attachment domain (PRAD)
PrEP trials, 86
Prescription opioid (PO), 95–96
Proline-rich attachment domain (PRAD), 190
Protein engineering and biological half-life
  amino-acid mutations to stabilize oligomer structure, 215–217
  fusion proteins, 217
  posttranslational modifications and pegylation, 214–215
Protein vaccines, 296
6-PrOxyHap conjugates, 409–410
Pseudomonas aeruginosa exoprotein A (rEPA), 405
Public Health Service Act, 435

Q
Quantum mechanical/molecular mechanical (QM/MM) calculations
  chemical reaction pathway, 194–195
  and QM/MM-FE calculations, 197–198

R
Rat PK model, 20
RBP-8000, 213
Reckitt Benckiser Pharmaceuticals, 3
Recombinant BChE, 189
Recruitment chains, 97
Resiquimod (R848)
  bearing nanoparticles, 261
  cytokine production (*see* Cytokines)
  innate and adaptive immune cells, 261–262
  systemic inflammatory cytokines production, 265–267
Respondent-driven sampling (RDS), 96
RV144 case-control study, 79

S
Self-assembly DNA nanostructures, 282–283
Self-healing microthermal zones (MTZ), 315
Severe combined immunodeficiency (SCID) mice, 111
Skin vaccination against nicotine addiction
  adjuvant-incorporated ID nicotine vaccination, 316–317
  adjuvants for
    conventional adjuvants, 312–313
    laser vaccine adjuvant (LVA), 314
    non-ablative fractional laser (NAFL), 315–316
  anti-nicotine antibodies (NicAb), 310
  delivery technologies
    ID immunization, 318–319
    lesion-free skin vaccination, 319–322
  easy-to-use delivery technologies, 311
  immunogenic skin vaccination, 311–312
  low-nicotine Quest cigarette, 310
  nicotine amount, 310
  smokers, tolerability and safety, 310
  vaccine-induced memory T and B cells, 310
Stability enhancement, hapten design
  cocaine
    benzoyl ecgonine, 353, 354–355
    binding affinity, 353–354
    bioisosteric replacement, 353
    brain concentration, 353–354
    C2 stabilization, 353
    nitrogen-promoted hydrolysis, 352
    primary active species, 351–352
    rat, cocaine self-administration relapse, 353
  heroin, 351–352
  nonenzymatic ester hydrolysis, 350
Stimulator of interferon genes (STINGs), 284
Structural flexibility, affinity enhancement, 348–349
Substance abuse vaccines. *See also* Adjuvants
  adjuvants, 415
  hapten–protein conjugates, 403
  toll-like receptors (TLRs), 296–297
Succinyl methamphetamine (SMA), 68
Succinyl norcocaine (SNC), 28
SVP. *See* Synthetic vaccine particle (SVP)
Synergistic effects, cocaine-HIV vaccine, 98
Synthetic vaccine particle (SVP). *See also* Nanoparticle design
  anti-nicotine antibodies, 271–273
  anti-nicotine response, 271, 273
  design criteria, 255–256
  hapten selection, 257–258
  local lymphadenopathy induction, 261–262
  in mouse and non-human primate models, 271–272
  production of, 268–269
Systematic virtual screening, transition states
  free energy barrier, 202–203
  human BChE mutants, 201–202
  hydrogen bonding (HB) interactions, 203
  hypothetical BChE mutants, 201–202
  integrated computational–experimental effort, 201
  overall interaction energy, 203

Systematic virtual screening, transition states (*cont.*)
QM/MM-FE calculations, 201
total hydrogen bonding energy (tHBE), 203
transition-state structure, 201
Systemic lupus erythematosus (SLE), DNA molecules, 285

T
TA-CD cocaine vaccine, 2
antibody levels, 28, 29
anti-cocaine IgG, 30–31
cholera toxin B, 31
cocaine-free urines, 32
human dosing, 29
mean antibody levels, 30
phase IIa outpatient trial, 30
phase I trial, 29
plasma antibody levels, 30
systemic adverse effects, 29
vaccination, 30
T-cell antigen (TCHP), 18
T-cell-dependent antibody response, carrier proteins, 403
T cell-dependent B cell generation
activation-induced deaminase (AID), 371
antigen-specific B cells, 371
B lymphocyte-induced maturation protein 1 (blimp-1), 371
germinal center (GC), 370–371
secondary lymphoid organs, 370–371
signal transducers and activators of transcription (STAT), 371
Tetanus toxoid (TT), 68, 402–403
T helper peptide development
anti-nicotine antibody induction, 269, 272
B cells, 267
CD4 central memory T cell recall response in human, 268, 270
dominant mouse T-cell epitope, 268
exogenous antigens, 267
memory epitopes, 268–269
MHC class II peptide S-320, 268, 271
ovalbumin, 267–268
S-320, 268–269
subpopulations, 267
SVP containing nicotine antigen, 268
T-cell helper peptide (TCHP), 268–269
TT830DTt, 268–269
Toll-like receptors (TLRs)
adjuvants, 68, 296–297
ligands, 281
Total hydrogen bonding energy (tHBE), 203
Transdermal vaccine delivery, 320
Treatment seekers, 425
Trex1, 285
Trinitrobenzenesulfonic acid (TNBS) assay, 408
Tryptophan amphiphilic tetramerization (WAT) domain, 190
TV-1380, 206–207, 217, 218, 434

U
Unimmunized mouse, 375
United Nations Office on Drugs and Crime (UNODC), 25

V
Vaccine(s)
active catalytic, 358–359
chronic noncommunicable diseases
B cell responses, 369
cancer-associated carbohydrate antigens, 368
cancer-associated mucin-type O-glycans, 368
for drug addiction, 368–369
immunogens, 367–368
synthetic glycan-based haptens, 368–369
T cell-dependent B cell activation, 368–369
T cell-independent antigens, 368
efficacy, 280
against drugs of abuse (*see* B cell mechanisms)
hapten-specific B cells, 379–380
individual variability in, 389–390
substance use disorders (SUD)
antidrug, 429–430
antigen–antibody complex, 429
applications, 430
brain, limited access to, 429
clinical benefit, 431
educational scheme, 431
HIV infection and, 430–431
immunosuppressed individuals, 429
in monkeys, 428–429
polyvalent, 430
psychiatric disorders, 431
relapse prevention, 429
requirements, 429
risks, 429–430
Vaccine-induced memory T and B cells, 310

Vaccines against drugs of abuse
  adjuvants (*see* Adjuvants)
  hapten design
    carriers, 397
    clinical therapeutics, 398–399
    DiAmHap-induced antibodies, 401
    faces, 398
    facial recognition, 401
    heroin, 398
    heroin/morphine surrogates, 399
    MorHap, 399, 401
    morphine, bridge nitrogen-linked haptens, 401
    nitrogen-linked haptens, 400–401
    6-PrOxyHap, 399
    stability, 397–398
  hapten–protein conjugates
    carrier proteins, 402–405
    conjugation chemistry, 405–406
    hapten density and conjugate yield, 407–410
    hapten–protein conjugate, 411–412
    linker, 410–411
Varenicline, 1, 8, 252, 310, 431
VaxGen trial, 78
Viral gene transfer, enzymes
  adenoviral vector, 169
  anti-drug proteins
    administration, 168
    BChE, 168
    immunoglobulins, 167
    limitations, 167
    liposomal nanoparticle, 168
    long-term delivery, 167
    mass production, 168
    naked protein, 169
    nicotine, 167
    viral vectors, 168
  clinical application, 169–170
  CocH (*see* Cocaine hydrolase (CocH))
  FDA
    addressing, 181–182
    species selection, preclinical studies, 182–183
    transgene expression product, 181
  inherited and life-threatening disorders, 169
  inon-integrating vectors, 170–172
  integrating vectors, 170
  long-term safety issues, 180–181
  SCID, 169
  therapeutic impacts, 169
  transduction durability, 172
  vector toxicity
    duration of expression, human, 178–179
    fatal outcomes, 177–178
    hdAD, 178–179
    hepatocytes, 177
    risk and obstacles, 179–180
    short term, 177
Viral subunit vaccines, 77
Virus-like particles (VLPs)
  adjuvants coadministration, 253
  antibodies production, 281
  antigenic determinants, 253
  antigens and adjuvants encapsulation, 251
  composition, 253
  CYT002-NicQb/Nic002, VLP-nicotine conjugate, 253–254
  neutralizing antibodies, 252
  particulate antigens, immunogenicity, 281
  pathogen-associated molecular pattern (PAMP) molecules, 281
  production and purification, bioprocess challenges, 253
  serum antibody, 254
  synthetic micro/nanoparticles, 281
  systemic IgG induction, 254
V1V2 glycoprotein, 79